P9-CCQ-524

PEDIATRIC NURSING

The Critical Components of Nursing Care

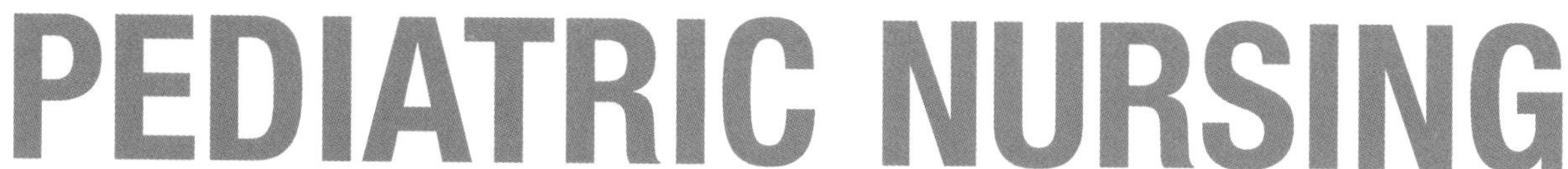

PEDIATRIC NURSING

The Critical Components of Nursing Care

Kathryn Rudd, MSN, RN, C-NIC, C-NPT
Clinical and Didactic Educator
Cuyahoga Community College
Case Western Reserve University
Cleveland, Ohio

Diane M. Kocisko, MSN, RN, CPN
Clinical Experience Coordinator
Cleveland State University
School of Nursing
Cleveland, Ohio

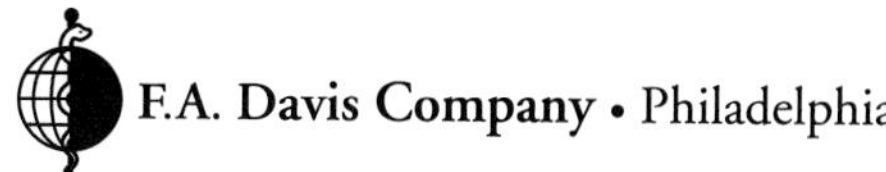

F.A. Davis Company • Philadelphia

F.A. Davis Company
1915 Arch Street
Philadelphia, PA 19103
www.fadavis.com

Printed in the United States of America

Last digit indicates print number: 10 9 8 7 6 5 4 3 2 1

Publisher, Nursing: Lisa B. Houck
Director of Content Development: Darlene D. Pedersen
Project Editor: Jamie M. Elfrank, M. A.
Electronic Project Editor: Katherine E. Crowley
Cover Design: Carolyn O'Brien

As new scientific information becomes available through basic and clinical research, recommended treatments and drug therapies undergo changes. The author(s) and publisher have done everything possible to make this book accurate, up to date, and in accord with accepted standards at the time of publication. The author(s), editors, and publisher are not responsible for errors or omissions or for consequences from application of the book, and make no warranty, expressed or implied, in regard to the contents of the book. Any practice described in this book should be applied by the reader in accordance with professional standards of care used in regard to the unique circumstances that may apply in each situation. The reader is advised always to check product information (package inserts) for changes and new information regarding dose and contraindications before administering any drug. Caution is especially urged when using new or infrequently ordered drugs.

Library of Congress Cataloging-in-Publication Data

Pediatric nursing: the critical components of nursing care / [edited by] Kathryn Rudd, Diane Kocisko. — 1st ed.
p. ; cm.
Includes bibliographical references.
ISBN 978-0-8036-2179-4 — ISBN 0-8036-2179-5
I. Rudd, Kathryn. II. Kocisko, Diane.
[DNLM: 1. Pediatric Nursing—methods. 2. Adolescent. 3. Child. 4. Infant. 5. Nursing Care—methods. WY 159]
RJ245
618.92'00231—dc23 2013005679

To my husband, Daniel Rudd,
and
my mother, Joan Antesberger, for their love and support.
Kathryn Rudd

To my mother, Kathleen Kocisko, for her love and inspiration.
Diane M. Kocisko

Preface

Pediatric Nursing: The Critical Components of Nursing Care is a pediatric nursing text that contains fundamental pediatric nursing content. This text was designed to address the contemporary changes in nursing education. Students are provided with the opportunity to investigate evidence-based practice and apply this knowledge to case scenarios. Developing knowledge in pediatric nursing is essential to all nurses, regardless of whether they ultimately become pediatric nurses. We all have children within our lives who may need care. Therefore, pediatric nursing is a life skill.

Most pediatric texts contain detailed information about every aspect of pediatric care. As pediatric nurses, we have found that this information can quickly become outdated. Today's technology provides the nurse with the opportunity to look up information within minutes. Within the text and on Davis*Plus*, we included multiple web links to encourage the reader to quickly validate and reference information. We recognize that student nurses must synthesize data from texts and life, laboratory, and clinical experiences to care for children. This text is organized to first present foundational information followed by complex information. Our concise outline format facilitates teaching pediatric nursing at all licensure levels and within varying time frames.

ORGANIZATION

The purpose of this text is to provide evidence-based practice and allow the student to apply this knowledge to the patient situation. Our focus is not to have the student memorize terms and data. We want the students to learn how to apply the information to the clinical setting. We encourage the use of electronic devices during the learning process. We believe that learning is not memorizing information for a test. Learning is the ability to apply new information to the clinical situation. For this reason, we have included special features within each chapter to facilitate the application of information.

FEATURES

This text is designed to include features that enhance the learning of the critical components in pediatric nursing:

- Objectives
- Key Terms
- Clinical Pearl feature
- Cultural Competence feature
- Critical Component feature
- Clinical Reasoning feature
- Evidence-Based Practice feature
- Medication Administration feature
- Promoting Safety feature
- Alternative Therapies (when applicable)

AUDIO BOOK

Chapters 1 through 20 have been recorded and are available as an audio book on Davis*Plus* Premium. This audio book meets the needs of those who learn best through audio, as well as the needs of adult learners who must multi-task when challenged by the multiple roles of life. The students can hear the chapters at any time of the day and in any available environment. The audio book can reinforce content learned in the classroom and clinical settings.

CRITICAL COMPONENTS

Our text is titled *Pediatric Nursing: The Critical Components of Nursing Care* because our aim is to provide the most crucial information in pediatric nursing. We have both worked within pediatrics and taught pediatric clinical. This experience enabled us to evaluate the learning needs of pediatric nurses. We strive to teach not just what is "normal" but to anticipate deviations from the norm. Early detection, especially in children, will lead to early interventions and improved outcomes.

CHAPTER ON DEATH AND DYING

We have included a pediatric-specific chapter on death and dying. This is not a topic that is covered in day-to-day conversation; at one time, discussion of death and dying in the pediatric context was considered taboo. We are dedicated to caring for children throughout their stages of life. Our goal is to provide information and a route to therapeutically care for terminally ill children. Within the interactive case scenarios, we have also included a scenario dealing with the death of a child.

REVIEW QUESTIONS

Each chapter includes 10 questions that cover information in the chapter to test student understanding. Answers to the review questions are available at the end of the text.

IMPORTANT FEATURES OF THE INSTRUCTOR'S RESOURCES ON DAVIS*PLUS*

Supplemental Instructor Materials for Theory Class Include:

- PowerPoint presentation covering the content of each chapter
- Two clicker questions within each PowerPoint presentation to encourage classroom engagement
- Instructor test bank with NCLEX-style questions is available on Davis*Plus*.
- Web links throughout each chapter to encourage students to seek up-to-date content

Supplemental Instructor Materials for Clinical Include:

- Each chapter includes a care plan exercise with NIC and NOC labels. Suggested answers are available for ease of grading.
- Interactive Clinical Scenarios allow your students to test their knowledge and practice their critical thinking skills.

Contributors

Kelly Betts, EdD (c), MNS (c), RN
Clinical Assistant Professor
Theory Coordinator Junior Pediatric Specialty
UAMS College of Nursing
Little Rock, Arkansas

Ludy Caballero, BSN, RN, EMTP
Clinical Nurse
MetroHealth Medical Center
Cleveland, Ohio

Irene Cihon Dietz, MD, FAAP
Assistant Professor of Pediatrics, Case Western Reserve University
MetroHealth Medical Center
Department of Pediatrics
Division of Comprehesive Care
Cleveland, Ohio

Suzanne M. Fortuna, Post MSN, RN, CNS, FNP, APN-BC
University Hospitals Case Medical Center/ Rainbow Babies and Children's Hospital/University Hospitals
Ahuja Medical Center
Cleveland, Ohio

Tina Goodpasture, MSN, RN, FNP
Cone Health Child Neurology
Greensboro, North Carolina

Mary Grady, MSN, RN
Assistant Professor
Lorain Community College
Lorain, Ohio

Bonnie Kitchen, MNS (c), RN, PNP, ACPNP
Arkansas Children's Hospital
General Pediatrics
1 Children's Way
Little Rock, Arkansas

Becky Loth Luetke, MSN, BA, RN
Associate Professor, Department of Nursing
Colorado Mountain College

Christina M. Mahovlic, MSN, APRN, FNP, CPNP
Digestive Disease Consultants
Brunswick, Ohio

Lauren G. McAliley, MSN , MA , RN, PNP-BC
Pediatric Nurse Practitioner, Child Advocacy & Protection
Associate Director, Rainbow Center for Pediatric Ethics
University Hospitals of Cleveland Case Medical Center
Cleveland, Ohio

Judith McLeod, DNP, RN, CPNP
Online Faculty
University of Phoenix

Anita Mitchell, PhD, APN, FNP
Associate Clinical Professor
College of Nursing
University of Arkansas for Medical Sciences
Little Rock, Arkansas

Jill Morinec, BSN, RN
Clinical Nurse
MetroHealth Medical Center
Cleveland, Ohio

Theresa L. Puckett, PhD, RN, CPNP, CNE
National Speaker/Author, PESI Healthcare
Clinical Nurse, Cleveland Clinic Foundation
EMR Consultant, Alego Health
Cleveland, Ohio

Daniel C. Rausch, BSN, RN
Sr. Pediatric Application Analyst
Advanced Clinical Nurse
Rainbow Babies and Childrens Hospital
University Hospitals
Cleveland, Ohio

Jill Reiter, MSN, RN
Assistant Professor
Lorain Community College
Lorain, Ohio

Andrea Warner Stidham, PhD, RN
Assistant Professor
Department of Nursing
Hiram College
Hiram, Ohio

Sheryl Stuck, MSN, RN, CNS,
Associate Professor
Department of Associate Degree in Nursing Program
Stark State College
Canton, Ohio

Ancillary Contributors

Cynthia Candow, BSN, RN

Barbara Cavender, MSN, RN, CNS, CNL

Holly Clark, MSN, RN, PNP

Judith Croasmun, MSN, RN

Sandi Duke, BSN, RN, CPN

Suzanne M. Fortuna, post MSN, RN, CNS, FNP, APN-BC

Diane M. Kocisko, MSN, RN, CPN

Julie Medas, MSN, RN, CNS

Anita Mitchell, PhD, APN, FNP

Jill Morinec, BSN, RN

Daniel C. Rausch, BSN, RN

Kathryn Rudd, MSN, RN, C-NIC, C-NPT

Terri Savage, MSN, RN

Michelle Smith, MSN, RN

Sheryl Stuck, MSN, RN, CNS

Reviewers

Vicky H. Becherer, PhD(c), RN
Assistant Teaching Professor
University of Missouri–St. Louis College of Nursing
St. Louis, Missouri

Elizabeth A. Berro, MA, RN, PNP
Clinical Instructor
Pace University
Pleasantville, New York

Glenda J. Bondurant, MSN, RN, CNE
Associate Dean for Allied Health and Sciences
Wilson Community College
Wilson, North Carolina

Patricia Brazell, MSN, RN
Instructor
Covenant School of Nursing
Lubbock, Texas

Margaret Bultas, PhD(c), MSN, RN, CPNP-PC
Assistant Professor
Goldfarb School of Nursing
Barnes Jewish College
St. Louis, Missouri

Nathania Bush, MSN, APRN, BC
Associate Professor of Nursing
Morehead State University
Morehead, Kentucky

Beth Desaretz Chiatti, RN, MSN, CSN, PhD candidate
Instructor, BSN2 Program Director
Eastern University
St. Davids, Pennsylvania

Jeanne N. Churchill, DNP, MSN, CPNP
Assistant Professor of Clinical Nursing
Columbia University
New York, New York

Sandra Clay, RN, MSN
Assistant Director, ADN Program
Pediatric Expert
Chaffey Community College
Rancho Cucamonga, California

Georgina Colalillo, MS, RN
Associate Professor, Nursing Department
Queensborough Community College (CUNY)
Bayside, New York

Thomas W. Connelly, Jr., PhD, RN
Director of Nursing Programs
Anna Maria College
Paxton, Massachusetts

Renee Courtney, MSN, FNP-BC
Nursing Instructor
Macomb Community College
Warren, Minnesota

Wendy Darby, PhD, CRNP
Associate Professor
University of North Alabama
Florence, Alabama

Lana K. Davies, MSN, RN, CPNP
Assistant Professor
Research College of Nursing
Kansas City, Missouri

Fredi de Yampert, PhD, MSN, RN
Professor, Nursing Department Chair
Finlandia University
Houghton, Minnesota

Karen R. Ferguson, PhD, RNC
Assistant Professor
Martin Methodist College
Pulaski, Tennessee

Roseann M. Flyte, MSN, RN
Nursing Faculty
Cedar Crest College
Allentown, Pennsylvania

Mary Jo Gay, RN, BSN, MSN, PhD
Associate Professor
Missouri Western State University
St. Joseph, Missouri

Yolanda Green, RN, MSN
Associate Professor of Nursing
Chattanooga State Community College
Chattanooga, Tennessee

Vicki Grubbs, MSN, RN, CPN
Associate Professor
Eastern Kentucky University
Richmond, Kentucky

Kathy L. Ham, RN, EdD
Assistant Professor of Nursing
Southeast Missouri State University
Cape Giradeau, Missouri

Paula M. Hayes, RN, MSN
Nursing Instructor
Maria College
Albany, New York

Jill Holmstrom, EdD, RN
Associate Professor
Concordia College
Moorhead, Minnesota

Beth Ann Kenney, RN, MSN
Assistant Professor
Blessing-Rieman College of Nursing
Quincy, Illinois

Mary Jo Konkloski, RN, MSN, ANP
Nursing Instructor
Finger Lakes Health College of Nursing AD Program
Geneva, New York

Sarah Jaynes Kulinski, RN, MA, MSN, Certification Mental Health Nursing
Assistant Professor, School of Nursing
Lenoir Rhyne University
Hickory, North Carolina

Lynx Carlton McClellan, RN, DSN
Clinical Associate Professor
University of Alabama–Huntsville
College of Nursing
Huntsville, Alabama

Kelly McGovern Lu, MSN, CPNP
Certified Pediatric Nurse Practitioner
University of Vermont
Fletcher Allen Health Care
Burlington, Vermont

Lisa Miller, MN, RN
Nursing Instructor
Everett Community College
Everett, Washington

Teak Nelson, MS, RN, NP-C
Assistant Professor of Nursing
Department of Nursing
Truman State University
Kirksville, Missouri

Helen Papas-Kavalis, RNC, BSN, MA
Professor of Nursing
Bronx Community College of the City
University of New York
Bronx, New York

Ramona Ann Parker, PhD, RN
Associate Professor
University of the Incarnate Word
School of Nursing and Health Professions
San Antonio, Texas

Beverly Rowe, RN, MSN
Associate Professor of Nursing
College of Coastal Georgia
Brunswick, Georgia

Gerilyn Rush, CNE, MSN
Nursing Faculty
Arapahoe Community College
Littleton, Colorado

Judy A. Scott, MSN, RN
Professor of Nursing, Clinical Coordinator
College of Southern Nevada
Las Vegas, Nevada

Heather Holland Snell, RN, MSN, CPNP
Clinical Instructor
Certified Pediatric Nurse Practitioner
The University of Texas at El Paso
El Paso, Texas

Kathleen E. Snider, RN, MSN, CNS
Professor of Nursing
Los Angeles Valley College
Valley Glen, California

Linda A. Strong, RN, MSN, CPNP, CNE
Assistant Professor of Nursing
Cuyahoga Community College
Cleveland, Ohio

Laurel R. Talabere, PhD, RN, AE-C
Professor Emerita (retired)
Adjunct Professor
Capital University
Columbus, Ohio

Nancy M. Thomas, RN, MSN
Assistant Professor
Cleveland State Community College
Cleveland, Tennessee

Jeannie Weston, BSN, MS
Clinical Instructor
Emory University
Decatur, Georgia

Dr. Sarah Whitaker, DNS, RN
Nursing Program Director
Dona Ana Community College at New Mexico State University
Las Cruces, New Mexico

Irish Patrick Williams, PhD, RN, MSN, CRRN
Nursing Instructor
Hinds Community College
Jackson, Mississippi

Acknowledgments

I am grateful to my husband, Daniel Rudd, and my children, Ashley, David, Matthew, and Mary Kathryn, for their continued love and support throughout this long project.

Thanks to my colleagues at Cuyahoga Community College, Huron School of Nursing, and Frances Payne Bolton Case Western Reserve University for their suggestions and support.

Thanks to my teachers and mentors Alice DeWitt, RN, and Rosemary Bolls, RN, at St. Alexis School of Nursing, who instilled in me a love of nursing and education.

I am thankful for my mother, Kathleen Kocisko, for her ongoing encouragement, prayers, and support.

Thanks to my teachers and mentors Maureen Mitchell, EdD, RN, and Marylin Weitzel, PhD, RN, for their encouragement, instilling in me the love of nursing education, pediatrics, and developing students.

I would like to thank my colleagues at Cleveland State University, MetroHealth Medical Center, and Cleveland Clinic for their ongoing support of this project.

Thanks to our F.A. Davis team—Lisa Houck, Robin Bushing, Jamie Elfrank, Padraic Mahoney—for their guidance.

Thanks to our contributors for sharing their expertise and taking on the task of writing these chapters despite their continued workload.

Brief Contents

Contents

UNIT 1 Pediatric Nursing: An Overview

1 Issues and Trends in Pediatric Nursing

Theresa Puckett, PhD, RN, CPNP, CNE
Christina Mahovlic, MSN, APRN, FNP-C, CPNP

OBJECTIVES

- ☐ Define *pediatric nursing.*
- ☐ Describe the differences between nursing care of infants, children, and adolescents versus care of the adult population.
- ☐ Describe the health of America's children.
- ☐ Identify models of care applied to pediatric nursing.
- ☐ Describe the history of pediatric nursing.
- ☐ Describe the roles of the pediatric nurse.
- ☐ Identify the different fields of nursing and the education required for each.
- ☐ Identify current issues and trends in pediatric nursing practice, education, and research.
- ☐ Identify evidence-based resources available for pediatric nurses.

KEY TERMS

- Family-centered care
- Relationship-based care
- Culturally sensitive care

INTRODUCTION TO PEDIATRIC NURSING

The nursing care of children from birth through adolescence includes health promotion, disease prevention, illness management, and health restoration (**Figure 1-1**).

How Providing Nursing Care for Children Differs from Caring for Adults

- These populations require assessment and evaluation tools that are unique to infants, children, and adolescent populations.
- Pediatric nurses need to assess attainment of developmental milestones (see Chapter 6).
- Pediatric nurses need to monitor growth and development, including the following:
  - *Physical maturation*
    - Development and mastery of gross and fine motor skills
    - Linear growth
    - Height, weight, and head circumference, tracked via growth charts; growth charts adapted for specific populations (e.g., Down syndrome)
    - Physical maturation of each body system (see Chapters 8–10)

Don't have time to read this chapter? Want to reinforce your reading? Need to review for a test? Listen to this chapter on DavisPlus at davispl.us/rudd1.

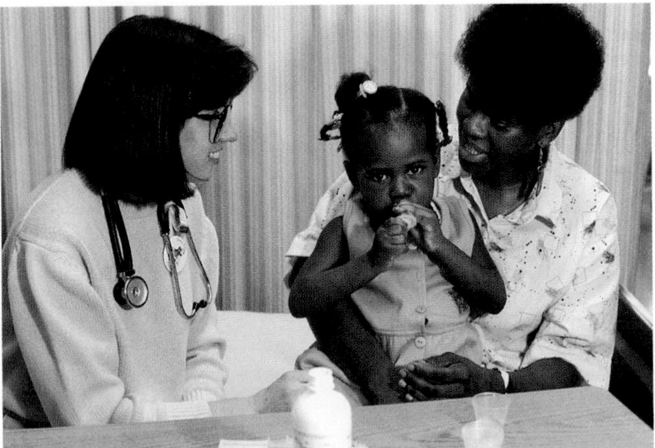

Figure 1–1 Nurse engaged with a child requiring health care.

- Onset of puberty, including Tanner Scales
- Immunizations
- *Cognitive maturation (see Chapter 6)*
  - Erikson's stages of psychosocial development
  - Piaget's stages of cognitive development
  - Freud's psychosexual stages of development
  - Kohlberg's stages of moral development
  - Language development
  - Assessment for presence of learning and developmental disabilities, where indicated

CRITICAL COMPONENT

Caring for children is not just caring for "little adults."

THE HEALTH OF AMERICA'S CHILDREN

- Causes of U.S. infant mortality in 2010, per 100,000 (Centers for Disease Control and Prevention [CDC], 2011):
  - *Birth defects: 136.3*
  - *Prematurity/low birth weight: 113.1*
  - *Sudden infant death syndrome (SIDS): 54.4*
  - *Complications of pregnancy: 41.2*
  - *Unintentional injury: 26.2*
- Causes of U.S. child and adolescent mortality in 1997 through 2007, ages 10 to 17, per 100,000 (CDC, 2011):
  - *Unintentional injury: 12.6*
  - *Homicide: 3.3*
  - *Suicide: 2.8*
  - *Cancer: 2.6*
  - *Heart disease: 1*
  - *Birth defects: 0.9*
  - *Influenza and pneumonia: 0.8*
  - *Sepsis: 0.2*
  - *Asthma: 0.03*
- Causes of U.S. child hospital admissions (data from Agency for Healthcare Research and Quality [AHRQ] Healthcare Cost and Utilization project KID database; U.S. Department of Health and Human Services, 2011):
  - *Children account for 18% of all hospital admissions.*
  - *Children have a 29% shorter stay than adults.*
  - *Two-thirds of child hospital stays are by children less than 30 days old; 95% of those problems/complications after birth.*
  - *Children account for one-third of hospital stays.*
  - *Child admissions: 45% are nonemergency; 55% are through the emergency department (ED).*
  - *The two most common reasons for hospitalization of children are respiratory problems and infections.*
  - *Asthma is the number-one reason for hospitalization among children.*
  - *Mental health problems account for 7% of child admissions (depression is the number-one mental health reason).*
  - *The most common procedures that children undergo are circumcision (59% of all males) and appendectomy.*

MODELS OF CARE IN PEDIATRIC NURSING

Family-centered care and **relationship-based care** are two models of care used in the delivery of nursing care to children. In both models, the importance of the family to the child is emphasized.

CRITICAL COMPONENT

In pediatric nursing, the unit of care is the child and the caregiver(s).

- Core concepts of family-centered care include the following:
  - *Dignity and respect for the child and family*
  - *Information sharing with the family*
  - *Participation in care by the family*
  - *Collaboration with the family to plan and provide care*
- Core concepts of relationship-based care include the following:
  - *The child and family remain the focal point in the plan of care.*
  - *The nurse makes an effort to develop a relationship with the child's family members and provides one-to-one time for conversations with the child and family on each shift.*
  - *Care is individualized to meet the specific needs of the child, based on issues that arise in the one-to one conversations with the child and family.*
  - *All staff members strive to respect, understand, and address the child's and family's concerns.*
  - *Children and families are actively engaged in all aspects of care, including decision making.*
  - *Open communication must occur between child, family, and staff.*
  - *The child's well-being and dignity must be safeguarded in all aspects of communication and care.*

HISTORY OF PEDIATRIC NURSING

- Before pediatrics became a specialty, newborns were delivered by midwives and cared for in the home (**Figure 1-2**).
- The first pediatric hospital was the Children's Hospital of Pennsylvania, founded in 1855.
- As early hospitals became more industrialized, the following were commonplace practices in infant and child care:
  - *Nursing care was geared toward preventing the spread of infectious disease, and was often cold and rigid.*
  - *Parents were unable to visit or stay at the bedside of their children, and relinquished all care responsibility to the staff.*
  - *Including the family in the plan of care was believed to be detrimental to patient outcomes.*
  - *The emotional and psychological needs of children were not considered in care planning.*
- In the late 19th and early 20th centuries, nurses became involved in many public and private health promotion initiatives, including the care of children (**Figure 1-3**).
- As the field of pediatric nursing progressed, efforts were made to improve nursing education.
- In 1917, the "*Standard Curriculum for Schools of Nursing* (*Standard Curriculum*) stated that classes on pediatric nursing were to include lectures on social issues and psychology, infectious diseases, orthopedic and surgical conditions, and information about infant feeding and child development to give a good sound basis for later work in connection with milk depots [breast milk donation sites], baby welfare, school-nursing and other fields of work where knowledge and skill in children's nursing are of essential importance" (Taylor, 2006).
- Research conducted in the mid-20th century indicated the negative effects of separating parent from child, resulting in a subsequent push toward more family-centered care.
- The early field of pediatric nursing influenced the later development of advanced practice roles (e.g., neonatal nurse practitioner, pediatric nurse practitioner).
- Pediatric nurse practitioners were the first nurse practitioners.
- In the later half of the 20th century, the nursing profession continued to define itself through:
  - *Development and publication of professional standards of practice*
  - *Availability of certification programs*
  - *Formation of professional organizations*
  - *Continued nursing research*
  - *Continued educational opportunities*

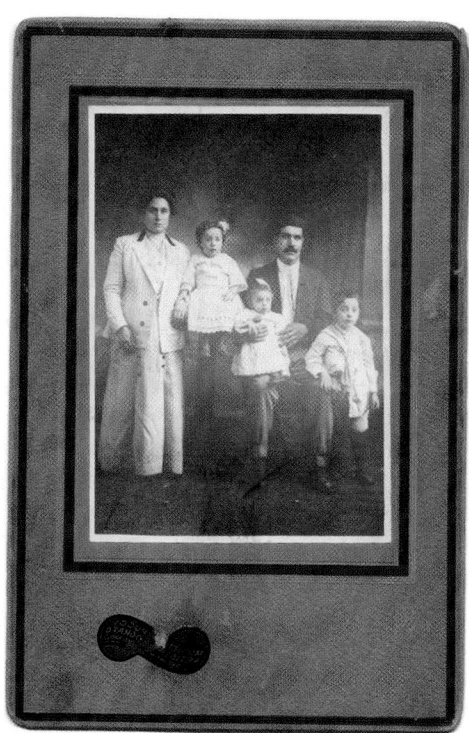

Figure 1-2 Family in early 1900s. *(Courtesy of D.M. Kocisko.)*

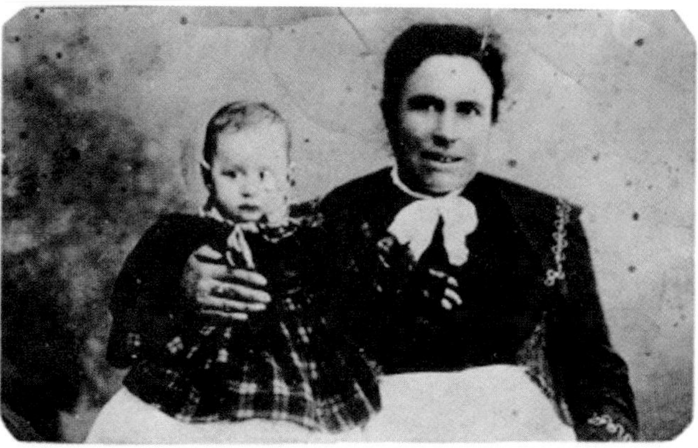

Figure 1-3 Child from the late 19th century. *(Courtesy of D.M. Kocisko.)*

ROLE OF THE PEDIATRIC NURSE

- Roles of the pediatric nurse include the following:
  - *Incorporates knowledge of human growth and development when providing care to children*
  - *Recognizes the physiological differences between children and adults*
  - *Provides care in a developmentally appropriate manner, in order to promote the optimal physical, psychological, and social well-being of children*
  - *Recognizes the integral role of family in a child's health, and thus incorporates the family in the plan of care*
  - *Provides* ***culturally sensitive care*** *by integrating knowledge of cultural and religious practices into the plan of care*
  - *Implements models of care that are specifically applicable to infants, children, and adolescents*

WHERE PEDIATRIC NURSES WORK

- Pediatric nurses with undergraduate preparation may be employed in the following settings and capacities:
  - *Acute care—bedside nurse*
  - *Certified pediatric nurse*
  - *Hospital nurse manager (BSN or MSN required for some positions)*
  - *Hospice and palliative care*
  - *Surgical care*
  - *Ambulatory care*
  - *Outpatient care*
  - *Home care*
  - *School nurse*
  - *Camp nurse*
  - *Travel nurse*
  - *Day-care consultant*
  - *Community educator*
  - *Public health nurse*
  - *Research trial coordinator*
- Pediatric nurses with master's degree preparation may be employed in the following settings and capacities:
  - *Pediatric nurse practitioner (inpatient/outpatient)*
  - *Family nurse practitioner (inpatient/outpatient)*
  - *Neonatal nurse practitioner*
  - *Clinical nurse specialist (inpatient)*
  - *Nurse educator (hospital/college or school of nursing)*
- Pediatric nurses with doctoral preparation may be employed in the following settings and capacities:
  - *Development and implementation of research programs (hospital/college or school of nursing)*
  - *Clinical practice in area of nursing doctorate (inpatient/outpatient)*

ADDITIONAL TRAINING AND CERTIFICATION AVAILABLE

- Neonatal Resuscitation Program (NRP)
- Pediatric Advanced Life Support (PALS)
- End of Life Nursing Education Consortium—PEDS (see also Chapter 5 on death and dying)
- Pediatric nursing certification (see http://www.pncb.org for more information):
  - *Certified Pediatric Emergency Nurse (CPEN)*
  - *Certified Pediatric Nurse Practitioner (CPNP; acute and primary care)*
- Certified Pediatric Oncology Nurse (CPON) (see http://www.oncc.org for more information)
- Neonatal/pediatric and critical care nurse certification (CCRN) (see http://www.aacn.org for more information)
- S.T.A.B.L.E. Program (post-resuscitation and pre-transport stabilization care of sick infants)
- Advanced practice certification:
  - *Certified Pediatric Nurse Practitioner (CPNP; acute and primary care) (see http://www.nursecredentialing.org for more information)*
  - *Certified Neonatal Nurse Practitioner (NNP-BC) (see http://www.nccwebsite.org for more information)*
  - *Certified Clinical Nurse Specialist (CCNS; neonatal or pediatrics) (see http://www.aacn.org for more information)*
  - *Certified Clinical Nurse Specialist (PCNS-BC; pediatrics) (see http://www.nursecredentialing.org for more information)*

ISSUES IN PEDIATRIC NURSING

- A decrease in the number of pediatric nurses has led to a current nationwide shortage in the field of pediatric nursing.
  - *The shortage is especially acute in the field of pediatric home-care nursing, resulting in children staying in the hospital longer than necessary while a home-care nurse is found and educated in the child's care.*
- The changing economy will affect pediatric health-care delivery in ways not yet known.
- Ethical considerations in pediatric nursing research that impact clinical practice include the following:
  - *As a result of the lack of research studies using infant, child, and adolescent participants, the indications of research results from studies with adult participants are often applied to children in clinical practice.*
  - *As a result of the lack of research studies using ethnically and culturally diverse participants, the indications of research results from studies with participants of one ethnic/cultural group are often applied to infants, children, and adolescents of another ethnic/cultural group in clinical practice.*
- As the number of chronically ill children continues to increase, the issue of continuity of care between hospital, home, and school must become more prominent.
- Maintaining communication with families and caregivers has become more challenging with the increased number of divorced parents, blended or reconstituted families, and grandparents who are the primary caregivers.
  - *Special issues in working with foster parents, extended families, single-parent families, gay/lesbian families, cohabitating families, and families with adopted children must be considered.*
- Ensuring adequate health education and follow-up services for children and families is a primary responsibility of nurses, and this becomes more challenging when working with children and families with limited health literacy and those for whom English is a second language.
- As health-care costs continue to increase, families' adherence to recommended therapy and treatments may be negatively affected by lack of insurance or being underinsured; families may not be able to afford follow-up care.
- The age of consent for children can present special issues (see also Chapter 2, Standards of Practice and Ethical Considerations)
  - *Discrepancies between what a child may want versus what the parent/caregiver may want*
  - *The child's ability to provide informed consent*

TRENDS IN PEDIATRIC NURSING PRACTICE

- Increased numbers of children requiring mental health services
- Increased numbers of children becoming ill as a result of antibiotic-resistant organisms
- Increased usage of blood conservation techniques for hospitalized children
- Increased emphasis on provision of safety education (e.g., Internet safety, dealing with bullying)
- Increased admissions based on environmental risk factors, such as dangerous living environments, unstable households, and risky behaviors
- Increased admissions based on deficient knowledge base of caregivers, such as not following or understanding the treatment regimen
- Increased admissions based on lack of primary care access
- Earlier onset of puberty and its ramifications for adolescent sexual health
- Shift in the focus of medical/nursing care from disease treatment to health promotion and disease prevention
- Provision of health education in the school system
- Increased incorporation of families in the overall care of children
- Increased numbers of children requiring home-care provision
- Increased prevalence of autism spectrum disorders and childhood depression, requiring more education and research in these areas
- Increased childhood incidence of the following conditions:
  - *Obesity*
  - *Hypertension*
  - *Diabetes*
  - *Asthma*

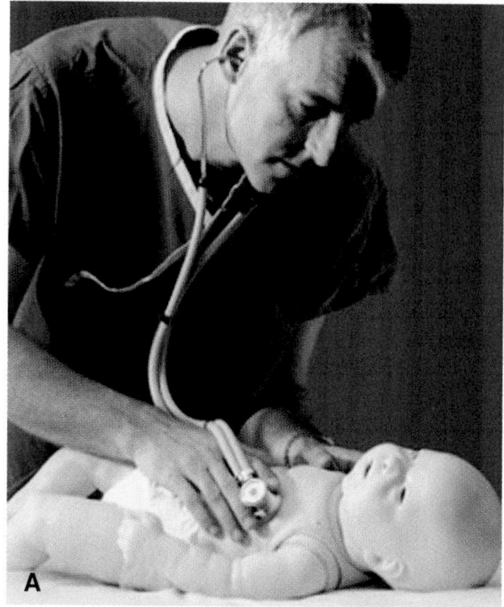

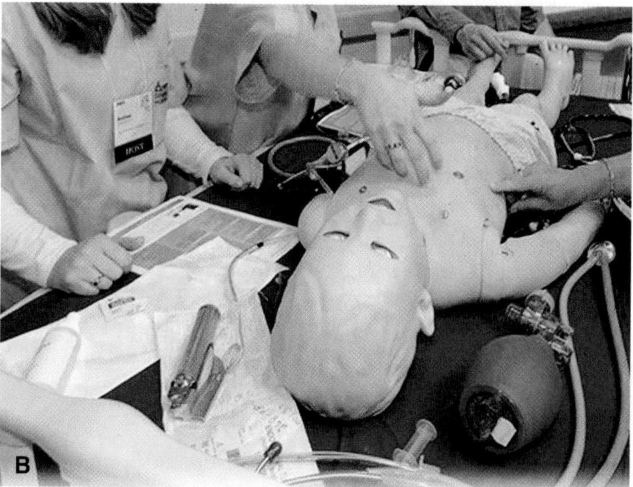

Figure 1–4 Infant and child patient simulators. *(PediaSIM pediatric simulation photo courtesy of CAE Healthcare. © 2011 CAE Healthcare.)*

CRITICAL COMPONENT

More children are experiencing health complications related to lifestyle, such as obesity.

TRENDS IN PEDIATRIC NURSING EDUCATION

- Use of child and infant human patient simulators (**Figure 1-4**)
- Inclusion of multicultural care topics and family theory in nursing programs
- Incorporation of growth and development concepts into nursing curricula
- Use of clinical-site experience in acute care, community, school, and well-care settings
- Increased focus on health promotion and disease prevention in nursing programs (e.g., screenings and preventive education)
- Increased focus on bringing nursing education into the community (e.g., health fairs, screenings, etc.)

TRENDS IN PEDIATRIC NURSING RESEARCH

- In 2007, the U.S. Congress reauthorized the Best Pharmaceuticals for Children Act, the Pediatric Research Equity Act, and the Pediatric Medical Device Safety and Improvement Act.
- These laws require that medications, medical devices, and interventions be tested on children if they are intended for use in children.
- This represents a new direction for research, as children were rarely used as research subjects prior to the passage of these laws.

- Because research studies now more frequently involve child participants, interventions will be safer for children as a result of being based on data from actual children, rather than adult, response to treatment.

RESOURCES FOR PEDIATRIC HEALTH DATA

- Child Stats (http://childstats.gov)
- CDC Wonder (http://wonder.cdc.gov/)
- Data Resource Center for Child and Adolescent Health (http://www.childhealthdata.org/content/Default.aspx)
- National Database of Nursing Quality Indicators (http://www.nursingquality.org)
- National Children's Study (http://www.nationalchildrensstudy.gov/Pages/default.aspx)
  - *The study is intended to determine how environmental factors influence health and development.*
  - *Participants in the study will be tracked from birth until age 21.*

RESOURCES FOR EVIDENCE-BASED PEDIATRIC NURSING PRACTICE

- Pediatric nursing journals:
  - *Journal for Specialists in Pediatric Nursing (Journal of the Society of Pediatric Nurses)*
  - *Journal of Child Health*
  - *Journal of Pediatric Nursing*
  - *Pediatric Nursing*
  - *Journal of Child and Adolescent Psychiatric Nursing*
  - *Society of Pediatric Nurses*
  - *The American Journal of Maternal/Child Nursing (MCN)*
- Online resources for pediatric nursing:
  - *American Academy of Pediatrics (AAP), Bright Futures: Guidelines for Health Supervision of Infants, Children, and Adolescents, 3rd edition (2008) (http://brightfutures.aap.org/3rd_Edition_Guidelines_and_Pocket_Guide.html)*
  - *Agency for Healthcare Research and Quality (AHRQ) resources:*
    - Innovations Exchange, a review of innovations and quality tools (http://www.innovations.ahrq.gov/)
    - Research updates (http://www.ahrq.org)
    - National Quality Measures Clearinghouse (http://www.qualitymeasures.ahrq.gov/)
  - *Food and Drug Administration (FDA), information on pediatric pharmaceuticals (http://www.fda.gov/cder/pediatric)*
  - *National Guideline Clearinghouse, information on evidence-based clinical practice (http://www.guideline.gov)*
  - *National Institute of Child Health and Human Development (NICHD; http://www.nichd.nih.gov)*
  - *National Institute of Nursing Research (http://www.ninr.nih.gov)*
- Pediatric professional organizations:
  - *AAP (http://www.aap.org)*
  - *Academy of Neonatal Nursing (http://www.academyonline.org)*
  - *Association of Camp Nurses (http://www.campnurse.org)*
  - *Association of Child Neurology Nurses (http://www.accn.org)*
  - *Association of Pediatric Oncology Nurses (http://www.apon.org)*
  - *National Association of Neonatal Nurses (http://www.nann.org)*
  - *National Association of Pediatric Nurse Practitioners (http://www.napnap.org)*
  - *National Association of School Nurses (http://www.nasn.org)*
  - *Society of Pediatric Nurses (http://www.pedsnurses.org)*

Review Questions

1. The leading cause of adolescent mortality in the United States is
A. asthma.
B. suicide.
C. unintentional injury.
D. cancer.

2. The most common cause of hospital admission among children is
A. traumatic injury.
B. asthma.
C. mental health.
D. surgery.

3. Pediatric nurses may monitor all of the following aspects of a child's physical maturation, *except*:
A. onset of puberty.
B. development and mastery of fine and gross motor skills.
C. height, weight, and head circumference, via growth-chart tracking.
D. progression through Piaget's stages of cognitive development.

4. The field of pediatric nursing gave rise to the first
A. nurse midwives.
B. nurse educators.
C. nurse anesthetists.
D. nurse practitioners.

5. Which of the following was the first children's hospital, founded in 1855?
A. Loma Linda Children's Hospital
B. Children's Hospital of Philadelphia
C. Children's Hospital of Providence
D. Boston Children's Hospital

6. Specialty certification in pediatrics allows the nurse to
   A. contribute to the nursing department's magnet status.
   B. meet the requirements of the Center for Medicare and Medicaid Services (CMS).
   C. continue to develop professionally.
   D. meet the requirements of the Joint Commission.
   E. enhance professional integrity and credibility.

7. In the United States, which of the following is the greatest cause of infant mortality?
   A. Unintentional injury
   B. Sudden infant death syndrome (SIDS)
   C. Complication of pregnancy
   D. Birth defects and/or prematurity

8. Pediatric nursing differs from adult nursing in that the nurse must (select all that apply)
   A. use unique pediatric assessment tools.
   B. evaluate developmental milestones.
   C. assess psychosocial needs.
   D. provide education regarding health-care needs.
   E. monitor growth and development.

9. Core concepts of family-centered care include which of the following? (select all that apply)
   A. Participation in care by the family
   B. Information sharing with the family
   C. Collaboration with the family to plan and provide care
   D. Responsibility for driving the plan of care resides with parents only
   E. Dignity and respect for the child and family

10. Pediatric nursing is the care of children from birth through adolescence and includes which of the following? (select all that apply)
    A. Health promotion
    B. Disease prevention
    C. Illness management
    D. Tutoring
    E. Health restoration

References

Centers for Disease Control and Prevention (CDC). (2011). Vital stats. Retrieved from http://www.cdc.gov/nchs/hdi.htm

Taylor, M. K. (2006). Mapping the literature of pediatric nursing. *Journal of Medical Library Association*, *94*, E128–E136. Retrieved from http://www.ncbi.nlm.nih.gov/pubmed/16710459

U.S. Department of Health and Human Services. (2011). Databases and related tools from the Healthcare Cost and Utilization Project, fact sheet. Retrieved from http://www.ahrq.gov/data/hcup/datahcup.htm#Recent

Standards of Practice and Ethical Considerations

2

Lauren G. McAliley, MSN, MA, RN, PNP-BC

OBJECTIVES

- ☐ Identify and describe sources of standards of practice that are of relevance to the day-to-day practice of pediatric nurses.
- ☐ Identify and elaborate on the key themes relating to pediatric nursing standards of practice.
- ☐ List the 6 standards of practice and 10 standards of professional performance highlighted in the Pediatric Nursing Scope and Standards of Practice (American Nurses Association, 2008b) and discuss associated measurement criteria.
- ☐ Describe the value and functions of the Code of Ethics for Nurses (American Nurses Association, 2001, 2008a).
- ☐ Identify the nine provisions of the Code of Ethics for Nurses and relate them to practical situations encountered in the day-to-day practice of pediatric nursing.
- ☐ Identify ethics controversies commonly encountered in the practice of pediatric nursing and discuss relevant principles, duties, rights, and virtues.
- ☐ Differentiate "consent," "permission," and "assent," and discuss how the process of promoting the best interest of children in the issue of consent differs from obtaining informed consent from a competent adult.

KEY TERMS

- Compassion
- Advocacy
- Codes of ethics
- Standards of practice
- Standards of professional performance
- Accountability
- Professional boundaries
- Therapeutic relationship
- Family-centered care
- Best-interest standard
- Autonomy
- Beneficence
- Nonmaleficence
- Justice
- Veracity
- Fidelity
- Utility or consequentialism
- Substituted judgment
- Consent
- Assent
- Permission
- Cultural diversity

INTRODUCTION

- The care of children and their families requires the application of the nursing process in accordance with accepted standards of practice, professional performance, and ethics. Quality pediatric care is
  - *developmentally appropriate,*
  - *family centered,*
  - *culturally sensitive, and*
  - *evidence based.*
- **Compassion**, **advocacy**, care coordination, continuity of care, and a holistic approach are additional hallmarks of quality care, and together these themes provide the context for standards that direct the practice of pediatric nurses.
- There is no universal consensus as to what constitutes a profession, but many definitions include the following elements:
  - *Body of science specific to the profession*
  - *Self-governance*
  - *Licensing/certification or other forms of credentialing or privileging*
  - ***Codes of ethics***
  - ***Standards of practice***
  - ***Standards of professional performance***
- Codes of ethics and standards of practice and professional performance serve as benchmarks of quality and **accountability**, providing protection for the public and guidance for professionals.
- Although "The Code of Ethics for Nurses with Interpretive Statements" (American Nurses Association [ANA], 2001)

Don't have time to read this chapter? Want to reinforce your reading? Need to review for a test? Listen to this chapter on DavisPlus at davispl.us/rudd1.

and the Pediatric Nursing Scope and Standards of Practice (ANA, 2008b) must be considered primary, the sources of standards relevant to the practice of pediatric nursing are actually many and varied. **Table 2-1** provides a representative listing of just a few of these sources.

- Familiarity with standards fosters the following:
  - *Decisiveness*
  - *Consistency*
  - *Empowerment*
  - *Accuracy*

TABLE 2–1 SOURCES OF STANDARDS THAT INFORM PEDIATRIC PRACTICE

Types and Sources of Standards		Select Examples
LAWS RULES OF LAW POLICIES CODES OF ETHICS POSITION STATEMENTS PROFESSIONAL STANDARDS PRACTICE STANDARDS CLINICAL STANDARDS ADMINISTRATIVE STANDARDS	International Federal Legislation and Regulatory Agencies	• UN Convention on the Rights of the Child • Department of Health and Human Services (DHHS): *Healthy People 2010* • Food and Drug Administration (FDA) • Centers for Disease Control and Prevention (CDC) • Health Insurance Portability and Accountability Act (HIPAA) • Patient Self-Determination Act (PSDA)
	State and Local Legislation and Regulatory Agencies	• Nurse practice acts • State boards of nursing • State pharmacy boards • State chapters of the American Hospital Association (AHA)
	NGOs/NFPs* and Public Advocacy Groups	• Joint Commission (formerly Joint Commission on the Accreditation of Hospitals) • National Association for Children's Hospitals and Related Institutions (NACHRI) • National Association for Children's Hospitals (NACH; NACHRI policy affiliate) • National Institute for Children's Healthcare Quality (NICHQ) • 5 Million Lives Campaign: Institute of Healthcare Improvement (IHI) • Institute for Safe Medication Practices (ISMP) • The Leapfrog Group
	Professional Associations	• American Nurses Association (ANA) • Society of Pediatric Nurses (SPN) • National Association of Pediatric Nurse Practitioners (NAPNAP) • National Association of Neonatal Nurses (NANN) • National Association of Neonatal Nurse Practitioners (NANNP) • National Association of School Nurses (NASN) • American Professional Society on the Abuse of Children (APSAC) • American Academy of Pediatrics (AAP)
	Hospitals and Other Health-Care Settings	• Institutional review boards that approve and monitor research • Institution-specific policies (clinical and administrative)

*NGOs/NFPs = nongovernmental organizations/not-for-profits.

- Moral considerations naturally attach to the key themes and standards; thus, pediatric nurses must develop an understanding of basic principles of ethics and acquaint themselves with the following:
  - *Types of dilemmas they are likely to encounter in practice settings*
  - *A process for resolving ethical problems*
  - *Resources available for consultation regarding ethical issues*

CLINICAL PEARL

Public Perception of Nursing

Nursing is a highly trusted profession. As of December 2010, nursing was ranked in first place in 11 out of 12 years in the annual Gallup survey of professional honesty and ethics. The only time the profession was ranked in second place was following the terrorist attacks of 9/11 in 2001 (see the "Additional Chapter Resources" section for a link to this study). This is largely a testament to the relationships nurses develop with patients and their families, as well as the principles, values, and standards by which they aspire to conduct themselves.

"THE CODE OF ETHICS FOR NURSES WITH INTERPRETIVE STATEMENTS": A BRIEF OVERVIEW

- The Code of Ethics for Nurses with Interpretive Statements (ANA, 2001) outlines and elaborates on the values and moral standards that should guide nurses in the course of carrying out their roles and is a formal and public declaration of the principles of good conduct expected of members of the profession.
- The ANA Code of Ethics for Nurses can be characterized as:
  - *A foundation for all we do, serving as a source of guidance for and empowerment of individual nurses and for the profession as a whole*
  - *A public affirmation—an exquisitely written covenant between the profession and the patients nurses serve*
  - *A reflection of key ethics philosophies, principles, rights, duties, and virtues as they apply to interactions with patients, their families, and the broader community, as well as colleagues and other stakeholders in the promotion and facilitation of quality health care*
  - *An evolutionary document that responds to and anticipates a constantly changing health-care delivery environment, emergent scientific knowledge and technological capabilities, the demands of increasingly better-educated and outcome- and quality-focused health-care consumers, and the realities of resource availability.*
- The Code of Ethics for Nurses has a comparatively short history and yet has undergone significant change over time (**Table 2-2**). The "legacy and vision" (Ellenchild Pinch & Haddad, 2008) of the Code are instructive, motivating, and deserving of exploration in greater detail than possible here, but a brief history is as follows:
  - *1893: The Nightingale Pledge, based largely on the Hippocratic Oath, was an early predecessor of today's Code and was often* unofficially *referred to as the code of ethics for the profession.*
  - *1950: The first formally sanctioned version of the Code, which included 17 provisions, appeared.*
  - *1976: The debut of the Code in its current format, which includes interpretive statements that elaborate on and clarify the provisions.*
  - *Present day: The Code's provisions have been reduced in number, from 17 in 1950 to 9 today, and modified in terms of content, emphasis, language, and format.*

CLINICAL PEARL

The Code of Ethics: A Source of Nursing Character and Strength

The ANA Code of Ethics is so fundamental to our practice and so richly developed that every nurse should own and periodically reread a copy. The Code takes on new meaning as the nurse gains in professional experience, and thus each rereading has the potential to reveal nuances that further enlighten personal practice. Dr. Barbara Daly, ethicist and chair of the task force that rendered the latest revision of the code, suggests that each time a nurse signs the initials "RN" after her or his name, it should amount to a reminder of and a recommitment to the promise of the code. The Code of Ethics for Nurses serves as a source of both inspiration and professional pride (ANA, 2001; used with permission).

CRITICAL COMPONENTS

Living Reflections of Elements of the Code of Ethics for Nurses

In view of the fact that the ANA Code of Ethics for Nurses is the underpinning for all we do as health-care professionals, an ongoing emphasis on Code provisions on the part of nursing leadership is essential in any workplace. This ensures the Code "comes alive" for practitioners and puts everyone in a better position to "walk the talk." A review of the provisions and the associated interpretive statements suggests a multitude of opportunities to formally highlight and incorporate elements of the Code within the scope of nursing employment, including the following:

- Hiring interviews
- Ongoing education classes
- Administrative policies
- Program development
- Role descriptions
- Peer-review tools
- New building design
- Employee recognition
- Orientation programs
- Annual appraisals
- Promotion criteria

TABLE 2–2 THE NINE PROVISIONS OF THE ANA CODE OF ETHICS FOR NURSES

1. The nurse, in all professional relationships, practices with compassion and respect for the inherent dignity, worth, and uniqueness of every individual, unrestricted by considerations of social or economic status, personal attributes, or the nature of health problems.
2. The nurse's primary commitment is to the patient, whether an individual, family, group, or community.
3. The nurse promotes, advocates for, and strives to protect the health, safety, and rights of the patient.
4. The nurse is responsible and accountable for individual nursing practice and determines the appropriate delegation of tasks, consistent with the nurse's obligation to provide optimum patient care.
5. The nurse owes the same duties to self as to others, including the responsibility to preserve integrity and safety, to maintain competence, and to continue personal and professional growth.
6. The nurse participates in establishing, maintaining, and improving health-care environments and conditions of employment conducive to the provision of quality health care and consistent with the values of the profession through individual and collective action.
7. The nurse participates in the advancement of the profession through contributions to practice, education, administration, and knowledge development.
8. The nurse collaborates with other health professionals and the public in promoting community, national, and international efforts to meet health needs.
9. The profession of nursing, as represented by associations and their members, is responsible for articulating nursing values, for maintaining the integrity of the profession and its practice, and for shaping social policy.

PEDIATRIC NURSING SCOPE AND STANDARDS OF PRACTICE

- Standards are statements that carry varying degrees of authority, impose responsibilities, outline correct processes, identify target outcomes, specify acceptable levels of performance, and/or define desirable professional attributes and qualifications.
  - *A distinction can be made between "standards" and "guidelines," but for the purposes of this chapter, the terms will be used interchangeably.*
  - *Standards may be labeled as such or may be embedded, with more or less subtlety, in laws, rules, policies, position statements, and codes of ethics, among others (see Table 2-1).*
  - *Many standards of practice and professional performance are derived from and/or reflect principles embodied in codes of ethics. In some instances, to separate discussions of standards from discussions of ethics is to draw an artificial distinction.*

A Primary Source of Standards

- Although far from being the *only* source of standards of practice for nurses who care for children and their families, the ANA publication *Pediatric Nursing Scope and Standards of Practice* (2008) is a definitive and primary source. This compilation of standards:
  - *Results from a collaborative effort between the National Association of Pediatric Nurse Practitioners, the Society of Pediatric Nursing, and the American Nurses Association, modifying and unifying previously distinct documents*
  - *Is of relevance to nurse generalists and to advanced practice nurses*
  - *Reflects key themes and trends that are relevant to our times and to all pediatric health-care settings, and that provide the framework for the emergence of specific standards*
  - *Specifies 6 standards of practice and 10 standards of professional performance (**Table 2-3**), elaborating on both with meaningful measurement criteria*
- The reader is advised to review the measurement criteria for the first six standards of practice (those referencing the nursing process) in the ANA publication and note that key modifiers or themes (e.g., *family centered, developmentally appropriate, culturally sensitive, evidence based, holistic, coordinated*) appear in association with each.

THERAPEUTIC RELATIONSHIPS AND PROFESSIONAL BOUNDARIES

Nature

- In pediatrics, as in other nursing specialties, the relationship formed between the nurse and the patient/family provides the framework for care delivery.
- **Professional boundaries** must be respected but can, at times, be difficult to define.
- Characteristics of **therapeutic relationships** include the following:
  - *Goal directed*
  - *Mutual respect and trust*
  - *Empathy*
  - *Advocacy*
  - *Avoidance of the extremes of the relationship continuum (i.e., enmeshment and disengagement)*
  - *Resultant empowerment of the patient/family (McAliley, et al., 1996)*

Clinical Reasoning

Rights of the Child and Standards of Practice: Shared Themes

Review a copy of "Pediatric Nursing: Scope and Standards of Practice" and compare it with the content from the United Nations (UN) Convention on the Rights of the Child highlighted in **Table 2-4**.

- Identify the shared themes and language.
- Tie specific nursing standards and measurement criteria with specific articles of the UN document.
- Are there any rights specified by the highlighted selections from the UN document that are not captured by the pediatric nursing standards?
- Which of the rights/standards mentioned in either document may be difficult for some countries and/or some health-care facilities or practice settings to implement fully? Why?
- Why should pediatric nurses in North America be concerned about the rights of children in other parts of the world, and how can they serve as effective advocates?
- What specific aspects characterize the UN rights and the measurement criteria for the first six standards of practice as distinctly "pediatric"? Are there any rights or standards and measurement criteria that do *not* apply equally well to human rights in general and adult health-care delivery?

Therapeutic Relationship Challenges in Pediatric Care Settings

- Infants and children are innately vulnerable, and this vulnerability increases in circumstances where parents or guardians are unable to be present and participate in the care of the child.
- The nature of some pediatric experiences and the vulnerability of children may move the nurse toward distancing or toward overinvolvement, especially in the following cases:
  - *Child abuse and neglect*
  - *Dying children*
  - *Children with chronic conditions such as cystic fibrosis, cancer, or sickle cell anemia who have repeated admissions to the hospital and stay for long periods or have frequent visits to the clinic and/or the emergency department (ED), becoming well known to the staff*
  - *Tough, street-wise adolescents who challenge everything and everyone*
  - *Noncompliant or nonadherent patients and families*
  - *Chronically ill children in long-term care facilities whose parents may not visit for months at a time*
  - *Children with parents who are diagnosed with borderline personality disorder or other types of mental illness and engage in manipulative and disruptive behaviors*

TABLE 2–3 PEDIATRIC NURSING STANDARDS OF PRACTICE AND PROFESSIONAL PERFORMANCE

PRACTICE	
#1	Assessment: The pediatric nurse collects comprehensive data pertinent to the patient's health or the situation.
#2	Diagnosis: The pediatric nurse analyzes the assessment data to determine the diagnoses or healthcare issues.
#3	Outcomes Identification: The pediatric nurse identifies expected outcomes for a plan of care individualized to the child, family, and the situation.
#4	Planning: The pediatric nurse develops a plan of care that prescribe strategies and alternatives to attain expected outcomes.
#5	Implementation: The pediatric nurse implements the identified plan of care.
	5a Coordination of Care and Case Management: The pediatric nurse coordinates care delivery.
	5b Health Teaching and Health Promotion, Restoration, and Maintenance: The pediatric nurse employs strategies to promote health and a safe environment.
	5c Consultation: The pediatric nurse provides consultation to healthcare providers and others to influence the identified plan of care for children, to enhance the abilities of others to provide health care, and to effect change in the health-care system.
	5d Prescriptive Authority and Treatment: The advanced practice pediatric nurse utilizes prescriptive authority, procedures, referrals, treatments, and therapies in providing care.
	5e Referral: The advanced practice pediatric nurse identifies the need for additional care and makes referrals as indicated.
#6	Evaluation: The pediatric nurse evaluates progress towards attainment of outcomes.
PROFESSIONAL PERFORMANCE	
#7	Quality of Practice: The pediatric nurse systematically enhances the quality and effectiveness of nursing practice.
#8	Professional Practice Evaluation: The pediatric nurse evaluates one's own nursing practice in relation to professional practice standards and guidelines, relevant statutes, rules and regulations.

Continued

TABLE 2–3 PEDIATRIC NURSING STANDARDS OF PRACTICE AND PROFESSIONAL PERFORMANCE—cont'd

PROFESSIONAL PERFORMANCE

#9	Education: The pediatric nurse attains knowledge and competency that reflects current nursing practice.
#10	Collegiality: The pediatric nurse interacts with and contributes to the professional development of peers and colleagues.
#11	Collaboration: The pediatric nurse collaborates with the child, family, and others in the conduct of nursing practice.
#12	Ethics: The pediatric nurse integrates ethical considerations and processes in all areas of practice.
#13	Research, Evidence Based Practice and Clinical Scholarship: The pediatric nurse integrates research findings into practice and, where appropriate, participates in the generation of new knowledge.
#14	Resource Utilization: The pediatric nurse considers factors related to safety, effectiveness, cost and impact on practice in planning and delivering patient care.
#15	Leadership: The pediatric nurse provides leadership in the professional practice setting and the profession.
#16	Advocacy: The pediatric nurse is an advocate for the pediatric client and family.

Reprinted with permission from the National Association of Pediatric Nurse Practitioners, Society of Pediatric Nurses, and American Nurses Association, *Pediatric Nursing Standards of Practice and Professional Performance*,

TABLE 2–4 UNITED NATIONS (UN) CONVENTION ON THE RIGHTS OF THE CHILD: SELECTED ARTICLES

The UN Convention on the Rights of the Child (CRC) is an international advocacy instrument with legal (as of 2000) and moral standing specifying societal responsibilities toward children the world over.

- The United States and Somalia are the only countries that have not ratified it. (Somalia has not signed because of the lack of a defined and stable government. The United States has established "signatory" status indicating good-faith intent to ratify the CRC—give it the force of law—once detailed study has been completed.).
- There are 54 articles (42 detailing the rights of children and 12 detailing implementation measures).
- Some rights/articles of special interest to pediatric health-care professionals include but are not limited to the following:
  - The best interests of children must be the primary concern in making decisions that may affect them. (#3)
  - Children have a right to live with their parents unless it is bad for them. (#9)
  - When adults are making decisions that affect children, children have the right to say what they think should happen and have their opinions taken into account. (#12)
  - Children have the right to get and share information, as long as the information is not damaging to them or others. (#13)
  - Children have the right to privacy. (#16)
  - Children have the right to be protected from being hurt and mistreated, physically and mentally. Forms of discipline are generally up to the parents but should be "nonviolent, appropriate to the child's level of development and take the best interests of the child into consideration." (#19)
  - "Children who have any kind of disability have the right to special care and support . . . so they can live full and independent lives." (#23)
  - Children have the right to good quality health care—the best health care possible—and information to help them stay healthy. (#24)
  - Minority or indigenous children have the right to learn about and practice their own culture, language, and religion. (#30)
  - "Protection against use of harmful drugs . . . involvement in drug trade . . . all forms of sexual exploitation and abuse . . . abduction and trafficking . . . and other forms of exploitation that could harm their welfare and development." (#32, #33, #34, #35, #36)
  - These rights should be made known to adults and children. (#42)

Adapted from United Nations Convention on the Rights of the Child. Comprehensive copy of document retrieved from http://www.unicef.org/crc/files/Rights_overview.pdf.

- As in any field of nursing, the cultural background, life experiences, and values of the nurse can result in biases and blind spots—especially when they differ from those of the patient/family.

CLINICAL PEARL

Therapeutic Relations, Family-Centered Care, and Relationship-Based Nursing: A Cautionary Note

The elements of family-centered care and relationship-based nursing are key to quality care, but are also associated with potential hazards, the avoidance of which requires very thoughtful analysis and application of self as the nurse works toward developing a therapeutic alliance. Issues include the following:

- Some may be of the belief that an interaction or intervention that feels "warm and fuzzy" and makes patients and families happy must be therapeutic and laudable when, in fact, some warm-and-fuzzy moments can result in boundary violations and staff splitting, may create unrealistic expectations of staff on the part of the family, and may interfere with achievement of key outcome goals.
- There is a distinction between being a friend and being a friendly professional.
- There is a distinction between being a parent substitute and being a caring, nurturing professional.
- There is a distinction between using good nursing judgment and being prejudiced or judgmental.

Recognizing these distinctions and acting accordingly is where some of the "art" of nursing comes into play, and can be particularly challenging in the pediatric setting.

Professional Boundaries and Personal Authenticity

- Provision 2.4 of the ANA Code of Ethics for Nurses acknowledges the challenge of "maintaining authenticity and expressing oneself as an individual, while remaining within the bounds established by the purpose of the relationship" (ANA, 2001).
  - *Very few treatises on the subject of boundaries provide specifics as to where the boundaries should be drawn.*
  - *Discovering and respecting professional boundaries and the keys to a therapeutic relationship are lifetime pursuits.*
  - *Policies and rules are sometimes counterproductive—professional judgment and collaborative decision making are necessary in such situations.*
  - *Articulating a* shared *concept of what constitutes a therapeutic relationship and identifying explicit guidelines for interactions with patients, families, and colleagues in the workplace are both prudent.*
  - *Individuals should commit to holding themselves and their colleagues accountable to maintaining boundaries and should revisit agreements as problems arise or staff turnover occurs.*

Clinical Reasoning

Therapeutic Relations: Sorting out Boundaries

Engage in a discussion with fellow students or colleagues about boundaries and potential guidelines regarding:

- Sharing/disclosure of personal information with patients/families
- Accepting gifts from patients/families
- Giving clothing or gifts or bringing home-cooked foods to patients/families
- Loaning money to patients/families
- Offering a child's family member a ride home at the end of the shift
- Babysitting for or socializing with patients/families outside the workplace
- Assignments and patient contact when a patient or family member is a relative, friend, or acquaintance
- Visiting the patient when admitted or transferred to another clinical location
- Visiting the patient or calling for patient updates on personal time
- "Good-bye" or "graduation" parties for patients discharged or transferred after a long stay or upon completion of courses of chemotherapy, or other milestones
- Funeral attendance when children pass away

Criteria for Analysis:

- What objectives do these actions meet, and whose needs do they serve?
- What are the potential impacts on other patients/families/staff?
- What might the impacts be with respect to identified outcome goals?
- How do these relate to workplace mission/vision/values/policies?
- Are these activities in keeping with the nurse's personal and professional philosophy and values?
- What safeguards must be put in place to avoid foreseeable negative consequences?
- Are there better alternatives for achieving the same goals if the goals are worthy?
- Would you do the same with or for every patient/family in your care under similar circumstances (universalizability)?
- When nursing judgment suggests the usual standard may or should be ignored, what are the issues that should be considered, and who else (if anyone) needs to be involved in the decision? (McAliley, Lambert, Ashenberg, & Dull, 1996)

The Roots of Challenging Patient and Family Behaviors

- Because of the fiduciary nature of the relationship, the nurse bears greater responsibility than the family for promoting and sustaining a therapeutic relationship; however, this does not imply that the patient and family have no responsibility or that the nurse has total control over the outcome.
- Nurses should avoid the use of labeling and instead use assessment skills to determine the roots of a problematic relationship, which will
  - *Reduce the impulse to personalize the patient/family behavior*

- *Help maintain compassion*
- *Avert a defensive or adversarial response*
- *Leave those involved open to addressing personal contributions to the situation*
- *Provide insights regarding appropriate intervention*

- Once contributing factors have been identified, the nurse must use judgment with respect to whether the primary focus should be on addressing the underlying factors, more directly addressing the disruptive behaviors, or taking a combined approach (***Table 2-5***).

FAMILY-CENTERED CARE

- **Family-centered care** recognizes the centrality of families to the well-being of children as well as the impact a child's illness may have on the family, and promotes partnering between patients, families, and health-care professionals to the benefit of all.
- The presence and involvement of the family can be as important to the child in some respects as any medication or treatment.
- "Family" may be defined in a variety of nontraditional ways.
  - *Nurses should be prepared to accommodate single-parent families, adoptive families, foster families, blended families, second-generation (grand parenting) families, same-sex partners or marriages, families involving mixed cultures or religions, and other family configurations (see also Chapter 3).*

TABLE 2–5 POTENTIAL CONTRIBUTING FACTORS TO CHALLENGING FAMILY BEHAVIORS
• Anxiety regarding child's condition/prognosis, unexpected changes in condition, the risks and burdens of treatment, transfers to a new environment, etc.
• Guilt over child's condition
• In possession of inadequate information or of misinformation
• Fear of loss of control (common among people with professional/leadership backgrounds)
• Unmet expectations (realistic or otherwise)
• Competing work/family/financial worries/concerns
• Altered thought process (mental health, substance abuse)
• Previous bad hospital experience or fears inspired by national focus on hospital errors and hospital-acquired infections
• Conflicting communications from professionals involved in the child's care
• Delays in availability of care/equipment—failures/errors of health-care team
• Environmental issues (dirty, lack of parental accommodations and privacy, noisy)
• Staff rude, impatient, slow to respond to need for assistance
• Unreasonably inflexible hospital/unit rules that fail to permit individualized care

Clinical Reasoning

Family-Centered Care Plans

Standard 4 of the Pediatric Nursing Scope and Standards of Practice (ANA, 2008b) refers to development of a family-centered plan of care and notes the following considerations:

- Practically speaking, what is meant by a plan of care that is "family centered"?
- What is the difference between a plan of care that is *family focused* and one that is *family centered* (the broader and more inclusive of the two terms)?
- Look at the plan of care for a current or recent patient and identify the family-centered elements as well as any opportunities for enhancing a family-centered approach to the development or content of the plan. For example:
  - How does the structure of the family (e.g., single parent, blended families, foster families, etc.) have an impact on the development of the plan?
  - How do the family's cultural and spiritual beliefs and practices influence the plan?
  - What are some of the barriers to development of a family-centered plan of care?

Child Life Specialists: Key Contributors to Family-Centered Care

- Child life specialists, like nurses, are key proponents of family-centered care, and their presence in inpatient settings, clinics, EDs, intensive care units, rehabilitation settings, procedural planning, and other areas is of incalculable value.
- They possess expertise in the field of child development.
- They can help promote effective coping, ongoing development, and normalization for children and families by:
  - *preparing children and families for and supporting them through procedures.*
  - *providing therapeutic play and self-expression opportunities.*
  - *helping design and maintain child- and family-friendly environments, as well as a host of other strategies.*
- In some settings they work closely with art and music therapists and are liaisons with hospital- and community-based school teachers.

Rewards of Family-Centered Care

- The costs of family-centered care are usually more than offset by the benefits:
  - *Decreased levels of patient and family stress*

CRITICAL COMPONENTS

Overview of Family-Centered and Family-Focused Strategies

- Consider the involvement of parents in medical rounds, nursing change-of-shift reports, and in the development, implementation, and evaluation of the child's plan of care.
- Adapt schedules, as possible, to suit the patient/family's routines and preferences.
- Implement noise-reduction efforts (see the Clinical Pearl feature):
  - Consider acoustic wall panels and flooring when designing new buildings or updating/refreshing older ones.
  - Consider quieter models when replacing existing ventilators, suction equipment, feeding pumps, IV pumps, and other equipment.
  - Use staff locator badges rather than overhead paging.
  - Set pagers on vibrate mode.
  - Implement dress code requirements for soft-soled shoes.
  - Install "Yacker Trackers" to sensitize staff to the noise level in the environment and encourage them to effectively contribute to noise reduction (for more information, enter the key word "Yacker Tracker" in an Internet search engine).
  - Plan periods of "quiet time" when diagnostic and therapeutic intrusions are limited to accommodate children in need of naps.
- Consider a hotel "room service" model for meals.
- Implement programs that provide free or reduced-cost food for breastfeeding mothers.
- Provide access to refrigerators and the means to prepare and heat food brought in from home for rooming-in family members or to stimulate the appetite of the hospitalized child.
- Provide dedicated family space in patient rooms, as well as laundry and lounge facilities for rooming-in parents.
  - Post signs on doors that remind health-care providers and visitors to knock and wait for permission to enter so that family privacy is respected.
  - Provide lockable family storage space in patient rooms.
- Create staffed "Family Resource Centers" with library and computer services to facilitate access to medical educational information, health-care support groups, and special services, and that permit patients/families to keep in touch with other family members, friends, and business associates via telephone or computer.
- Create staffed "Family Learning Centers" where families can learn procedures such as blood glucose testing and administration of insulin injections, or how to suction and change a tracheotomy tube or insert a nasogastric tube administer an enteral feeding, or how to recognize the need for and then administer infant cardiopulmonary resuscitation, for example. The center should include:
  - Dedicated instructors
  - Formal teaching modules and videos
  - Simulated, hands-on practice with anatomically correct dolls
  - Consistent educational practices

In addition, the center should afford parents the opportunity to develop competence and confidence under comparatively low-pressure circumstances prior to the need to perform these procedures on their children.

- Create "Family and Patient Advisory Councils" that permit input into policies, programming, building renovation or design, food services, or other areas.
- Create "Foster Grandparent" or "Special Visitor" programs that provide visitors for children who do not have family members rooming-in or visiting with frequency.
- Consider programs of other organizations, and whether similar programs could be adopted in your workplace. For example, for over 35 years, Ronald McDonald House Charities (RHMC), funded primarily by the McDonald's restaurant chain, has sponsored a variety of initiatives to better the status of children and families in many cities and countries across the world. Many of these initiatives are in line with the principles of family-centered care, such as:
  - RHMC provides family members who must travel a distance to the hospital an inviting, home-like place to stay near the hospital at very little cost (sometimes free, depending upon circumstances and charitable resources).
  - In some children's hospitals, RMHC sponsors "Ronald McDonald Family Rooms," which provide free access to a living room environment and host/hostess services that permit families to escape the constant sickroom focus while being only minutes away from their child. Many hospitals offer their own version of a hospitality center.

- *Enhanced patient/family learning of new information and skills*
- *Increased likelihood of adherence to plans of care*
- *Reduced likelihood of medical error*
- *Improved patient/family sleep and nutrition*
- *Decreased disruption of normal patient/family routines and responsibilities*
- *Increased patient and family satisfaction*
- *Those looking for a starting place for additional information about family-centered care are advised to visit the website of the Institute for Family Centered Care and the Family Voices website (see the "Additional Chapter Resources" section for links).*

DEVELOPMENTALLY APPROPRIATE CARE

- Children are not simply mini-adults—they are in the process of developing in the physiological, motor, cognitive, psychosocial, psychosexual, moral, and spiritual realms.
- It must also be recognized that families go through stages of development. (See Chapters 3 and 6 for overviews of family and child development theories.)
- A complex interplay of genetic, experiential, and environmental factors influences the developmental course and outcomes of a given child and family.

Clinical Reasoning

Family-Centered Care Scenarios

- What can be done to keep in touch with parents and support their involvement in decision making if they cannot visit often?
- What practical steps might be taken to support a relationship between a premature infant in the neonatal intensive care unit and his 7-year-old brother who is not permitted to visit during respiratory virus season?
- How can daily medical rounds and nursing change-of-shift reports be structured to include families when they are present, without becoming prohibitively time consuming?
- How can we accommodate unmarried minor parents who want to room-in and who need to learn the details of the complex care of their child but also have to keep up with school attendance and homework?
- As peers are critical in the life of adolescents and are, in a sense, part of their "family," how can we keep them "in touch" during hospitalizations? What can we do for hospitalized teens who miss out on important school events, such as the high school senior who will miss her prom or the injured basketball player who will miss out on the championship game?

- Familiarity with developmental theories, principles, and milestones enables:
  - *effective communication and support that maximizes cooperation and minimizes anxiety.*
  - *developmentally appropriate and effective assessments, goals, plans of care, and education.*
  - *safely structured environments, routines, and procedures.*
  - *facilitation or minimal disruption of ongoing development.*

Child Development and Pain Management

- Prompt and effective pain management is an absolute moral imperative, and there are definite developmental implications for the assessment and management of discomfort in children. Children differ from adults in the following respects:
  - *Physiologic responses to/manifestations of pain*
  - *Ability to describe, localize, and quantify pain*
  - *Tolerance of and response to medications*
- Many tested tools are available for assessing the need for and response to pain management interventions in children of different ages or stages of development (see **Table 2-6**).

CLINICAL PEARL

A Family-Centered Care Tool: Ethical Considerations

There is now a proliferation of web-based communities that permit families of hospitalized children and/or children with rare or chronic conditions to create personalized, interactive web pages where they journal their health-care journeys and/or communicate with others experiencing the same challenges they face. Benefits of such communities include the following:

- They enable parents to update all concerned friends and families at once, thus eliminating the stress of making or fielding numerous phone calls.
- Friends and families can respond immediately, but parents are able to tap into the thoughts, prayers, and offers of assistance at times that are convenient for them.
- The computerized journaling involved can be therapeutic for the parent.
- Parents may learn of helpful coping strategies, support groups, and service delivery resources by viewing the pages created by other families.

Despite the potential benefits and the safeguards that may be built in, ethical issues regarding these online communities also deserve attention, such as the following:

- Parents may share huge amounts of specific and very personal information regarding their children and families—some of it unintentionally shared as a result of what people read between the lines. The children thus have little or no say about what goes out into the "computer universe." Even anonymously posted details can be used to help identify individual children, and at some point (whether as youth or adults) children may come to regret or resent what was made public.
- Some of the health information and recommendations put out by families may be unreliable but may still have a cache of respect and the ability to influence others.
- The course of one child's illness may be very different than that of another child with the same condition, and yet families may feel their children are receiving inferior care if they do not receive the same tests or the same treatments that the parents of other children have reported. This can result in requests for and sometimes administration of unnecessary diagnostic or therapeutic interventions and can also result in "doctor/hospital shopping."
- Despite the many safeguards, those who want unauthorized access to family sites may be able to hack through to them. Vulnerable families may become the targets of unscrupulous individuals seeking to take advantage of them (e.g., advertising of useless "cures" and equipment, etc.).
- What staff read on these sites about patients/families may bias the care they provide in ways that are sometimes subtle and sometimes quite overt.

Pediatric nurses are in a good position to help parents anticipate and sort through some of the ethical issues potentially associated with these web-based communities, and pediatric hospitals would be wise to assess their sponsorship of such sites and the formal guidance they might provide.

TABLE 2-6 OVERVIEW OF SELECT PAIN ASSESSMENT SCALES

BEHAVIORAL AND PHYSICAL INDICATOR SCALES			
PIPP: Premature Infant Pain Profile (Stevens, 1996)	**NIPS:** Neonatal Infant Pain Scale (Lawrence et al., 1993)	**CRIES** (Krechel & Bildner, 1995; Taylor et al., 2006)	**FLACC** (Merkel et al., 1997)
Neonates (28–40 weeks of gestation)	Preterm and full-term neonates	Preterm and full-term neonates	2 months to 7 years of age
0–3 points each for gestational age, behavioral state, heart rate, O_2 saturation, brow bulge, eye squeeze, nasolabial furrow	0–1 (2 for cry) points each for facial expression, cry, breathing patterns, arm movements, leg movements, state of arousal	0–2 points each for cry, requires O_2, increased vital signs, expression, sleeplessness	1–3 points each for face, legs, activity, cry, consolability
SELF-REPORT SCALES			
FACES (Wong-Baker referenced but there are others) (Hockenberry & Wilson, 2009)	**Oucher (Byer, 2009)**	**VAS: Visual Analogue Scales (variety of scales and descriptors)**	**Adolescent Pediatric Pain Tool** (multidimensional) (Savedra & Crandall, 2005)
3 years through adolescence	3 years and older	6 years and older	8–17 years
Six line drawings of faces with expressions from happy to neutral to crying, each associated with a number from 1 to 6	Series of photographs of facial expressions from neutral to crying (Caucasian, Hispanic, African American, First Nation, Asian) associated with ratings of 0 to 10	Horizontal or vertical line with linguistic pain descriptors and equidistant markings associated with numbers (usually 0 to 10)	Body outline (draw location of pain); word-graphic scale (mark on a line closest to the intensity descriptor); word list (circle the sensory, affective, and evaluative words that apply)

- Assessment tools can be classified as behavioral observation scales (infants) or self-report rating scales (young child through adult).
- Infant behavioral scales rely on specifically defined indicators, such as vital signs, need for oxygen, breathing patterns, facial expressions, presence and nature of crying, and movement of extremities.
- Self-report rating scales may require a child to:
  - *Point to drawings or photos of facial expressions reflecting varying degrees of pain*
  - *Pick up a number of poker chips correlated with the amount of pain*
  - *Point to a spot on a visual scale that is associated with a number (usually 0–10) and/or words describing pain feelings*
- Use of infant behavior observation tools requires staff training and achievement of interobserver reliability (similar results obtained by different observers.
- Success in using the self-report rating scales necessitates preliminary teaching with the child and family and assessment of the child's readiness to use a specific tool.
- Growth and developmental status also influence choice of pharmacologic and/or nonpharmacological pain management techniques.
  - *In the first few months of life, swaddling, nonnutritive sucking, and/or the administration of small amounts of 24% sucrose solutions have been demonstrated to be effective in reducing the physiologic and behavioral responses to pain and to hasten the recovery from simple procedural pain.*
  - *Distraction (e.g., toys, television, video games) can work to some extent with children of almost all ages who are experiencing pain at the lower ends of the pain scales.*
  - *Hypnotherapy, biofeedback, and other complementary and alternative treatment approaches may be suitable for children able to follow instructions and use their imaginations.*
  - *Medication dosages are calculated based upon weight or body surface area, and the formulations of oral medications depend upon the child's ability to swallow pills versus liquid.*

- *Most children's pain medications are flavored to increase acceptance, but some may need to be disguised further with foods or flavorings.*
    - Compounding pharmacies prepare formulations of medications that are palatable to children and suitable to their dosage requirements and developmental abilities. (American Academy of Pediatrics, Committee on Fetus and Newborn, 2006; Dlugosz, Chater, & Engle, 2006; Doyle & Colleti, 2006; Greco & Berde, 2005; Huang, 2003; Johnston et al., 2003; Kemper & Gardiner, 2003; Morash & Fowler, 2004; Taylor et al., 2006)

Child Development and Patient and Family Education

- The child should be provided with developmentally appropriate and culturally sensitive health-care education, employing a variety of learning modalities:
    - *Video*
    - *Educational comic books*
    - *Reader-friendly diagrams and handouts*
    - *Computer-assisted learning*
    - *Hands-on experience with anatomically correct dolls and actual materials/equipment*

Educational Role of the Pediatric Nurse

- The nurse provides children and their families with learning opportunities relating to health maintenance and promotion, illness and injury management, and decision making and coping. In the role of patient educator, the nurse is responsible for:
    - *Assessing learning preference styles (parents may have helpful information)*
    - *Assessing learning readiness (interest and motivation; freedom from pain, anxiety, distractions).*
    - *Provision of accurate, useful information that is developmentally appropriate and culturally sensitive; education that is tailored to the needs of the individual*
    - *Assessment of understanding and retention of information, and of the need for reinforcement and/or additional education*
    - *Documentation of all of the above*

Child Development, Privacy, and Confidentiality

- Privacy and confidentiality are related but distinct concepts that must be addressed from a developmental perspective and that give rise to challenges of an ethical nature in the pediatric setting.
- Standards require that we give increasing respect to the needs for privacy and confidentiality as children get older.
- As they mature, children become increasingly more involved in providing their own medical history, and they begin to approach health-care professionals with agendas of their own.
- Older children cannot be expected to provide reliable information or request education or services with respect to sensitive subjects if not provided with privacy and some assurance of confidentiality. Such sensitive subjects include the following:
    - *Family violence*
    - *Substance use/abuse*
    - *Depression and suicidal thoughts*
    - *Struggles with weight or eating disorders*
    - *Gender identity issues and sexual activity*
- Privacy measures also need to be taken with respect to the physical exam, and the older child or adolescent may request confidentiality with regard to some clinical findings and even diagnoses.

Evidence-Based Practice: Adult Literacy and Readability of Health-Care Education Materials

The 2003 National Assessment of Adult Literacy surveyed 19,000 U.S. individuals age 16 and older. Results: 14% had "no more than the most simple and concrete literacy skills" for prose literature (fifth-grade level and lower), and another 29% "can perform simple and everyday literacy activities" (between fifth- and eighth-grade level). This translates into an estimated 93 million American adults who perform at or below the basic literacy level. In this study, performance below the basic level had strong associations with poverty, English as a second language (not started prior to school entry), noncompletion of high school, and the presence of multiple disabilities (Greenberg, Jin, & White, 2007).

Multiple studies have demonstrated correlates between low literacy and poor health-care behaviors and outcomes, such as increased frequency of emergency care visits and hospital admissions, decreased compliance with medications, improper use of metered-dose inhalers, incorrect installation of infant car seats, failure to seek screening and later diagnosis of cancer, and poorer glycemic control, to name a few examples (Merriman, Ades, & Seffrin, 2002; Schillinger et al., 2002; Williams, Baker, Honig, Lee, & Nowlan, 1998).

- It is suggested that health education materials intended for *adults* be created at a reading level no higher than eighth grade, although most exceed this standard.
- A popular approach to assessing and adjusting readability is the SMOG (Simple Measure of Gobbledygook) approach:
    - Count the number of three-syllable words in three separate sets of 10 sentences and apply a simple mathematic equation.
    - Greater detail and a SMOG calculator are available through a website belonging to originator, Harry McLaughlin (see the "Additional Chapter Resources" section for a link.)

Privacy and Confidentiality: Conflicting Duties to Child and Parents

- Respecting privacy and confidentiality may create some tension for the nurses when they experience a sense of conflict with respect to duties owed the child and those owed the parent.
- It is the parent's duty to instill values and provide for the health and safety of the child, yet this can be difficult to

CRITICAL COMPONENTS

The Use of Chaperones

Although their presence can be viewed as a barrier to ensuring privacy and confidentiality, an offer of a medical chaperone is highly advisable under potentially sensitive circumstances such as the following:

- Any exam or procedure involving exposure and/or touching of breasts or anogenital areas
- Exams involving children/parents known to be anxious, suspicious, seductive, mentally or cognitively impaired, and/or litigious
- A medical history that requires detailed questions of a sensitive nature that could be misinterpreted as inappropriate by the patient (for example, when obtaining a history specific to sexual abuse)

Chaperones are an equally wise precaution for nurses as for physicians, and they afford protection for both the patient and the professional.

- It does not matter whether the patient and professional are of the opposite sex or of the same sex; concerns about heterosexual and homosexual improprieties are prevalent, and children become sensitive to these concerns at increasingly early ages.
- Parents make effective chaperones in most cases with infants and young children but are often not acceptable to older children and adolescents (privacy reasons).
- Chaperones must be aware of their responsibilities to witness safe/appropriate care delivery and to maintain privacy and confidentiality.
- The presence and identification of the chaperone should be documented in the medical record.
- If the offer of a chaperone is declined, the professional should use judgment as to whether the exam/procedure should take place without one or be cancelled or deferred to someone else. When possible, the wishes of the patient/family should be honored. The offer and the refusal should be documented.

The patient/family and chaperone should have full explanation of the nature and purpose of the exam or procedure so that surprises, misperceptions, and charges of impropriety are less likely. They should also be informed that the same confidentiality safeguards apply to the chaperone as to the examining physician/nurse.

do if the parent is unaware of matters requiring momentous decisions and/or exposing the child to risk.

- It is important to have discussions with parents and older children/adolescents about privacy and confidentiality interests.
  - *How they relate to the normal developmental tasks of achieving identity and autonomy*
  - *How they will be supported by the health-care provider*
- It is also important to specify practical limitations and legal exceptions.
  - *Encourage frank and open discussion about sensitive matters between adolescents and their parents.*
  - *Realize that there are times that such discussions will not happen and perhaps, in select cases, times when honest discussion could be dangerous for the child.*
  - *When unable to convince the child to disclose to parents or to permit the professional to disclose for or with the child, confidentiality will be maintained to the degree practical and legal. (See the Clinical Pearl regarding practical and legal exceptions.)*
  - *Information may sometimes be withheld from parents, but the professional should not lie on behalf of the child.*

Confidentiality and HIPAA

- Among other things, the Health Insurance Portability and Accountability Act of 1996 (HIPAA) requires standards for electronic health-care transactions and mandates provisions for the security and privacy of personal health information.
- HIPAA imposes obligations with respect to how we dispose of personal health information, how we shield information on computer screens from the view of others, how we afford privacy when registering a patient at a desk in a public lobby or when obtaining a medical history, what we talk about in hospital elevators and hospital cafeterias, and how and where we give change-of-shift nursing reports or make patient rounds.
- HIPAA has implications for policies regarding what we can do and say in front of grandparents who are visiting, how we respond to a telephone caller claiming to be a parent, what we do when a patient asks for an update regarding another patient with whom he or she is friendly and shares information, and how we protect parts of the record the patient wishes to remain confidential.

Child Development and Health-Care Decision Making

- To what extent and in what manner can children of various ages be involved in their own medical decision making?
  - *This is the source of an abundance of ethics controversies and angst in clinical settings, and the concepts, principles, and legalities involved deserve serious attention.*
  - *Some familiarity with bioethics basics will be helpful, as described in the Critical Components feature.*

CHALLENGES PRESENTED BY THE BEST-INTEREST STANDARD

- The **best-interest standard** sounds good in principle, but in practice presents all sorts of challenges for pediatric health-care providers. There are two major concerns:
  - *Who gets to decide what is in a particular patient's best interest?*
  - *What are the criteria that should be taken into consideration when deciding what is in a patient's best interest?*

CLINICAL PEARL

Practical Limitations and Legal Exceptions Regarding Confidentially

Practical considerations such as the following may preclude confidentiality.

- Parental right to access medical records:
  - Some confidential information may be omitted by the nurse in the course of documenting histories and exams.
  - Some information of a sensitive nature must be documented (to justify care given, direct the care of others, document responses to treatment, and as otherwise required by law or professional standard).
- Parental financial responsibility:
  - Parents have no obligation to pay for nonemergency care for which they did not provide consent.
  - Children without access to money or to a free clinic or other such service that might waive a charge face a very practical barrier to confidentiality.
  - When insurance is used, parents may receive billing information that discloses the nature of the visit/condition.
- Pregnancy contraindications to diagnostic or therapeutic procedures or medications:
  - Some important diagnostic procedures and treatments or medications require testing for pregnancy and may have to be withheld or significantly modified if the test results are positive.
  - Adolescents and their parents must be informed of the need for the pregnancy testing and told what will be done with the results before the test is actually performed.

In a few circumstances, the health-care provider is required by law to break confidentiality:

- Professionals have legal and moral obligations to disclose "reasonable concerns" that the child is going to intentionally harm her- himself or someone else or suspicions that the child may be the victim of any form of abuse.
- Child should be given the option to participate in telling parents if that is the professional's intended course of action.
- Health-care providers should anticipate, prepare the child for, and help mitigate potential fallout from disclosure to family.
- In the case of suspected abuse, a report must be made to a child protective services agency and/or to law enforcement (depending upon local requirements).
  - There is no need to have *proof* when reporting suspicions, and the individual making the report is immune from liability no matter what the outcome of the investigation is, as long as it can be shown that the report was made in good faith and not frivolously or maliciously.
  - If it is the policy of the workplace that the reports are filed by a social worker, the nurse must confirm that the patient's record contains documentation of the report, as only then is the nurse's obligation fulfilled as a mandated reporter.

Clinical Reasoning

Privacy and Confidentiality Scenario

A 15-year-old girl with type I diabetes asks the nurse for education about various birth control options and resources for obtaining them without parental knowledge. The nurse is aware that the girl is sexually active, although her mother believes she is not. Furthermore, the mother is devoutly religious. Per her orthodox religion, sexual intercourse is only appropriate between married individuals and for the purpose of procreation. There is a religious prohibition regarding the use of contraception other than abstinence.

- How might the nurse respond to the girl's request?
- What contribution (if any) does the diagnosis of diabetes make to your decision?
- Does it matter whether this comes up during the course of a hospital admission or during a clinic visit?
- Suppose the mother had made it clear at some point prior to the patient's inquiry that she did not want professionals providing her daughter with any information regarding sexually related topics because she views it as purely a parental prerogative. Would your answers to the previous questions change?

CLINICAL PEARL

Privacy Passwords

- At admission, have parents select a personalized password.
- Instruct them to share this password only with persons with whom they permit staff to share the patient's personal information. Remind them they will need to remember the password when calling from outside the hospital.
- Record this password in an easily retrievable section of the medical record and in a protected area at workstations.

Best Interest: Who Gets to Decide?

- When the patient is a minor, the parent or legal guardian makes the decisions, although this "default position" is not without limits.
- Parental decision-making rights should never be revoked casually, and the burden of proof should rest with those challenging those rights. The following are circumstances that may warrant revocation:
- *The parents are making decisions based on the interests of someone other than the child or might even be experiencing an apparent conflict of interest.* Example: *the profoundly brain-injured child with no prospect of recovery or of a meaningful interactive life was the victim of abuse. Removal of life support would result in the parent being charged with murder instead of child endangerment and other lesser crimes; thus the parent refuses to give permission for withdrawal of life-sustaining interventions.*
- *The parents are insisting on unduly burdensome interventions with very little hope of any benefit and that would result in a quality of life that the average person or most people would find intolerable.*
  - Individuals may sometimes be misguided in attempts to thwart nature—resulting in prolonging death rather than preserving life.

CRITICAL COMPONENTS

Key Principles of Biomedical Ethics

The following principles are commonly viewed as primary to the analysis and resolution of bioethics dilemmas:

- **Autonomy**: The right for the competent adult to accept or refuse any medical treatment based on his or her own values, priorities, and preferences, regardless of potential outcome, including death. This is the basis for privacy, confidentiality, and informed consent and refusal policies.
- **Beneficence**:* The duty of health-care providers to do things that are beneficial or good.
- **Nonmaleficence**:* The duty of health-care providers to do no harm.
- **Justice**: Fair access to and distribution of resources—treat patients with like needs in like ways.
- **Veracity**: This may be seen as the duty to tell the truth or may merely be viewed as the duty not to lie. The distinction is significant.
- **Fidelity**: The duty to keep promises (some promises are implied in the context of a nurse–patient relationship rather than expressly stated).
- **Sanctity of life**: Do not kill.

*It is often not possible to benefit patients without causing harm (for example, if the patient has bone cancer, it may not be possible to cure the cancer without subjecting the child to amputation and toxic chemotherapy and radiation). Beneficence and nonmaleficence are therefore often combined and treated as one principle, that of **utility or consequentialism**: do things that provide *proportionately greater good than harm* and avoid doing things that are disproportionately burdensome. The focus is on consequences or outcomes and brings quality-of-life considerations into play. Outcomes can be difficult to predict with confidence, and quality of life can be very subjective (Beauchamp & Childress, 2001; Fox & DeMarco, 2008; Veatch, 2003).

- Most people would agree there are fates that are worse than death, although not necessarily agreeing on where to draw that line.
- *To the clear detriment of the child, the parents are refusing interventions that have a high likelihood of success and benefit, are associated with limited burden, and would be favored by the average person or most people.*
- *The parents do not demonstrate the capacity to understand the factors involved in or the implications of the decision they are being asked to make.*

- It is critical to note that overruling parental or patient preferences (whether or not child protective agencies or the courts are involved) should not equate to total disregard for those preferences.
  - *Make authentic attempts to understand the family's wishes and the priorities and values behind them.*
  - *Make any partial accommodations or compromises that are possible.*
  - *Continue to update the parents about the child's condition and give them the opportunity to be involved in ongoing planning and care of the child.*
- The wishes of the child matter, and for some decisions and at some points in time may be the determinate factor. For example:
  - *A 15-year-old with acute appendicitis who is very fearful of and actively resisting the surgery will generally be taken to the operating room, even against his wishes, but a 15-year-old who is fearful of scoliosis surgery and who is not willing to deal with the recovery process need not be taken for the procedure against his wishes—there is time to work with him so that he might come to understand the benefits of the procedure.*
  - *An 8-year-old refusing blood because of religious beliefs will generally be given the transfusion anyway if all else fails, but a 16-year-old's informed, passionate, and insistent refusal of the same on religious grounds may be*

CRITICAL COMPONENTS

Standards of Ethical Decision Making and Relationship to Child Development/Capacity

- **Gold Standard—Autonomy**: Competent individual makes informed choice based on personal priorities and values and free of coercion. Applies to most adults.
  - Primarily a negative right: the right to be left alone
  - No right to care that is futile or exceedingly and disproportionately burdensome or fails to meet recognized standards of practice and care
- **Silver Standard—Substituted Justice:** A surrogate stands in for a *previously competent* individual who is currently unable to express personal preferences.
  - The surrogate chooses what he or she has *good reason to believe* (based on prior written instructions or past conversations or observations of the way the patient lived his or her life and made other relevant choices) the patient him- or herself would have chosen.
  - Applies to previously competent adults who may now suffer dementia; be comatose, intubated, or sedated; be under the influence of mind-altering drugs; and so forth.
- **Bronze Standard—Best Interest**: A surrogate makes the decision on behalf of an individual who *is not and never was competent* (or who may have been competent in the past but for whom there is no friend, relative, document to tell us what his or her preferences might have been).
  - Decisions are based on what is judged to be in the *patient's* best interest.
  - Applies to infants, young children, and most adolescents most of the time as well as to significantly cognitively impaired and/or mentally ill adults. (Beauchamp & Childress, 2001; Veatch, 2003).

CLINICAL PEARL

Strategies for Achieving Concordance Between Family and Health-Care Team

Prior to overruling parental decisions, the following strategies should be employed, assuming the child's condition permits the time required:

- Tincture of time/repeated discussions—goal/outcome focused.
- Family spends lots of time at bedside so reality of child's situation and experience is apparent
- Care conferences with all involved specialists, family members, and key family support persons—goal/outcome focused
- Ethics consultation

persuasive, given what we understand of the stages of spiritual development.

- Children should be involved in decision making even if the ultimate choice is not theirs to make.
  - *Developmentally appropriate education regarding condition, treatment options, and rationale for choices*
  - *Solicitation of preferences and reasons for preferences*

Best Interest: What Criteria Count?

- How do we decide what factors should be taken into consideration and how much weight should be assigned to any given factor?
  - *Reasonable Person Standard: The usual standard is to go with what the "average person" or "most people" or the "reasonable person" would choose.*
    - In any group of 10 people are debating over a true bioethical dilemma, it is likely there will be a diversity of opinion, and yet it is just as likely that all 10 individuals would think of themselves as the "reasonable person"—each likely believes his or her choice represents what "most people" would tend to choose.
  - *Consensus or Majority Standard: Some would suggest taking a vote.*
    - Must there be 100% agreement, a clear and convincing majority, or just a simple majority of 1?
    - Majority support (even 100% agreement) is not, by itself, sufficient to prove something is right (at points in history, the vast majority thought the sun circled the earth, the earth was flat, ownership of slaves was acceptable, etc.)
- *Should decisions be made based strictly on medical criteria?*
  - Is there such a thing as "strictly medical" best interest?
  - What role should religion play?
  - What about finances, resource distribution and utilization, and impact on marriage and family and/or careers?

TEMPLATE FOR PEDIATRIC DECISION MAKING

- Not infrequently, pediatric health-care providers are confronted with situations where the parents disagree with each other, the parents disagree with the child (children should be given an increasingly stronger role in decision making as they mature), and/or the parents disagree with the health-care team.
- **Figure 2-1** provides a generic template for decision making in such circumstances.

Role of Parental Religion in Best-Interest Determinations

- With few limitations, parents have the right to raise their children according to the tenets of their religion and in keeping with the practices of their culture.
- Health-care professionals have a responsibility to make an authentic attempt to understand the religious and cultural beliefs of the child and family, must respect the

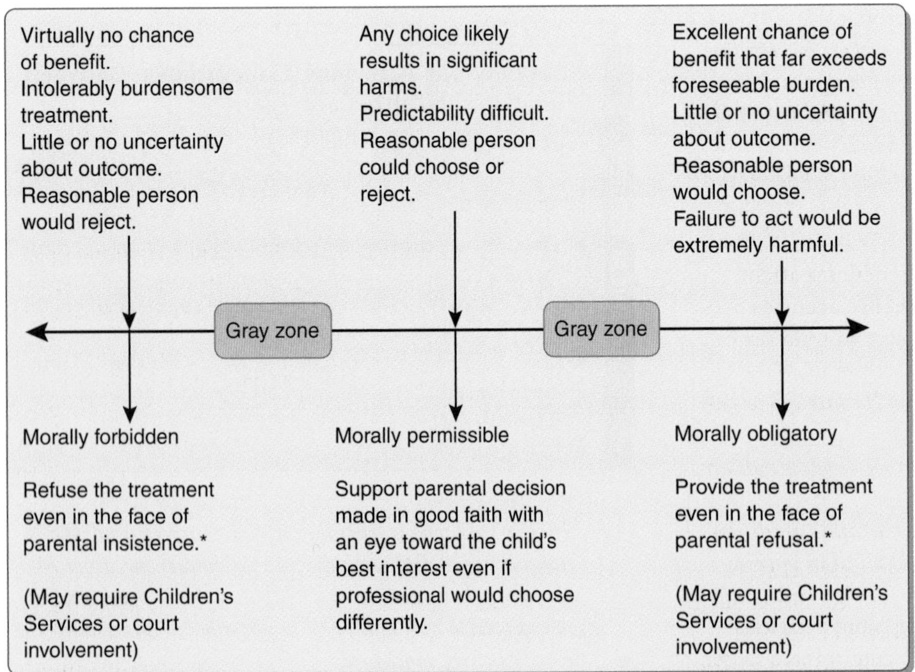

Figure 2-1 The best interest of the child: A generic paradigm.

right for individuals to have and express those beliefs (not the same as condoning them), and should attempt to honor them to the extent that is feasible and safe.

- Paraphrasing a famous legal quote from the Supreme Court decision in the case of *Prince v. Commonwealth of Massachusetts* (1944), parents are free to martyr themselves based on their own religious beliefs but may not make martyrs of their children, who do not yet have the capacity to make the same decisions in an informed and freely chosen manner.
- Parental religious beliefs and cultural practices that expose children to significant, reasonably imminent, and avoidable harm, suffering, or death should not be honored.

Partnering with Children in Decision Making

- As children grow up and their capacity for decision making develops and matures, they can and should become more actively involved in promoting their own health care.
- There are specific circumstances when some adolescents are accorded autonomy by law for their health-care choices.
- Gradually increasing the minor's responsibility for providing his or her own medical history, making his or her own appointments, making sure his or her prescriptions do not run out, contributing to the development of his or her own plan of care, and so forth are crucial for the transition from pediatric to adult health care.

Parental Consent Exception: Emancipated Minor Statutes

- Approximately 32 states have emancipated minor statutes, although terminology may differ among states.
  - *Pennsylvania has applicable statutes in some counties but not in others.*
  - *There is variability with respect to minimum age requirements, the application process, and the rights afforded to the emancipated minors.*
- In general, it is required that the minor live outside of the parental home and be self-supporting.
- Being legally married and/or employed by the military may be qualifiers.
- Among those states that do recognize emancipated minor status, some grant the status to minors who are parents, whereas others do not.
- Emancipated minors generally qualify to sign contracts, own property, retain their own earnings, and make their own health-care decisions—but again, there can be some variation.

Parental Consent Exception: Mature Minor Doctrine

- Minors 14 or over (for some purposes, 16 or over) who demonstrate the ability to understand their condition and their treatment options along with associated risks and benefits and who can demonstrate an ability to personalize the information and articulate their reasoning should be permitted to accept or refuse care on their own.

CRITICAL COMPONENTS

Consent, Assent, and Permission

Informed **Consent**: An individual with presumed (or demonstrated) adult decision-making capacity agrees to (or refuses) diagnostic or treatment interventions for him- or herself or may accept or reject participation in a clinical research trial.

- In the United States, the age of consent for most medical decision making is 18 years.
  - "Emancipated minor" status and the "mature minor doctrine" provide for exceptions to the 18-year-old age requirement (see following discussion).
  - In parts of Canada, the age of consent for medical decision making is 14 years.
  - In parts of the United States, teenage parents may make medical decisions for their babies that they are not in the same legal position to make for themselves, and this can be the source of confusion and frustration for those adolescents, for health-care providers, and for the grandparents of the babies.

Informed **Assent**: A child or other individual thought not to have full capacity to make freely chosen and informed decisions is asked his or her thoughts about treatment or participating in a research trial (if parent or guardian has provided prior approval).

- Basic information about the child's condition and proposed treatment is provided at the level of the child's ability to comprehend it, and his or her support is sought.
- If the child refuses, the following possibilities exist:
  - Treatment may be modified until it is acceptable to the child.
  - Treatment may not be provided at all.
  - Treatment may be delayed to permit further discussion until the child is in agreement.
  - Treatment proceeds and the child is given developmentally appropriate explanations as to why the plan is going ahead despite his or her expressed rejection.
- Research assent is requested as young as 7 years of age.
  - Standards are stricter for child participation in research, as the child is generally being exposed to risks with little or no hope of benefit for him- or herself or, as in the cases of some cancer treatment protocols, there is the hope of benefit but the risks are significant and the outcomes are very uncertain.

Informed Parental Permission: A parent or guardian makes an informed and freely chosen decision to permit (or refuse to permit) the treatment or research participation the professional has recommended for the child. If we are to be precise in our use of terminology, individuals provide consent to their own care but surrogates provide **permission** for the care of others.

- The less consequential the decision, the less likely this doctrine will be challenged.
- Only a few states have formalized this doctrine into law, but the fact that a particular state is silent on the subject does not mean the health-care provider cannot

use professional judgment concerning applying the doctrine.

- Documentation of the rationale for and the evidence of mature capacity is important.

Specified Clinical Exceptions to Parental Consent Requirements

- Some states have statutes that permit minors who are not emancipated to independently consent to diagnosis and/or treatment of specific conditions.
- There is a good deal of variability from state to state regarding the specific conditions, the age minimums that apply, and whether or not parents must be notified even though their permission is not needed.
- Depending on the specific laws of the states where they reside, minors may consent to:
    - *diagnosis and treatment of sexually transmitted infections,*
    - *contraceptive services,*
    - *prenatal services,*
    - *diagnosis and management of substance use/abuse,*
    - *limited mental health treatment (exclusive of medications),*
    - *placing of children for adoption, and*
    - *health care for their own children.*
- Consent to abortion services is formalized into law in some states; when it is, limiting stipulations are usually attached. States may require
    - *parental notification,*
    - *consent of one or of both parents, or*
    - *judicial bypass procedures.*

> **CLINICAL PEARL**
>
> **Source of Information Regarding State Parental Consent Requirements**
>
> The Allen Guttmacher Institute is a research, policy analysis, and public education organization with the stated aim of advancing sexual and reproductive health on a worldwide basis. Regularly updated state-by-state summaries of adolescent consent regulations are available through its Web site, along with fact sheets, research articles, policy updates, media kits, slide shows, and other educational aids. Materials for and about adolescents are available. (See the "Additional Chapter Resources" section for link.)

Decision Making and the Patient Self-Determination Act (PSDA)

- The Patient Self-Determination Act (PSDA) is an amendment to the Federal Omnibus Budget Reconciliation Act of 1990 that, strictly speaking, applies to those who are 18 or older but has implications with respect to participation of adolescents in decision making regarding end-of-life care. (See the "Additional Chapter Resources" section for link.)
    - *The PDSA requires Medicare and Medicaid facilities and health care providers to inform competent adults of their right to accept or refuse treatment and to express their preferences through advance directives such as a living will (LW) or durable power of attorney for health care (DPAHC).*
    - *Young adults with chronic childhood conditions may continue to receive care in pediatric inpatient and ambulatory care settings, and therefore pediatric nurses must be familiar with policies and their role regarding advance directives.*
- The PSDA also has some applicability to emancipated minors and mature minors.
- With respect to the PSDA, minors are not qualified by law to draw up formalized advance directives (LW, DPAHC) that have guaranteed legal standing. Nonetheless, discussions concerning advance directives should be held from time to time with older school-age children and adolescents who have chronic and/or life-threatening conditions.
- Conversations regarding advance directives are of clinical, ethical, and legal importance even if without *automatic* legal standing. They can carry significant weight with parents, health-care professionals, and, if necessary, with courts in times of crisis and/or conflict.
- Waiting until those times of crisis or conflict occur to have these discussions adds to the stress experienced by all involved and may hamper good and thoughtful decision making.
- A frequent and frustrating circumstance encountered by ethics consultants is that of undocumented conversations concerning advance directives nature.
    - *An opportunity to convincingly influence the family's decision and their confidence in their decision has thus been lost.*
    - *The same holds true with regard to influencing the courts or a guardian ad litem, if it should come to that.*

Advance Directives Are More Than Mere Legal Documents

- They foster and reflect a process of discussion over time between health-care professionals and their patients and between patients and their families and loved ones.
- Though the discussions can be quite emotional, they can also be relationship-building experiences.
    - *Encouraging children and their parents to have these discussions together and providing them with the guidance and support so that they handle the discussions sensitively and comfortably can be part of the pediatric nurse's role.*
    - *Even though another member of the child's medical team sees these discussions as his or her prerogative or has had the task formally assigned, children and families may seek out the nurse as the person spending the most time at the bedside. (See Chapter 5 for further discussion.)*

SAFETY IN THE PEDIATRIC SETTING

- Health-care safety concerns have been receiving much attention from within the health-care industry and by educated consumers and watchdog agencies. These

CLINICAL PEARL

Approaching Children About Advance Directives

Discussions with children about advance directives do not have to be formal, lengthy, or directed toward specific end-of-life issues.

- They generally are not conducted in a single setting but take place over time.
- The discussions may be planned and initiated by the health-care provider, or they may be impromptu and initiated by the patient or the provider.
- Some questions that may help determine values, priorities, and preferences include:
  - What things are most enjoyable and most important to you in life?
  - What do you hope to accomplish during your life?
  - What, if anything, would make life seem intolerable to you?
  - What things worry you?
  - What things do you believe worry your parents?

The health-care provider can capitalize on situations the child or adolescent has seen other patients encounter or has read about/seen in the news, and ask questions such as the following:

- Is that something you've ever thought about/worried about?
- If you were in that situation, what do you think you would want?"
- What do you think your parents would want for you?
- Have you ever discussed this with them?
  - If yes: How did they react and how do you feel about the discussion you had?
  - If no: What keeps you from having this discussion, and what do you think would happen if you brought it up?
  - We've helped other children like you talk with their parents—would you like some help from someone here to have this kind of discussion with your family?

If discussions are based on the direct experiences of the patient, questions similar to the following are appropriate:

- You were in the intensive care unit last month and you were supported with a ventilator for several days. What was that like for you?
- If you were to require the support of a ventilator again, what would you think about that?
- What would you want if it was determined that you could not be successfully weaned from the ventilator but would need it for the remainder of your life?

concerns have spawned a multitude of studies and standards concerning the following:

- *Medication errors*
- *Hospital-acquired infections*
- *Wrong-surgery/wrong-site incidents*
- *Patient falls*
- *Skin breakdown in bedridden patients or those with limited mobility*
- *Patient abduction (in pediatric facilities)*

CRITICAL COMPONENTS

Documenting Advance Directive Discussions

- Context (who raised the topic and how)
- Specific topics and/or scenarios discussed
- Specific options introduced and preferences expressed
- Underlying values and priorities the patient might reveal. This last element can be difficult to elicit from children, but it is helpful information to seek, as one cannot anticipate all possible scenarios and options.
  - In the event of something unforeseen, it can provide everyone a sense of direction if the child's values and priorities are known.
  - Sometimes reflecting on decisions a person has made and actions a person has taken can provide a sense of the values and priorities that guided that individual (McAliley, Hudson, Gunning, & Rowbottom, 2000).

National Patient Safety Goals (NPSGs)

- NPSGs are issued by the Joint Commission (formerly known as the Joint Commission on Accreditation of Healthcare Organizations, or JCAHO) and updated on an annual basis.
- The Joint Commission is a private, not-for-profit (NFP) organization that accredits hospitals and other health-care organizations.
  - *Accreditation is a voluntary process that promotes health-care safety and quality based on hundreds of benchmark standards.*
  - *Among the standards are the NPSGs that are singled out annually to receive nationwide priority attention.*
  - *Some NPSGs are so critical or in need of such constant reinforcement that they are carried over from year to year for priority attention.*
  - *As is the case with other standards of all kinds and sources, some of the NSPGs require adaptation in the pediatric setting. (See the "Additional Chapter Resources" section for link.)*
- Two NPSGs that were focuses for previous years and require pediatric adaptation or considerations are the requirement for the use of two patient identifiers and the requirement for implementation of a program aimed at the reduction of patient falls, both of which are discussed next.

NPSG: Two Patient Identifiers

- The identifiers must be checked every time a patient is admitted, transported, transferred, or discharged; every time a medication or blood product is administered; every time a lab specimen is obtained; and every time a procedure is performed, no matter how long the patient has been known to the nurse or admitted to the facility.
- The room or bed number may not be one of the identifiers.
- In most inpatient settings, the identifiers are the patient's first and last name and the patient's medical record number.

- Both are manually read from a patient ID band or scanned with a bar code wand.
- In ambulatory care settings where patients may not wear ID, the most common identifiers are name and birth date.
- In some settings, children are tagged with ID equipment that sets off alarms if the children are removed from the setting in an unauthorized manner.
- It can be difficult to keep ID bands or labels on children.
  - *Premature infants are so tiny that it is difficult to fit them, and their fragile skin may be too easily irritated.*
  - *Older infants and toddlers find ingenious ways to remove ID bands that adults have a hard time removing.*
  - *Teens may not like the idea of being identified as patients and may remove the IDs when their friends are visiting.*
- Children in outpatient settings who may be old enough to tell their names may still not be able to provide their birthdates.
- When parents are not present and an ID has been removed from a child or infant who cannot provide his or her own ID, there must be a standard in place for verifying who the child is before applying a new ID.
- Child identification is not the only challenge; parent identification is also a big safety issue. This can be especially true when the children are at the center of custody disputes.
- Many children's hospitals take the precaution of locking all entrances and exits from patient care units and require all visitors to wear ID at all times.
- Photo IDs for family and visitors are becoming the trend.
- The manner in which all of these safety precautions are presented to patients and families is critical.
  - *Parents may become insulted or frustrated by insistence that the ID be worn at all times and checked every time a treatment or medication is administered, even though the staff members know the child and family very well.*
  - *It is also crucial that* everyone *is held accountable for following ID safety standards all the time, or parents will lose trust in the staff and children will be at risk of being misidentified and receiving the wrong care or being removed by noncustodians.*

NPSG: Patient Falls Reduction Standards

- Health-care settings are required to implement programs designed to reduce the number of patient falls and to evaluate the effectiveness of those programs.
- There must be a process to identify patients who are at risk for falls and to make sure everyone encountering the high-risk patients knows of the risk.
- There must be standardized strategies for addressing the risks and documentation that those strategies are being continuously applied.
- A process for educating staff and educating families is also necessary.
- Children present special challenges:
  - *Older infants and toddlers who are learning to walk frequently fall (although not very far and usually without sustaining any injuries).*
  - *Preschool children run as much as they walk and are not particularly safety conscious.*
  - *Cribs, infant seats, beds, exam tables, wheelchairs, and high chairs present their own safety challenges if children are not secured or monitored appropriately or equipment is not maintained properly.*
- Until recently, most of the data and literature addressing falls risk factors and reduction strategies was specific to adult patients and adult care settings. Statistics are now being compiled and risks are being evaluated in pediatric health-care settings.
  - *Miami Children's Hospital has evolved a pediatric falls reduction program that is beginning to see widespread implementation and evaluation in other settings across the country (see Clinical Pearl on Humpty Dumpty™).*

CLINICAL PEARL

Humpty Dumpty Falls Prevention Program™

Miami Children's Hospital has developed and tested a pediatric falls reduction program that is now commercially available in the form of a teaching module. The teaching module includes:

- Risk Assessment Scale
- Prevention Protocol
- Educational materials for staff and for patients and families
- Room signage and patient ID stickers
- Access to onsite or teleconference training sessions

The program is customizable, and in addition to providing tools for promoting safety, it provides a basis for quality monitoring. Additional detail and ordering information is available through the link provided in the "Additional Chapter Resources" section at the end of the chapter.

Medication Safety Standards

- Medication safety standards that emanate from the Joint Commission and other sources are usually quite generic and apply to adults as well as children, so it is often up to the pediatric health-care setting to tailor them to reflect regard for the special vulnerability and needs of children. For example:
  - *Children's medication dosages are largely based on formulas involving the child's weight and/or body surface calculations. This adds opportunities for error in dosing: wrong weight or height, wrong formula, math errors.*
  - *Children's medications come in a variety of formulations and strengths, presenting additional opportunities for error in preparation and dispensing.*
  - *Infants and young children will not recognize that the wrong medication is being given, and some older children who suspect something is wrong may not feel they can challenge adults by questioning why the pill is a different color or why there are three pills instead of two.*

- *Most medications we give to children have never been researched using child subjects. Furthermore, children may be unable to communicate symptoms of adverse reactions; thus they must be monitored closely for more objective signs.*

Sampling of Medication Safety Precautions

- Reconciliation of medications given at home with those given in the hospital and reconciliation of medications given in one setting of the hospital with those given in another setting when the child is transferred
- Computer order entry to ensure use of standardized formulas, reduce human calculation errors, and prevent mistakes due to difficulty reading handwriting
- Special labeling and storage of look-alike and sound-alike medications
- The banning of medication order abbreviations and careful attention to guidelines for placement of decimal points in numbers
- Special labeling and two-person verification of high-risk or "high-alert" medications (see the "Additional Chapter Resources" section for link)
- Labeling of all medications and medication containers (including medicine cups and syringes) as they are drawn up/poured
- Use of unit-dose dispensing
- Use of pumps with built-in, customizable software to prevent errors in infusion of IV fluids and medications
- Careful labeling of all patient lines so that medications are not administered via the wrong route or mixed in solutions with which they are not compatible

CLINICAL PEARL

Valuable Source of Current and Archived Information on Medication Safety

The Institute for Safe Medication Practices (ISMP) is an invaluable resource for nurses. The ISMP has as its singular goal the education of health-care professionals and health-care consumers alike with respect to safe medication practices. The ISMP's site is a premier Web site for medication safety (see the "Additional Chapter Resources" section for link), and any nurse can readily subscribe to regular e-mail updates. Learning from the errors and benefiting from the best practices of others is one of the best assurances of error prevention.

- The ISMP sponsors a national medication error reporting program that is voluntary and confidential. The ISMP also assists with analysis and recommendations and publishes case studies and alerts so that others do not make the same mistakes.
- The ISMP provides newsletters, educational programs, consultation services, and dozens of medication safety tools and resources, including the following:
  - High-Alert Medication List
  - Error-Prone Abbreviation List
  - Do Not Crush List
  - Confused Drug Name List

CRITICAL COMPONENTS

Links to Sources of Practice Standards

The following nongovernmental, not-for-profit organizations (NGO-NFP) originate and/or facilitate implementation of standards of practice and standards of care that have relevance for pediatric nurses.

- National Association of Children's Hospitals and Related Institutions (NACHRI) and its public policy affiliate, the National Association of Children's Hospitals (NACH) (see the "Additional Chapter Resources" section for link)
- Institute of Healthcare Improvement (IHI) 5 Million Lives (see the "Additional Chapter Resources" section for link)
- National Initiative for Children's Healthcare Quality (NIHCQ) (see the "Additional Chapter Resources" section for link)

STANDARDS OF PRACTICE AND CULTURALLY SENSITIVE CARE

- Living and working in a society with a broad mix of ethnic and **cultural diversity** is both enriching and challenging.
- Culture is multidimensional.
  - *Culture of origin (usually referring to ethnicity)*
  - *Culture of poverty*
  - *Religious culture*
  - *Culture associated with gender and with sexual preferences*
  - *Culture associated with age*
  - *Culture associated with workplaces, professional organizations, hobby and special interest groups, and so on*
- The nurse is obligated by standards of practice and ethics to make an authentic attempt to understand the cultural beliefs and practices of patients and their families and to accommodate them to the extent feasible and safe and in keeping with standards of practice and care. Cultural sensitivity may require the following considerations:
  - *Dietary accommodations*
  - *Interpreters for those who speak little or no English or who are deaf and use sign language*
    - Children and their family members should generally not be asked to serve as interpreters.
    - Use of interpreters involves issues of privacy and confidentiality, capacity to understand medical matters, and willingness and ability to accurately and fully translate.
  - *Scheduling accommodations: To the extent possible, schedule around prayer times for Muslims and be aware of Sabbath restrictions such as the use of electricity and phones and cars for orthodox Jewish families, for example.*
  - *Treatment accommodations: Jehovah's Witness adults may refuse life-saving blood for themselves but not for their children. Still, much can be done to avoid the need to give blood to their children, and having a comprehensive blood conservation program or knowing of a program that can be consulted is appropriate.*
  - *Muslim women are not supposed to alone with or seen by men who are not their husbands. Attempts should be made to provide female caretakers, but care should be taken not to make such a promise if staffing will not permit it.*

- *Home-care accommodations: For example, the Amish family going home with a technologically dependent family member will probably not have electricity or a phone and may need arrangements made for a generator and for installation of a phone just off their property or for the use of a neighbor's phone.*
- *Knowledge of and tolerance for complementary and alternative medicine approaches (CAM): Reiki, acupuncture, hypnotherapy and biofeedback, homeopathy, and the use of herbs and supplements are but a few examples.*

- There must be a balance between respecting the beliefs and practices of other cultures and keeping children safe–making sure the benefits outweigh the risks and burdens.
- Some CAM treatments may be helpful. Some may be ineffective but harmless, whereas others may be harmful themselves or interact in harmful ways with elements of traditional or Western medicine being administered.
  - *Nurses should routinely ask in an open-minded way about CAM treatments when taking a history.*
- Some cultural practices (such as coining, spooning, cupping, and perhaps even some carefully applied forms of moxibustion) that are minimally painful and cause damage of a temporary nature may be acceptable, whereas others, such as female genital circumcision, would be considered painful and harmful to the extent of being classified as abuse.
  - *Some scarring and tattooing rituals have religious or cultural significance, but both have been used abusively as well.*
  - *Even when intent is "good," the extent or nature of scarring or tattooing may be considered abusive.*
  - *Judgment is called for and lines can be difficult to draw.*
- Families may be encouraged and supported in praying for their child's recovery from pneumococcal meningitis, acute appendicitis, or leukemia, but health-care providers are obligated to advocate on behalf of the children when the antibiotics, appendectomy, or chemotherapy are being rejected in favor of simply putting faith in God.
- It can be helpful to invite (with the family's permission) respected pastors or elders from the religious or ethnic community to participate in decision-making discussions.
- Geographic medicine departments of medical schools or large medical centers that serve international clientele may have experts available to consult with health-care professionals in local practices. (For further discussion of cultural issues, see Chapter 4).

TRUTH-TELLING STANDARDS AND PEDIATRIC NURSING

- Veracity is a principle that implies a duty to tell the truth or at least not to tell a lie. Truth-telling contexts in the clinical setting include but are not limited to the following:
  - *Disclosing diagnosis and/or prognosis*
  - *Withholding some or disclosing all treatment options*
  - *Adequately informed and noncoerced consent*
  - *Conflicts arising from confidentiality requests*
  - *Consideration of the use of placebos in the course of treatment or research*
  - *Disclosures regarding medical errors*
  - *Fudging the qualifications of patients who otherwise would not receive health-care services or, for example, breaks on their utility bills to keep the home heated and the aerosol and suction machines and feeding pump running*
  - *The nurse overhears a parent lying to a child about whether a procedure will hurt—does the nurse become an accomplice?*
    - If not, how does the nurse correct the information the child was given without compromising the parent?
- Children prefer the truth and may develop distrust for health-care providers in general when just one health-care provider deceives them.
  - *They generally do not have the same appreciation adults may have for the subtle moral distinctions we sometimes make between lying and other forms of distinction, such as withholding information, sharing partial truths, using euphemisms, and so forth. Good intentions may not matter.*
  - *What children anticipate or imagine is sometimes far worse than the truth.*
  - *When children ask questions, it is important to figure out exactly what they really want to know before anguishing over how to reply and how much detail to provide. The traditional example is the 4-year-old who comes home and asks where babies come from. He is probably not asking about sperm and ova and intercourse—he may just want to know which hospital.*
- When parents or patients prefer to simply trust the recommendations of the team and avoid getting into all the details, this desire can sometimes be respected as an "informed choice"; it depends to some extent on the nature of the decision and the risks and burdens involved.
  - *If the recovery process will be arduous and burdensome and require ongoing motivation and cooperation on the part of the patient and/or family in order to realize a successful outcome, the patient/family must have that information.*
- Culture may play a role with respect to truth telling.
  - *Some individuals with traditional Navajo beliefs, for example, do not want to hear potential risks because hearing them spoken out loud is synonymous with inviting them to occur (Carrese & Rhodes, 1995).*
  - *One cannot assume that anyone of a particular culture subscribes to all of its traditionally held beliefs and should be prepared to explore the possibilities.*

Truth Telling and Medical Errors

- Prompt disclosure and transparency along with sincere apologies and attempts to repair and make up for damages in the event of medical errors may help maintain trust in health-care professionals and may lessen the likelihood of lawsuits.

- It can also be prudent and therapeutic to spell out for patients and families what changes will be put in place as a result of the error in order to prevent the same thing from happening to other patients.
- Most health-care settings will have policies regarding who in the institution is to be informed of medical errors, the nature of the investigation that is to take place, who should disclose to the family and in what manner, and what contact, if any, the person(s) most directly involved in the error should continue to have with the patient/family.

ADVOCACY

- Advocacy entails speaking up on behalf of those who cannot speak for themselves and helping to further empower those who do have a voice.
- Advocacy involves the championing of care as much as it does the actual provision of care.
- Children are vulnerable to varying extents from developmental and political perspectives and are particularly in need of surrogate voices.
- Nurses advocate for safe and quality care on a daily basis on behalf of patients and families within the practice setting.
- Nurses may engage in advocacy efforts on a broader scale on behalf of the rights and health of all children on a local, national, or international level.
- Advocacy may require risk taking, organizational sensitivity, political savvy, and activism. Good communication skills are essential.
- Advocacy is not an option; it is an obligation that is reflected in the ANA Code of Ethics for Nurses and in the Pediatric Nursing Scope and Standards of Practice.
- The UN Convention on the Rights of the Child (see Table 2-4) and versions of Pediatric Patient Bill of Rights and Responsibilities that can be found in most children's health care settings (**Table 2-7**) highlight the rights that direct many pediatric nursing advocacy efforts.

TABLE 2–7 PEDIATRIC PATIENT AND FAMILY BILL OF RIGHTS

- Many versions of the Pediatric Patient and Family Bills of Rights are available
- The now defunct Association for the Care of Children's Health (ACCH) is generally credited with a national push to document and respect pediatric patient and family rights
- Each hospital, clinic, or professional organization modifies the document to capture its mission, vision, and values and to appeal to its constituents
- Commonly expressed rights include the right to:
  - Respectful interactions with health-care team
  - Quality, individualized, professional care that meets or exceeds national standards
  - Prompt and ongoing assessment and management of pain and other discomforts
  - Confidentiality
  - Understandable, comprehensive, accurate information regarding condition, prognosis, and diagnostic and treatment options
  - Participation in the development of the plan of care
  - Parent/guardian or surrogate rooming-in
  - Identity of any and all persons involved in care delivery
  - Safe environment
  - Second opinions/specialty consultations
  - Respect for religious and cultural beliefs and practices and provision of interpreters or signers as needed for communication purposes
  - Informed participation in medical research as appropriate and available
  - Knowledge of hospital services, mission, vision, values, and rules
  - Prompt attention and response to concerns
  - Knowledge of hospital charges and access to financial counseling
- Commonly expressed responsibilities of patients/families include the responsibilities to:
  - Interact respectfully with health-care team
  - Provide comprehensive and accurate information regarding health status, medical history, and response to treatment
  - Collaborate in the development of the plan of care, including requirement for parents to be readily available in person or via phone when decisions need to be made
  - Comply with plan of care or discuss difficulties and renegotiate
  - Keep appointments and be on time or provide prompt notification when appointment must be canceled
  - Respect hospital rules and safety measures
  - Report complaints and/or compliments to the appropriate individuals
  - Make good-faith arrangements to meet financial responsibilities

Advocacy and Child Maltreatment

- A major advocacy focus is that of prevention, detection, and treatment of child maltreatment.
- Physical Abuse: An injury is inflicted that results in or poses the risk of significant physical harm or death. Even if intent was not to harm, if the damage was reasonably predictable and avoidable, due care and protection were not afforded the child.
- Sexual Abuse: "The engaging of a child in sexual activities that the child cannot comprehend, for which the child is developmentally unprepared and cannot give informed consent and/or that violate the social and legal taboos of society" (Kellogg & the Committee on Child Abuse in Children, 2005).
- Emotional Abuse: "Systematic, psychologically destructive behavior that attacks a child's development of self and social competence" (Brodeu & Monetleone, 1994).
- Medical Abuse (also referred to as "pediatric condition falsification," or PCF): The child is needlessly exposed to diagnostic and therapeutic interventions for symptoms or conditions that have been exaggerated, totally fabricated, or purposefully induced. The person lying about or inducing the symptoms can be the patient, but in pediatrics, it is most commonly a caretaker (usually although not always the mother or mother figure) (Roesler & Jenny, 2008).
- Neglect: Failure to provide for basic needs to the extent that the child is harmed or put at significant risk of harm. Deficits might be in the areas of food, shelter, clothing, education, health care, and/or safe supervision.
- Pediatric nurses must be familiar with risk factors (**Table 2-8**), possible medical and behavioral indicators of maltreatment (**Table 2-9**), effective interventions, and the availability of resources.

TABLE 2–8 CHILD MALTREATMENT RISK FACTORS AND AT-RISK POPULATIONS

- Young, immature parents with unrealistic expectations
- Parents with unmet emotional needs
- Economic crises
- Domestic violence
- Lack of parenting knowledge
- Parental depression or other mental health problems
- Substance abuse
- Families with premature and/or chronically ill children
- Families with children with attention deficit hyperactivity disorder (ADHD) or mental health disorders such as oppositional defiant disorder (ODD)
- Families with the presence of a nonbiological father or maternal boyfriend (sexual abuse)

Sources: Giardino & Alexander, 2005; Reece & Christian, 2008; Roesler & Jenny, 2008.

- All health-care providers are mandatory reporters of child maltreatment and cannot be held liable for good-faith reports, but could suffer legal penalties for failing to report to law enforcement or the appropriate children's service agency.

Ethical Issues and Child Maltreatment

- Issues of ethics emerge in dealing with cases of possible child maltreatment:
  - *Professionals may not have a high enough index of suspicion regarding abuse with families that seem "nice" or "respectable" and may be disproportionately suspicious of those who are poor or are members of minority groups.*
  - *It can be difficult to decide how much of a concern is enough to warrant making a formal report to the authorities when there is not clear proof.*
    - Even if a family is cleared following the medical or social services investigation, the fact that a report was made remains on the books—it is a serious step to make a report and should not be undertaken lightly.
  - *The question frequently comes up as to whether the family should be informed of the report before it is made.*
    - Honesty and advance notice are usually the best choices.
    - The only time the report should be made without the knowledge of the family is in the rare circumstance when there is good reason to believe the child or staff will be in danger.

Child Advocacy Strategies and Skills

- Though advocacy usually begins with the efforts of one lone player, it is most effective when engaged in as a team sport. For those who are interested in advocacy beyond the boundaries of the practice setting, a multitude of opportunities and avenues exists.
  - *Membership in professional organizations can include involvement in the development of position statements and participation on legislative affairs councils. Even if there is no time for active participation, the simple paying of dues facilitates the advocacy efforts of such organizations.*
  - *Letters to legislators and participation in campaign efforts for those supportive of children's health and welfare and on behalf of ballot issues that impact children*
  - *Participation in local initiatives to get smoke detectors in every home, supply families with car seats, supply children with bike helmets and cycling safety education, improve immunization rates, and so forth*
  - *Community education regarding child health and welfare issues; hospital newsletters and websites that highlight hot topics; speaking engagements; and so forth*

CLINICAL PEARL

The Power of Child Advocates

"Never doubt that a small group of thoughtful, committed citizens can change the world. Indeed, it is the only thing that ever has."

—Margaret Mead

TABLE 2–9 POTENTIAL MEDICAL AND BEHAVIORAL INDICATORS OF CHILD MALTREATMENT

The presence of one or two isolated indicators does not necessarily portend child maltreatment, and developmental factors must always be taken into consideration.

NONSPECIFIC INDICATORS

These are general indicators of stress or distress that might be observed in a variety of circumstances that include but are not restricted to child maltreatment. They could be a reflection of a move to a new neighborhood, parent out of work and/or financial woes, new baby in the family, parent in jail, parental discord, substance use/abuse within the household, bullying, death in the family, and other factors. When reflections of maltreatment, they could be indicative of physical abuse, sexual abuse, emotional abuse, or neglect.

- Sudden personality changes
- Mood swings (emotionality, aggression)
- Depressed, disinterested, withdrawn
- Change in appetite/eating habits
- Sleep disturbances
- Problems with concentration
- Sudden change in school performance/behavior
- Excessive absences from school
- Regressive behavior
- Stuttering
- Run-away behavior or threats
- Cruelty to animals
- Self-injury
- Suicide threats or attempts
- Low self-esteem
- Too eager to please
- Fearful of going home
- Destruction of homework, books, learning aids, or favorite toys

PHYSICAL ABUSE

- Frequent injuries ("accident prone")
- Injuries inconsistent with explanation or explanation changes over time
- Placing blame for infant's injuries on siblings—too young to speak up for themselves
- Delays in seeking medical attention for significant injuries
- Injuries to sites that aren't commonly injured accidentally (e.g., neck, back of shoulders and upper arms, lower back, buttocks, back of thighs)
- Patterned injuries (e.g., belt, brush, cigarette lighter, cords, heating grates, curling irons, irons)
- Parents are rejecting, ignoring, belittling
- Child is hypervigilant; startles easily; shrinks from adults (or from males or females)

SEXUAL ABUSE

- Genital pain/itching/swelling/discharge/lesions; diagnosed sexually transmitted infections (STIs)
- Difficulty walking or sitting comfortably
- Frequent/painful and/or bloody urination; painful and/or bloody bowel movements
- Stained or bloody underclothing
- Seductive, sexualized behaviors: touches other people; humping behavior with other people or with objects; tongue kissing; making sexual sounds (moaning , sighing, heavy breathing)
- Excessive/public masturbation; inserting of fingers or objects in anal or genital area
- Excessive/age-inappropriate curiosity about sex; drawing of sexually explicit pictures
- Seems concerned about homosexuality

Continued

TABLE 2–9 POTENTIAL MEDICAL AND BEHAVIORAL INDICATORS OF CHILD MALTREATMENT—cont'd

NEGLECT

- Poor hygiene; bad body odor
- Inadequately dressed for weather; tattered, improperly sized, and/or unclean clothing
- Poor growth pattern
- Developmental lags
- Constant hunger; stealing and/or hoarding of food; rooting through garbage for food
- Constant fatigue
- Destruction of homework, books, learning aids, or toys
- Unattended medical needs (e.g., lack of immunizations, gross dental problems, needs glasses/hearing aids, untreated illnesses/injuries)
- Frequently left unsupervised for long periods of time (may come to school early and hang around late or always wants to go home with another child)
- Infants/toddlers: bald spots, listlessness, self-stimulation behaviors, rocking, head banging, lack of interest/curiosity

MEDICAL ABUSE/PEDIATRIC CONDITION FALSIFICATION

- Unexplained, persistent, or recurrent condition or one that is unusually unresponsive to therapy
- Symptoms and signs for which the onset has not been witnessed by anyone other than the parent/caretaker, or that do not occur when the parent/caretaker has no access to the child
- Caretaker observations that are not in keeping with health-care provider observations
- The patient reportedly doesn't tolerate the treatment regime
- Finding of unexpected drug in blood, urine, or stool or finding of blood that is not of the same type as the child in emesis, urine, or stool
- Polymicrobial infections or infections with organisms not commonly associated with site
- Alternate diagnoses included in the differential are very uncommon, even in the experience of a specialist
- Frequent change in medical providers and expensive/extensive evaluations in more than one medical center
- Repeated parental requests for invasive and/or risky diagnostic tests or treatments
- Feeding tubes and central lines that provide easy means to introduce infection/toxins

Sources: Giardino & Alexander, 2005; Reece & Christian, 2008; Roesler & Jenny, 2008.

Review Questions

1. The ANA Code of Ethics for Nurses
   A. is a set of practice guidelines that nurses are free to employ or reject.
   B. is a static and set document of tried-and-true ethical principles.
   C. covers not only nursing but the entire medical profession.
   D. is an evolutionary document that covers what nurses do.

2. A primary source of pediatric nursing scope and standards of practice includes which of the following?
   A. Results from a collaborative effort among National Association of Pediatric Nurse Practitioners, the Society of Pediatric Nursing, and the American Nurses Association
   B. Results from a collaborative effort among the National Pediatric Nurses Association, the state boards of nursing, and the American Medical Association
   C. Results from studies of pediatric health-care settings and private health-care settings
   D. Results from a collaborative effort among state boards of nursing, the American Academy of Pediatrics, and the Association of Pediatric Nurse Practitioners

3. A therapeutic relationship with pediatric patients and their families does which of the following?
A. Maintains professional boundaries and utilizes sympathy with those patients
B. Maintains professional boundaries, utilizing empathy
C. Maintains professional and interpersonal relationships that extend beyond the health-care setting
D. Maintains professional relationships through the nurse advocating and making the health-care decisions for the family unit

4. The Ronald McDonald House does which of the following? (select all that apply)
A. Provides healthy meals to families visiting the health-care setting
B. Provides lodging and meal services to out-of-town families visiting the health-care setting
C. Provide a local resource center for out-of-town patients and families
D. Provides families that must travel a distance to the hospital an inviting, home-like atmosphere

5. Which of the following is a role of the child life specialist? (select all that apply)
A. Promote effective coping, ongoing development, and normalization
B. Promote healing through play and goal setting
C. Promote distraction from unpleasant situations
D. Provide mental health counseling to distressed patients

6. The role of family-centered care in the inpatient hospital environment is to
A. alter the patient's and family's control over all aspects of health-care delivery.
B. eliminate the stress experienced by patients and families.
C. eliminate incidents of medical errors.
D. enhance patient and family learning and adherence to the plan of care, as well as increase patient satisfaction.

7. Chaperones in the pediatric health-care setting are a wise precaution not only for physicians but also for nurses because of which of the following?
A. Parents as chaperones are acceptable for all ages, and chaperones are needed even when the care provider is the same sex as the patient.
B. A chaperone is not needed if the child does not request one.
C. A chaperones is not needed if the caregiver is the same sex as the child.
D. Parents as chaperones are acceptable for infants and young children and should be offered to all children and families.

8. The gold standard as it applies to ethical decision making and relationship to child development or capacity is
A. beneficence.
B. utility.
C. autonomy.
D. fidelity.

9. Emanicpated minor laws have the following stipulations:
A. It is a legally recognized statute in all 50 states
B. Statutes guarantee those rights to children who are also parents
C. Minors can sign their own contracts and make their own healthcare decisions
D. Minors must be married or in the military to qualify as emancipated.

10. National Patient Safety Goals mandated by Joint Commission and updated annually refer to:
A. Two patient identifiers, falls reduction and prevention, and medication administration and reconciliation.
B. Cobedding, medication administration, and staffing ratios
C. Infection control, two patient identifiers upon admission to the healthcare setting
D. Falls prevention and elimination, medication reconciliation

References

American Academy of Pediatrics, Committee on Fetus and Newborn. (2006). Prevention and management of pain in the neonate: An update. *Pediatrics, 118*, 2231–2241. doi: 10.1542/ peds.2006-2277

American Nurses Association. (2001). *Code of Ethics for Nurses with Interpretive Statements*. Silver Spring, MD: nursebooks.org.

American Nurses Association. (2008a). *Code of Ethics for Nurses*. Spring Hill: nursesbooks.org.

American Nurses Association. (2008b). *Pediatric Nursing Scope and Standards of Practice*. Silver Spring, MD: nursesbooks.org.

Beauchamp, T., & Childress, J. F. (2001). *Principles of biomedical ethics*. New York: Oxford University Press.

Brodeu, A. E., & Monetleone, J. A. (1994). *Child maltreatment: A clinical guide and reference* (2nd ed.). St. Louis, MO: G.W. Medical Publishers, Inc.

Byer, J. (2009). The Oucher: A summary. Retrieved from http://www.oucher.org/the_scales.html

Carrese, J., & Rhodes, L. A. (1995). Western bioethics on the Navajo Reservation. *Journal of the American Medical Association, 274*, 826–829. doi: 10.1001/jama.274.10.826

Dlugosz, C., Chater, R. W., & Engle, J. P. (2006). Appropriate use of nonprescription analgesics in pediatric patients. *Journal of Pediatric Health Care, 20*, 316–325. doi: 10.1016/ j.pedhc.2006.07.001

Doyle, L., & Colleti, J. E. (2006). Pediatric procedural sedation and analgesia. *Pediatric Clinics of North America, 53*, 279–292. doi: 10.1016/j.pcl.2005.09.008

Ellenchild Pinch, W. J., & Haddad, A. M. (2008). *Nursing and health care ethics: A legacy and a vision.* Silver Spring, MD: nursesbooks.org.

Fox, R. M., & DeMarco, J. P. (2008). *Moral reasoning.* Mason, OH: Cengage Learning.

Giardino, A. P., & Alexander, R. (2005). Child maltreatment. St. Louis, MO: G. W. Medical Publisher.

Greco, C., & Berde, C. (2005). Pain management for the hospitalized pediatric patient. *Pediatric Clinics of North America, 52*, 995–1027. doi: 10.1016/j.pcl.2005.04.005

Greenberg, E., Jin, Y., & White, S. (2007). *2003 National Assessment of Adult Literacy.* Institute of Education Sciences & National Center for Education Statistics, U.S. Department of Education. Washington, DC: U.S. Department of Education.

Hockenberry, M., & Wilson, D. (2009). *Wong's essentials of pediatric nursing.* St. Louis, MO: Mosby.

Huang, C. (2003). Comparison of pain responses of premature infants to the heelstick between containment and swaddling. *Journal of Nursing Research, 12*, 31–40. Retrieved from http://www.ncbi.nlm.nih.gov/pubmed/15136961

Johnston, C., Stevens, B., Pinelli, J., Gibbins, S., Filion, F., Jack, A., . . . Veilleux, A. (2003). Kangaroo care is effective in diminishing pain response in preterm neonates. *Archives of Pediatrics and Adolescent Medicine, 157*, 1084–1088. doi: 10.1001/archpedi.157.11.1084

Kellogg, N., & the Committee on Child Abuse in Children. (2005). The evaluation of sexual abuse in children. *Pediatrics, 116*, 506–512. doi: 10.1542/peds.2005-1336

Kemper, K., & Gardiner, P. (2003). Complementary and alternative medical therapies in pediatric pain treatment. In N. Schechter, C. B. Berde, & M. Yaster (Eds.), *Pain in infants, children and adolescents* (pp. 449–461). Philadelphia, PA: Lippincott.

Krechel, S., & Bildner, J. (1995). CRIES: A new neonatal postoperative pain measurement score. Initial testing of validity and reliability. *Pediatric Anesthesia, 5*, 53–61. doi: 10.1111/j.1460-9592.1995.tb00242.x

Lawrence, J., Alcock, D., McGrath, P., Kay., J., MacMurray, S. B., & Dulberg, C. (1993). The development of a tool to assess neonatal pain. *Neonatal Network, 12*, 59–66. Retrieved from http://www.ncbi.nlm.nih.gov/pubmed/8413140

McAliley, L. G., Lambert, S., Ashenberg, M. D., & Dull, S. M. (1996). Therapeutic relations decision making: The rainbow framework. *Pediatric Nursing, 22*, 199-203. Retrieved from http://www.ncbi.nlm.nih.gov/pubmed/8717837

McAliley, L., Hudson, D., Gunning, R., & Rowbottom, L. (2000). The use of advance directives with adolescents. *Pediatric Nursing, 26*, 471–480. Retrieved from http://www.ncbi.nlm.nih.gov/pubmed/12026336

Merkel, S., Voepel-Lewis, T., Shayevitz, J. E., & Malviya, S. (1997). The FLACC: A behavioral scale for scoring postoperative pain in young children, *Pediatric Nursing, 23*, 293–297. Retrieved from http://www.ncbi.nlm.nih.gov/pubmed/9220806

Merriman, B., Ades, T., & Seffrin, J. R. (2002). Health literacy in the information age: Communicating cancer information to patients and families. *CA: A Cancer Journal for Clinicians, 52*, 130–133. doi: 10.3322/canjclin.52.3.130

Morash, D., & Fowler, K. (2004). An evidence-based approach to changing practice: Using sucrose for infant analgesia. *Journal of Pediatric Nursing, 19*, 366–370. doi: 10.1016/j.pedn.2004.05.016

Prince v. Commonwealth of Massachusetts, 321 U.S. 158 (1944).

Reece, R. M., & Christian, C. W. (Eds.). (2008). *Child abuse: Medical diagnosis and management.* Elk Grove Village, IL: American Academy of Pediatrics.

Roesler, T. A., & Jenny, C. (2008). *Medical child abuse: Beyond Munchausen syndrome by proxy.* Elk Grove Village, IL: American Academy of Pediatrics Press.

Savedra, M., & Crandall, M. (2005). Multidimensional assessment using the adolescent pediatric pain tool: A case report. *Journal for Specialists in Pediatric Nursing, 10*, 115–123. doi: 10.1111/j.1744-6155.2005.00023x

Schillinger, D., Grumbach, K., Plette, J., Wang, F., Osmond, D., Daher, C., . . . Bindman, A. B. (2002). Association of health literacy with diabetes outcomes. *Journal of the American Medical Association, 288*, 475–482. doi: 10.1001/jama.288.4.475

Stevens, B. (1996). Premature infant pain profile: Development and intial validation. *Clinical Journal of Pain, 12*, 13–22. doi: 10.1097/00002508-199603000-00004

Taylor, B., Robbins, J. M., Gold, J. I., Logsdon, R. R., Bird, T. M., & Anand, K. S. (2006). Assessing post operative pain in neonates: A multicenter observational study. *Pediatrics, 118*, 992–1000. doi: 10.1542/peds.2005-3203

Veatch, R. M. (2003). *The basics of bioethics.* Upper Saddle River, NJ: Prentice Hall.

Williams, M., Baker, D. W., Honig, E. G., Lee, T. M., & Nowlan, A. (1998). Inadequate literacy is a barrier to asthma knowledge and self-care. *Chest, 114*, 1008–1015. doi: 10.1378/chest.114.4.1008

Additional Resources

2010 Gallup Poll concerning trustworthy professionals

http://www.gallup.com/poll/145043/Nurses-Top-Honesty-Ethics-List-11-Year.aspx

Institute for Family Centered Care

http://www.familycenteredcare.org/

Family Voices Organization

http://www.familyvoices.org/

SMOG website

http://www.harrymclaughlin.com/SMOG.htm

Guttmacher Institute

http://www.guttmacher.org/

GOA review of implementation Patient Self-Determination Act and

http://www.legistorm.com/showFile/L2xzX3Njb3JlL2dhby9wZGYvMTk5NS84/ful25813.pdf

Current year's NPSGs (Click on "Patient Safety" and then click on "National Patient Safety Goals")

http://www.jointcommission.org/

Humpty Dumpty Falls Protection Program™ Site

http://www.mch.com/content.aspx?PageID=2257

Institute for Safe Medication Practice

http://www.ismp.org/

ISMP High-Alert Medications Tool

http://www.ismp.org/Tools/highalertmedications.pdf

National Association for the Care of Children in Hospitals & Related Institutions (NACHRI)

http://www.childrenshospitals.net

Institute for Health Improvement

http://www.ihi.org/ihi

National Institute for Children's Healthcare Quality

http://www.nichq.org

Psycho-Social-Cultural Assessment of the Child and the Family

UNIT 2

Family Dynamics and Communicating with Children and Families

3

Kathryn Rudd, MSN, RN, C-NIC, C-NPT
Diane Kocisko, MSN, RN, CPN
Jill Reiter, MSN, RN

OBJECTIVES

- ☐ Define key terms.
- ☐ Describe the process of normal communication.
- ☐ Describe family dynamics.
- ☐ Describe family theories.
- ☐ Identify family function roles.
- ☐ Describe family structures and the approaches to communication within each structure.
- ☐ Identify age-specific approaches for communicating with parents, families, toddlers, school-age children, and adolescents.
- ☐ Explain various influences in communication, including body language, tone, pitch, and environment.
- ☐ Describe strategies for incorporating communication into assessment.
- ☐ Describe communication with families during periods of emergency care.
- ☐ Identify the role of family-centered care in caring for the hospitalized child.

KEY TERMS

- Communication
- Family
- Extended family
- Blended family
- Single-parent family
- Same-sex partner family
- Cohabitating family
- Family of origin
- Adoptive family
- Dyad family
- Forming stage
- Storming stage
- Norming stage
- Performing stage
- Adjourning stage
- Triangulation
- Dyad

Don't have time to read this chapter? Want to reinforce your reading? Need to review for a test? Listen to this chapter on DavisPlus at davispl.us/rudd1.

COMMUNICATION AND FAMILIES

- **Communication** is a two-way process by which information is exchanged between individuals with a common use of language, mannerisms, behaviors, or symbols.

Principles of Communication in Families

- The manner of communication used by families provides information about the family style, as well as the structure and function of family relationships.
- Communication influences the decision-making process.
- Communication is based on trust factors.
- Dysfunctional communication inhibits nurturing and results in a decrease in self-esteem and self-worth in communication partners.
- Ill and hospitalized children may regress to a lower level of communication than is typical of their communication pattern.
- Communication is influenced by culture, and the nurse needs to have cultural awareness to facilitate effective communication (see Chapter 4).

Process of Communication in Families

- Bidirectional process: needs both sender and receiver
- Constantly in motion
- Transactional
- Irreversible
- Learned through culture and society
- Denotation: the dictionary meaning of a word
- Connotation: the meanings and feelings associated with a word based on an individual's past experiences

Components of the Communication Process

- Verbal:
  - *Spoken words—choose clear, concise language; avoid distancing language such as assigning gender; don't use avoidance language, such as euphemisms (e.g., "passed on" instead of "died").*
  - *Written words—written communication can be in the form of utilizing storybooks that highlight certain information, encouraging journaling for adolescents; don't write directions above the reading level of the child, use complex wording, or medical jargon.*
- Nonverbal:
  - *Body language—an open stance is welcoming; crossed arms indicate coldness or displeasure.*
  - *Gestures*
    - Confirming behaviors such as nodding of your head, restating what you hear
    - Nonconfirming behaviors such as tapping your foot, standing in the doorway, looking at your watch
- Paralanguage—includes pitch, volume, and pausing
- Children are very aware of anxiety and fear in their caregivers, which can be conveyed through both nonverbal and verbal behaviors.
  - *Speak slowly.*
  - *Be mindful of long pauses.*
- Effective listening is the key to successful communication and requires that the individual be actively involved in the communication process.
- Silence is a critical tool.
- Empathy enhances the communication process. Empathy is an understanding of a person's feelings—not sympathy, which is not therapeutic.
- Responding positively to an individual helps develop communication skills, language, self-esteem, and trust.
- Typically, children will communicate in a manner consistent with their developmental level (see Chapter 6 for growth and development information).
- The importance of establishing good communication cannot be overstated, as it affects all aspects of patient care.

Health and Communication Issues Within Families

- Children learn health habits from their families.
- However, this does not occur in a vacuum and is influenced by the community and the environment.
  - *In 2007, the National Coalition on Healthcare sought to provide the framework for health education in the community through the schools.*
  - *The framework established eight initiatives focusing on health education, health promotion, reducing health risks, and addressing healthy behaviors.*
  - *In addition, the framework focused on decision-making and goal-related skills to enhance the community, the family, and the individual (American Cancer Society, 2007).*
- Access to health care varies among U.S. families.
- Uninsured—individuals or families lacking health insurance.
  - *In 2010, 49.1 million Americans did not have health insurance (U.S. Census Bureau, 2011).*
- Underinsured—individuals or families with insurance but inadequate coverage.
  - *In 2010, 25 million Americans did not have adequate insurance (Kaiser Commission on Medicaid and the Uninsured, 2011).*
- Uninsured or underinsured families and individuals may forgo treatment until the condition becomes worse.
- The insurance status of uninsured or underinsured families affects their health-care practices:
  - *Many do not have primary care physicians, and instead utilize emergency rooms as primary care outlets.*
  - *Many do not follow up at appointments due to transportation or employment issues.*
  - *Many do not have the resources to obtain needed medication for acute or chronic conditions.*

Communicating with Families: Nurse's Role

- Provide appropriate introductions for the nurse, caregivers, and family members. Identify the stakeholders and the caregivers, including the child in the process.
- Record all telephone calls during office hours and after, and log all incoming and outgoing calls, advice given, and questions answered. Include date, time, and who was involved in the communication process (Poole, 2005).
- Identify your role.
- Establish an appropriate setting to communicate information.
- Ensure privacy.

CLINICAL PEARL

Health Insurance Portability and Accountability Act (HIPAA)

In 1996, the Health Insurance Portability and Accountability Act (HIPAA) was enacted to protect a patient's privacy as it relates to the patient's health records and information. The privacy law protects "individually identifiable health information" (U.S. Department of Health & Human Services, 2003). It also limits access to health information in any format (e.g., written, oral, facsimile, social media) to authorized individuals who have a right to know. Deviations from this federal law can result in imprisonment and fines for the offending individual or institution.

- Provide anticipatory guidance—this critical communication strategy improves care and supports competence in caregiving by providing information, guidance, and education for caregivers.

Barriers to Effective Communication

- Physical abnormalities such as cleft lip or cleft palate
- Physiological alterations such as hearing or visual impairment (**Table 3-1; Figure 3-1**)

CLINICAL PEARL

Protection for Individuals with Hearing Disabilities

"Title III of the Americans with Disabilities Act (ADA) prohibits discrimination against individuals with disabilities by places of public accommodation" (42 U.S.C. §§ 12181-12189). Private health-care providers are considered places of public accommodation. As noted by the National Association of the Deaf (2011), "the U.S. Department of Justice issued regulations under Title III of the ADA at 28 C.F.R. Part 36. Health care providers have a duty to provide appropriate auxiliary aids and services when necessary to ensure that communication with people who are deaf or hard of hearing is as effective as communication with others. 28 C.F.R. § 36.303(c)."

CLINICAL PEARL

Hearing Screenings

Hearing screenings are performed on all newborn infants born in the hospital prior to the infant's discharge. This screening is completed to evaluate any deviations in hearing that would produce a potential for the infant to not meet developmental milestones, such as turning the head toward a sound, being soothed by the voice of a caregiver, and mimicking sounds heard by the child. These primary skills of communication must be obtained prior to the development of the communication process. Infections passed from the mother and the antibiotics used to treat such infections may cause ototoxicity and alter hearing. Additionally, chronic ear infections can cause limitations in hearing.

- Cognitive barriers
- Avoidance or distancing language (Hockenberry, 2004)
- Environmental noise
- Cultural differences—the sender does not focus on the beliefs, values, goals, and outcomes of the child and family (see Chapter 4 for further cultural factors).

CULTURAL AWARENESS: Communication

- Include family members in interactions.
- Be an active listener.
- Observe verbal and nonverbal cues.
- Note that family responses to wellness and illness strongly influence behaviors.
- Learn culturally appropriate interactions, such as whether or not to use eye contact, and be mindful of pauses.
- Repeat important information more than once, and speak slowly.
- Avoid medical jargon, and use terms family members can understand.
- Allow time for questions.
- Information should be given in the family's native language, with the use of interpreters as necessary.
- Address intergenerational needs.

- Language barriers—need for interpreters and use of interpreter phones, individuals approved for medical interpretation, preprinted educational materials available in multiple languages
- Psychological alterations
- Sender and receiver biases or barriers
- Closed-ended, yes-or-no questions
- Ignoring of family and psychosocial issues (Levetown, 2008)

Promoting Safety

The 1964 Civil Rights Act states that no person should be denied the benefits of or experience discrimination in any program receiving federal assistance based on an individual's race, color, gender, or natural origin. The Supreme Court determined that discrimination based on language amounts to discrimination based on natural origin. This relates to health-care institutions maintaining language accessibility for their patients. Many states, such as California, New Jersey, and Washington, have enacted health-care interpreter certification as directed by the National Council on Interpreting in Healthcare, which advocates for the development and implementation of national standards of practice for interpreters in health care (Chen, Youdelman, & Brooks, 2007). Not utilizing trained medical interpreters in health-care settings puts children and families at risk and is a form of discrimination.

TABLE 3–1 BARRIERS TO COMMUNICATION

BARRIERS TO COMMUNICATION WITH CHILDREN AND FAMILIES
1. Closed-ended questions with yes-or-no answers
2. Prejudiced or preconceived messages based on race, age, ethnicity, culture, gender, lifestyle, wealth, appearance, or status
3. Preconceived messages based on the practitioner's beliefs of what constitutes *correct* family structure, function, or roles
4. Unaddressed fears of the child or the caregiver
5. Child, family, or caregiver not being treated with respect
6. Insufficient information
7. Not answering minor questions, such as those related to diet
8. Failure to include parents in the care plan
9. Parents not being treated as partners in their child's care
10. Failure of nurses to understand parent–child relationships
11. Failure to meet the developmental needs of the child
12. Failure to take into account cultural aspects or speaking in nuanced language that is specifically culturally based

Communication with Family Members Undergoing Stress

- Families undergoing stress associated with health care may be preoccupied with family concerns, such as the following:
  - *Overwhelming concern for the child*
  - *Feelings of neglect of other children and family structure*
  - *Loss of income*
  - *Impact on social status*

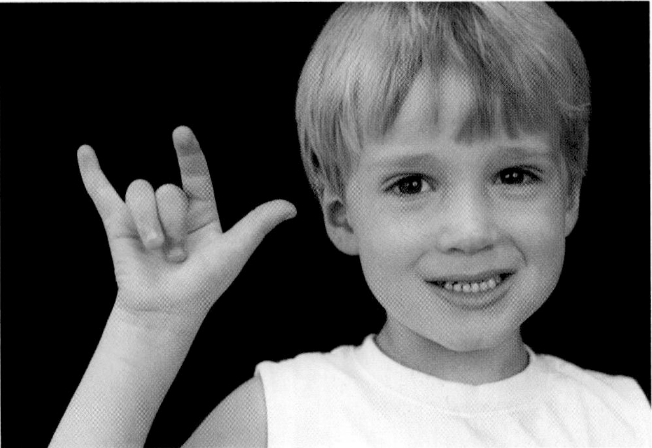

Figure 3–1 Child using American Sign Language for the word "love."

Communication with Family Members During Emergencies

- Provide a quiet environment to communicate.
- Communicate slowly.
- Avoid medical jargon.
- Sit down and look caregivers in the eyes.
- Allow plenty of time for questions.
- Avoid giving false hope.
- Allow for repetition of what caregivers have heard to ensure understanding.
- Be empathetic and sincere. (Browning, 2003)

CRITICAL COMPONENT

Emergencies

Critical components and interventions during emergencies include:

- Provide clear and concise information.
- Do not make promises.
- Inform family members that the physician will speak with them as soon as possible.
- If possible, give them a private environment.
- Call clergy, child life specialists, and social workers if available to offer support.

DEFINITION OF A FAMILY

- A **family** consists of two or more members who interact and are dependent upon one another socially, financially, and emotionally.
- Nuclear families (husband, wife, and child/children) were norm until the early 1960s (**Figure 3-2**).
- **Extended families**, families in which multiple generations live together, became more common during the

CLINICAL PEARL

Diversity of Families

Family is also defined as the structure or the relationship between individuals that provides the financial and emotional support needed for social functioning (Friedemann, 1989). Nurses should not be judgmental when caring for patients and families. We must remember that every family acts as a unique unit.

Great Depression, as a result of economic necessity (**Figure 3-3**).

- In the 1960s, **blended families**, those consisting of remarried parents and the children of their former marriages, began to be shown in the media, and media portrayals later included **single-parent** and **same-sex-partner families**.

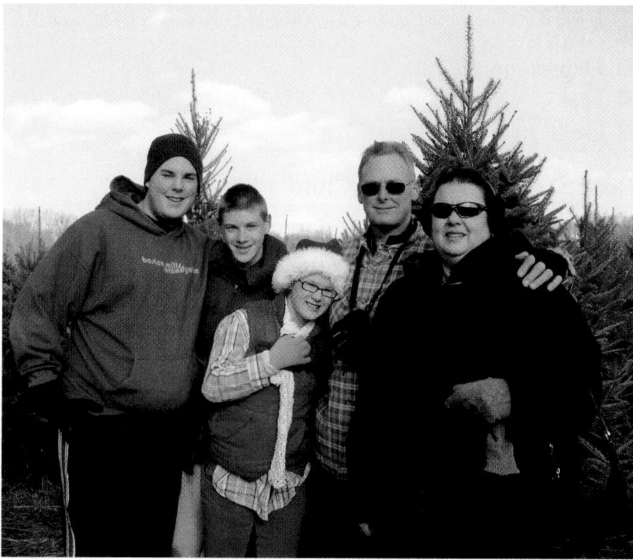

Figure 3–2 A nuclear family (mother, father, child or children).

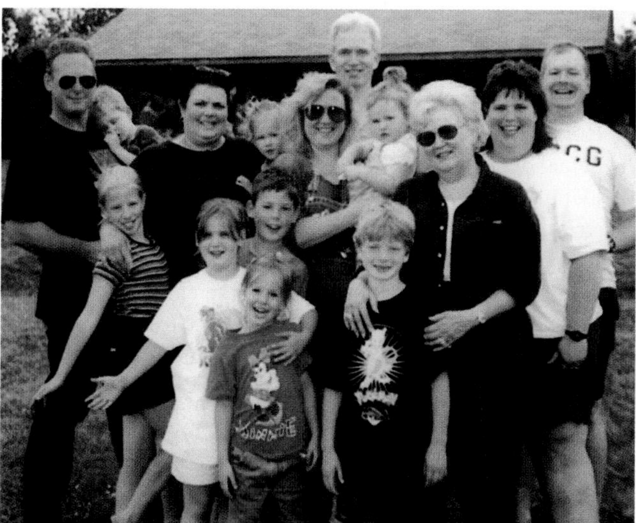

Figure 3–3 An extended family may have three generations of a family living together.

- Divorce rates have stabilized since the 1990s, but have led to fundamental changes in family structure.
- Children are more likely to be living in a single-parent family or a **cohabitating family** (consisting of unmarried adults and the children of one or both adults) at some time in their lives.
- Available family resources such as goods, services, information, and influences have an impact on the child's health, development, and adaptation to disease and illness.
- Race, ethnicity, and immigrant status also influence families and children.
- Nurses must be aware of these influences and assist in strengthening the family structure to maintain the parenting and family process.

Family Types and Functions

- **Family of origin**—family that raises the child.
- Family of choice—family formed through marriage or cohabitation.
- Nuclear family—male and female parents and their children living separately from grandparents.
- Extended family—usually includes three generations of family members living within the same house. Children are influenced by and have interactions with all of the adults living in the home.
- Married—family consists of married parents and their biological or adoptive children.
- Nontraditional families–single-parent families, grandparents functioning in the role of parents, same-sex-partner families, and blended families are some examples.
- Single-parent family—family headed by a divorced, widowed, or unmarried biological or adoptive parent.
- Same-sex-partner family—family headed by lesbian or gay partners (**Figure 3-4**).
- **Adoptive family**—family includes a nonbiological adopted member; can be a subset of other family types (**Figure 3-5**).

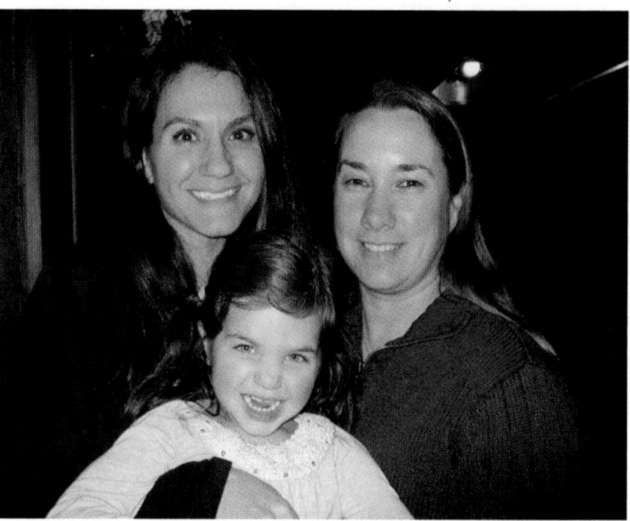

Figure 3–4 This nontraditional family represents the diversity in family types.

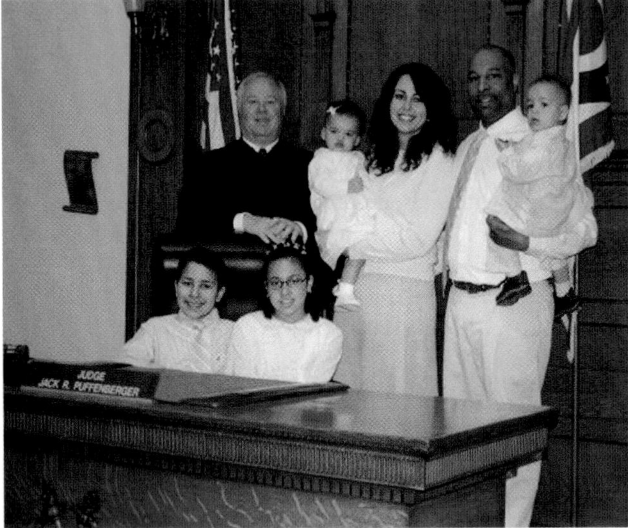

Figure 3-5 Adoptive family.

- Blended family—family consisting of members of two or more prior families; can be a result of death or divorce, as well as other factors.
- Cohabitating family—family in which the parents are unmarried.
- Solely extended family or no-parent family—a family in which children are cared for by other relatives, such as grandparents or aunts and uncles, rather than parents.
- **Dyad family**—A couple living together without children.

> **Clinical Reasoning**
>
> **Who Is the Primary Caregiver?**
>
> Children will typically refer to the adult(s) living with and caring for them as "mom" or "dad." This can be confusing for the medical staff when identifying a child's primary caregiver or legal guardian.
>
> 1. How can the health provider obtain this information without offending the adult accompanying the child?
> 2. Depending on the child's age, what are some of the barriers for obtaining an accurate health history from the child's care provider?
> 3. How does the health-care provider decide which adult can and cannot receive medical information regarding the child?

Stressors on Families

- Employment constraints, unemployment, underemployed
- Insurance issues—underinsured, uninsured, catastrophic illness or injuries
- Poverty
- Homelessness
- Mental illness or chronic physical illnesses
- Addition of family members, increasing the amount of finances that are needed to maintain the home
- Lack of support systems
- Seriousness of the family member's disease or illness
- Previous experience with illness or the hospital environment
- Cultural and religious constraints
- Inadequate coping skills
- Societal pressures, HIV, suicide, public education
- Diminished numbers of nuclear families; nontraditional families with special needs
- Time at work necessitating the use of day care and non-family care providers

Reaction of Family to Child's Illness

- Disbelief
- Frustration
- Worry
- Anger
- Denial
- Anxiety
- Depression
- Fear
- Guilt

Reaction of Siblings to Child's Illness

- Isolation
- Fear
- Feelings of being responsible because they had bad feelings about the sibling
- Disruption in family roles and routines
- Problems in school
- Acting-out behaviors
- Sibling rivalry or jealousy

Roles and Developmental Tasks of the Family

- Families provide for a child's physical needs, such as shelter, food and water, and clothing, as well as economic needs.
- Families provide nurturing, including provider roles and health-care provider roles.
- Families provide a sense of belonging and feeling loved.
- Families provide financial organization and boundary management.
- Role strain and time constraints due to dual-career demands present problems for families.
- Coping strategies are needed to help families deal with stresses of life and provide a nurturing environment.
- Communication may need to be expanded to meet the emotional and behavioral needs of the child.
- Socialization of the family is necessary to meet the demands of society and facilitate the assumption of values, morals, and socially acceptable behavior. (Duvall, 1985)

Family Dynamics

- Family members interact and participate in activities with one another.
- Sibling rivalry may occur (**Figure 3-6**).

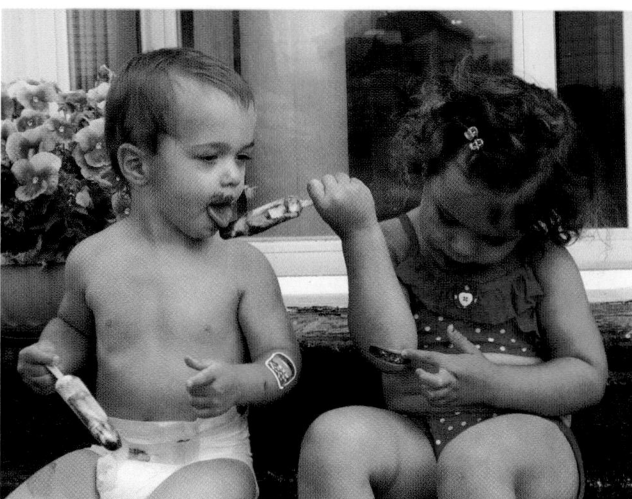

Figure 3-6 Sibling rivalry.

- A single adult may function as the disciplinarian.
- Children in the home interact and learn skills from each other.
- The birth order of children may influence communication patterns.
- A same-sex parent and child or opposite-sex parent and child may interact with stronger alliances.

> **CLINICAL PEARL**
>
> **Legal Custody/Legal Power of Attorney**
>
> With the increase of nontraditional family types, nurses must be aware of who has legal custody and who has legal power of attorney. These questions must be asked upon admission to the hospital.

COMMUNICATION THEORY

Healthy Families

- Give clear, congruent, and consistent verbal and nonverbal cues.
- Assist child in moving forward in the decision-making process.
- Foster the child's attainment of autonomy through support and guidance (Mitnick, Leffler, & Hood, 2010).
- Encourage interactions and consistently interact in a positive manner.
- Members derive pleasure, companionship, kinship, and love (**Figure 3-7**).

Unhealthy Families

- Give inconsistent, noncongruent verbal and nonverbal messages
- Humiliate, intimidate, or control communication

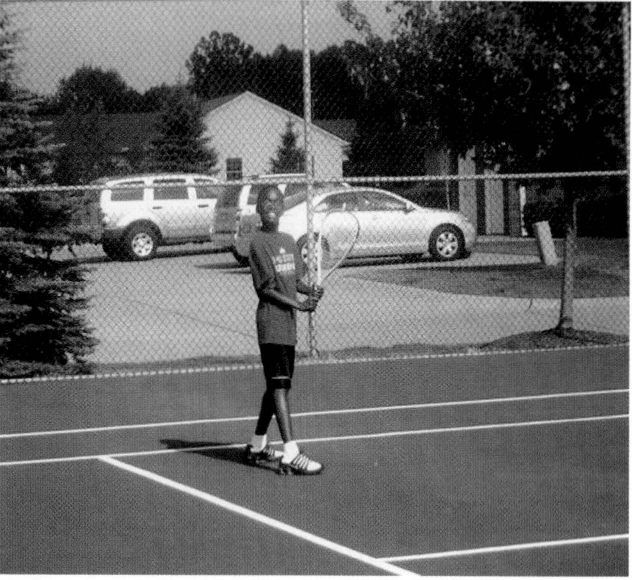

Figure 3-7 Family members sharing activities together form healthy bonds.

- Do not promote decision making through communication
- Neglect interactions due to lack of knowledge, time, or interest of the caregiver in the child, as well as other barriers

FAMILY THEORY

Group theory is applied to the family unit:

- **Forming stage**—marriage or cohabitation, birth or adoption of children
- **Storming stage**—two or more personalities realize their differences, such as emotional clashes with teenagers
- **Norming stage**—adjustment to individual members and rules; parental rules are imposed; children agree to obey rules
- **Performing stage** —family or group accomplishes goals and produces results
- **Adjourning stage**—death, divorce, or children leave to form their own families

Family Systems Theory

- Changes that occur in aspects of one family member's life affect the entire family.
- The family shares an unique identity.
- The family is characterized by the concepts of wholeness and the interdependence of the parts of the family (**Figure 3-8**).
- The family is dynamic.
- Interactions with work, church, school, and friends encouraged, but family boundaries remain intact.
- Subsystems within a family may form, such as alliances between siblings or with one parent.
- Families strive to maintain balance during a crisis.

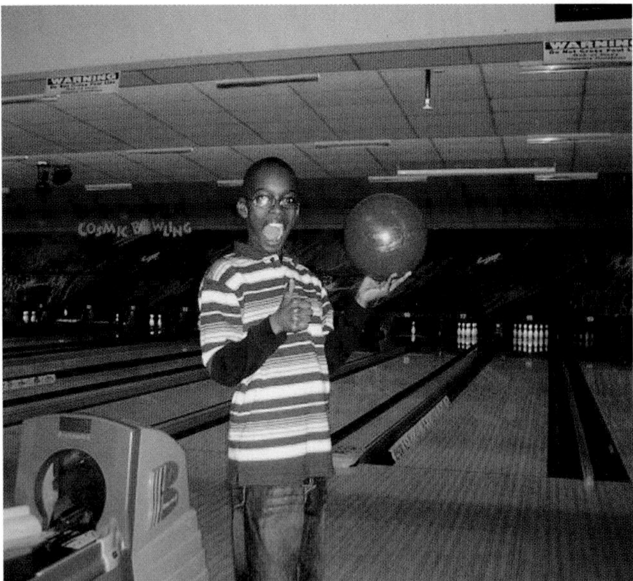

Figure 3-8 Bowling together with his family gives this child a sense of belonging.

Resiliency Model of Family Stress, Adjustment, and Adaptation

- Family's ability to adjust during times of stress and crisis
- Family's ability to adjust to members who are physically or mentally disabled
- Focuses on family strengths and capabilities (McCubbin, Thompson, & McCubbin, 1996)
- Affects all members of the family, as well as family functions and goals

Murray Bowen and Family System Theory

- Psychiatrist Murray Bowen developed the family system theory.
- The theory is based on human behavior and sees the family as an emotional unit, as family members are connected emotionally.
- The theory helps to identify family problems that can be a result of failure to communicate or teach values that are important to the family.
- The theory describes the interactions of the family unit as interdependent: A change in one member's role or functioning will impact the functioning and roles of the other members.
- Interdependence assists in promoting cohesiveness and cooperation of the family members (Bowen Center, 2010).
- Eight interrelated concepts:
  1. Triangles—a three-person relationship is the smallest stable relationship.
  2. Differentiation of self—whether good or bad, feelings of self will influence family relationships.
  3. Nuclear family emotional system
  4. Marital conflict
  5. Dysfunction in one spouse
  6. Impairment of one or more children
  7. Emotional distance (Bowen Center, 2010)
  8. Multigenerational transmission process—small differences between parent and sibling transfers over generations. Individuals choose mates with concepts of self that are similar to their own (Bowen Center, 2010).
- Emotional cutoff system—how individuals manage their unresolved emotional issues with family members
- Family projection process
- Sibling position—birth order affects behavior and development
- Societal emotional process—promotes progressive and regressive periods in the family (Bowen Center, 2010)

Virginia Satir and Family Therapy

- Satir was key in the development of family therapy.
- Satir believed that a healthy family was one that was open and reciprocal in sharing love, support, and ideas.
- Love and nurturance are key concepts of family healing and health (Caflisch, 2011).

Duvall and Family Development Theory

- The family is described as a small group.
- The family is portrayed as a semi-closed system that interacts with a larger social system.
- The family unit changes over time. Members must move through earlier developmental stages before moving on to the later stages, and the role of the health-care practitioner changes with each stage.
- Beginning family—practitioner aids in identifying a common goal, choosing career paths, planning for children.
- Childbearing stage—practitioner aids in preparing for and adjusting to life with children.
- Preschool stage—practitioner notes evolving parenting skills and is alert for signs of abuse or neglect.
- School-age and adolescent stages—practitioner aids in health promotion, including providing information on drugs and sex.
- Launching, middle-age, and retirement stages—family comes full circle to return to the self and couple building; practitioner roles vary. (Duvall, 1985).
- The family's life-cycle stages are based on changes in the structure, function, and roles within the unit. The age of the oldest child serves as a marker for stage transition.
- Understanding the stage of development the family is currently in can assist the nurse in identifying areas where education and anticipatory guidance may be needed.

- The eight stages are based on Erickson's developmental stages (California State University, Northridge, n.d.).

Eight Stages of Family Growth

- **Stage1**: Marked by marriage, joining of families, and development of an independent home
- **Stage 2:** Integration of an infant into the family unit
- **Stage 3**: The family unit with preschoolers
- **Stage 4:** The family unit with school-age children
- **Stage 5:** The family unit with teenagers
- **Stage 6**: The family unit contains young adults with independent identities. Young adults are ready to start their own careers and families
- **Stage 7**: Middle-age family unit that contains in-laws and grandchildren
- **Stage 8**: Aging family unit/a shift back to the original unit that started in stage 1 (Duvall, 1985)

CULTURAL AWARENESS: What Makes a Family Unit?

The family unit of today varies. Family members do not have to be related by blood to be considered a unit. Families of today can be nuclear, extended, single-parent, blended, and adoptive. Parents can be of different sexes or the same sex. One family unit is not better than another. The most important thing is for children to be in a positive environment so that they can grow and develop to their highest potential.

Neuman's System Theory

- The family is viewed as a target that should be assessed and to which nursing interventions should then be applied.
- All members express themselves differently, and this influences the group as a whole.
- The goal in this theory is to keep the family structure stable in its environment. (Application of Betty Neuman's System Model, 2011)

Family-Focused Care

CLINICAL PEARL

Benefits of Family-Focused Care

Family-focused care benefits the child and the family. The benefits for the child include decreased anxiety, reduced need for pain medication, and improved coping during hospitalization (American Academy of Pediatrics, Committee on Pediatric Workforce, 2004). As for the family, members participate in care conferences, participate in the child's care, and may feel empowered by being included in the decision-making process, which allows them to develop the skills needed to care for and support the child. It also decreases feelings of stress and dependency on others. The nurse's role is one that supports the family and provides members with the knowledge needed for self-care.

- The philosophy is based on the belief that a patient receives the best quality care when health-care providers work with the parents and family.
- The family is a constant in the life of a child.
- Acknowledge diversity, differences in family backgrounds, and support systems.
- Families assist children in meeting their psychosocial and developmental needs.
- In acute care settings stress should be placed on family communication patterns.
- Family members and health-care professionals work as a team to promote quality care for the child.
- Maintain the support system for the child by having parents and family members involved in the child's care.
- Focus on family relationships, values, coping strategies, and perceptions.
- Enable caregivers by encouraging them to room-in with the child.
- Nurses can empower and assist families to make informed choices.
- Provide families with a place to spend quality time with the child.
- When appropriate, allow the family to spend time talking and playing with the child in the absence of medical staff.
- Encourage and support the family to make decisions and implement care.
- Caregivers are the experts in caring for their child.
- Recognize that the illness or injury of a child affects the entire family (Institute for Family-Centered Care, 2008).
- Needs of all family members should be assessed.
- Provide siblings with age-appropriate information and encourage visitation.
- Offer specific needed support and education to the different family members.

CLINICAL PEARL

Separation Anxiety

Nurses need to take in to account that separation anxiety occurs during the toddler years (1 to 3 years of age), but can begin as early as 6 months of age (see Chapters 7 and 8 for further details). Separation from caregivers is stressful for toddlers, and can be even more stressful if the child is hospitalized. Care should be given to include the parents in any procedures that need to be done to the child.

Structural-Functional Theory

- Focuses on the functioning of the family to promote family function
- Provider role
- Housekeeper
- Child-caregiver
- Socializer and recreational organizer
- Sexual partner

- Therapist
- Kinship (Kafka, 2008)

King

- The family is a social system.
- The nurse, patient, and family communicate information, set goals together, and then apply interventions to achieve these goals.
- Goal attainment theory—personal system, interpersonal system, and social system involved in goal attainment.
- Nurse utilizes the nursing process to assist the child and the family in achieving their goals through action, reaction, and interaction (Nursing Theorists, 2011).

Roy Adaptation Model

- The model was formulated by Sister Calista Roy, a nurse theorist.
- God and humans have a relationship with the environment, and humans are an adaptive system.
- The model has four components:
  - *Psychological mode*
  - *Self-concept mode*
  - *Role function mode*
  - *Interdependence mode*
- The model demonstrates how stressors can be dealt with.
- People are viewed as individuals, but can also be viewed as existing within groups, families, or populations.
- Systems strive to maintain balance.
- Responses to adaptations can be healthy or unhealthy.
- Nurses promote adaptation for groups, families, or populations. (William F. Connell School of Nursing, 2010)

FAMILY ASSESSMENT

- Family resources and processes are primary influences on the child's health and development.

Family Size and Shape

- Family structure, socioeconomic status, resources, physical and mental health, and identity are influential factors.
- Average family size has decreased as compared to a generation ago.
- Family structure is very diverse.
- Family members are not necessarily blood related.
- Families may be defined differently by the child and the parent. (Ward & Hisley, 2009)

Parenting Styles

- Parenting style influences a child's developmental outcomes. Children view their parents as powerful (access to resources), as protectors, and as problem solvers.
  - *Authoritarian-dictatorial parenting*
    - Absolute rules, strict expectations
    - Children have little decision-making power
    - Punishment by withdrawal of approval
    - Children may become shy, sensitive, loyal, and honest.
  - *Permissive parenting*
    - Children control their environment and make their own decisions.
    - Few rules to follow
    - Children may have difficulty following rules that are expected in the public environment.
    - Children may grow up to be irresponsible, disrespectful, and aggressive.
  - *Authoritative or democratic parenting*
    - Combination of authoritarian and permissive styles, drawing on the positive aspects of each
    - Firm rules but allow some freedom
    - Children are taught the correlation between actions and the consequences of those actions.
    - Children may become self-reliant, assertive, and display high self-esteem. (Ward & Hisley, 2009)

Religious, Cultural, and Socioeconomic Orientation

- Religious beliefs may influence family relationships and the relationship with the environment.
- Many cultures place emphasis on the extended family and having respect for one's elders.
- Communication patterns may be influenced by culture (see Chapter 4).
- Socioeconomic status will influence living arrangements, which will further influence family interactions.
- Socioeconomic status will have an impact on the preventative and maintenance health care that the child receives.
- The ideas of health and wellness are defined differently by various cultures and religions.

Communication Patterns

- How families exchange information, values, and emotional connections
- Are messages supporting or attacking?
- Does nonverbal communication stifle verbal communication?
- Are love and support withheld when differences of opinion are shared?

Roles and Relationships

- Observe the delegation of tasks.
- Note clothing and personal hygiene.
  - *Is personal hygiene congruent between the caregiver and the child?*
- Note the condition of the home.
- Observe household chore delegation.
  - *How is good and bad work rewarded/punished?*
  - *Are traditional sex roles observed?*

Tools for Assessment

- Observation, questionnaires, assessment tools, surveys

- Assessment tools are designed to evaluate the strengths and protective components of the family unit (Ward & Hisley, 2009). Conduct the assessment in a comfortable environment after a relationship has been established with the child and the family.

Genogram

- Pictorial representation of the family unit (**Figure 3-9**)
- Diagrams health concerns and behavioral patterns

Kinetic Family Drawing

- Child draws a picture of the family unit (**Figure 3-10**).
- The picture depicts the child's view of the family.
- The picture can reflect the family's health and distress.

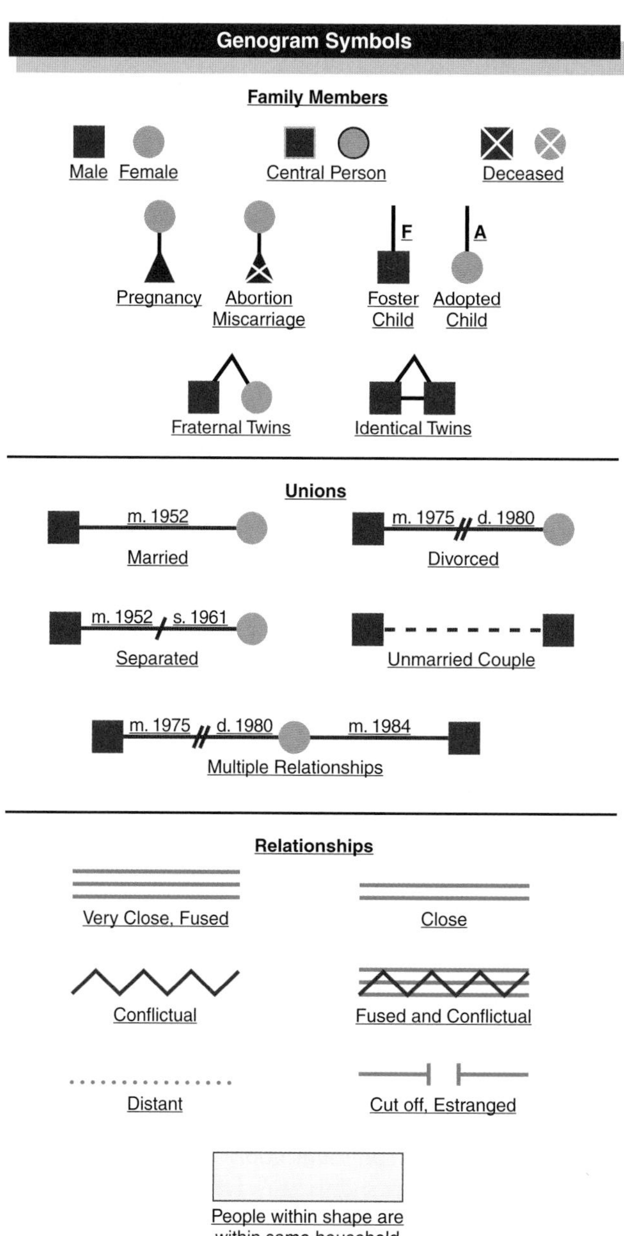

Figure 3-9 Example of a genogram template.

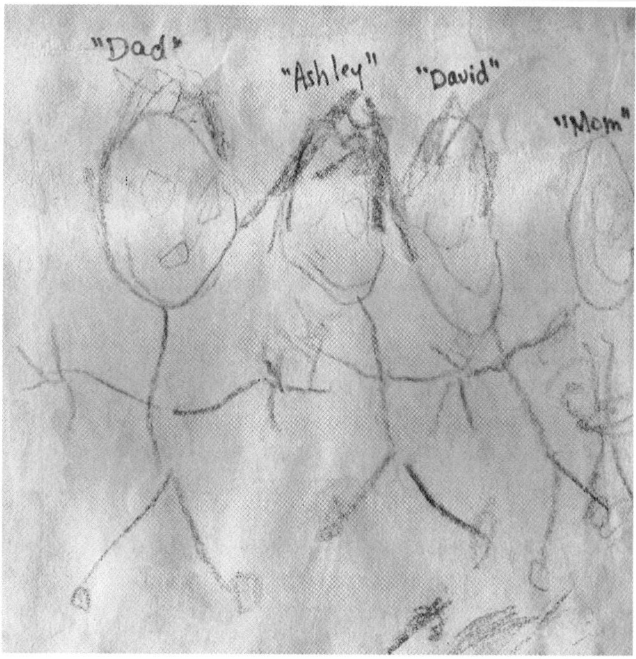

Figure 3-10 A kinetic drawing illustrates the family unit.

Structural Family Assessment

- Who lives in the home?
- What is the social, economic, cultural, and religious makeup?
- What is the family composition?
- What are the occupations and education levels of family members?
- Accomplished through interviews and questionnaires (McLendon, 2005)

Family Developmental Stage

- Assessed by interview, observation, tools, and surveys
- The family can exist in a variety of stages, such as having a preschooler and sending a child off to college.
- Tasks must be met for each child at each stage.
- Children will go through the stages of development noted by Eric Erikson.
- The success in meeting the tasks of the various stages of development will influence the communication demonstrated by the child.

Family Rituals

- Family rituals consist of the routines or activities taught by the family to maintain stability.
- The nurse assesses, through observation or surveys, the importance of these rituals.
- The nurse needs to maintain or allow these rituals to be maintained as much as possible for the continuity and stability of the family unit.
- When possible, permit families to share meals together.
- When possible, maintain regular nap times and nighttime rituals.
- When appropriate, permit families to maintain involvement in the child's routine care.

Triangulation

- **Triangulation** occurs when two or more family members team up against a third family member. It can also occur when one family member will not speak to another family member but communicates through a third family member. This places the third family member in a triangular relationship.
- A **dyad** is the formation of a two-person bond or subsystem within the family unit, such as a husband-and-wife dyad or a twin-to-twin dyad.

Functional Family Assessment

- Interviewing family and observations
  - *Who has the power or does the decision making in the family?*
  - *What characterizes family interactions and roles?*
  - *What communication methods are used, and are they successful?*
- Develop cultural sensitivity in recognizing cultural factors that shape family perceptions (see Chapter 4).
- Develop cultural competence as a nursing assessment tool (see Chapter 4).
- Subroles of the nurse:
  - *Stranger*
  - *Resource person*
  - *Teacher*
  - *Leader*
  - *Surrogate*
  - *Counselor (Child Welfare Group, n.d.)*

Family APGAR Five-Item Questionnaire

- The APGAR questionnaire is used to determine family members' satisfaction with the functional status of the family (**Table 3-2**). It is usually completed in an outpatient or home environment and consists of the following five items:
  - *A—Adaptation: the ability to use resources for problem solving in a crisis.*
  - *P—Partnership: the ability to share responsibilities and nurturing roles in a crisis.*
  - *G—Growth: the ability to achieve physical or emotional growth.*
  - *A—Affection: the ability to demonstrate love and attention to family members.*
  - *R—Resolve: the ability to devote time to other family members in the nurturing process.*
- Results are scored numerically from 0 to 20 as highly functional, moderately dysfunctional, or highly dysfunctional family. Higher scores indicate higher family satisfaction (Gallo, Knafl, & Angst, 2009; Smilkstein, 1978).

TABLE 3–2 EXAMPLES OF FAMILY NURSING DIAGNOSES

Any North American Nursing Diagnosis Association (NANDA) diagnosis may be appropriate for describing an individual family member's health status. A family diagnosis is intended to describe the health status of the family as a whole. Examples of family diagnoses include the following:

- Caregiver role strain (actual and risk for)
- Dysfunctional family processes: Alcoholism
- Family coping: Compromised
- Family coping: Disabled
- Impaired parenting (actual and risk for)
- Ineffective family therapeutic regimen management
- Readiness for enhanced family copying
- Readiness for enhanced parenting
- Risk for parent-infant-child attachment
- Social isolation
- Spiritual distress

Nursing Outcomes Classification (NOC) designations specifically for families as units are included in the NOC domain "Family Health." This category includes the following classes: family caregiver status; family member health status; family well-being and parenting. Outcomes from other domains may also apply. Nursing Intervention Classification (NIC) designations for families as units are included in the NIC domain "Family." This category includes the following classes: childbearing care; childrearing care; life-span care.
From Ward, S. L., & Hisley, S. M. (2009). *Maternal-child nursing care* (revised reprint). Philadelphia: F.A. Davis; original sources Carpenito-Moyet (2006); Wilkinson & Van Leuven (2007).

COMMUNICATING WITH THE FAMILY

- Encourage parents to talk openly regarding their concerns.
- Use open-ended questions.
- Use careful, nonjudgmental statements.
- Men may prefer a focus on cognitive, problem-solving talk.
- Females may prefer a focus on the process rather than the outcome.
- Be aware and considerate of generational differences.
- Incorporate active listening skills.
- Be aware and considerate of cultural differences.
- When communicating, use silence, empathy, respect, genuineness, and trust as nursing interventions.
- Communication can be tricky with nontraditional and noncustodial parents. Follow the established policies and procedures the hospital has in place.
- Remember to observe and record nonverbal communication factors, such as tone of voice, body language, and facial expression. Be aware of your own nonverbal communication factors and make sure you are not communicating unintended messages.
- Allow family members to voice their understanding of the current situation.
- Clarify or provide teaching points to decrease misunderstandings.

Communicating with Children

- The majority of the communication will take place between practitioners and parents. However, the child cannot and should not be excluded.
- Make sure to incorporate active communication strategies with the pediatric patient as well. Incorporate an

understanding of growth and development when communicating with the pediatric patient.

- Observe body language, facial expressions, and other nonverbal gestures.
- Incorporate play into nursing assessments and interactions where appropriate (**Figure 3-11**).
- Use special toys or games to assist with assessments (**Figure 3-12**).

Methods of Communication with Children

- Verbal—words, face-to-face interactions; infants cry, coo, and respond to their environment; parents and caregiver need to learn the cues of the infant or child (see Chapter 7).
  - *Be mindful of long pauses, rapid speech, and engaging the appropriate individuals in the communication process.*
  - *Gear communication to the cognitive and developmental level of the child.*
- Nonverbal—gestures, body language, posture, eye contact. Be aware of cultural factors (see Chapter 4).
  - *Visual—can include signs, photos, and illustrations.*
  - *Play—allows children to express feelings and concerns in a nonverbal manner (**Figure 3-13**).*
- Decision should be made as to who will speak to the child about the health-care issue—the practitioner, the caregiver, or a combination of the two.
- Child health decision making is a result of family health-care decision making (Traugott & Alpers, 1997).
- Children base their views on the relationships and experiences within their daily lives.
- Infants and children with altered hearing may have delayed communication.

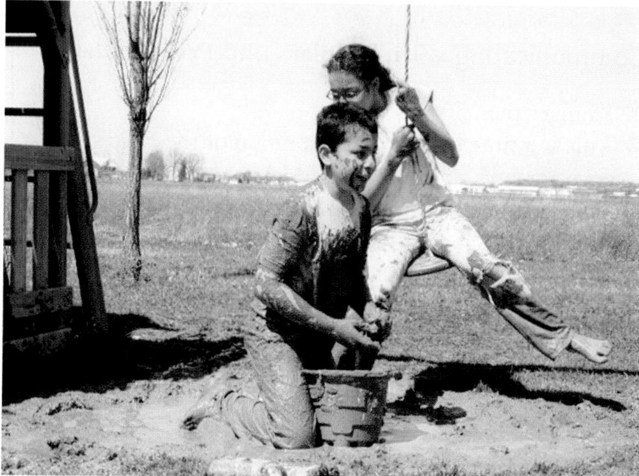

Figure 3-11 Incorporate play into family assessments.

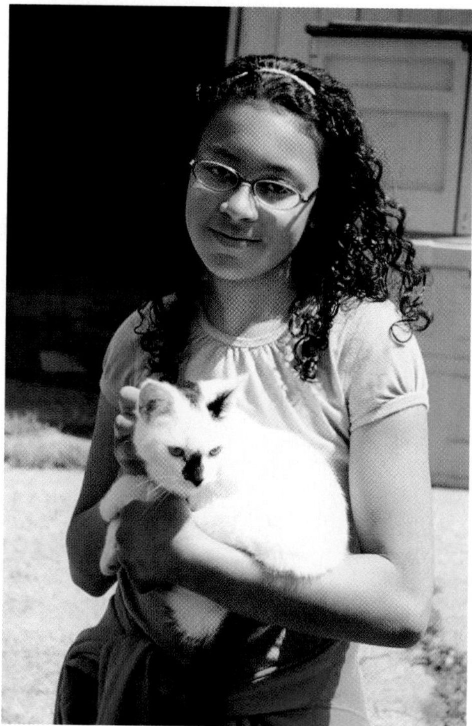

Figure 3-12 Use special toys or games to assist with assessments.

Communicating with Infants

- Newborn to 12 months
- This is a time of rapid physical and developmental growth. The body systems are maturing, and skill development is taking place.
- Social development is influenced by the infant's environment and the attachment developed with their parents and caregivers.
- Infants are unable to verbalize needs, concerns, and discomforts.
- Nonverbal behaviors, such as smiling, promote socialization.
- Infants display crying and cooing.
- Infants cry when they are hungry, when their diapers need to be changed, when feeling pain or discomfort, and when feeling lonely or wanting to be held.
- Infants coo when they are content or happy.

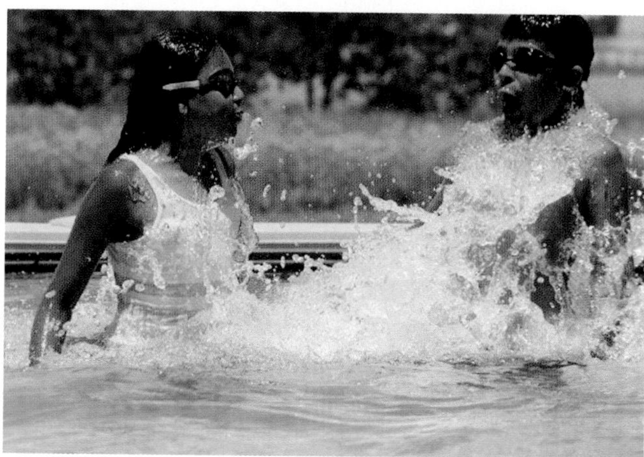

Figure 3-13 Play allows children to express feelings and concerns in a nonverbal manner.

- Infants are often quiet, observing the environment around them.
- Infants respond to the nonverbal behaviors of adults: touch, sound, and tone of voice.
- Observe parents and child caregivers' interactions and handling of the infant:
  - *Separation anxiety*
  - *Fear of strangers*
  - *Temperament and disposition*
- If the child has attained understanding of object permanence, he or she will know when a parent is missing (see Chapter 6).

Nursing Interventions for Infants

- Communicate primarily with parents and/or caregivers.
- Learn the infant's routines—feeding, changing, sleeping schedule—and incorporate them into nursing care.
- Use gentle touch when handling the infant to provide a sense of security and comfort.
- Allow the infant to suck on the pacifier to promote stress relief and relaxation.
- Talk to the infant when providing care to console the infant.
- Use music and sounds to assist in soothing the infant.
- Quickly respond to the infant's crying by feeding, diapering, or picking up the infant, all the while talking to the infant about what you think the infant is communicating (**Figure 3-14**).
- Use sing-song approaches to communication—singing and music can quickly gain the infant's attention. Wide-eyed, high-pitched communication also garners the infant's attention (Gable, 2003).
- Incorporate visual, auditory, tactile, and kinesthetic stimulation into nursing care and activities.
- If the hospital utilizes child care specialists who come and provide interaction, include such specialists in the provision of the child's care.
- Incorporate continuance of care so that the same nurses (as much as possible) are providing care. The infant will become familiar with the nursing staff.
- Incorporate consistency in nursing care and contact to allow the infant to develop trust.
- Consistent nursing staff will allow the nurse to better interpret the nonverbal communication patterns of the infant.
- To decrease problems with temperament and disposition, incorporate as much of the infant's normal routine as possible in care provision.

Communicating with Toddlers and Preschoolers

- Younger than 5 years old
- This is a time of intense exploration of the child's environment. The young child learns more of his or her environment while also exhibiting some negative behaviors, including tantrums.
- This time can be overwhelming and challenging for parents and caregivers but is an important period of development for the child. Much cognitive, social, psychosocial, and biological growth and development is occurring.
- Children of this age are typically egocentric, or unable to think from another person's point of view.
- Use statements such as "good job" instead of "good boy/girl."
- The child is unable to separate his or her actions from the origin of his or her pain.
- Children of this age need to feel and touch the things around them to gain knowledge of and experiment with unknown environments (**Figure 3-15**).

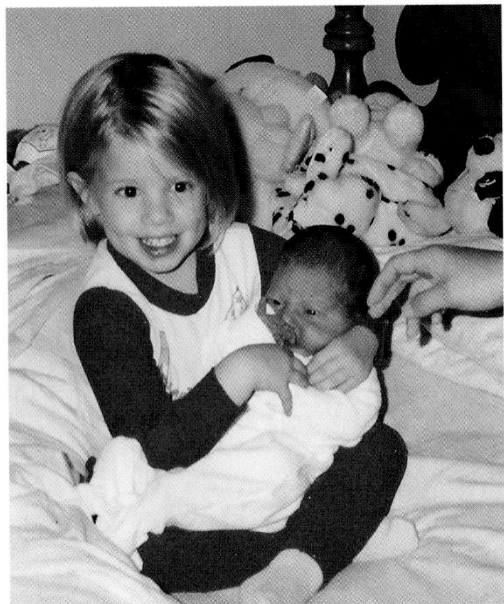

Figure 3-14 Quickly respond to the infant's crying by feeding, diapering, or picking up the infant.

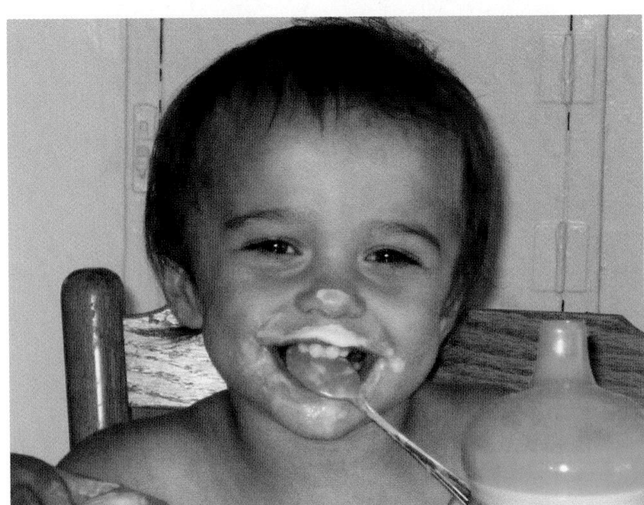

Figure 3-15 Infants need to feel and touch the environment around them.

- Medical play may be useful in demonstrating how a procedure will take place.
- The child may practice or pretend that a doll is having a procedure done.
- If appropriate, allow the child to handle a stethoscope, pulse oximeter, and blood pressure cuff and explore these items in a nonthreatening environment.
- Children of this age are very concrete and literal, and are often unable to conceptualize that one word may have more than one meaning.
  - *"IV" means "intravenous" to the nurse, but may be translated as "ivy," a known plant, by the young patient (**Figure 3-16**).*
  - *"Stick" or "poke" refers to a needle insertion for the nurse, but the young patient views a stick as a small piece of wood found in the yard.*
- Bleeding may be perceived as a child's "insides leaking out." Young children are often comforted by an adhesive bandage used to cover an open area.
- When having an x-ray procedure, the child may smile when getting his or her "picture" taken.
- Children assume that inanimate objects feel and act as humans do. For example, they might think that something inanimate could bite them.

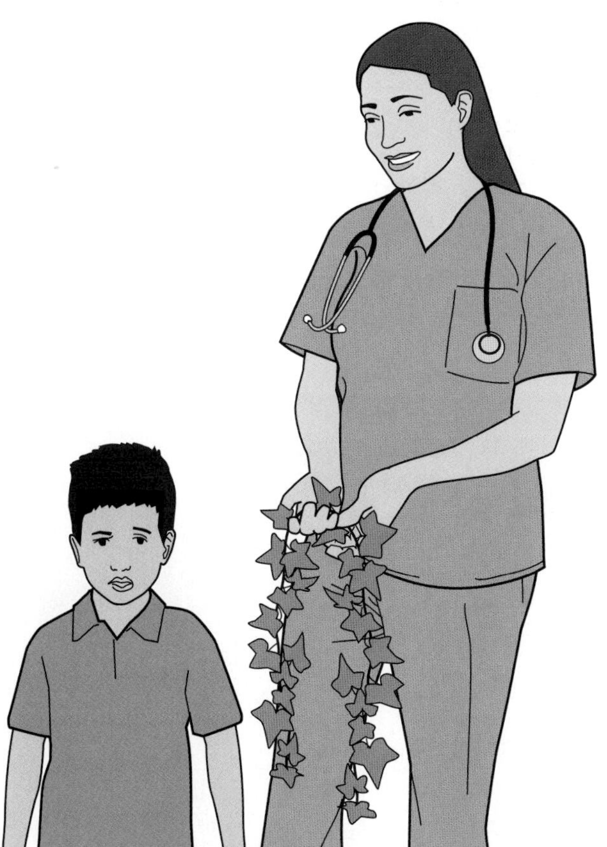

Figure 3–16 Toddlers are very concrete and literal, and are unable to conceptualize that one word may have more than one meaning.

- The child may call an instrument "bad" if it has caused pain or discomfort to them.
- They are fearful of unfamiliar objects and environments.
- When possible, allow the child to tour a facility or treatment room prior to the actual treatment.
- Preschoolers begin to develop skills in fantasy and pretend play.
- This is a period of social, language, and behavioral development.
- Children of this age are developing a sense of autonomy (**Figure 3-17**; see also Chapter 6).

Nursing Interventions for Communicating with Toddlers and Preschoolers

- Use simple terminology. Young children are unable to understand certain concepts. Those concepts need to be discussed in concrete terms that the child can understand.
- Do not use phrases such as "a small stick in the arm," which may be misunderstood.
- Assume the same position the child is in. If the child is sitting in a small chair, sit in a chair at his or her eye level.
- Keep equipment that is not being used out of the room until it is time for the equipment to be used.
- Utilize the treatment room for painful procedures so that the assigned patient room is a safe haven.
- Label the child's emotions to validate any feelings of fear and anxiety.
- Have toys available to use during procedures. Allow the child to perform the procedures on the toy so he or she can understand more of what will occur. Supporting pretend and fantasy play with the child allows for opportunities to express fears and anxieties.
- Utilize the parents and caregivers to interact and assist with providing care and communication.
- Support preschoolers who self-talk, as it encourages the alignment of thought patterns (Gable, 2003).
- Prepare the child for the procedure just prior to the procedure, not days in advance.

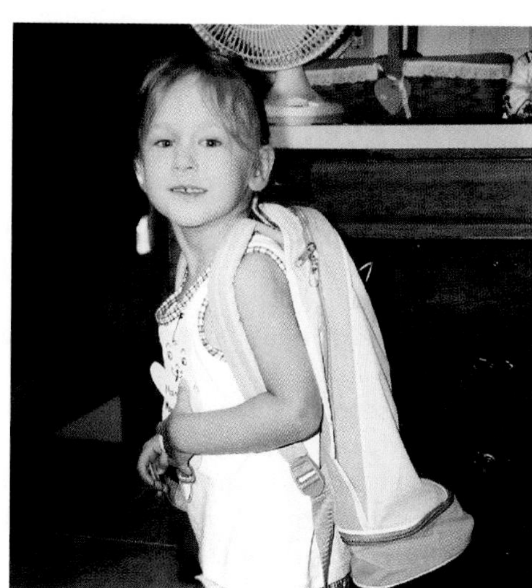

Figure 3–17 Developing a sense of autonomy.

Communicating with School-Age Children

- Ages 6 to 12 years
- This period of physical and psychosocial development includes many milestones, such as entering school, communicating independently, and beginning to conceptualize the environment.
- Communication directly with children of this age is equally important as communicating with their parents.
- School-age children are energetic and want answers to the questions they have. They want to develop connections and ties with information learned and ask themselves and others why certain things occur and happen. The pediatric nurse must be aware of this in his or her communication with the school-age child.
- Curious
  - *Used to asking questions in school when they cannot understand*
  - *Want to know why or how things happen or occur*
- Gain knowledge by experience and by understanding what is occurring
  - *Enjoy having a job or task to complete*
    - Eager to please, and want to complete a task independently
    - Work well with positive feedback
  - *Tell the child that he or she is part of the medical team that will help to get him or her well.*
    - Assign daily jobs, such as an exercise or a task, so that the child can assist with care.
- Concrete
  - *Unable to think abstractly*
  - *Examples should be given in a physical context in which the child can see, feel, or hear a result.*
  - *May overreact if feeling threatened*
  - *Able to verbalize thoughts, feelings, or concerns*
- Encourage children to ask questions.
- Older children may wish to journal their experiences.
- Other children may serve as a support group.
  - *Need play time*
  - *Playing will allow the child to communicate thoughts or feelings in a nonthreatening environment.*

Nursing Interventions for Communicating with School-Age Children

- When appropriate, offer the child choices so that control can be maintained (e.g., do you want water or juice after you swallow your medicine?)
- Explain the why and how in simple, nondescript, and nonfearful terms.
- Remember that abstract thinking has not yet been accomplished at this age.
- Allow the child to participate in procedures (if safe and not harmful), such as taking off an adhesive bandage or depressing a blood pressure cuff.
- Allow the child to voice his or her concerns.
- Answer questions honestly and simply, in concrete verbiage.
- Allow the child to have time to play, explore questions, and have fun (**Figure 3-18**).

Communicating with Adolescent Children

- Ages 13 to 18
- This is a time of developing independence and maturity. The adolescent child focuses more on social networks and friends.
- The adolescent child may seek counsel and feedback from sources other than parents and caregivers.
- Sexual development, including menstruation and emission, has already occurred.
- Behavior may fluctuate between adult and childlike.
- Adolescents are independent with activities of daily living, but still require adult supervision and input (**Figure 3-19**).

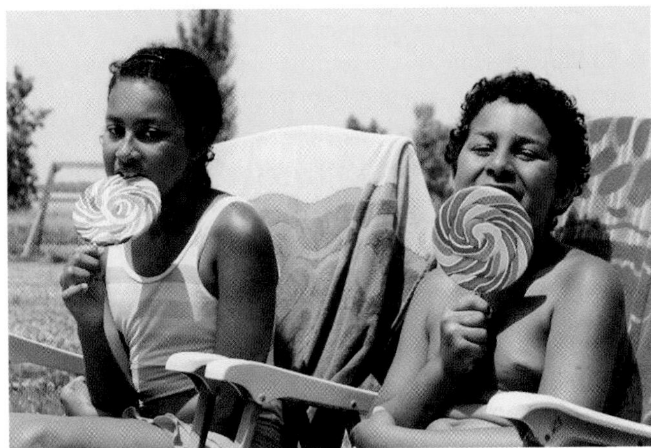

Figure 3–18 Allow the school-age child to be an active participant in care.

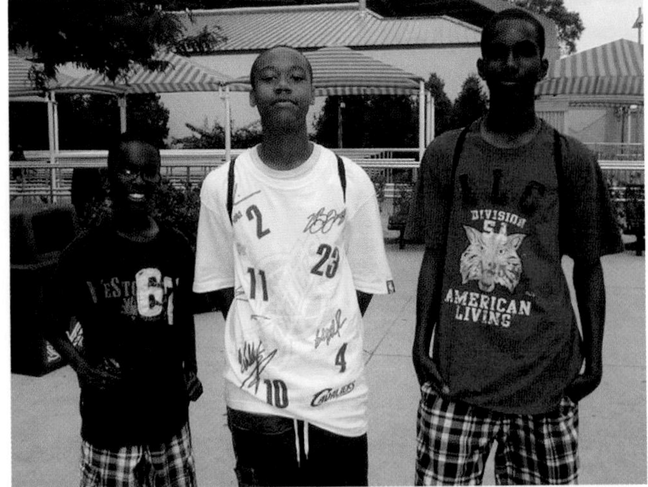

Figure 3–19 Adolescents are becoming more independent, but still require adult supervision and input.

- Social networking and friends are extremely important to their functioning.
- Trust is extremely important in their relationships and influences the extent of communication.
- Adolescents may have their phones to text message friends while in the hospital—consult with caregivers as to whether adolescents are allowed to make and receive phone calls.
- Adolescents tend to develop their own language and culture, which may be different from those of parents and caregivers.
- Medical decisions may be influenced by the adolescent's peer group.

Nursing Interventions for Communicating with Adolescent Children

- Use opened-ended questions.
- Encourage the patient to express his or her feelings and concerns.
- Provide privacy, as many adolescents will not be honest if interviewed in the presence of parents or caregivers.
- Explain to the adolescent patient the limits of confidentiality.
- Clarify differing opinions and/or reports from parents and child.
- Incorporate genuineness, trust, active listening, respect, and rapport skills into nursing care.

COMMUNICATING WITH THE ALTERED FAMILY UNIT

- Families may be affected by situational crises such as hurricanes, tornados, floods, loss of job, or loss of a family member, as well as developmental crises such as those experienced by adolescents.
- Substance abuse
  - *Negatively affects the family*
  - *Abuser often enabled as a result of denial, pride, or embarrassment*
  - *Roles shift to enable the abuser to continue to abuse substances:*
    - Responsible member role
    - Hero member role
    - Scapegoat role
    - Lost child role
- The family unit is codependent.
- There may be an inability to communicate with outsiders—secret keepers.
- Coercive family processes:
  - *Members are critical and punitive.*
  - *Punishment is used inconsistently.*
  - *Child's behavior is ignored by the family.*
  - *Rewards are coerced.*
- Physical, emotional, or sexual abuse:
  - *Secrets are kept within the family unit, preventing a resolution.*
  - *The nonabuser parent may ignore or cover up the abuse, or may take up the role of a sexual, emotional, or physical competitor against the abused.*
  - *Usually one member of the family is singled out for abuse.*
  - *Nurses are legally bound to report suspected abuse in any form.*
- Chronic physical or mental illness:
  - *Nurses need to educate families on the physical and emotional care needed by members who experience chronic illnesses.*
  - *Educate the patient and the family unit on the need to follow the prescribed treatment regimen, schedule of follow-up appointments, and administration of medications.*
  - *Empower the affected member and family unit by discussing options and alternatives.*
  - *Refer the family unit to other specialists or departments as questions arise related to financial resources, such as Social Security, Medicaid, or other resources related to paying for medications.*
  - *Educate the family unit concerning techniques to assess for deficits, strategies for interventions, and when to call for help (Ward & Hisley, 2009).*
  - *Provide suggestions, options, and resources available for respite care when caregiver issues arise.*
- Hospitalization:
  - *Often triggers a crisis situation*
  - *Adaptation of the family unit dependent upon past experiences, coping skills, and resources available to the family unit*
  - *Nurses may need to coordinate resources in the community or the home to facilitate the transition from the hospital to the home.*
- Death of a family member:
  - *The developmental stages of family members affect their responses to death.*
  - *Stages of grief vary from family member to family member and from family unit to family unit (**Table 3-3**; see Chapter 5 for further details).*

TABLE 3–3 THE GRIEVING PROCESS AS DESCRIBED BY VARIOUS THEORISTS

Kübler-Ross's Stages of Grieving	Rodebaugh's Stages of Grieving	Harvey's Phases of Grieving	Epperson's Phases of Grieving	Rando's Reactions of Bereaved Parents
Denial (shock and disbelief)	Reeling (stunned disbelief)	Shock, outcry, and denial (external response to loss)	High anxiety (physical response to emotional upheaval)	Avoidance (confusion and dazed state, avoidance of reality of loss)
Anger (toward God, relatives, the health-care system)	Feelings (emotionally experiencing the loss)	Intrusion of thoughts, distractions, and obsessive reviewing of the loss (internal response, isolation)	Denial (protective psychological reaction)	Confrontation (intense emotions, anger, sadness, feeling the loss)
Bargaining (trying to attain more time, delaying acceptance of the loss)	Dealing (taking care of the details, taking care of others)	Confiding in others to emote and cognitively restructure (integration of internal thoughts and external actions to move on)	Anger (directed inwardly, toward another family member, or toward others)	Reestablishment (intensity declines, and the parents resume their lives)
Acceptance (readiness to move forward with newfound meaning or purpose in one's own life)	Healing (recovering and reentering life)		Remorse (feelings of guilt and sorrow)	
			Grief (overwhelming sadness)	
			Reconciliation (adaptation to existing circumstances)	

Source: Ward, S. L., & Hisley, S. M. (2009). *Maternal-child nursing care* (revised reprint). Philadelphia: F.A. Davis.

Review Questions

1. Discharge planning begins
   A. on the morning of discharge.
   B. at the time of admission.
   C. at the beginning of every shift.
   D. only when the family asks for it.

2. Open communication involves which of the following?
   A. Asking yes-or-no questions
   B. Taking into account cultural, religious, and ethnic background considerations
   C. Finding out from the caregiver what the patient likes to eat
   D. Talking to the child about social issues

3. Nonverbal communication involves which of the following?
   A. Pictures, gestures, facial expressions, and body position
   B. Gestures, facial expressions, tone, and attitude
   C. Written materials, tapes, and brochures
   D. Pamphlets, the use of props, gestures, and volume of speech

4. Which of the following is stated in Duvall's family theory?
   A. All families are interactive and progress through five main stages.
   B. The predictable patterns and developmental tasks of families are accomplished through the eight stages of the family life cycle.
   C. The age of the children is the determinant of the family stage, and there are six stages of the family life cycle.
   D. The family life cycle divides the family into four main stages over the life span.

5. Family-centered care
   A. is not possible in pediatric intensive care units.
   B. directs the family through the hospital process.
   C. allows only the family to make the decisions in the care delivery model.
   D. integrates the family, child, and caregivers into the decision-making and care delivery model.

6. Which of the following describes triangulation in a family?
   A. The family is involved with another family at social events.
   B. Members of the family pair off into groups of threes to effect a change.
   C. Certain members of the family form a bond within a group of three.
   D. Two members of a family unit team up against a third family member.

7. The nurse should display the following characteristics when working with a family?
   A. Empathy
   B. Sympathy
   C. Disgust
   D. Judging

8. Anticipatory guidance with a 2-year-old would include which of the following?
   A. Providing safety information to the child related to riding a two-wheeled bike and bike helmets
   B. Providing parental education related to the psychosocial development of the 2-year-old
   C. Providing parental education related to separation anxiety
   D. Providing safety education to the child related to friends and interacting with peers

9. Healthy families provide
   A. few interactions, so as not to interfere in the child's social development.
   B. limited intrusion into school activities, except for homework.
   C. clear, concise, and consistent verbal and nonverbal cues.
   D. clear rules and boundaries, with serious and immediate consequences for deviations.

10. The primary role of the family includes providing all of the following, *except*
   A. nurturing, food, support, clothing.
   B. financial support.
   C. emotional support and feelings of belonging.
   D. an iPod, cell phone, and a car at the age of 16.

References

American Academy of Pediatrics, Committee on Pediatric Workforce. (2004). Ensuring culturally effective pediatric care: Implications for education and health policy. *Pediatrics, 114,* 1677–1685. doi: 10.1542/peds.2004-2091

American Cancer Society. (2007). *National health education standards.* Retrieved from http://www.cancer.org/Healthy/MoreWaysACSHelpsYouStayWell/SchoolHealth/national-health-education-standards-2007

Application of Betty Neuman's System Model. (2011). *Nursing theories: A companion to nursing theories and models.* Retrieved from http://currentnursing.com/nursing_theory/application_Betty_Neuman%27s_model.html

Bowen Center. (2010). *Bowen theory.* Retrieved from http://www.thebowencenter.org/pages/theory.html

Browning, D. (2003) To show our humanness—relational and communicative competence in pediatric palliative care. Initiative for pediatric palliative care. *Bioethics Forum, 18,* 23–28. Retrieved from http://www.ippcweb.org/display.asp?filename=hand5_1_eap.pdf&type=pdfd

Caflisch, N. (2011). *An application of Satir's systematic brief therapy. Pei Li Yeo ePortfolio.* Retrieved from http://peiliyeo.wordpress.com/2011/08/13/an-application-of-satirs-systematic-brief-therapy/

California State University, Northridge. (n.d.). *Family development theory.* Retrieved from http://www.csun.edu/~whw2380/542/Family%20Developmental%20Theory.htm

Chen, A. H., Youdelman, M. K., & Brooks, J. (2007). The legal framework for language access in healthcare settings: Title VI and beyond. *Journal of Internal Medicine, 22,* 362–365. doi: 10.1007/s11606-007-0366-2

Child Welfare Group. (n.d.). *The functional family assessment process.* Retrieved from http://www.childwelfaregroup.org/documents/FunctionalAssessmentProcess.pdf

Duvall, E. (1985). *Marriage and family development.* New York: Harper & Row.

Friedemann, M-L. (1989). The concept of family nursing. *Journal of Advanced Nursing, 14,* 211–216. doi: 10.1111/j.1365.2648.1989.1601527.x

Gable, S. (2003). *Communicating effectively with children. GH6123. Information from human environmental sciences extension.* Retrieved from http://extension.missouri.edu/explorepdf/hesguide/humanrel/gh6123.pdf

Gallo, A. M., Knafl, K. A., & Angst, D. B. (2009). Information management in families who have a child with a genetic condition. *Journal of Pediatric Nursing, 24,* 194–204. doi: 10.1016/j.pedn.2008.07.010

Hockenberry, M. J. (2004). *Wong's essentials of pediatric nursing* (6th ed.). St. Louis, MO: Elsevier, Mosby.

Institute for Family-Centered Care. An excerpt from *Partnering with Patients and Families to Design a Patient- and Family-Centered Health Care System: Recommendations and Promising Practices,* (2008). Available at: http://www.familycenteredcare.org/tools/downloads.html

Kafka, P. (2008). *Structural family therapy.* Retrieved from http://pauline-kafka.suite101.com/structural-family-therapy-a61267

Kaiser Commission on Medicaid and the Uninsured. (2011*).* Five facts about the *uninsured.* Retrieved from http://www.kff.org/uninsured/upload/7806-04.pdf

Levetown, M. (2008). Communicating with children and families: From everyday interactions to skill in conveying distressing information. *Pediatrics, 121,* e141–e1460. doi: 10.1542/peds.2008-0565

McCubbin, H. I., Thompson, A. I., & McCubbin, M. A. (1996). *Family assessment: Resiliency, coping and adaptation: Inventories for research and practice.* Madison: University of Wisconsin Publishers.

McLendon, D. (2005). Family-directed structural therapy. *Journal of Marital and Family Therapy, 31,* 327–339. Retrieved from http://www.familydirectedstructuraltherapy.com/articles

Mitnick S., Leffler, C., & Hood V. L. (2010). Family caregivers, patients and physicians: Ethical guidance to optimize relationships. *Journal of General Internal Medicine, 25,* 255–260. doi: 10.1007/s11606-009-1206-3

National Association of the Deaf. (2011). *Questions and answers for health care providers*. Retrieved from http://www.nad.org/issues/health-care/providers/questions-and-a answers

Nursing Theorists. (2011). *Imogene King*. Retrieved from http://nursing-theory.org/nursing-theorists/Imogene-King.php

Poole, S. R. (2005). *The complete guide to developing telephone triage and advice systems in a pediatric office practice: During office hours or after hours.* Elk Grove Village, IL: American Academy of Pediatrics.

Smilkstein, G. (1978). The family APGAR: A proposal for a family function test and its use by physicians. *Journal of Family Practice, 6,* 1231–1239. Retrieved from http://www.ncbi.nlm.nih.gov/pubmed/660126

Traugott, I., & Alpers A. (1997). In their own hands: Adolescents' refusals of medical treatment. *Archives of Pediatric and Adolescent Medicine, 151,* 922–927. doi:10.1001/archpedi.1997.02170460060010

U.S. Census Bureau. (2011). *Health insurance*. Retrieved from http://www.census.gov/hhes/www/hlthins/hlthins.html

U.S. Department of Health & Human Services. (2003). *OCR privacy brief. Summary of the HIPPA privacy rule.* Retrieved from http://www.hhs.gov/ocr/ privacy/hipaa/understanding/summary/index.html

Ward, S. L., & Hisley, S. M. (2009). *Maternal-child nurse care: Optimizing outcomes for mothers, children and families.* Philadelphia, PA: F. A. Davis.

William F. Connell School of Nursing. (2010). *The Roy Adaptation Model.* Retrieved from http://www.bc.edu/schools/son/faculty/featured/theorist/Roy_Adaptation_Model.html

Cultural, Spiritual, and Environmental Influences on the Child

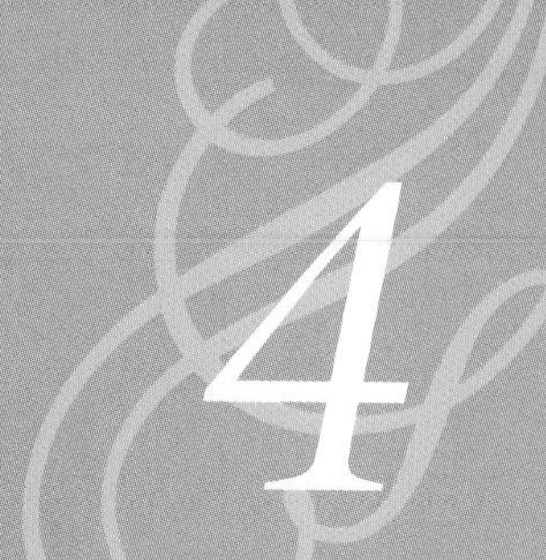

Diane Kocisko, RN, MSN, CPN

OBJECTIVES

- ☐ Define key terms.
- ☐ Identify individual cultural bias.
- ☐ Discuss Leininger's theory and how this theory can be used to plan patient care.
- ☐ Identify effective communication, body language, nurse–patient relationships, and multidisciplinary relationships between the caregiver and the pediatric patient.
- ☐ Identify tips for overcoming language barriers and describe the importance of overcoming such barriers.
- ☐ Identify and describe the characteristics that are determined by culture.
- ☐ Describe the components involved in performing a cultural assessment.
- ☐ Identify environmental considerations when caring for a pediatric patient.

KEY TERMS

- Culture
- Cultural bias
- Cultural assessment
- Cultural competency
- Transcultural nursing
- Cross-cultural nursing
- Spiritual concerns

CULTURALLY COMPETENT CARE

- Nurses must be aware of their own belief system and identify the belief systems of the client and caregiver.
- Be careful not to stereotype different **cultures**; each family and individual is unique.
- Family members of the same culture may apply and interpret this culture in different ways.
- Nurses must identify how their own belief system will impact their care.
- **Cultural bias** may occur when the nurse places his or her own values before the values of a different culture.
- Culture will impact both verbal and nonverbal communication.
- Not all cultures are open to communicating with individuals outside of their culture. Some families may have a spokesperson or person of authority who will make medical decisions for the patient.
- Culture may change with time, and may be interpreted differently among generations of the same culture.
- Culture serves as a template for evaluating the patient's psychosocial needs. When these needs are met, the client is better able to participate in care and focus attention on individualized health education.
- The parents or caregivers serve as role models and teachers in demonstrating how culture is applied to everyday living and how illness is perceived (**Figure 4-1**).
- Parents or caregivers may dictate the child's cultural needs. The child's age and stage of development will also influence the child's ability to recognize and articulate cultural needs.
- Recognizing cultural differences will impact the health disparities of minority populations and encourage minorities to seek medical attention (University of Nevada Las Vegas, Center for Health Disparities Research, 2009).

CULTURAL AWARENESS: Self Awareness

The following are introspective questions all nurses should ask themselves:

1. What do I believe in?
2. Am I familiar with the patterns of care for children within different cultures?
3. What have been my past experiences with those of different cultures?
4. Am I treating all caregivers and patients in a way that shows respect for and inclusion of their cultural values and beliefs?
5. Have I asked the caregivers for input to better understand their beliefs and demonstrate cultural competency to the pediatric patient?
6. How do I view cultures that are different than my own?

Don't have time to read this chapter? Want to reinforce your reading? Need to review for a test? Listen to this chapter on DavisPlus at davispl.us/rudd1.

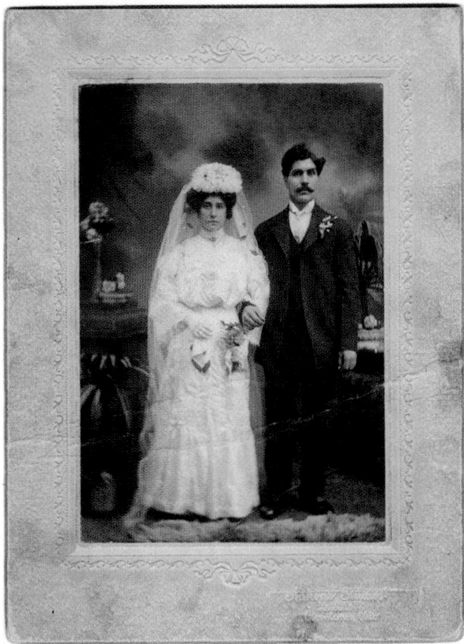

Figure 4–1 Parents are role models and teachers of culture. *(Courtesy of D.M. Kocisko.)*

Cultural Assessment

A **cultural assessment** should evaluate the following areas that impact health care and may differ by culture:

- Religious beliefs
- Perceptions of the client's current health status
- Food preferences
- Typical schedule that is followed

In addition, consider the following:

- Will an interpreter be required to communicate?
- Who is responsible for making the health decisions for the client?
- Will health-care interventions interrupt or interfere with any cultural or spiritual beliefs?
- Does the patient or caregiver need you to contact a spiritual leader for assistance in care?
- What are the patient and caregiver's perceptions of the cause of the disease?

Transcultural Assessment Model

- Giger and Davidhizer (2002) note that individuals are unique and provide a transcultural assessment model that consists of evaluating the following six aspects:
  - ***Communication,*** *how thoughts and feelings are expressed*
  - ***Space*** *between the individuals who are communicating*
  - ***Biological variations,*** *such as appropriate weight and development*
  - ***Time,*** *both the perception of time in general (e.g., fast-paced, time-centered lifestyle vs. more leisurely lifestyle) and when daily events should occur (e.g., meal times)*
  - ***Environmental control,*** *identified as internal or external and concerns the degree to which individuals feel they can influence or control their environment or experiences*
  - ***Social organizations*** *that the patient and family are a part of (e.g., family, religious affiliation, social groups)*

Agency Policy

The agency's policies steer the overall care, including visitation and diet, for the client. The nurse should investigate an agency's policies concerning these practices prior to applying for a job at the agency. If this is not done, the nurse may be challenged in adhering to his or her own cultural and spiritual beliefs as well as in providing culturally competent care. Consider the following policies:

- Visitation
  - *Parent or caregiver and grandparent visitation is unrestricted*
  - *Other visitors able to visit during the child's waking hours*
  - *Other visitors are free of communicable diseases or disease prevention strategies are maintained*
  - *Opportunity for the client to get appropriate rest*
  - *Good hand-hygiene practices for all visitors*
  - *Family privacy allowed during visitation*
  - *Patient allowed to be held and cared for by family members*
  - *Proper seating and space for socialization provided*
  - *When possible, family allowed to take patient out of the room*
  - *Play items and items used for diversion techniques available*
- Family-centered care
  - *Some normalcy is brought into the patient's day.*
  - *The patient has the opportunity to play with other children and siblings.*
  - *Caregivers have the opportunity to room in.*
  - *Caregivers have a place to maintain hygiene and eat meals.*
  - *Caregivers have unlimited access to the patient.*
  - *Whenever possible, caregivers are given the opportunity to provide care.*
  - *Caregivers are encouraged to provide input into the plan of care.*
  - *The health-care team listens to caregiver suggestions.*
- Dietary needs
  - *Caregivers are encouraged to bring familiar cultural foods from home. (Check for any medical dietary restriction.)*
  - *Food preparation and options are adequate and appealing.*
  - *Vegetarian meal options are available.*
  - *Patients and caregivers may select from a variety of foods available.*
  - *Nutritious food selections are available and encouraged.*
  - *Patient's restricted food items are documented and diet restrictions are enforced.*
  - *Cultural and spiritual food restrictions are documented and enforced.*

Education of Staff

The agency's policy and procedures will drive the type of information that is provided to the nursing staff. Each individual nurse has the professional responsibility to appraise the cultural differences and concerns of the patient. It should be the goal of every health professional to tailor care to meet the holistic health needs of the patient.

- Staff must strive for **cultural competency**, knowledge of and effectiveness in interactions with individuals of different cultures.
- Annual education to maintain current knowledge and understand new and evolving practices in culturally competent care should be provided and sought.
- Staff should identify cultural groups predominant in the organization's practice and examine the beliefs and values of these cultures that may affect care.
- Staff should ideally be provided with theory and tools necessary to perform culturally competent care for all children and their caregivers.
- Staff should seek information on any unfamiliar cultures.
- Leininger's Cultural Care Theory
  - ***Transcultural nursing*** *is the nurse incorporating the patient's culture into the care the nurse is providing (Leininger, 2009).*
  - ***Cross-cultural nursing*** *is delivering care in manner proven to be appropriate to the patient's culture.*
  - *Environmental context refers to the setting that care is delivered in.*
  - *Identify family values.*
  - *Identify family beliefs.*
  - *Identify family lifestyles.*
  - *Evaluate how an individual's culture might impact health and perceptions of health.*
  - *Culture, religion, and environment all affect the care of the child.*

CRITICAL COMPONENT

Cultural Care Theory

Madeline Leininger's Cultural Care Theory considers the complexity and interrelatedness of an individual within an environment and the community to which he or she belongs. Dr. Leininger has been termed the founder of cultural care nursing (Leininger, 2009). Dr. Leininger's theory has been able to capture and articulate how culture affects health. Dr. Leininger's Web site, www.madeleine-leininger.com, provides samples of her work and educational materials helpful to both instructors and students.

- The FICA tool is used to identify the patient's spiritual and religious history (**Table 4-1**; Puchalski, 2006; Puchalski & Romer, 2000).
  - *Easy-to-remember FICA acronym reminds nurse of components of tool; F-Faith, I-Importance, C-Community, A-Address*
  - *Provides nurse with baseline patient data*
  - *Provides nurse with data to individualize care*
  - *Offers opportunity to identify spiritual distress and collaborate with other disciplines*
  - *Identifies* ***spiritual concerns****, those issues that the patient and family describe as important. Only the patient and caregiver can describe their perceptions and beliefs.*

TABLE 4–1 FICA SPIRITUAL ASSESSMENT TOOL
F – FAITH AND BELIEF "Do you consider yourself spiritual or religious?" or "Do you have spiritual beliefs that help you cope with stress?" If the patient responds "No," the health-care provider might ask, "What gives your life meaning?" Sometimes patients respond with answers such as family, career, or nature.
I – IMPORTANCE "What importance does your faith or belief have in your life? Have your beliefs influenced how you take care of yourself in this illness? What role do your beliefs play in regaining your health?"
C – COMMUNITY "Are you part of a spiritual or religious community? Is this of support to you? If so, how? Is there a group of people you really love or who are important to you?" Communities such as churches, temples, and mosques, or a group of like-minded friends, can serve as strong support systems for some patients.
A – ADDRESS IN CARE "How would you like me, your health-care provider, to address these issues in your health care?"
As with any other part of the patient interview, the spiritual histories should be patient-centered. Thus, the tool is meant to create an environment of trust by indicating to the patient that the physician or other health-care professional is open to listening to the patient about his or her spiritual issues, if the patient wants to talk about those issues. There are ethical guidelines to which the physician or health-care provider should adhere when taking a spiritual history. Health-care professionals are encouraged not to use the FICA tool as a checklist, but rather to rely on it as a guide to aid in open discussion of spiritual issues.
Sources: Puchalski & Romer, 2000; George Washington Institute for Spirituality & Health, 2009.

  - *Ensures that nurse obtains a complete health history*
  - *Provides additional information for the nurse to better understand the patient's viewpoint when health decisions are made*
  - *Allows the patient and caregiver the opportunity to provide input into the plan of care*

Clinical Reasoning

Pediatric Spiritual and Cultural Assessments

Health-care providers are challenged by time constraints, financial constraints, and knowledge deficits regarding the cultural and spiritual needs of a child.

1. How can the health-care provider include a spiritual and cultural assessment in routine care?
2. What are some barriers to obtaining an accurate spiritual and cultural assessment?
3. How old must the child be to contribute to his or her own health assessment?

Evidence-Based Practice

Bull, A., & Gillies, M. (2007). Spiritual needs of children with complex healthcare needs in hospital. *Pediatric Nursing, 19,* 34–38.

Bull and Gillies (2007) identified that minimal research has been done to study the spiritual needs of children with conditions requiring complex medical care. The only three research studies identified by these authors took place in the United States. The small number of available articles on studies of this subject demonstrates that little research attention has been directed toward children and spirituality. Even though young children are concrete thinkers, they still have values and beliefs.

The study by Bull and Gillies (2007) was performed in the United Kingdom with five children age 8 through 11, and utilized pictures to prompt storytelling. Only five children were involved in this study; therefore, generalizations cannot be drawn. However, four main themes were identified: relationships, hospital environment, coping with invasive procedures, and belief (Bull & Gillies, 2007). The researchers concluded that health-care providers need to evaluate and meet the spiritual needs of children when providing care.

CROSS-CULTURAL COMMUNICATION

CLINICAL PEARL

Health assessments, in the United States, are typically made in a private setting and contain direct questions that anticipate direct answers. This process may not be well received by individuals from other cultures. Health-care providers need to treat patients and caregivers with respect and communicate in a manner that will reap accurate health information.

- Communication is influenced by the relationship of the individuals, the culture of origin, and the individual interpretation of the receiver.
- Communication is provided with words, tone, body language, and rate of speech.
- Effective cross-cultural communication can be accomplished by communicating in a manner that is well received within a given culture.

Effective Communication

- Learn about interacting with diverse cultures.
- Know who is responsible for making health decisions for the patient.
- Identify the patient and caregiver's perceptions of the cause of the illness or health alteration.
- Determine if the gender of the care provider will impact the patient's care.
- Communicate in a language that is understood by the person who is receiving the information.
- Ensure written communication is legible and in the language that the receiver can easily understand.
- Determine the literacy level of the individual who is receiving information and making health-care decisions, and explain information at a level that can be understood and is appropriate for the level of the receiver.
- Do not interrupt; allow the patient or caregiver time to articulate descriptions of or feelings about care.
- Speak in a tone that is appropriate for the situation.
- Provide undivided attention to the patient and caregiver.
- Silence can mean different things in different cultures.
- Be aware of your body language:
  - *Eye contact (direct or indirect)*
  - *Sitting or standing*
  - *No crossing arms*
- Know what body language is acceptable to individual cultures.
- Consider appearance (neat or disheveled) and the values/beliefs of the individual's culture.
- Maintain appropriate distance between the individuals who are communicating.
- Avoid hand and arm gestures when possible, as they mean different things in different cultures.

Nurse–Patient Relationship

- Information is kept confidential.
- The relationship is developed on mutual respect.
- Recognize that you are developing a new relationship within a different culture.
- Recognize appropriate boundaries and maintain those boundaries.
- By law, all nurses must report suspicion of and actual child abuse or neglect. These "secrets" cannot be kept.
- Patients are treated as unique individuals.
- All patients are treated equally.
- Relationships are kept within the boundaries of the care setting.
- When appropriate, provide the patient with opportunities to make choices.

Multidisciplinary Relationships

- Health-care providers work as a team and share information, as appropriate.
- Individuals will have different perspectives and different experiences.
- Respect differences of opinion.
- Respect does not equate to agreement.
- Support each other.
- The patient's best interest is kept in mind by all care providers.
- Ethics consultations should take place when differences are identified between care providers or families and care providers.

CRITICAL COMPONENT

Developing a new relationship with a patient from a different culture may feel uncomfortable. This discomfort is likely due to your own uncertainty and the mental strain involved in interpreting and understanding the culture in a manner that is organized or makes sense for you.

Clinical Reasoning

You are assigned to care for a child who belongs to a culture that is different from your own. It has been noted that the family does not comply with the visitation policy of the unit.

1. How will you address this issue with the family?
2. Identify some of the obstacles to providing culturally competent care.
3. How will you resolve the visitation issue with the family and caregivers?

Language Barriers

- Barriers include any circumstance in which the sender of communication and/or his or her message is not accurately understood by the intended receiver of communication.
- Both sender and receiver may become frustrated.
- Feelings of frustration may lead to anger.
- Remain calm and contact an interpreter.
- Patients and families with language barriers are to receive the same information, education, and support as those without language barriers.
  - *Contact interpreters*
    - Avoid using "charades" to communicate; wait for the interpreter.
    - Pictures can be used to communicate ideas when an immediate interpreter is not available.
    - Family members may serve as an interpreter, but take caution that interpretation is accurate to the message that is being conveyed by the care providers.
    - Document the name of the interpreter used.
    - Interpreter services are available free of charge to the patient.
    - Interpreter services should be readily available to clients.
    - The Internet can sometimes aid in interpretation; ensure only reputable sites are used.

CLINICAL PEARL

Tips for Communicating with Individuals with Language Barriers

1. Remain calm and provide support via body language.
2. Contact an interpreter.
3. Hand gestures mean different things in different cultures, so avoid their use if possible.
4. When appropriate, allow parents to remain with their child.
5. When appropriate, use touch and facial expressions to communicate concern.
6. Utilize family members who may be able to interpret.
7. Use pictures that may be able to accurately depict concepts.
8. Pictures are only a temporary intervention and should be used when an interpreter is not available.
9. You and the patient/caregiver point at pictures to communicate if immediate interventions are needed.
10. Utilize the Internet for basic interpretation of words and phrases.
11. Do not provide elective procedures without the consent of the caregiver.

Clinical Reasoning

A family enters your facility and is unable to speak English. No one in your work area is able to understand or communicate with this family. The female caregiver appears frantic and is pointing to her child. You look at the child, and she appears to be having difficulty breathing.

1. Do you treat the patient?
2. How will you communicate with the child and caregiver?
3. Which nonverbal communication techniques are best to use?

Characteristics and Behaviors Determined by Culture

- Individuals will act and respond as they have been taught to act and respond.
- Children may "pretend" by responding in the way that their caregivers would respond, or by responding in an acceptable way rather than one that accurately communicates their feelings.
- Social skills are acquired through an individual's normal interactions.
  - *Full disclosure is needed in the following areas:*
    - Individual medical history
    - Family history
    - Description of symptom
    - Length of symptom occurrence
    - Potential embarrassment and disgrace of having the disease/condition
  - *Personal space*
    - Your interpretation of personal space may be different from the interpretation of other cultures.
    - Know what space between communicators is expected, and respect that space in personal discussions.
  - *Eye contact*
    - Know the etiquette of eye contact among different cultures—some may prefer direct eye contact, whereas others may not.
    - Provide eye contact if unsure if it is appropriate.
  - *Diet*
    - Most children do not have control over what food is stored in the home.
    - Processed foods are cheaper than fresh foods.
    - Fresh fruits and vegetables can be costly.
    - Most nutritious foods cost more than non-nutritious foods.
    - Children will more likely eat foods they are familiar with.
    - Home eating times should be maintained as much as possible during the hospital stay.
    - Encourage parents to eat meals with their child to promote normalcy and socialization.
    - Food storage practices may require two separate refrigerators.
  - *Time*
    - Perceptions of time may be different among individuals of varying cultures.
    - Personal time may be required for prayer.
    - Preferred times for visitation may not be consistent with visiting hours, presenting difficulties.

- *Touch*
  - Touch with communication may be offensive to patients and caregivers.
  - It can be interpreted differently and may be dependent on the care environment.
  - Touch also may be interpreted differently between genders.
- *Use of alternative medicine*
  - Herbs may have drug interactions.
  - Treatments or remedies may be called "old wives' tales."
  - A family leader may dictate how to treat symptoms.
  - Treatments should be accepted as long as they will not harm the patient.
  - Alternative treatments and medicines, proposed or being used, should be discussed with the multidisciplinary team.

CULTURAL ASSESSMENT

- Mechanism to receive subjective data that helps to identify beliefs and values associated with the patient's culture
- Assures the patient that the care provider is interested in the patient's values
- Allows the care provider to individualize care and incorporate cultural beliefs and values
- Provides data to incorporate subjective and objective information into holistic assessment
- This aspect of a patient assessment usually comes last and has inaccurately been perceived as having less importance than other assessment data.

CLINICAL PEARL

Questions to Ask or Consider During the Cultural Assessment

1. What culture do you consider yourself to belong to?
2. Are your cultural beliefs important to you?
3. Are you an immigrant?
4. How long have you been in this country?
5. Are you having difficulty meeting your health-care needs?
6. Do you have a social support system within your cultural community?

See **Table 4-2** for a description of cultures and their beliefs.

TABLE 4–2 CULTURES AND SELECTED CHARACTERISTICS OR BELIEFS INFLUENCING HEALTH CARE

African American	Higher risk for heart disease due to diet and genetics (Purnell & Paulanka, 2008)
American Indian	Believe they are one with nature May be "now" oriented and do little planning for future events.
Asian	Believe in the balance of hot and cold in the body (Jenko & Moffitt, 2006) Health status influenced by the amount of time individuals have been in the United States
European American	A curse called the Maloic may cause illness Family is important and visitors are expected to show respect
Latino and Hispanic	Family and extended family may visit without regard to time and may talk within a close proximity (Jenko & Moffitt, 2006)
Pacific Islander	Have unique ideas of what health means to them (Purnell & Paulanka, 2008)

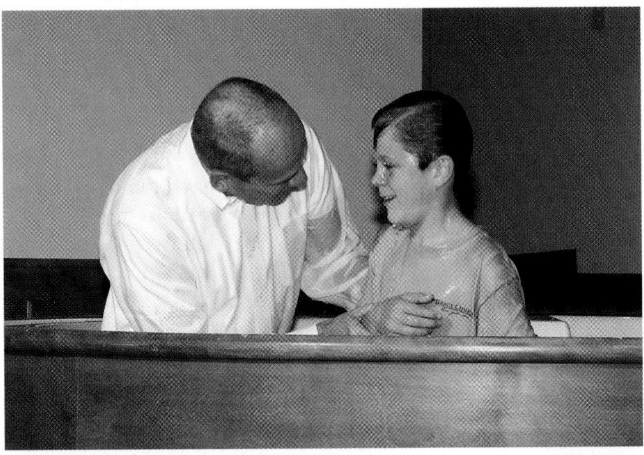

Figure 4–2 Water baptism of a child. *(Courtesy of Grace CMA Church.)*

SPIRITUALITY

- Belief in a greater being that has impact on daily living and views of the afterlife
- Concept of where and how the human race began
- Feeling of a greater being having control over world events
- Individual definition of God

See **Figure 4-2**, an example of a spiritual rite of passage in one religion.

Religious Affiliations

- Group or formal community of individuals with shared spiritual beliefs
- Individuals are not to be stereotyped; all individuals within a religious group are unique.
- Individuals may accept most, but not all, of a religion's beliefs.
- Health-care providers must acknowledge religious affiliations and alter care as appropriate (see **Table 4-3**).

CLINICAL PEARL

Nurses should become familiar with the religious beliefs of the patient and caregiver. Information about a particular religious affiliation can be obtained from the patient, caregiver, books, or caregiver-suggested Internet sites. Patient and caregiver beliefs should be respected, regardless of the beliefs of the care provider.

ENVIRONMENTAL CONSIDERATIONS

- Influences how care is delivered
- Influences the temperature of the home
- Influences the type of food that may be available
- Influences how medications are stored

TABLE 4–3 RELIGIOUS AFFILIATIONS AND NURSING CONSIDERATIONS

Religious Affiliation	Beliefs	Nursing Considerations
Atheism	No belief in God	Care should be provided in ways that make the patient and care provider feel comforted
Buddhism	Buddha taught Four Noble Truths Life is one of suffering Karma is what affects health May pray to ancestors to promote good karma.	May pray to a Buddha idol kept in the room May be vegetarian or have other dietary restrictions Use forms of meditation to promote well-being Promote conservation due to belief that man and earth are one May practice yoga
Christian	Believe that God created the Earth and is omnipotent Bible is the religious book that is followed Believe God is a trinity (God the Father, God the Son, and God the Holy Spirit)	Salvation comes from the belief that Jesus Christ died on the cross for all sins and transgressions Salvation comes from this path alone Prayer and sacraments such as baptism are related to health
Jehovah's Witnesses	Read the *Watch Tower* publication Believe they belong to God's government Read a translation of the Christian Bible called The New World Translation	Will not salute the American flag or say Pledge of Allegiance. May not accept blood transfusions. Reservation should be kept with frequent blood draws
Jewish	Religious leader is called a rabbi Day of rest is called the Sabbath and occurs from sundown Friday to sundown on Saturday	May have dietary considerations with food preparation and storage (kosher foods) No pork in diet No gelatin products in diet (may come from different animal parts that are not acceptable)
Mormonism: The Church of Jesus Christ of Latter-Day Saints	Believe that they will become a god with their own planet to oversee Believe in more than one god	Ask how care can be provided to support the patient and caregiver Discourage the use of caffeine and other stimulants
Muslim	Common religion in the Middle East Pray five times a day while facing Mecca Call God "Allah" Believe Muhammad was a prophet The Quran is the religious book that is followed	Fast from dawn to dusk during Ramadan (ill Muslims are not required to fast) May state that "Allah's will be done" May not verbalize that a child has a chronic illness May need assistance with "ablution," which is a process of washing prior to saying prayers Allow women to cover their heads or wear scarves No pork in diet Handle food with the right hand; the left hand is considered to be unclean
New Age	Believe in karma Believe in yin/yang forces Believe in reincarnation	May want room rearranged to bring about optimum health

- Influences degree to which personal space is respected (privacy)
- Witnessed communication between individuals in the home may influence the child or adolescent's communication style or way of handling unfamiliar circumstances.
- The number of children in the home may influence the time and amount of attention given to each member.
- Living arrangements may be unstable.
- Members of the home may be staying within close quarters.
- Family is defined by the individual child and caregiver(s), and family members are not necessarily biological.
- Factors differing among families include the following:
  - *Family composition*
    - Married male and female with children
    - Unmarried male and female with children
    - Single-parent household
    - Extended family (e.g., aunts/uncles) raising children
    - Grandparent or other family member raising children
    - Group home or foster home
    - Two women or two men raising child
    - Blended families (containing stepparents, stepsiblings, or half siblings)
  - *Socioeconomic status*
    - Both parents working (children may attend day care or be watched by other caregivers)
    - Single working parent (adequate or limited income)
    - No working adult in the home
    - Low-income home with limited resources
  - *Community dangers*
    - Adequate sidewalks to walk on; safe areas for play
    - Lead in soil or lead-based paint chipping off of house
    - Safe drinking water
    - Living near a nuclear power plant
    - Adequate medical help during emergency situations
    - Adequate police coverage to protect neighborhood
    - Gas and chemicals released from local industries
    - Available Level 1 trauma center to care for the critically ill or injured pediatric patient

CLINICAL PEARL

A family is defined by who the child and caregiver say is the family. Families are not necessarily blood or legally related. Many times, a child may have a sitter or care provider who spends an extended amount of time with that child. The child may be more familiar and comfortable with the non-blood-related care provider than an actual family member. A parent or grandparent figure may also play an important role in the child's life.

Review Questions

1. Culturally competent care includes
   A. treating others exactly how you would like to be treated.
   B. seeing each individual as unique.
   C. treating individuals within the same cultural group the same.
   D. providing care without concern for your own values.
2. A nurse is caring for a 12-year-old patient who has recently been hospitalized. Which statement by the patient proves that the nurse did not perform a complete cultural assessment?
   A. "I'm glad that my prayer times work around my care."
   B. "I feel better when my mom stays with me."
   C. "I'm not allowed to eat pork, and it is on my lunch tray."
   D. "My mom doesn't like it when my room is messy."
3. Which of the following characteristics should pediatric visitation include? (select all that apply)
   A. Available 24 hours/day for parents and grandparents
   B. Semi-structured available times for visitors other than parents and grandparents
   C. Time provided for socialization and playing
   D. All of the above
4. A nurse promotes family-centered care when
   A. caregivers can room in and provide care to the child.
   B. the nurse provides the care as the physician orders.
   C. care is provided when the family steps out of the room.
   D. visitation guidelines are strictly followed.
5. When utilizing an interpreter, which item does *not* need to be documented?
   A. Name of the individual interpreting
   B. Primary language of the patient and caregiver
   C. Pictures used to communicate an idea
   D. Understanding of the patient and the care provider
6. A nursing student understands pediatric cultural dietary needs when she tells the parent of her patient:
   A. "You can bring in food from home."
   B. "The hospital food should be adequate."
   C. "I don't know how the food is prepared."
   D. "Food from home will only make your child miss home."

7. Staff education should include which of the following? (select all that apply)
   A. Education on cultures commonly receiving care in their organization's practice
   B. Annual updates and reviews
   C. Self-reflection on care providers' own values and beliefs
   D. All of the above

8. Spiritual assessments should be performed
   A. during every contact with health-care providers.
   B. during hospitalizations.
   C. annually.
   D. as needed.

9. Effective communication can be confirmed when the
   A. patient or caregiver asks questions.
   B. patient or caregiver does not ask questions.
   C. receiver of the messages understands the information as the provider intended the message to be received.
   D. receiver of the message speaks the same language as the person giving the message.

10. When performing an initial assessment, the FICA spiritual assessment tool will
   A. help the care provider to include spiritual needs in the care plan.
   B. complete the questionnaire in the chart.
   C. be answered by the parent or care provider.
   D. only be answered by the patient.

References

Bull, A., & Gillies, M. (2007). Spiritual needs of children with complex healthcare needs in hospital. *Pediatric Nursing, 19*, 34–38. Retrieved from http://www.pediatricnursing.org

George Washington Institute for Spirituality & Health. (2009). FICA for self-assessment. Retrieved from http://www.gwumc.edu/gwish/clinical/fica.cfm

Giger, J. N., & Davidhizar, R. (2002). The Giger and Davidhizar Transcultural Assessment Model. *Journal of Transcultural Nursing, 13*, 185–188. doi: 10.1177/10459602013003004

Jenko, M., & Moffitt, S. R. (2006). Transcultural nursing principles: An application to hospice care. *Journal of Hospice and Palliative Nursing, 8*, 172–180. Retrieved from http://journals.lww.com/jhpn/pages/default.aspx

Leininger, M. (2009). Madeleine-Leininger.com FAQ. Retrieved from http://www.madeleine-leininger.com/en/faq-1.shtml

Puchalski, C. (2006). Spiritual assessment in clinical practice. *Psychiatric Annals, 36*, 150–155. Retrieved from http://www.psychiatricannalsonline.com

Puchalski, C., & Romer, A. L. (2000). Taking a spiritual history allows clinicians to understand patients more fully. *Journal of Palliative Medicine, 3*, 129–137. Retrieved from http://www.liebertpub.com/products/product.aspx?pid=41

Purnell, L. D., & Paulanka, B. J. (2008). *Transcultural health care: A culturally competent approach* (3rd ed.). Philadelphia: F.A. Davis Company.

University of Nevada Las Vegas, Center for Health Disparities Research. (2009). What are health disparities? Retrieved from http://chdr.unlv.edu/index2.htm

5 End-of-Life Care

Rebecca Loth Luetke, MSN, RN, BA

OBJECTIVES

- ☐ Define key terms.
- ☐ Understand causes of infant and pediatric death.
- ☐ Understand and describe appropriate communication with the patient and family in end-of-life care.
- ☐ Understand and describe appropriate communication within the multidisciplinary care team in end-of-life care.
- ☐ Define the role of family-centered care and culturally competent care in end-of-life care.
- ☐ Define and describe palliative care, including the role of the nurse and multidisciplinary team.
- ☐ Discuss assessment and treatment of pain in the palliative care of an infant or pediatric patient.
- ☐ Understand and explain the role spiritual and cultural care have within end-of-life care.
- ☐ Define and compare the stages of grief.
- ☐ Understand and describe role of nursing education in end-of-life care.
- ☐ Define and understand withdrawal of care in infant and pediatric end-of-life care.
- ☐ Define and describe the role of the nurse in infant and pediatric end-of-life care.
- ☐ Understand and describe organ donation and procurement.
- ☐ Define and describe legal aspects of infant and pediatric end-of life-care.

KEY TERMS

- Family-centered care
- Palliative care
- Grief
- Bereavement
- Anticipatory grief
- Denial
- Anger
- Bargaining or negotiations
- Depression or depressed mood
- Acceptance
- Legal considerations
- Withdrawal of care
- Terminal

OVERVIEW OF END OF LIFE

- Death is the end of sustainable life; for infants and pediatric patients, death is the end of a short life, caused by disease or trauma.
- Routine nursing care in pediatrics differs from end-of-life care in pediatrics.
  - *End-of-life care differs from routine pediatric nursing in that it is based on the palliative needs of the patient and family rather than a diagnosis or disease.*
  - *The goal of end-of-life care differs from that of routine care in that the goal is a natural death versus continuation of a healthy life.*
- A terminal diagnosis or disease is one that will end the life of the patient.
- A terminal diagnosis categorized as being the result of either trauma or physiologic causes.
  - *Trauma: caused by outside forces*
    - Accidental: car accident, drowning
    - Nonaccidental: intentional injury, abuse
  - *Physiologic: caused by physiologic forces within the body*
    - Disease: cancer
    - Congenital defect: Edwards syndrome

COMMUNICATION IN CARE OF THE DYING PATIENT

- Communication with family
  - *Family assessment needed for all families to determine how the family unit functions*

Don't have time to read this chapter? Want to reinforce your reading? Need to review for a test? Listen to this chapter on DavisPlus at davispl.us/rudd1.

CRITICAL COMPONENT

Causes of pediatric death in the United States in 2006 varied by age range, as noted in the following list (Centers for Disease Control, 2010):

1–4 years of age

- Number of deaths: 4,631
- Deaths per 100,000 population: 28.4
- Leading causes of death
  - Accidents (unintentional injuries)
  - Congenital malformations

5–14 years of age

- Number of deaths: 6,149
- Deaths per 100,000 population: 15.2
- Leading causes of death
  - Accidents (unintentional injuries)
  - Cancer

Promoting Safety

- Accidents or unintentional injuries are the leading cause of death in pediatrics (National Institutes of Health, 2009).
  - Parents of newborns and infants up to 1 year need safety education regarding the "back to sleep" campaign for prevention of sudden infant death syndrome (SIDS).
  - SIDS remains one of the leading causes of death for infants 1 month to 1 year of age (**Figure 5-1**). The peak time for SIDS deaths is 2 to 4 months of age (American Academy of Pediatrics, n.d.).
  - Instances of SIDS are reduced by 50% by putting babies down to sleep on their backs (National Institutes of Health, 2009).

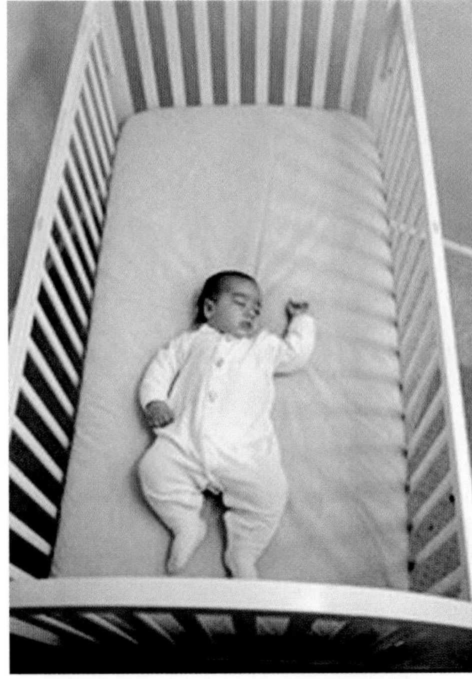

Figure 5-1 Always educate parents to put their infants on their backs to sleep to help prevent sudden infant death syndrome. *(Photo courtesy of the Back to Sleep campaign, Eunice Kennedy Shriver National Institute of Child Health and Human Development, National Institutes of Health and Human Services, www.nichd.nih.gov/sids.)*

  - *Determination of communication needs by looking at family assessment and how much information the family seems to desire*
  - *Assessment of cognitive level of family to provide education at appropriate level*
  - *Assessment of family educational needs considering the determination of communication needs and assessment of cognitive level, as well as overall understanding of patient's diagnosis and potential outcome*
- Determination of legal guardians necessary to know whom information can be released to (See Chapter 3 for further details on communicating with the family.)

Family-Centered Care in End of Life

- **Family-centered care** is the basis for all interactions with the family of a patient receiving end-of-life care.
- Communication
  - *With family: is cognitively appropriate, is based on family assessment, and utilizes family-centered care.*
  - *With patient: is developmentally appropriate; is compassionate.*
  - *Culturally appropriate: considers culture of patient and family in all communications.*
  - *Developmentally appropriate: considers developmental level of siblings when communicating with them and in front of them.*
  - *Compassionate: all aspects of end-of-life care are kind and compassionate.*
  - *Informative: when appropriate, informative communication includes details regarding the diagnosis and death and dying process.*
  - *Honest: in end-of-life care, care providers must be honest when discussing the outcome of death with the family and patient; do not give false hope.*

Clinical Reasoning

Your patient is an 8-year-old child who has a terminal diagnosis. The family only speaks Mandarin Chinese, and the child is fluent in English and Chinese.

1. How do you best communicate with this family in an effective manner?
2. How do you provide family-centered care to this family?

- Communication within multidisciplinary care team takes place in rounds or through charting.

- Communication with each member of the care team on an individual basis takes place to ensure optimum care of the patient and family.
- Nurses have an important communication role in end-of-life care; within the multidisciplinary care team, the nurse has the most contact with the patient and family and acts as an advocate and voice for them to provide optimum care.
- Communication within the palliative care team can be different than communication within the routine multidisciplinary care team; understand the role of palliative care to provide professional education (**Figure 5-2**).

Clinical Reasoning

Your assigned patient is 12 months old and is in the end stage of Tay-Sachs disease. When you walk into the patient's room, the child is being read to by a man who appears to be the same age as the mother. When you introduce yourself to the mother, the man stops what he is doing and directs his attention toward you while reaching out to put his arm around the mother. You read in the patient report that the father is not involved with the family. You then proceed to get written consent for a bedside procedure scheduled for later that afternoon. The man takes the consent form and begins to sign consent for the child.

1. How do you determine the relationship of the man in the room to the child?
2. What do you tell the mother and the man in the room regarding the need for legal guardians to sign for consent?

PALLIATIVE CARE

- Definition of **palliative care**: care provided at end of life to promote patient comfort and family involvement.
- When palliative care is appropriate: at end of life, within 6 months of death.

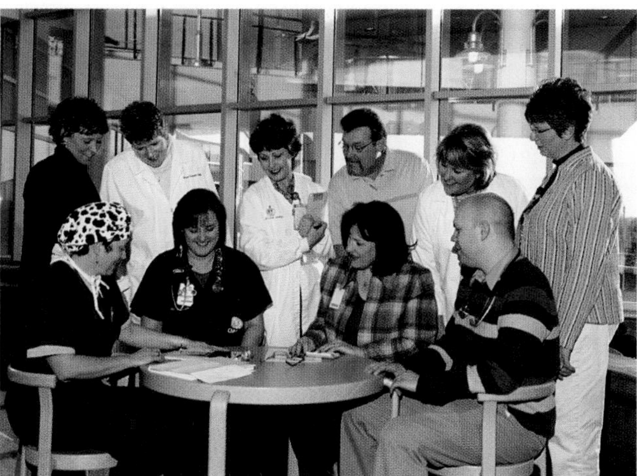

Figure 5-2 The multidisciplinary health-care team provides communication, support, and guidance during the death of an infant or child.

- What makes palliative care different: it promotes a graceful, natural death rather than attempting to prevent death.
- What palliative care offers to family: compassionate care that focuses on the comfort of the patient and inclusion of the family.
- What palliative care offers to patient: comfort; compassionate care with as few invasive devices and procedures as possible.
- Home versus hospital palliative care: palliative care can occur in the hospital in any unit or at home with visiting nurses and care aids.
- Roles of multidisciplinary team members within palliative care
  - *Nursing role and responsibility within pediatric palliative care is as patient advocate and bedside patient care provider.*
  - *Pharmacy role and responsibility within palliative care is to provide medications to increase comfort and medications in appropriate route for patient.*
  - *Nutrition role and responsibility within palliative care is to provide desired diet and food choices for patient as needed.*
  - *Social work role and responsibility within palliative care is to work with the family to ensure that the other needs of the family, such as housing and employer notification, are taken care of.*
  - *Chaplain or pastoral care role and responsibility within palliative care is to care for the spiritual and religious needs of the patient and family.*
  - *Child-life specialist role and responsibility within palliative care is to provide age- and developmentally-appropriate toys and environment for patient and siblings.*
  - *Physician role and responsibility within palliative care is to lead care and order medications and interventions while providing patient and family with education regarding diagnosis.*

CLINICAL PEARL

Child-life therapists are specially trained therapists who are experts in how children play, socialize, and develop (**Figure 5-3**). Children's hospitals generally have a child-life department dedicated to the proper development of hospitalized children.

- The goals of palliative care are to provide for comfortable and graceful end-of-life care.
- Initiation of palliative care is generally done by the physician with input from the multidisciplinary care team.
- Family-centered care in palliative care
  - *Family communication with staff needs to be an important aspect of all daily care.*
  - *Sibling care is necessary in the care of the family.*
  - *Outcomes of using family-centered care include a more cohesive family unit during the death of a child and possibly promoting healing after death.*

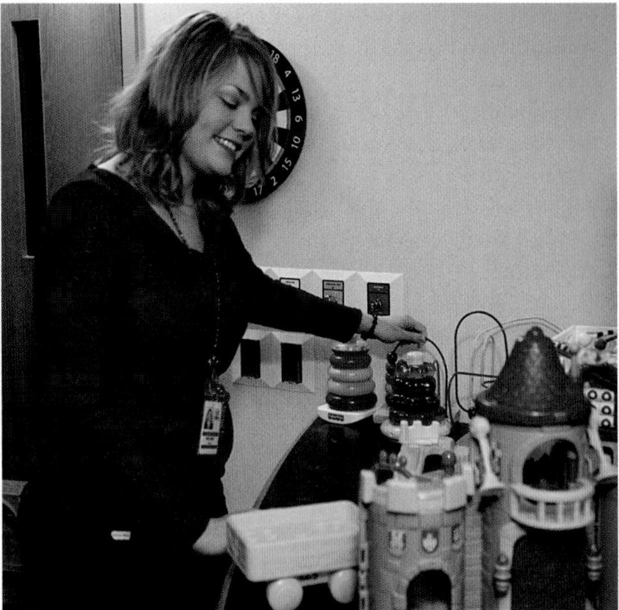

Figure 5-3 A child-life therapist provides developmentally appropriate interventions for patients and siblings.

- Pain control is an important aspect of the definition of palliative care and is the job of the nurse, physician, and pharmacist.

Pediatric Pain Control

- Definition of pain in end-of-life pediatric care: any uncomfortable feeling that prevents patient relaxation or rest.
- Pediatric pain can manifest very differently than adult pain, and pediatric pain symptoms can be very different than adult pain symptoms.
- Pediatric pain assessment techniques include using vital signs, positioning, and parent/caregiver input.
- Pain interventions include pain medication and other therapies to increase comfort and decrease anxiety, promoting relaxation.
- Involvement of family in determination of pain is an important aspect of pediatric pain control; parents/caregivers can be excellent judges of their child's comfort level.
- The multidisciplinary care team members involved in pain control include the physician, nurse, pharmacist, and child-life specialist.
- Involvement of family in alternative pain treatments includes having the parents discuss and suggest other options, such as the following:
  - *Distraction therapy: distracts the patient from the intervention that is causing pain.*

CLINICAL PEARL

Many pediatric hospitals offer a pain team as part of the multidisciplinary care team. The pain team is generally headed by an anesthesiologist, and the primary purpose of the team is to assess and alleviate a patient's pain. The pain team is responsible for writing and ensuring follow-through on all pain-related medical orders and interventions.

Medication

Administration

When administering end-of-life pain medication, various routes are available, including inhaled, topical, oral, intravenous, and rectal. The various routes of administration allow for the child to be free of most invasive devices at the time of death. An example is morphine, a pain medication often given intravenously. If a patient does not have an IV the medication can be given orally; if the patient cannot swallow the medication it can be given via nebulizer in an inhaled form. The inhaled form generally provides for good pain relief without the use of invasive administration techniques.

  - *Relaxation therapy: helps the child relax; techniques include massage, music, holding, and positioning.*
  - *Play therapy: distracts the patient from the pain; generally consists of calm developmentally appropriate activities, such as puzzles and coloring.*

Cultural and Religious Care During End of Life

- Cultural considerations for pediatric end of life include respecting the cultural beliefs of the family and patient. (See Chapter 4 for further details.)
- Providing culturally competent care requires the nurse to incorporate the cultural beliefs of the family and patient into the daily care of the patient.
- The spiritual needs of family and patient require the nurse to incorporate the spiritual beliefs of the family and patient into the daily care of the patient (**Figure 5-4**).
- Family-centered care within cultural care encourages the nurse to incorporate the cultural needs of the family into the care of the patient and family.

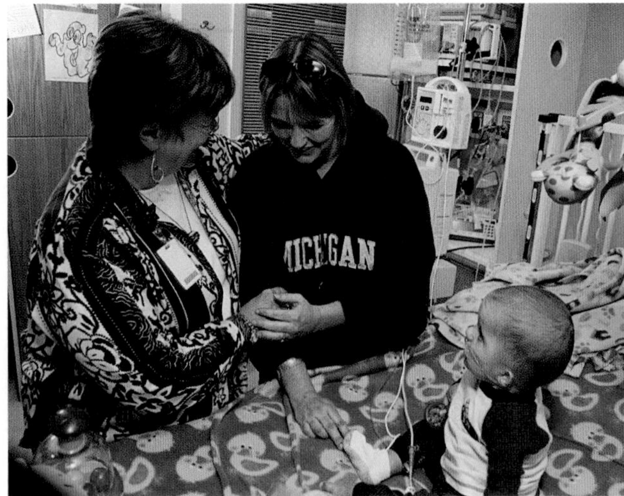

Figure 5-4 The hospital chaplain or spiritual care staff can provide support to the patient and family.

CHILD DEVELOPMENT

- An understanding of overall child development and how it relates to a child's view of death is necessary to provide competent care. (See discussions of development in Chapters 7–10.)
  - *A child's view of life is created from his or her life experiences and also depends on developmental level.*

Clinical Reasoning

One of your patients is a 3-year-old girl who has just passed away from a terminal cancer diagnosis; the physician has declared death and signed the death certificate. The coroner has just called and stated that due to his discussions with the attending physician, the child does not need an autopsy. The family is Amish and is requesting to take the child back to the family property for burial using the family's horse-drawn buggy.

1. How do you respond to this request?

-
  - *If a child is dying from a congenital condition or disease, his or her developmental level may be lower than expected for age; developmental delays must be considered in the developmental assessment.*
- A child's view of death is based on developmental stage and life experiences, so expect varied behavior and opinions related to death (**Table 5-1**).
- The developmental level of siblings is a consideration in family-centered care.
  - *In providing family-centered care, the nurse needs to incorporate care of the siblings at the appropriate developmental level.*
- Nursing interactions with children at the end of life should be based on the developmental level and cultural needs of the child.
- Child behavior at end of life may be abnormal based on the stress and confusion of death and dying.

Clinical Reasoning

You are caring for a 5-year-old girl dying from a progressive osteosarcoma; in recent days she has begun to wet her bed. There is no medical explanation for her lack of bladder control, and her mother is very angry and scolding the child.

1. How do you help the patient's mother to understand that the child's lack of bladder control is related to stress?
2. What is the best way for the family and nursing staff to deal with this child's behavior?

- Parent and family education related to the child's developmental stage is important so that the parents and family understand how their dying child and any siblings understand death.

GRIEF

- There are many theories on **grief**, or **bereavement**, including those of Kübler-Ross, Bowlby, Engle, and Worden.
- Most theories have a common theme of stages of grief, theorizing that individuals progress through their grief on an individual timeline but through similar stages.
- Kübler-Ross (2009) is a respected grief theorist who defined the common stages of grief (**Table 5-2**).
- **Anticipatory grief** occurs before the stages of grief and is common in infant and pediatric death, when the

TABLE 5–1 CHILD'S VIEW OF DEATH BASED ON DEVELOPMENTAL STAGE AND LIFE EXPERIENCES

Age Group	Emotional Development	Conceptual View of Death
Infants and toddlers (birth to 35 months)	Fear and anxiety over separation	No or little understanding of death (Brown & Warr, 2007)
Preschoolers (3–5 years)	Magical thinking, formation of peer relationships, gender identification	Death is something that happens to others Death is not a permanent state; death is reversible Curious about dead animals and flowers (Brown & Warr, 2007)
Early childhood (6–12 years)	Enthusiasm for learning and work Developing strong interpersonal relationships Building self-esteem	Death is final Death is universal Death is only in the distant future (Brown & Warr, 2007)
Preadolescents and adolescents	Identity formation Development of complex cognitive skills	Understand death in a logical manner Death is permanent (Brown & Warr, 2007)

family of a patient with a terminal diagnosis prepares for death prior to the dying process (Kübler-Ross, 2009).

- Stages of grief
  - ***Denial:*** *Following anticipatory grief is denial, which is a refusal to believe that an infant or child is dead or dying (Kübler-Ross, 2009).*
  - ***Anger:*** *Anger concerning death results in feelings of wrath or indignation; it will often manifest as anger toward the disease, the cause of death of the infant or child, or even the medical staff and caregivers of the child (Kübler-Ross, 2009).*
  - ***Bargaining or negotiations:*** *These are an attempt to create a change in the situation through an agreement for services exchanged (Kübler-Ross, 2009).*
  - ***Depression or depressed mood:*** *This stage of grief is often manifest as the loss of interest in life and normal activities, along with feelings of guilt or low self-worth (Kübler-Ross, 2009).*
  - ***Acceptance:*** *Acceptance is to receive or agree with what is offered. In pediatric grief, it is when the parents or family come to terms with the event and the associated loss.*
- Family members may grieve at different stages; everyone will not grieve in the same manner at the same time. The family should be educated that this may occur and is normal.
- Staff feelings of grief over the loss of a patient are common and should be expected.

TABLE 5–2 KÜBLER-ROSS STAGES OF GRIEF

Common Stages of Grief	Expected Behaviors from Family Members
Denial	Unwillingness to accept diagnosis, lack of trust in medical staff (Kübler-Ross, 2009)
Anger	Anger or aggression toward staff or family members; verbal arguments and confrontations are common (Kübler-Ross, 2009)
Bargaining	Reliance on a higher power to prevent death, belief that promises of future behavior will prevent death of the child (Kübler-Ross, 2009)
Depression	Crying, withdrawal from family and friends, loss of appetite (Kübler-Ross, 2009)
Acceptance	Statements of understanding of the loss, positive outlook, discussion of the future (Kübler-Ross, 2009)

NURSING EDUCATION IN END-OF-LIFE CARE

- Education for patient (when appropriate for age and development)
  - *Provide explanation of cause for terminal diagnosis, with details regarding how the disease will cause death.*
  - *Provide explanation of current medical interventions needed, with descriptions of what to expect related to the interventions.*
  - *Expected interventions: discuss and educate parents as to possible medical interventions and reasons for those interventions.*
  - *Explain the dying process, with appropriate explanation of what to expect of the child and staff.*
- Education for parents
  - *Disease process (when appropriate): give details of how the disease process affects the child.*
  - *Current medical treatments available for patient diagnosis: provide parents with all information possible concerning available treatment options.*
  - *Discuss potential outcomes from the disease, with discussion of time frame when possible.*
  - *Explain what to expect during the dying process—in terms of the child, siblings, and other family members.*
  - *Discuss what to expect at the time of death, such as how the child will look, the involvement of the staff, and whom the family wants in the room.*
  - *Discuss what to expect after death, such as caring for and disposition of the body and funeral arrangements.*

WITHDRAWAL OF CARE

- Withdrawal of care is to stop all life-saving measures and allow the infant or child to die naturally.
- Parental rights in withdrawal of care allow them to give consent to stop interventions and determine when the interventions will be stopped; they also have the right to change their minds and continue care.
- Withdrawal of care allows for the patient to die in a natural way with the family at the bedside, versus in an end-of-life attempted resuscitation with the child surrounded by medical staff.
- Parent and family education regarding withdrawal of care—how it is done and what to expect in the response of the child—is important to prevent misunderstandings.
- When appropriate, educate the siblings and patient regarding withdrawal of care and what to expect.
- Initiation of withdrawal of care is determined by the condition of the patient, the physician's opinion, and parent/caregiver desires.

- Outcomes of withdrawal of care need to be discussed with the family so that they know what to expect.
- Nursing interventions in withdrawal of care include turning off the monitor, disconnecting all invasive lines, and creating a comfortable, peaceful, and private environment for the family.
- Family presence in pediatric code situations is handled differently in all hospitals, and you need to know the protocol of the facility you are working in.
  - *Positive aspects of family presence in pediatric code situations include the family knowing that everything was done to attempt to save the patient.*
  - *Family involvement in pediatric code situations provides family-centered care in a very stressful situation.*
  - *A negative aspect of family presence in pediatric code situation is that the family sees the child in the worst situation possible.*
  - *The family may attempt to be at the bedside, which can be inappropriate with specific interventions.*

Promoting Safety

In recent years families have been invited to remain with the patient during resuscitation (Calvin et al., 2004). Research has demonstrated that presence during resuscitation was beneficial for the family members, and they often felt that being present was both a right and an obligation (Meyers et al., 2004).

During a pediatric code situation, it is very important to provide for the safety of the patient's family.

- Ensure that a staff member is assigned to be with the family during the entire code event.
- Ensure that family members are not touching the bed or medical equipment during cardiac shock delivery.
- Ensure that family members are not in the way of medical staff.
- Ensure that family members are not in the way of medical equipment.
- If family members are unsteady on their feet, ensure that they are given a place to sit.

  - *The desired outcome of family-centered care in pediatric code situations is to create greater communication and decrease confusion for the family.*

NURSING ROLE IN CARE OF THE DYING CHILD

- Creation of mementos and keepsakes for the family of dying infants and children provides them with a tangible memory of their child (**Figure 5-5**).
  - *Handprints and footprints are created using molds or ink and can be very valuable to the parents and family.*

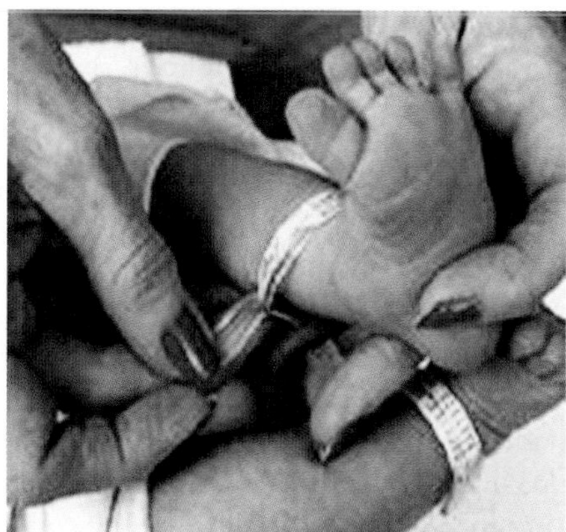

Figure 5-5 A patient's name band is often kept as a keepsake by the family. *(From the National Institute of Child Health and Human Development. Retrieved from http://www.nichd.nih.gov/sids/.)*

  - *A lock of hair is often cut to give to the parents; ensure the hair is put in a secure envelope or bag to prevent loss.*
  - *Pictures are very common and provide wonderful tangible images for the family who has lost an infant or child; some hospitals provide a camera for the staff to take digital photographs, and some professional photographers take end-of-life pictures as a gift for the family.*
- Family needs should be considered and included in the daily nursing care of the dying patient; caring for the family's needs allows the parents to care for their child.
- Family involvement in the child's care will be different for all families, but when appropriate the family should be involved in all aspects of the care of the dying infant and child.
- Bathing and dressing of the infant or child will depend on the desires of the parents. When appropriate, have the parents choose the clothing for the child and assist with the bathing and dressing.
- Accommodating for visitors despite unit visitation rules is the role of the nurse and should be done in an appropriate way while respecting the needs of the other patients on the unit.
- Accommodations needed for any religious or spiritual ceremonies needs to be included in the bedside care of the dying patient. When appropriate, assist hospital pastoral care in meeting the spiritual needs of the family and patient.
- Allow family time to say goodbye to child and have time alone with the child.
- When possible/desired, allow family to hold the child or lay in the bed next to the child.

- Follow hospital protocol for declaration of death; this will vary based on facility policies, so be sure to follow the policies and protocols of the facility you are working in.
- Follow hospital protocol for disposition of the body. Depending on the cause of death, the body will go to the coroner or funeral home; be sure to properly label the body and respect the body at all times.
- Follow state regulations and hospital protocol for autopsy. Some patients will require an autopsy, and it is generally at the discrimination of the local coroner. Follow facility protocol related to patient death and contacting the coroner.
- Proper documentation at time of death is the responsibility of the nurse. Ensure that all care, nursing interventions, and patient outcomes are charted.

ORGAN DONATION

- Organ donation is the giving of viable organs from a dying patient to a patient in need of a specific organ.
- Pediatric organs can be transplanted into adult and pediatric patients.
- A patient is considered a viable donor when the organs needed are not damaged by disease, diagnosis, or medication.
- Protocols for organ donation
  - *When a child is considered a viable candidate for organ donation the family is approached by an organ donation approach team.*
  - *An approach team is a multidisciplinary team of healthcare providers and ancillary staff who are specially trained in approaching families to request that they donate the patient's organs.*
- Consent is needed from the legal guardians for organ donation.
- Once consent is given, blood is drawn from the patient to determine who on the transplant list is going to be the best match for the organs available.
- Procurement of organs is done by the transplanting surgical team. The team travels to the site of the organ donor and the patient is taken to the operating room to remove the organs.
  - *Parents and family members should say goodbye to the patient prior to transfer to the operating room; the patient will die in the operating room.*
- Family education regarding donation is very important and should include:
  - *Information regarding how the patient will be kept alive via medical intervention until the procurement surgeon arrives*
  - *Details of how the infant or child will pass away in the operating room and the fact that the family cannot be in the operating room*
  - *The benefits of organ donation to the recipient*

CULTURAL AWARENESS: Organ Donation

The Gypsy (Romani) culture does not approve of organ donation; be sure to know the cultural beliefs of the family prior to notifying the approach team for organ donation.

- Federal regulations governing organ donation: There is a national government-funded organ donor branch of the federal government that oversees and acts as a watchdog for organ donation.
  - *The Organ Procurement and Transplantation Network (OPTN) is the unified transplant network established by the U.S. Congress under the National Organ Transplant Act (NOTA) in 1984 (U.S. Department of Health and Human Services, 2009).*
  - *The OPTN oversees the federal laws related to organ donation and procurement and ensures that organs are distributed fairly and are given to patients based on diagnosis, stage in life, and matching percentage (U.S. Department of Health and Human Services, 2009).*
  - *The OPTN facilitates organ matching and placement through the use of a computer system and fully staffed organ center operating 24 hours a day that works in conjunction with individual state organ donation networks (U.S. Department of Health and Human Services, 2009).*
- Organ donation is generally a closed process; the donating family will not know who has received their child's organs (U.S. Department of Health and Human Services, 2009).

LEGAL ASPECTS OF PEDIATRIC END OF LIFE

- It is the responsibility of the nurse to understand and adhere to the nursing scope of practice.
- When caring for a dying child, the nurse must include any **legal considerations** in the plan of care.
- Determination of legal guardians
- Obtaining consent
- **Withdrawal of care**

See Chapter 2 for legal and ethical considerations.

CLINICAL PEARL

The nursing practice act of each individual state guides nursing practice; these acts vary from state to state. You can locate the nursing practice act for the state you practice in by contacting the State Board of Nursing.

- Autopsies can be requested by the family, the physician, and the coroner; note that autopsy policies and procedures differ by state and facility.
  - *Families may request an autopsy if they wish to know the exact cause of the death of their child; if the coroner*

does not agree that an autopsy needs to be performed, the family may be responsible for the cost of the autopsy.
  - *The physician may request an autopsy if the patient's cause of death is not known; if the coroner does not agree with the need for an autopsy, the family may need to give consent.*
  - *The coroner has the legal right to request an autopsy in any death and does not need consent of the family if it is considered legally necessary.*
- Some **terminal** children will have a do not resuscitate (DNR) order, and just as in adult medicine, this order must be respected.
  - *All facilities will have specific policies relating to DNR orders; be sure to follow facility policies when caring for a patient without a DNR order.*
  - *Only the legal guardians can determine a minor patient's DNR status.*
  - *A DNR order can be reversed at any time by the legal guardians.*
  - *DNR orders can differ in regard to provision of no life-sustaining interventions to provision of partial or limited life-sustaining interventions.*
  - *Parents or legal guardians need to be fully educated on all aspects of a DNR order.*
  - *If you are the nurse caring for a terminal child, it is your responsibility to know if the child has a DNR and the limitations within the specific DNR.*
  - *When a patient has a legal DNR order, it is the responsibility of the health-care team to follow the DNR order.*
- In the death of a child from suspected abuse or intentional injury, the legal aspects can become very important and need to be considered.
  - *Understand the facility policies and state laws when caring for a child who is the suspected victim of abuse.*
  - *Ensure when you are caring for any child that information is only released following the protocols and laws outlined in the Health Insurance Portability and Accessibility Act (HIPAA).*
  - *All aspects of nursing care require proper documentation and charting, and this includes the death of a child.*
  - *If you were involved in the care of an infant or child in which the infant or child's death included resuscitation attempts, ensure that everything is documented in the proper form according to hospital policy.*
- Determination of legal guardian
  - *The person who is legally able to give consent for the child needs to be determined upon admission based on facility policies and state laws.*
  - *Many types of family units exist within U.S. society, and people in the patient's life who function as a family unit are not always legally seen as a family unit.*
  - *Some pediatric patients are able to give self-consent, depending on the laws of the state or individual legal rulings making the minor independent.*
  - *Every state has individual laws that determine the age of consent, or the age at which a child is considered legally an adult and able to sign for his or her own medical care.*
  - *When you are caring for any infant or pediatric patient, you must ensure that the people who are giving consent for treatment are the legal guardians.*
  - *In cases of abuse or patients who are a ward of the state, it is essential that the consent for any and all procedures is only obtained from the legal guardian(s).*
  - *Always utilize social work staff for any unclear family units to ensure that the legal guardian is giving consent.*
  - *Proper documentation: as with all nursing care, ensure that you document the determination of legal guardian and who is able to sign consent for the patient.*

Review Questions

1. A mother of a 3-year-old diagnosed with a terminal grade 4 neuroblastoma with side effects of balance and hearing issues asks the nurse about an appropriate activity that is safe for the child. Which of the following is an appropriate response from the nurse?
   A. "No playing is good—the child should remain in bed."
   B. "Play groups with children in the neighborhood are recommended."
   C. "Age-appropriate gymnastic classes are a good choice."
   D. "Quiet play with minimal stimuli is appropriate, such as puzzles or books."

2. The nurse is aware that there are two causes of pediatric death:
   A. psychological and physiologic
   B. trauma and physiologic
   C. trauma and psychological
   D. physiologic and external

3. A nurse in a maternity unit is providing emotional support to a client and her husband who are preparing to be discharged from the hospital after the birth of a stillborn full-term infant. Which statement if made by the client indicates a component of the normal grieving process?
   A. "We would really like to attend a support group."
   B. "We are okay; we are going to work on having another baby now."
   C. "We never want to have a baby again or talk about our loss."
   D. "We are filling out the paperwork to adopt a baby."

4. A nursing instructor asks a nursing student the leading causes of death for pediatric patients. Which of the following statements demonstrates that the student is aware of the leading causes of death for pediatric patients?
   A. "Disease and terminal cancer are the leading causes of death for pediatric patients."
   B. "Abuse and SIDS are the leading causes of death for pediatric patients."
   C. "Accidents such as unintentional injuries are the leading causes of death for pediatric patients."
   D. "Accidents and congenital defects are the leading causes of death for pediatric patients."

5. Which, if any, of the following circumstances might incline a nurse to become disengaged or enmeshed rather than therapeutically engaged with a patient/family?
A. Five-year-old child dying of cancer
B. Six-month-old infant in a vegetative state secondary to inflicted head injury
C. Dying 10-day-old neonate with anencephaly whose parents do not visit
D. All of the above

6. The nurse is aware that the purpose of pediatric palliative care is to
A. speed up the process of death and decrease suffering.
B. promote patient comfort and family involvement.
C. increase patient comfort and decrease environmental stimuli.
D. prevent disease and promote overall health.

7. The nurse is creating a care plan for palliative care for a terminal 6-year-old child in the hospital and is aware that an essential intervention and assessment that needs to be included is which of the following?
A. Pain
B. Developmental needs
C. School needs
D. Discharge

8. Which of the following pain interventions is appropriate for a palliative care pediatric patient?
A. Assess the patient's pain using a developmentally appropriate pain scale.
B. Ask the patient's family to participate and provide input into the patient's pain assessment.
C. Use a combination of prescribed medications, distraction, and positioning to provide comfort and decrease pain.
D. All of the above are appropriate.

9. The nurse is preparing to assess a 4-week-old infant who is suffering from shaken baby syndrome. The most appropriate pain scale to use in this situation is the
A. CHOPS.
B. Numerical Scale.
C. VAS.
D. NIPS.

10. When a child is at the end stage of life, the nursing priority should be
A. restoration of health.
B. health education.
C. patient comfort.
D. developmental assessment.

References

American Academy of Pediatrics. (n.d.). SIDS handout. Retrieved from http://www.healthychildcare.org/Doc/SIDSexercise1.doc

Brown, E., & Warr, B. (2007). *Supporting the child and the family in pediatric palliative care.* Philadelphia: Jessica Kingsley Publishers.

Calvin, A., Clark, A. P., Eichorn, D. J., Gizzetta, C. E., Klein, J. D., Meyers, T. A., & Taliaferro, E. (2004). Family presence during invasive procedures and resuscitation: The experience of family members, nurses, and physicians. *Topics in Emergency Medicine, 26* (1), 61–73.

Centers for Disease Control. (2010). Child health, data for the United States health status. Retrieved from http://www.cdc.gov/nchs/fastats/children.htm

Kübler-Ross, E. (2009). *On death and dying: What the dying have to teach doctors, nurses, clergy and their own families* (40th anniversary ed.). New York: Routledge.

National Institutes of Health. (2009). Back to Sleep education campaign. Retrieved from http://www.nichd.nih.gov/sids/

U.S. Department of Health and Human Services. (2009). Organ procurement and transplantation network. Retrieved from http://optn.transplant.hrsa.gov

UNIT 3 Growth and Development of the Child

6 Growth and Development

Mary Grady, MSN, RN and Jill Reiter, MSN, RN

OBJECTIVES

- ☐ Describe general principles of growth and development.
- ☐ Discuss cognitive growth and development according to Jean Piaget.
- ☐ Discuss psychosocial growth and development according to Eric Erikson.
- ☐ Discuss psychosexual growth and development according to Sigmund Freud.
- ☐ Discuss social-moral growth and development according to Lawrence Kohlberg.
- ☐ Discuss the theory of nature versus nurture.
- ☐ Explain the effects of Family Theory, as described by Murray Bowen and Virginia Satyr, on the child who is ill.
- ☐ Apply principles of family-focused care in approaches toward the child.
- ☐ Analyze factors that affect growth and development.
- ☐ Understand nursing applications of growth and development theories.

KEY TERMS

- Growth
- Development
- Family-centered care
- Psychosexual
- Psychosocial
- Traditional family
- Nontraditional family

GENERAL PRINCIPLES OF GROWTH AND DEVELOPMENT

- Unique and highly individualized processes
- Interrelated and interdependent processes
- Ongoing from conception to end of life
- Influenced by factors such as genetics, environment, and nutrition
- **Growth**—increase in height and weight.

Clinical Reasoning

Failure to Thrive

Failure to grow and develop at an expected rate can mean that a child is failing to thrive. The diagnosis of failure to thrive (FTT) is given to children who fall below the 5th percentile ranges on height and weight charts. For infants, it usually presents first with an absence of weight gain or weight loss (Block & Krebs, 2005). There is then a drop in height that is followed by a drop in head circumference. This failure to grow can cause developmental delay.

Don't have time to read this chapter? Want to reinforce your reading? Need to review for a test? Listen to this chapter on DavisPlus at **davispl.us/rudd1.**

- **Development**—acquisition of skills and abilities.
- Developmental tasks (**Table 6-1**)
  - *Developmental tasks are the sets of skills and competencies that are unique to each developmental stage.*
  - *Certain tasks must be mastered in order for the child to progress to the next level.*
  - *Variation at different ages is due to specific body structure and organ growth.*
- Growth and development are characterized by periods of rapid growth and plateaus (spurts and lulls).
- Growth and development follow an orderly pattern.
  - *Cephalocaudal—starts at the head and moves downward. Example: The child can control its head and neck before it can control its arms and legs.*
  - *Proximodistal—starts in the center and processes to the periphery. Example: Movement and control of the trunk section of the body occurs before movement and control of the arms.*
  - *Differentiation—simple to complex progression of achievement of developmental milestones. Example: The child learns to crawl before learning to walk.*

TABLE 6–1 DEVELOPMENTAL MILESTONES

AGE	FINE MOTOR	GROSS MOTOR
3 months	Grasps toys, can open and close hands	Raises head and chest when lying on stomach Supports upper body with arms when lying on stomach Stretches legs out and kicks when lying on stomach or back
6–8 months	Bangs objects on table Can transfer objects from hand to hand Start of pincer grasp	Can roll from side to side Can sit unsupported by 7 or 8 months Supports whole weight on legs
1 year	Can hold crayon, may mark on paper	Pulls self up to stand Walks holding onto furniture May walk two or three steps independently
2–3 years	Learning to dress self Can draw simple shapes	Jumps Kicks ball Learning to pedal tricycle
4–5 years	Dresses independently Uses scissors Learning to tie shoes Brushes teeth	Goes up and down stairs independently Throws a ball overhand Hops on one foot

Source: Centers for Disease Control and Prevention, 2010.

Promoting Safety

Caregivers need to be aware of the different growth and developmental milestones so that they can prevent injury at the different stages. In early childhood, much care and consideration should be given to prevent falls, choking, and aspiration of food or objects. Childproofing the home to prevent injuries is important.

Five Stages in Childhood

- Infant—birth to 1 year
- Toddler—age 1 to 3 years
- Preschool—age 3 to 6 years
- School-age—6 to 12 years
- Adolescence—12 to 18 years

See **Table 6-2** for an overview of growth and development by age.

Physical Examination

Clinical Reasoning

Reflexes

Nurses need to know normal infant reflexes and recognize when they are not present. Reflexes that remain can be a sign of growth and developmental issues and delays (Hockenberry & Wilson, 2009). A few of the most common reflexes to watch for are as follows:

- Tonic neck/fencing reflex–disappears around 2 to 3 months
- Moro/startle reflex–disappears around 4 to 6 months
- Babinski's–disappears by 2 years of age

CLINICAL PEARL

Family-Centered Care

As part of **family-centered care**, nurses need to adapt their care and nursing interventions to the child's stage of growth and development. They will need to explain what is happening to a child in language and on a developmental level the family can understand. A child's caretaker should always be included in the child's care and interventions. Nurses need to remember that we are not caring for just a child, but for the entire family unit (Institute for Patient- and Family-Centered Care, 2010).

TABLE 6–2 OVERVIEW OF GROWTH AND DEVELOPMENT BY AGE

AGE	GROWTH FACTS
INFANT: Age birth to 1 year	**Weight:** -Doubles by 5 to 6 months -Triples by 1 year **Height:** -Increase of 1 foot by 1 year of age **Teeth:** -Erupt by 6 months -Has six to eight deciduous teeth by 1 year of age
TODDLER: Age 1 to 3 years	**Weight:** -Gains 8 oz or more a month from 1 to 2 years -Gains 3 to 5 lbs a year from 2 to 3 years of age **Height:** -From 1 to 2 years of age, grows 3 to 5 inches -From 2 to 3 years of age, grows 2 to 2.5 inches per year **Teeth:** -By 3 years of age, has 20 deciduous teeth
PRESCHOOL: Age 3 to 6 years	**Weight:** -Gains 3 to 5 lbs a year **Height:** -Grows 1.5 to 2.5 inches a year
SCHOOL-AGE: Age 6 to 12 years	**Weight:** -Gains 3 to 5 lbs a year **Height:** -Grows 1.5 to 2.5 inches a year
ADOLESCENCE: Age 12 to 18 years	**Variations** **Weight:** **Girls** -15 to 55 lbs **Boys** -15 to 65 lbs **Height:** **Girls** -2 to 8 inches **Boys** -4.5 to 12 inches

PSYCHOINTELLECTUAL DEVELOPMENT

Cognitive Development: Jean Piaget

- Lived from 1896 to 1980
- Swiss scientist who focused on child psychology
- Development is viewed as a sequential and orderly process.
- Cognitive acts occur as the child adapts to the surrounding environment.
- Child's experience with the environment naturally encourages growth and maturation.
- Moves from stages that are relatively simple to the more complex (**Table 6-3**).
- The child must accommodate to new or complex problems by drawing on past experiences.

Key Stages of Theory

- **Sensorimotor—birth to 2 years**
  - *The child learns through motor and reflex actions.*
  - *The child learns that he or she is separate from the environment and others.*
    - **Stage 1:** Reflexes—birth to 2 months
      - *Understands the environment purely through inborn reflexes such as sucking.*
    - **Stage 2:** Primary Circular Reactions—1 to 4 months
      - *Beginning to coordinate reflexes and sensations. For example, may find the thumb by accident, find pleasure in sucking it, then later repeat sucking it for pleasure.*
    - ***Stage 3:*** *Secondary Circular Reactions—4 to 8 months*
      - *Child focuses on environment, and begins to repeat actions that will trigger a response. For example, the child puts a toy rattle in his or her mouth.*
    - ***Stage 4:*** *Coordination of Secondary Schemata—8 to 12 months*
      - *To achieve a desired effect, the child will repeat the action. An example of this is the child repeatedly shaking a rattle to make the sound.*
    - ***Stage 5:*** *Tertiary Circular Reactions—12 to 18 months*
      - *The child begins trial-and-error approaches, for example, making a sound to see if it will get attention from the caregiver.*
    - ***Stage 6:*** *Inventions of New Means/Mental Combinations—18 to 24 months*
      - *The child learns that objects and symbols represent events, such as a bowl and spoon means dinner is coming.*

CLINICAL PEARL

Object Permanence

Object permanence is one of the most important developments in the sensorimotor stage. The child now knows that an object exists even when it cannot be seen or heard. This is a wonderful time to introduce the game peek-a-boo; by the end of this stage the child will understand that you did not disappear just because your hands are over your face.

TABLE 6–3 PIAGET'S FIVE STAGES OF COGNITIVE DEVELOPMENT

	SENSORIMOTOR STAGE	PREOPERATIONAL STAGE*	INTUITIVE THOUGHT PHASE	CONCRETE OPERATIONAL STAGE	FORMAL OPERATIONAL STAGE
AGE	Birth to 2 years **Stage 1:** Reflexes Birth to 2 months **Stage 2:** Primary Circular Reactions 1 to 4 months **Stage 3:** Secondary Circular Reactions 4 to 8 months **Stage 4:** Coordination of Secondary Schemata 8 to 12 months **Stage 5:** Tertiary Circular Reactions 12 to 18 months **Stage 6:** Inventions of New Means 18 to 24 months	2 to 4 years	4 to 7 years	7 to 11 years	11 to adulthood
CHARACTERISTICS	During this stage the child progresses from reflex activity to simple repetitive behaviors. The end result is behaviors that are imitative. By the end of the stage the following concepts should be mastered: -Object permanence -Understanding of cause and effect -Understanding of spatial relationships -Uses make-believe and pretend play	-Egocentric -Magical thinking -Increase in language development -Associates words with objects/ symbols	-Less egocentric -Thinks of others -Can think of one idea at a time -Words used to express thoughts	-Continues to become less self-centered -Thought process is more coherent and logical -Solves concrete problems -Still unable to think abstractly	-Adaptable and flexible - Use of rational thinking -Thinks abstractly -Reasoning is deductive

*The preoperational stage often includes ages 2 to 7 years.

- **Preoperational—2 to 7 years**
  - *Application of language*
  - *Use of symbols to represent objects*
  - *Ability to think about things and events that aren't immediately present*
  - *Oriented to the present, the child has difficulty conceptualizing time.*
  - *Thinking is influenced by fantasy.*
  - *Teaching must take into account the child's vivid fantasies and undeveloped sense of time.*

CLINICAL PEARL

The Procedure from the Child's Perspective

In this stage the child is egocentric, or unable to take the view of others. While the child is hospitalized, the nurse should introduce role playing and medical play therapy. The child needs to understand the procedure from his or her own perspective, such as by touching and playing with the equipment prior to it being used.

- **Concrete operational—7 to 11 years**
  - *Increase in accommodation skills*
  - *Develops an ability to think abstractly and to make rational judgments about concrete or observable phenomena*
  - *In teaching, give the opportunity to ask questions and explain things back to you. This allows the child to mentally manipulate information.*

> **CLINICAL PEARL**
>
> **Language to Use for Explanations**
>
> The hospitalized child often does not understand the terminology medical professionals may use. They have difficulty understanding abstract thoughts. A statement such as "This IV will feel like a bee sting" may cause the child to think there will a bee biting his or her arm. Remember to speak in clear terms and avoid comparing different experiences without explanation. For example, a better approach would be "Have you ever been stung by a bee? (wait for response; if the child has been stung, continue with this approach) Some kids say the IV feels like a pinch from a bee sting."

- **Formal operational—11 years to adulthood**
  - *This stage brings cognition to its final form.*
  - *The individual no longer requires concrete objects to make rational judgments.*
  - *Individuals are capable of hypothetical and deductive reasoning.*
  - *Teaching for adolescents may be wide ranging because they are able to consider many possibilities from several perspectives.*

> **CLINICAL PEARL**
>
> **Formal Operational**
>
> The child in this stage begins to consider that his or her actions will result in possible consequences. It is important to remember when caring for a patient in this stage that you should explain reasons for the hospitalization, the disease process, and possible outcomes, especially those related to the patient's behavior.

PSYCHOSEXUAL DEVELOPMENT

Psychosexual Development: Sigmund Freud

- Freud, a physician from Vienna, Austria, who lived from 1856 to 1939, proposed a theory of **psychosexual** development.
- He also developed an approach called psychoanalysis to explore the unconscious mind.
- His psychosexual theory is based on the belief that experiences from our early childhood form the unconscious motivation for the things we do later in life as adults.
- The theory proposes that sexual energy is stronger in certain parts of the body at specific ages.
- Fixation of development can occur at a specific stage if needs are not met or conflicts are not resolved.
- This theory views the personality as consisting of three parts: the id, the ego, and the superego (**Table 6-4**).
  - ***Id****—the basic sexual energy that is present at birth and drives the seeking of pleasure.*
  - ***Ego****—the realistic part of a person, which develops during infancy and searches for acceptable methods to meet impulses.*
  - ***Superego****—the moral and ethical system that develops in childhood and contains values as well as conscious thoughts.*
- Sexual feelings are present in different forms depending on age.
- Human nature has two sides
  - *Rational intellect—being able to think about others, and do what is right. Example: delayed gratification.*
  - *Irrational desires—following the unconscious mind, which is driven by uncontrollable instincts that are irrational and pleasure seeking. Example: getting what you want when you want it even if the timing is not right or others are affected negatively.*

Key Stages of Theory

- Oral—birth to 1 year
  - *Preoccupied with activities associated with the mouth*
  - *Sexual urges gratified with oral behaviors: sucking, biting, chewing, and eating*
  - *Children that do not have their oral needs met may become thumb suckers or nail biters.*
  - *In adulthood they may become compulsive eaters or smokers.*
  - *Normal development requires no depriving of oral gratification.*
  - *Examples of deprivation:*
    - Weaning too soon
    - Rigid feeding schedule
- Anal—1 to 3 years of age
  - *Preoccupied with the ability to eliminate*
  - *Sexual urges gratified by learning to voluntarily defecate*
  - *Sphincter muscles maturing*

> **CLINICAL PEARL**
>
> **Toilet Training**
>
> Nurses should explain to caregivers the basic biological characteristics that allow a child to be toilet trained. Freud believed that how a child is toilet trained can have lasting effects on personality. If toilet training is too rigid or scheduled, the child can develop behaviors that are hypercritical or meticulous later in life (Potts & Mandleco, 2007).

- Phallic stage—3 to 6 years
  - *The child is preoccupied with the genitals.*
  - *Curious about childbirth, masturbation, and anatomic differences*
  - *The phallus/penis—girls experience penis envy and wish they had one; boys suffer from castration anxiety, the fear of losing the penis.*
  - *Children develop strong incestuous desire for caregiver of the opposite gender.*
  - *Oedipal complex—attachment of boy to his mother.*

TABLE 6-4 FREUD'S DEFINITION OF PERSONALITY

THREE COMPONENTS OF PERSONALITY		
Id	Ego	Superego
Primitive rational -Requires immediate gratification -Inward-seeking behavior	Conscious and ideas Acts as a censor to the id	The person's conscience instincts

- *Electra complex—attachment of girl to her father.*
- *Children need to identify with caregiver of same gender to form male or female identity.*
- Latency stage—6 to 11 years of age
  - *Sexual drives submerged*
  - *Energy focus on socialization and increasing problem-solving abilities*
  - *Appropriate gender roles adopted*
  - *Oedipal or Electra conflicts resolved*
  - *Identifies with same-gender peers and same-gender caregiver*
  - *Superego developed to a point where it keeps id under control*
- Genital stage—begins at around 12 years of age and lasts to adulthood
  - *Struggle with sexuality*
  - *Sexual desires return and are related to physiological changes and fluctuating hormones*
  - *Changing social relationships*
  - *Dealing with struggle of dependence and independence issues with parents*
  - *Learning to form loving, appropriate relationships*
  - *Must manage sexual urges in socially accepted ways*

See **Table 6-5** for Freud's stages of development.

CLINICAL PEARL

Recognition of Cognitive and Emotional Differences

Children are different than adults. They grow in particular patterns, and their behavior develops in particular stages. Nurses need to recognize the cognitive and emotional features of children of varying ages, based on developmental principles (Berk, 2007).

PSYCHOSOCIAL DEVELOPMENT

Psychosocial Development: Erik Erikson

- Lived from 1902 to 1994
- Studied under Freud's daughter, Anna
- Erikson established his theory in 1959, which emphasizes **psychosocial** rather than psychosexual development.

TABLE 6-5 FREUD'S FIVE STAGES OF PSYCHOSOCIAL DEVELOPMENT

Age	Stage
Infancy (birth–1 yr)	**Oral Stage** Comforted through the mouth
Toddler (1–3 yrs)	**Anal Stage** Derives gratification from control of bodily excretions
Preschool (3–6 yrs)	**Phallic Stage** Becomes aware of self as sexual being Identifies with the parent of the opposite sex, but by the end of stage will identify with same-sex parent Oedipal complex: attachment of a boy to his mother Electra complex: attachment of a girl to her father
School Age (6–12 yrs)	**Latency Stage** Focuses on peer relationships Emphasis on privacy and understanding the body
Adolescent (12–18 yrs)	**Genital Stage** Focus on genital function and relationships

Key Stages of Theory

- Addresses development over the life span
- Consists of eight different stages of development
- Each stage has a crisis that exists; healthy personality development occurs as each crisis is resolved (**Table 6-6**).
- A person must master psychosocial crises in order to grow and progress to the next stage of development.
- An individual either meets the healthy needs or does not, and this will influence future social relationships.
- Challenges between the ego and social and biological processes are described as crises.
- Ego—part of personality that controls thoughts and behaviors.
- **Trust vs. mistrust (birth to 1 year). See Figure 6-1.**
  - *An infant requires that basic needs are met—food, clothing, touch, and comfort.*
  - *If these needs are not met, the infant will develop a mistrust of others.*
  - *If a sense of trust is developed, the infant will see the world as a safe place.*
  - *Play during this stage is referred to as solitary (Ball & Bindler, 2008).*

TABLE 6–6 ERIKSON'S FIVE STAGES OF PSYCHOSOCIAL DEVELOPMENT

Age	Stage	Comments
Infancy: **Birth to age 1**	Trust versus mistrust	The child learns to trust as needs are met by the caregiver
Toddler: **Age 1 to 3 years**	Autonomy versus shame and doubt	The child becomes more independent Frame of mind: "I am a big kid now" The child starts to have some control over body functions
Preschool: **Age 3 to 6 years**	Initiative versus guilt	Development of a conscience Learning right from wrong
School Age: **Age 6 to 12 years**	Industry versus inferiority	Rule-following behavior Forming social relationships is seen as important
Adolescent: **Age 12 to 19**	Identity versus role confusion	Changes in the body are great Preoccupied with appearance and what others think of them Peers are very important Working on establishing own identity

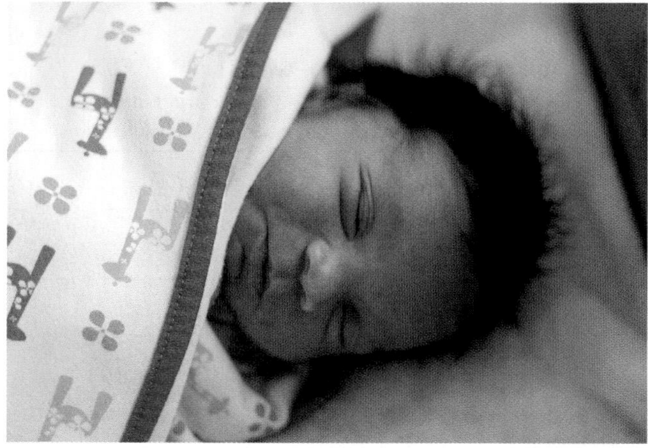

Figure 6–1 A newborn infant requires that basic needs are met—food, clothing, touch, and comfort.

- **Autonomy vs. shame and doubt (1–3 years). See Figure 6-2.**
  - *The child is learning to control bodily functions.*
  - *Independence starts to emerge.*
    Example: Toddlers control their world by deciding when and where elimination will occur.
  - *They vocalize by saying no to something, and direct their motor activity.*
  - *Children who are consistently criticized for showing independence and autonomy will develop shame and doubt in their abilities.*
  - *Toddlers also need to recognize the feelings and needs of others; excessive autonomy could lead to disregard for and an inability to play with others (Ball & Bindler, 2008).*
  - *Play during this stage is known as parallel (Ball & Bindler, 2008).*

CLINICAL PEARL

Age-Appropriate Toys

Toys that are age appropriate for toddlers and take into account their growth and development include: stuffed animals, building blocks, books, play dough, tricycles, small cars and trains, and pretend toys to play housekeeping, such as pots, pans, spoons, and cups.

- **Initiative vs. guilt (3–6 years). See Figure 6-3.**
  - *The preschool child is exposed to new people and new activities; the child becomes involved and very busy.*
  - *Learns about the environment through play*
  - *Learns new responsibilities and can act based on established principles*
  - *Develops a conscience*

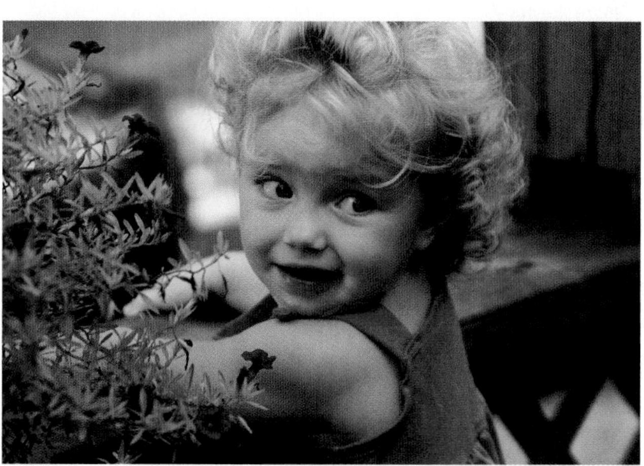

Figure 6–2 Toddlers experience the conflict of autonomy versus shame and doubt.

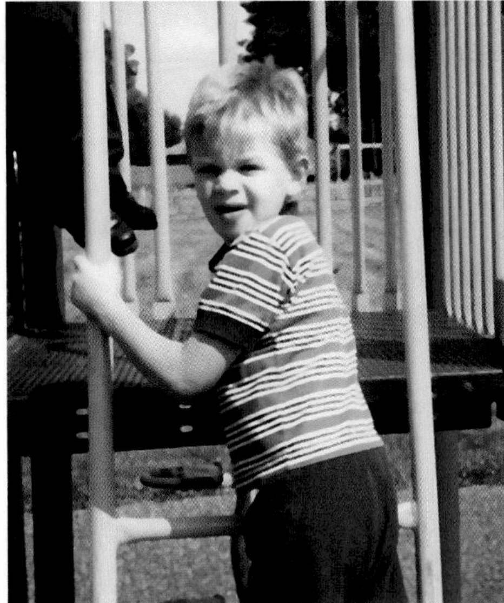

Figure 6–3 The preschool child learns about the environment through play.

- *If the child is constantly criticized for his or her actions, this can lead to guilt and a lack of purpose.*
- *Play at this stage is known as associative play (Ball & Bindler, 2008).*

- **Industry vs. inferiority (6–12 years). See Figure 6-4.**
  - *Developing interests and takes pride in accomplishments*
  - *Enjoys working in groups and forming social relationships*
  - *Enjoys projects*
  - *Follows rules and order*
  - *Developing a sense of industry provides the child with purpose and confidence in being successful.*
  - *If a child is unable to be successful, this can result in a sense of inferiority.*
  - *A child must learn balance, an understanding that he or she cannot succeed at everything, and that there is always more to learn.*
  - *Play during this stage is known as cooperative play (Ball & Bindler, 2008).*
- **Identity vs. role confusion (12–18 years). See Figure 6-5.**
  - *Preoccupied with how they are seen in the eyes of others*
  - *Working to establish their own identity*
  - *Trying out new roles to see what best fits for them*
  - *If they are unable to provide a meaningful definition of self, they are at risk for role confusion in one or more roles throughout life.*
  - *Some confusion is good and will result in self-reflection and self-examination.*

Promoting Safety

Adolescents feel that nothing bad will happen to them. Care should be given to educate this age group on safe practices, such as wearing a seat belt when driving.

SOCIAL-MORAL DEVELOPMENT

Social-Moral Development: Lawrence Kohlberg

- Children acquire moral reasoning in a developmental sequence.
- Kohlberg's theory was based on the cognitive-developmental theory of Piaget.
- The theory is based on the premise that at birth, we are void of morals or ethics.
- Moral development occurs through social interaction with the environment around us.

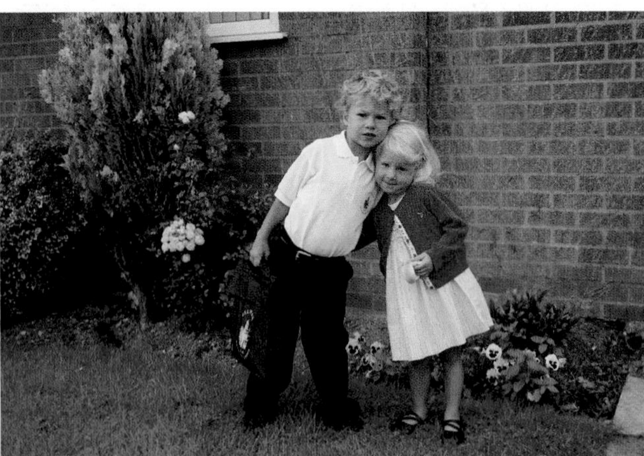

Figure 6–4 The school-age child develops a sense of industry that provides the child with purpose and confidence in being successful.

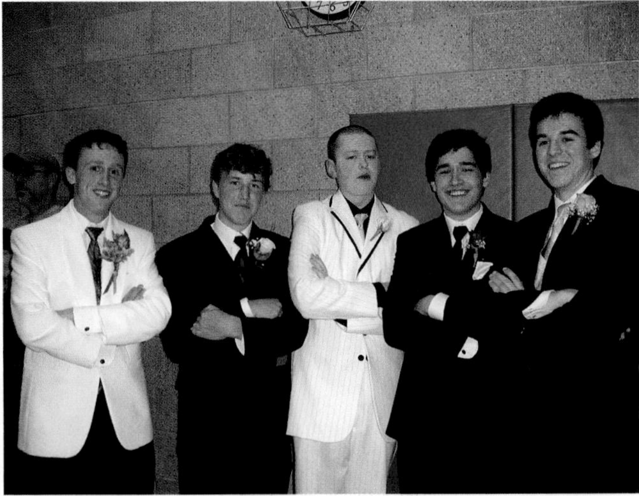

Figure 6–5 Teenagers are preoccupied with how they are seen in the eyes of others.

- Moral development can be advanced and promoted through formal education.
- Moral development includes three major levels. See **Table 6-7** for Kohlberg's theory of moral development.

NATURE VS. NURTURE

- To what extent do hereditary factors and environmental influence shape the various personal traits and characteristics of a child?
- This has been a debated topic in growth and development. The debate has also been called *heredity versus environment* or *maturation versus learning.*

Nature

- Traits, capacities, and limitations that a person inherits from parents at the moment of conception
  - *Examples: hair and eye color, body type, and inherited diseases*
  - *Possible examples: athletic or musical ability*

Nurture

- Environmental influences that occur after conception
- Influences begin with the mother's health before birth and the child's environment thereafter.

General Notes on Nature vs. Nurture

- Both play a part in shaping us to be who we are, though the extent of influence of each is debated.
- The interaction between the two is a critical influence in our development.
- Nurture takes what nature gives us and molds us as we grow and mature.

FAMILY

- **Traditional family** (or nuclear family)—comprised of a mother, a father, and a biological or adopted child or children.
- **Nontraditional families**—describes family forms other than traditional, such as single-parent homes, grandparents functioning in the role of parents, same-sex parents with a child or children, and blended families, in which families from divorce are joined together by remarriage. (See Chapter 3 for further details on the family.)

CLINICAL PEARL

Definition of "Family"

Family is defined as the structure or the relationship between individuals that provides the financial and emotional support needed for social functioning (Friedemann, 1995). Nurses should not be judgmental when caring for patients and their families. We must remember that every family acts as a unique unit.

BEHAVIORIST AND SOCIAL LEARNING THEORY

- Describe the importance of the environment and nurturing of a child
- Developed as a response to psychoanalytical theories
- Behaviorist theory was the dominant view from the 1920s through 1960s.
- John B. Watson, Ivan Pavlov, and B. F. Skinner are some of the most noted theorists.
- Behaviorist theories are based on observable behaviors.
- These behaviors arise from conditioning, either classical or operant conditioning.
  - *Classical conditioning—"a learning process that occurs through associations between an environmental stimulus and a naturally occurring stimulus" (Cherry, 2011).*
  - *Operant conditioning—a change in behavior based on rewards, reinforcement, and punishment (Cherry, 2011).*

CLINICAL PEARL

Growth Based on Experiences

Behaviorists believe that children are born with a "blank slate," and as they grow and develop they are changed based on their experiences. Nursing and child life specialists can use stickers, rewards, and praise to let children know they did a great job after a procedure such as an IV insertion or a blood pressure reading.

TABLE 6–7 KOHLBERG'S THREE STAGES OF MORAL DEVELOPMENT

Level	Preconventional Level	Conventional Level	Postconventional Autonomous Level
Stages	1: Obedience and Punishment Orientation 2: Individualism and Exchange	3: Good Interpersonal Relationships 4: Maintaining the Social Order	5: Social Contract and Individual Rights 6: Universal Principles
Age	2 to 7 years	7 to 12 years	Age 12 years and older
Characteristics	-Follows rules that are set by those in authority -Adjusts behavior according to good/bad and right/wrong thinking	-Seeks conformity and loyalty -Follows rules -Maintains social order	-Constructs a personal and functional value system independent of authority figures and peers

Social Learning Theory: Albert Bandura

- Children learn through observing others in their environment, as well as from rewards and punishments.
- Intrinsic reinforcements such as satisfaction and accomplishment leads to learning.
- Observing the actions of other people, children develop new skills and acquire new information.

FACTORS THAT AFFECT GROWTH AND DEVELOPMENT

> CLINICAL PEARL
>
> **Environment and Culture**
>
> A child's ability to master tasks and grow and develop in the proper way is affected by numerous factors. The environment and culture are two areas that should always be assessed. A child needs an appropriate environment and proper stimuli, or development may be delayed.

Intrauterine Factors

- The mother's health and nutritional status while pregnant affect the fetus.
- Poor nutrition in the mother can lead to low-birth-weight babies and babies with slow development, compromised neurological performance, and impaired immune status (Ball & Bindler, 2008).
- Low iron levels in the mother can result in anemia in the infant (Institute for Patient- and Family-Centered Care, 2010).
- Low-birth-weight infants are associated with maternal smoking.
- Ingestion of alcoholic during pregnancy may lead to delays and fetal alcohol syndrome.
- Substance and drug abuse prenatally may result in neonatal addiction, convulsions, hyperirritability, poor social responsiveness, neurological disturbances, and changes in the cognitive functioning of the child (Ball & Bindler, 2008).
- Prescription and nonprescription drugs may affect the unborn child.
- Certain maternal illnesses can harm the fetus, such as rubella.
- Exposure of the mother to environmental factors, such as chemicals or radiation, can harm the fetus.

Birth Events (Prematurity, Birth Trauma)

- Premature infants can experience delayed growth and development.
- Premature infants are expected to reach developmental milestones at the same age they would have reached them if they were born at normal gestational age.
- Age is adjusted for assessments: subtract the weeks/months that the infant was born prematurely from the current chronological age. The child should be reaching the adjusted age milestones.
- Most premature children have caught up with all the milestones/developmental tasks by the age of 2.

Illness and Hospitalization

- Illness and hospitalization are stressful events for a child and family.
- The family routine is disrupted, and the child and family are not able to do what they normally do.
- The possible separation of family members due to the child's illness adds to stress.

> CLINICAL PEARL
>
> **Play as a Stress Reducer**
>
> Play is what children do and should not be overlooked when a child is in the hospital. Play can be a diversional activity and a stress reducer. Play provides the hospitalized child with an opportunity to act out fears and anxieties. Many children's hospitals provide the ill child with a playroom and the services of a child life specialist who can assist the child in fostering growth and developmental needs through play. The child life specialist has a strong background in growth and development and can use this training to assist the medical team in preparing a child for hospitalization and procedures.

Chronic Illness

- A child's physical state of well-being can affect developmental levels.
- Illness may interfere with normal progression through developmental levels.
- Illness may cause the child to experience delays in acquiring the skills/competencies needed to progress to the next level.

> CLINICAL PEARL
>
> **Separation Anxiety**
>
> Nurses need to take in account growth and developmental stages when a child is hospitalized or ill. Toddlers fear separation from caregivers (separation anxiety), and preschoolers fear body mutilations, the dark, being left alone, and ghosts.

Environmental Factors

- Child may experience abuse or neglect
- Child may experience delays in learning to trust others.
- Child may experience disorders of attachment.
- Problems may occur in numerous areas of growth and development; examples of problem areas are sleeping and feeding disorders.

Abuse

- Can be physical, emotional, or sexual
- Physical
  - *Beatings, burns or, other physical injuries*

- Emotional
  - *Yelling at, ridiculing, or consistently putting a child down*
- *Sexual*
  - *Any sexual activity with a child under the age of 18*
  - *Commanding a child to perform sexual acts upon an adult or other child*

Neglect

- Can be medical, emotional, educational, or abandonment
- Medical
  - *Not providing common medical care*
  - *Not allowing a child who is ill to consult a health-care provider*
  - *Death of a child from an illness that is considered treatable by Western health care*
- Emotional
  - *Not attending to the child's emotional needs*
  - *Ignoring the child*
  - *Leaving the child alone for significant amounts of time*
- Educational
  - *not providing education for the child in any manner*
  - *not providing the child needed aids to encourage education (hearing aids, speech therapy, etc.)*
- Abandonment
  - *leaving a child to care for him- or herself*
  - *not providing adequate adult supervision for a child*

Promoting Safety

Nursing is one of the professions required by law to report any suspected child abuse or neglect. Circumstances, protocols, and paperwork may vary from state to state, but reporting to the authorities when you suspect or have reason to believe a child is in harm is necessary and mandated for the health-care professional. More information about mandatory reporting for the health-care professional can be found at the Child Welfare Information Gateway Web site, www.childwelfare.gov/systemwide/laws_policies/statutes/manda.cfm.

Home

CRITICAL COMPONENT

Physical Home Environment

A safe and healthy home environment is needed for normal growth and development to occur. The quality of housing and access to basic services—such as clean water, sanitation and waste disposal, fuel for cooking and heating, and ventilation—need to be addressed with the family. Exposure to lead paint, radon, and electromagnetic sources should also be assessed, as these can affect normal growth and development (Sly et al., 2009)

Genetics

- Inherited traits that are genetically passed on to each generation by the DNA found in our genes
- Examples of inherited traits: eye color, hair color, physical resemblances such as height or body size

BASIC NEEDS

Maslow's Hierarchy of Needs

- Basic needs at each level need to be met before a child can progress to the next highest level of growth and development.
- Number One: Physiological needs must be met first: food, rest, air, water.
- Number Two: Activity is needed for stimulation, novelty, and change.
- Number Three: The child has the need to be protected from harm and feel safe.
- Number Four: Feeling loved and part of a group.
- Number Five: Esteem needs to develop—the need to respect yourself and be respected by others.
- Number Six: Self-actualization, or becoming a complete person and reaching your greatest potential. (Price & Gwin, 2005)

CLINICAL PEARL

Sleep Deprivation

Children need more sleep than adults. Sleep deprivation can impact the growth and development of a child and cause delays. Preschoolers, for example, need 12 hours of sleep a day (Oskar & O'Connor, 2005)!

Family

Early Parent–Child Relationships

Pinto-Martin, J., Dunkle, M., Earls, M., Fliedner, D., & Landes, C. (2005). Developmental stages of developmental screening: Steps to implementation of a successful program. *American Journal of Public Health, 11,* 1928–1932. doi: 10.2105/AJPH.2004.052167

Early parent-child relationships have been shown to play a major role in a child's social-emotional development. This relationship also influences and is linked to cognitive development and learning patterns. Feeling loved and cared for can enhance development in these areas (Pinto-Martin, Dunkle, Earls, Fliedner, & Landes, 2005).

Socioeconomic Factors

- Lack of income can affect a child's health and development.
- Lack of income may result in less healthy food choices.
- Families may lack transportation to health facilities.
- Both parents may need to work and thus have little time to devote to children.

Cultural Background

> **CLINICAL PEARL**
>
> **Cultural Factors**
>
> Nurses need to take a child's cultural background into account when doing developmental testing. Children may not be familiar with particular games or activities used in the test if they were not exposed to them. There could also be possible language barriers that interfere with reliable testing.

- Cultural background influences how children are socialized and experience the world around them.
- Beliefs, customs, and values are learned from cultural surroundings. (See Chapter 4 for further discussion of cultural factors.)

> **CLINICAL PEARL**
>
> **Influence of Cultural Identity**
>
> Everyone is a product of their cultural background. Culture does more than shape our preferences; it is the foundation of our worldviews. The cultural identity of a child and the family is always relevant and must be considered in the care that we give (Oskar & O'Connor, 2005).

Review Questions

1. J. H., 20 months old, has to be sure that all of his toys are put in the right places before bedtime. This is an example of
A. dawdling.
B. negativism.
C. perfectionism.
D. ritualism.

2. The type of play that toddlers frequently engage in is
A. parallel.
B. solitary.
C. associative.
D. cooperative.

3. The oral stage of personality development described by Freud is
A. not important for the infant's physical and psychological development.
B. evidenced by the Moro reflex.
C. evidenced by the infant's desire to obtain pleasure through sucking.
D. of little significance to the pediatric nurse.

4. Piaget's theory of development
A. describes intellectual development.
B. describes psychosocial development.
C. describes sexual development.
D. is similar to Freud's theory and Erikson's theory.

5. A child is admitted for surgery. On your admission assessment, the mother tells you that her family is composed of herself, the patient (her son), her new husband, and her stepdaughter. What type of family is this?
A. Cohabitation family
B. Nuclear family
C. Foster family
D. Blended family

6. This theorist postulated that the personality is a structure with three parts called the id, the ego, and the superego.
A. Jean Piaget
B. Erik Erikson
C. Sigmund Freud
D. All of the above

7. Your neighbor Patty is concerned because her 7-month-old does not have any teeth yet, whereas her friend's 7-month-old does. What is the best advice you can offer her in regard to her child's growth and development?
A. Tell her that her child is falling behind on growth and development.
B. Tell her that her baby is normal and her friend's child has issues.
C. Tell her to take the child to the doctor as soon as possible.
D. Tell her that growth and development are unique and highly individualized processes.

8. You are caring for a 2-year-old child on the evening shift at the hospital where you work. Visiting hours are now over, but parents have arrived to visit their child. Which statement shows that you and your nursing peers understand the concept of family-centered care?
A. Tell the parents to go home and get some rest so that they can come back and visit tomorrow.
B. Encourage the parents to room in/stay with the child overnight at the hospital. Assure them that you will wake them up and include them in any care that needs to be provided to their child during the night.
C. Tell the parents that they can stay overnight with the patient if they stay out of the way of the nursing staff during the procedures that they need to perform on the child.
D. Tell the parents to go home and get some rest so that they will be of use to the child the next day. Let them know that they are welcome to call at any time during the night for information.

9. School-age children like to be involved in team sports. This is an example of what type of play?
A. Onlooker play
B. Associative play
C. Parallel play
D. Cooperative play

10. Which of the following factors can have an impact on a child's growth and development?
   A. Being born a month premature or having a low birth weight of 4 pounds, 4 ounces
   B. Mother's infection with rubella while carrying the child
   C. Mother's use of numerous nonprescription drugs while pregnant for her allergies
   D. All of the above

References

Ball, J. W. & Bindler, R. C. (2008). *Pediatric nursing: Caring for children.* Upper Saddle River, NJ: Pearson Prentice Hall.

Berk, L. E. (2007). *Development through the lifespan* (4th ed.). Boston, MA: Allyn and Bacon.

Block, R. & Krebs, N. (2005). Failure to thrive as a manifestation of child neglect. *Pediatrics, 116*, 1234–1237. doi: 10.1542/peds.2005-2032

Centers for Disease Control and Prevention. (2010). Learn the signs. Act early. Retrieved from http://www.cdc.gov/ncbddd/actearly/milestones/index.html

Cherry, K. (2011). Psychology theories. Retrieved from http://psychology.about.com/od/psychology101/u/psychology-theories.htm

Friedemann, M. L. (1995). *The framework of systemic organization: A conceptual approach to families* and *nursing.* Thousand Oakes, CA: Sage.

Hockenberry, M. J., & Wilson, D. (2009). *Wong's essentials of pediatric nursing.* St. Louis, MO: Mosby Elsevier.

Institute for Patient- and Family-Centered Care. (2010). Profiles for change. Retrieved from http://www.ipfcc.org

Oskar, G. J., & O'Connor, B. B. (2005). Children's sleep: An interplay between culture and biology. *Pediatrics, 115*, 204–216. doi: 10.1542/peds.2004-0815B

Pinto-Martin, J., Dunkle, M., Earls, M., Fliedner, D., & Landes, C. (2005). Developmental stages of developmental screening: Steps to implementation of a successful program. *American Journal of Public Health, 11*, 1928–1932. doi: 10.2105/AJPH.2004.052167

Potts, N. L., & Mandleco, B. L. (2007). *Pediatric nursing: Caring for children and their families.* Clifton Park, NY: Thomson and Delmar Learning.

Price, D. L., & Gwin, J. F. (2005). *Thompson's pediatric nursing.* St. Louis, MO: Elsevier Saunders.

Sly, P. D., Eskenazi, B., Pronczuk, J., Sram, R., Diaz-Barriga, F., Machin, D. G., . . . Meslin, E. M. (2009). Ethical issues in measuring biomarkers in children's environmental health. *Environmental Health Perspectives, 111,* 1185–1190. doi: 10.1289/ehp.0800480

7 Newborns and Infants

OBJECTIVES

- ☐ Define key terms.
- ☐ Describe the growth and development that occur during the newborn and infancy period.
- ☐ Describe the physical assessment approaches for the newborn and infant.
- ☐ Discuss the variations in nursing procedures related to the care of the newborn/infant.
- ☐ Describe the approaches to medication administration in the newborn and infant.
- ☐ Describe the health promotion functions necessary in an infant/newborn's family structure.
- ☐ Discuss the emergency care of the newborn/infant.
- ☐ Describe the specific characteristics of the care of the hospitalized newborn/infant.
- ☐ Discuss the chronic care of the newborn/infant.
- ☐ Describe the importance and function of play in the newborn/infant's life.
- ☐ Describe the safety measures needed to care for a newborn/infant in the home.
- ☐ Discuss alternative/complementary therapies for the family of the newborn/infant.
- ☐ Describe child abuse considerations in the newborn/infant population.

KEY TERMS

- Newborn
- Infancy
- Gestation
- Apgar
- Surfactant
- Brown fat
- Respiratory distress syndrome (RDS)
- Acrocyanosis
- Apnea
- Gasping
- Tachypnea
- Tachycardia
- Grunting
- Retractions
- Murmur
- Neutral thermal environment (NTE)
- Cold stress
- Kangaroo care (or skin-to-skin contact)
- Gluconeogenesis
- Conjugation
- Jaundice
- Kernicterus
- Coombs' test
- Meconium
- Hypospadias
- Epispadias
- Circumcision
- Pseudomenstruation
- Lanugo
- Milia
- Vernix caseosa
- Erythema toxicum
- Mongolian spots
- Molding
- Caput succedeneum
- Cephalhematoma
- Craniosynostosis
- Epstein pearls
- Cephalocaudal
- Proximodistal
- Microcephaly
- Colostrum
- Let-down reflex
- Respiratory syncytial virus (RSV)

INFANT/NEWBORN

The human infant less than 28 days old is a **newborn** or neonate. The term *newborn* refers to any preterm, term, or postmature child. The **infancy** period is that period from 1 month of age to 1 year of age.

- **Gestation** is the duration, in weeks, of pregnancy.
  - *Average full-term baby: born after 38 to 42 weeks of pregnancy*
  - *Preterm infant: born before 37 weeks of pregnancy*
  - *Postmature infant: born after 42 weeks of pregnancy*
- Care associated with the majority of full-term infants ≥38 weeks' gestation is primarily to protect and support the neonate during its physiological transition to extrauterine life.
  - *Delivery room and transitional care*
  - *Maintenance of thermoregulation*
  - *Newborn assessment with a review of the maternal history and a complete physical examination*
  - *Prophylaxis care to prevent disorders specifically related to respiratory function and decreasing risk for infections*
  - *Family education and discharge preparation related to caring for and feeding the newborn*

Don't have time to read this chapter? Want to reinforce your reading? Need to review for a test? Listen to this chapter on DavisPlus at davispl.us/rudd1.

- Immediate needs of the newborn: Nurses' predominant role is to assess the newborn in the transition period, protect the physical well-being of the infant, and promote a family-centered environment.
  - *Clearing of the airway: Wipe mouth and nose with the delivery of the head. If suctioning, suction mouth first, then nose to remove mucus and blood with bulb syringe. Depress bulb first and then insert into the orifice to remove secretions.*

CLINICAL PEARL

Inserting the Syringe for Suctioning

When inserting the bulb syringe, insert it in the corner of the mouth, not the center. Always suction the mouth first and then the nose. Suctioning the nose first may cause the infant to gasp and thereby force mucus deeper into the respiratory tract.

- Assign the Apgar score, based on the system developed in 1952 by Dr. Virginia Apgar (**Table 7-1**).
- **Apgar** scoring system
  - *Evaluates a neonate's ability to adapt during the birthing process*
  - *Determines the need for resuscitation, the effectiveness of the resuscitation, and the neonate's morbidity and mortality risks*
  - *Measures five areas: respiratory rate, heart rate, muscle tone, color, and reflex irritability*
  - *A higher score (rated from 0 to 10) indicates adequate adaptation.*
  - *The Apgar score at 1 minute indicates the neonate's ability to transition to extrauterine life, factors occurring during the birthing process, and whether resuscitation is needed.*
  - *The Apgar score at 5 minutes indicates the neonate's status and the effectiveness of resuscitative efforts, as well as neurological deficits and long-term morbidity and mortality.*
  - *In depressed infants, the scoring is repeated every 5 minutes.*
    - Numbers are assigned at 1 and 5 minutes.
    - Neonate is rated with a zero, one number, or two numbers for each category.
    - Total score of 0 to 2 = severely depressed
    - Total score of 3 to 6 = moderately depressed
    - Total score of 7 to 10 = good condition
- Maintain thermoregulation with immediate drying and removal of wet linens.
- Chilling increases oxygen consumption and metabolism by evaporation.
- Band infant with on-demand or barcode on arm and leg, with corresponding bands applied to the mother and significant other if present in the delivery room.

Promoting Safety

Alert staff to similar or identical last names on labor, delivery, and postpartum units. Alert staff to check the bands against the correct information, such as infant's name, mother's name, sex, medical record number, and date of birth. Many institutions utilize umbilical cord clamp bands and electronic tags that if removed from the infant's body will lock and shut down elevators and all doors. All infants should also have their own baby bands with their own unique identifiers of name, sex, date of birth, and medical record number. Limited human-readable data are present with on-demand and barcode information. Careful attention should be paid to the identification of multiples. Some institutions utilize footprints or photos of infants for additional identification.

- Baby prophylactic medications (**Table 7-2**)
  - *Vitamin K_1—newborns are born with a sterile intestinal tract and do not have the bacteria that is necessary for the production of vitamin K.*
  - *Therefore, newborns have decreased levels of vitamin K, the nutrient responsible for clotting and preventing hemorrhages.*
  - *Erythromycin eye ointment—prevents serious eye infections and should not be washed away.*
  - *Hepatitis B immunization to prevent hepatitis B*
- Protect the physical well-being of the newborn.
  - *Prevent the spread of infection through strict hand hygiene, limited traffic in the labor and delivery room suite, the use of scrub clothing by personnel to minimize infection exposure, and no artificial nails or nail polish.*

TABLE 7–1 NEONATAL APGAR SCORING

	SCORE		
Sign	0	1	2
Respiratory effort	Absent	Slow, irregular	Good cry
Heart rate	Absent	Slow, below 100 bpm	Above 100 bpm
Muscle tone	Flaccid	Some flexion of extremities	Active motion
Reflex activity	None	Grimace	Vigorous cry
Color	Pale, blue	Body pink, blue extremities	Completely pink

From Chapman, L., & Durham, R. (2010). *Maternal-newborn nursing: Critical components of nursing care.* Philadelphia: F.A. Davis.

TABLE 7–2 PROPHYLACTIC MEDICATIONS FOR NEWBORNS AND INFANTS

Baby Medication	Aquamephyton, Phytonadione, Vitamin K	Erythromycin, Tetracycline, Eye Ointment, Silver Nitrate	Hepatitis B, Enerix-B, Recombivax HB
Uses	Prevent hemorrhagic disease of the newborn by enhancing the liver's synthesis of clotting factors II, VII, IX, and X	Prevent transmission of infections of gonorrhea and chlamydial ophthalmia during passage through the birth canal	Prevent hepatitis B, a liver disease caused by the HBV virus that can cause serious chronic liver disease and cancer of the liver
Side effects	Pain at the injection site	Silver nitrate can cause eye irritation, goopy discharge of the eyes, or slight redness of the eyes	Pain at the injection site
Administration	Single dose of 0.5 (for preterm) to 1.0 mg (for full term) IM within 1 hour of birth Injection site is vastus lateralis muscle—lies lateral to the midline of the thigh	1-cm thin ribbon administered from inner canthus to outer canthus on lower eyelid	Vaccinate all newborns with monovalent vaccine before discharge—0.5 mL IM for first dose Given within 12 hours with hepatitis B immune globulin (HBIG) if mother is hepatitis-B positive or status is unknown; given at discharge if mother's status is known to be negative Massage area for dispersion of the drug Injection site is vastus lateralis muscle
Special considerations	Protect from light Mandated by state laws	Do not delay administration beyond 1 hour following delivery Mandated by state laws	Follow immunization schedule for administration; some parents defer to first pediatrician appointment Series of three doses, given in vastus lateralis

From Deglan, J. H., Vallerand, A. H., & Sanoski, C. A. (2011). *Davis's drug guide for nurses* (12th ed.). Philadelphia: F.A. Davis.

- *Provide baby prophylactic medications, cord care, circumcision care, strict hand hygiene, and infant bathing.*
- Foster parent–infant bonding; promote family-centered care.

MATERNAL HISTORY

- Review of prenatal history, including past pregnancies, complications, and genetic factors in both mother, father, and previous pregnancies
- Infections—prenatal as well as past exposures
- Screening tests and risk factors
- Labor and delivery problems or risk factors

TRANSITION TO EXTRAUTERINE LIFE

- Begins in utero as the fetus prepares to transition to extrauterine life

Intrauterine Changes

- Changes are dependent upon gestational age, maternal health factors, condition of the placenta, and/or defects and congenital abnormalities.

Evidence-Based Practice: Family-Centered Care

American Hospital Association. (2005). Resource guide: More information about the concepts of patient- and family-centered care. Retrieved from www.aha.org/aha/content/2005/pdf/resourceguide.pdf

- Dignity and Respect
  Health-care practitioners listen to and honor patient and family perspectives and choices. Patient and family knowledge, values, beliefs, and cultural backgrounds are incorporated into the planning and delivery of care.
- Information-sharing
  Health-care practitioners communicate and share complete and unbiased information with patients and families in ways that are affirming and useful. Patients and families receive timely, complete, and accurate information in order to effectively participate in care and decision making.
- Participation
  Patients and families are encouraged to participate in care and decision making at the level they choose.
- Collaboration
  Patients, families, health-care practitioners, and hospital leaders collaborate in policy and program development, implementation, and evaluation; in health-care facility design; and in professional education, as well as in the delivery of care (American Hospital Association, 2005).

- In utero, the lungs are filled with amniotic fluid and the placenta is the organ of respiration and waste removal.
- Fetus produces **surfactant** (at 34 weeks of gestation).
  - *Surfactant, a phospholipid, is produced in the alveoli of the lungs.*
  - *This phospholipid decreases surface tension and allows the alveoli sacs to remain partially open upon expiration.*
  - *This partial opening of the alveoli sacs permits a decreased amount of pressure and energy needed to take the next breath.*
    - Fetus practices breathing in utero.
    - Fetus has depositions of **brown fat** (vascular adipose tissue).
    - Fetus stores and converts glycogen to glucose in the liver to meet metabolic needs.

Respiratory System Transition

- Transition occurs when the umbilical cord is clamped and the infant takes the first breath. All body systems of the neonate transition to extrauterine life, but most significant are the respiratory and circulatory system transitions.
  - *Cord is cut and placenta is no longer the organ of respiration.*
  - *Several factors influence the first breath.*
    - Internal stimuli such as chemical changes due to hypoxia and increasing carbon dioxide levels
    - External stimuli such as thermal changes, sensory changes, or mechanical changes due to the delivery process (**Figure 7-1**; Ward & Hisley, 2009)
  - *The first breath begins to clear amniotic fluid and fill the lungs with oxygen, which does the following:*
    - Increases alveoli oxygen tension (Pa_{O_2}), which dilates the pulmonary artery, decreases pulmonary vascular resistance, increases pulmonary blood flow, and increases O_2 and CO_2 exchange (see Chapter 12).
  - *Alterations in this system's transition result from insufficient production of surfactant owing to prematurity, hypoxia, and acidosis, all of which increase pulmonary vascular resistance.*
    - Retained alveolar fluid can result in transient tachypnea of the newborn (TTN).
    - Insufficient surfactant production can result in collapsed alveoli and the development of **respiratory distress syndrome (RDS)**. RDS is a disease that results in poor lung compliance, loss of residual capacity, and chronic lung changes and is prominent in premature infants.
    - Failure of the normal drop in pulmonary vascular pressure can result in persistent pulmonary hypertension of the newborn (PPHN).
  - *These alterations require specialized medical care in neonatal intensive care units that support the neonate's respiratory system.*

Newborn Respiratory Assessment and Development

- Assess the nose for patency.
- Chest wall symmetry/asymmetry can be a result of pneumothorax.
- Respiratory pattern is normally very irregular, sporadic, shallow, and diaphragmatic.
- Respiratory rate decreases with age.
- Average rate at birth is 40 to 60 breaths/minute; count for a full minute (Acute Care of at-Risk Newborns Neonatal Society (ACoRN), 2009).
- Newborns are obligate nose breathers, but after several months they become nose-and-mouth breathers.
- **Acrocyanosis** (bluish color of hands and feet) is normal in the term infant in the first 24 hours. After 24 hours, this may be an indication of cardiac disease (see Chapter 12).
- In dark-skinned infants, cyanosis is better assessed through the mucus membranes.
- Older infants become diaphragmatic breathers.

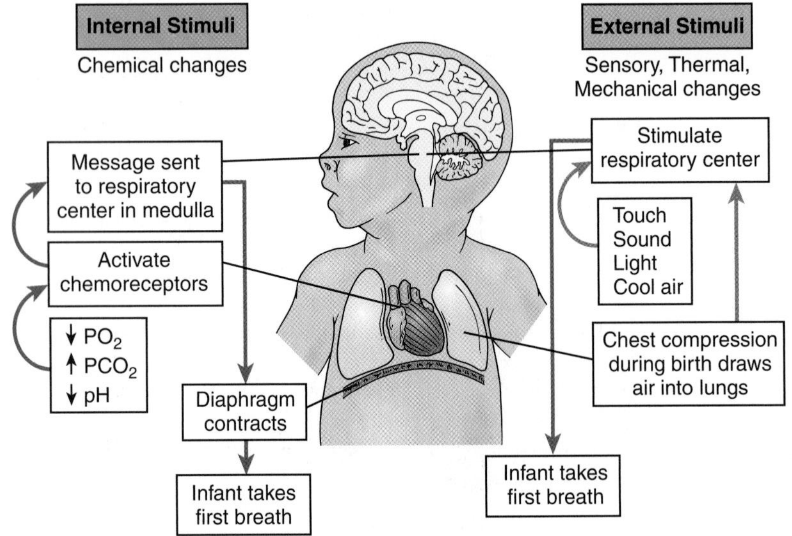

Figure 7–1 Stimuli that influence respirations.

CRITICAL COMPONENT

Signs and Symptoms of Alterations in Respiratory Transitioning

- Cyanosis
- **Apnea**—a cessation of breathing >20 seconds; may or may not be associated with change in color or heart rate
- **Gasping**—deep, slow, irregular terminal breaths (Acute Care of at-Risk Newborns Neonatal Society, 2009)
- Flaring—outward flaring movements of the nostrils on inspiration due to forced airflow
- Excessive mucus or drooling
- **Tachypnea**—respiratory rate >60 breaths/minute
- **Tachycardia**—heart rate >170 beats/minute
- Chest wall asymmetry
- **Grunting**—audible expiratory groaning heard on expiration due to a partial closing of the glottis (Acute Care of at-Risk Newborns Neonatal Society, 2009)
- **Retractions** of the ribs or substernal area—backward movements of the sternum or intercostals spaces of the ribs due to increased negative pressure
- Congenital abnormalities (see Chapter 11)

Circulatory System Transition and Assessment

- Transition occurs with the clamping of the cord and the first breath (**Figure 7-2**).
- The successful transition is directly influenced by the changes that occur in the respiratory and thermoregulation systems.
- Three fetal structures maintain fetal circulation: (1) the ductus arteriosus (PDA), between the pulmonary artery and the aorta; (2) the foramen ovale (or PFO, patent foramen ovale), the connection between the right and left atrium; and (3) the ductus venosus in the hepatic system (**Figure 7-3**).
- As pulmonary vascular resistance decreases, there is a decrease in placental secretion of prostaglandins (PGE_1), the fetal ducts close, and the transition occurs (see Chapter 12).
- Three vessels should be present in the umbilical cord: two arteries and one vein.
  - *The presence of only two vessel cords may indicate renal agenesis or lack of development.*
  - *Cord blood may be obtained from an Rh-negative mom or O blood group.*
  - *Blood gases may be obtained if O_2 levels are decreased or Apgar scores are depressed at 5 minutes of age.*
    - Heart rate decreases as infant ages.
    - Newborn heart rate averages 100 to 160 beats/minute at rest but can increase with crying. Count for a full minute.
    - Blood pressure increases with age (see Chapter 12).
    - Four extremity blood pressures are indicated with heart murmur (see Chapter 12).
    - **Murmur**—turbulent blood flow heard by a stethoscope as swooshing or whooshing.

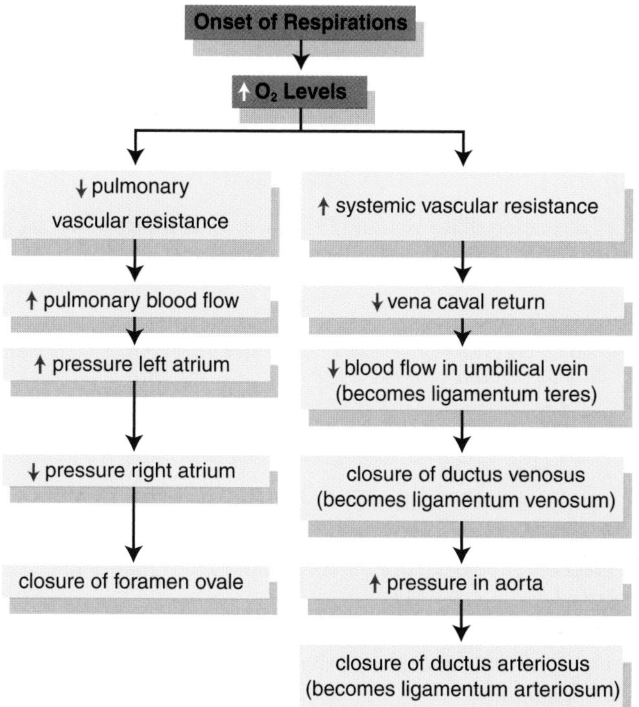

Figure 7-2 Transition from fetal to neonatal circulation.

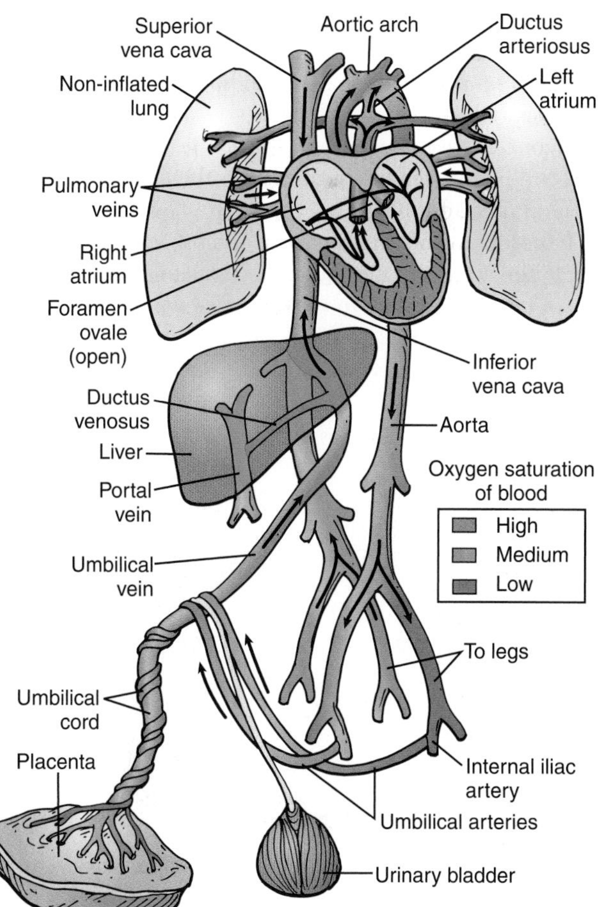

Figure 7-3 Fetal circulation.

- Murmurs may be present at birth and can be completely normal (see Chapter 12).
- Brisk capillary refill should be <3 seconds; abnormal is >4 seconds.
- Congenital abnormalities are related to failure of the fetal structures to close, structural abnormalities, or blood outflow problems (see Chapter 12).

Thermoregulatory System Transition and Assessment

- The thermoregulatory system is necessary for sustaining homeostasis.
- It is dependent on external and internal factors.
- **Neutral thermal environment (NTE)**—the temperature that the infant requires to minimize metabolic and oxygen needs, prevent metabolic acidosis, and arrest brown fat depletion.
- Normal neonatal temperature is 36.5°C to 37.0°C through axillary method (under the armpit).
- Normal rectal temperatures range from 36.5°C to 37.5°C; in many institutions these must be ordered and are performed with great care to avoid rectal injury.
- Gestational-age term infants have stores of brown fat located in the neck, intrascapular region, axillae, groin, and around the kidney area (**Figure 7-4**). Brown fat is utilized and burned for heat metabolism.
- Weight and prematurity affect the infant's ability to regulate body temperature owing to a decrease in brown and subcutaneous fat stores.
- Full-term infants have increased body surface area as compared with total body mass.
- Neonates have a higher metabolic rate.
- Term infants can lose heat even in the first few minutes and hours after birth.
- Exposure to cold in a newborn sets off alterations in physiological and metabolic processes to generate heat. An infant's response to cold includes the following:
  - *Peripheral vasoconstriction and chemical thermogenesis take place.*
  - *Newborns do not shiver.*
  - *The sympathetic nervous system responds by decreasing the temperature and stimulation of skin receptors, many in the face, to increase peripheral vasoconstriction.*
  - *Brown fat utilization breaks down fat into glycerol and fatty acids to produce heat.*
  - ***Cold stress**—excessive heat loss resulting in an increase in heart rate, respiratory rate, and oxygen consumption; metabolic acidosis; and depletion of glucose and surfactant levels, leading to respiratory distress; or*
  - *Rapid utilization of brown fat can result in metabolic acidosis, jaundice, infection, and poor weight gain due to thermogenesis, which increases oxygen demands and caloric consumption (**Figure 7-5**).*
    - Risk factors for development of cold stress include sepsis, prematurity, being small for gestational age, and hypoglycemia.

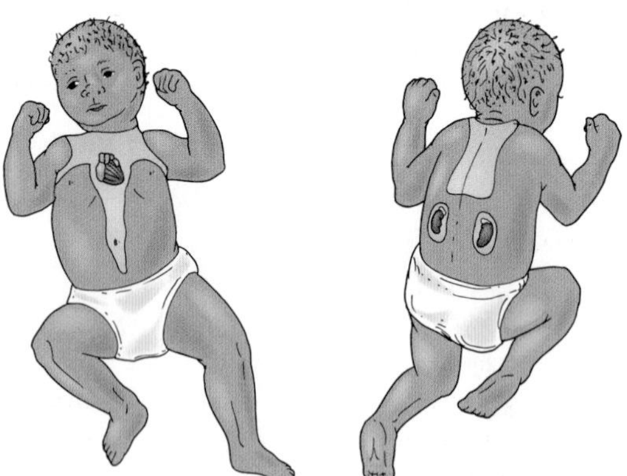

Figure 7-4 Sites of "brown fat" (brown adipose tissue stores) in the newborn.

CLINICAL PEARL

Signs and Symptoms of Cold Stress

- Jitteriness
- Tachypnea
- Grunting
- Hypoglycemia
- Hypotonia
- Pallor
- Lethargy
- Poor sucking reflex

CLINICAL PEARL

Heat Loss in the Newborn

- Radiation heat loss occurs when an infant is placed near a window or the cold walls of a single-walled isolette.
- Conduction–transfer of heat directly from the infant to a cooler surface or equipment. Place the infant on a warm surface, remove wet linens, and cover the infant's head.
- Convection–transfer of heat through drafts passing over the infant, such as from fans, air drafts, blowing oxygen, or air conditioners.
- Evaporation–transfer of heat when water on the surface of the infant's skin is converted to water vapor.

- Nursing interventions to prevent hypothermia
  - *Place infant skin to skin (kangaroo care) with mom or on a radiant warmer to rewarm.*
  - *Remove wet linens, which cause heat loss through radiation and conduction.*
  - *Maintain dry, warmed linen as the most effective means of rewarming an infant.*
  - *Delay the first bath until the infant has regulated and stabilized core body temperature.*
  - *Keep the infant's head (largest surface area) covered with a stocking cap to prevent heat loss due to radiation and conduction.*

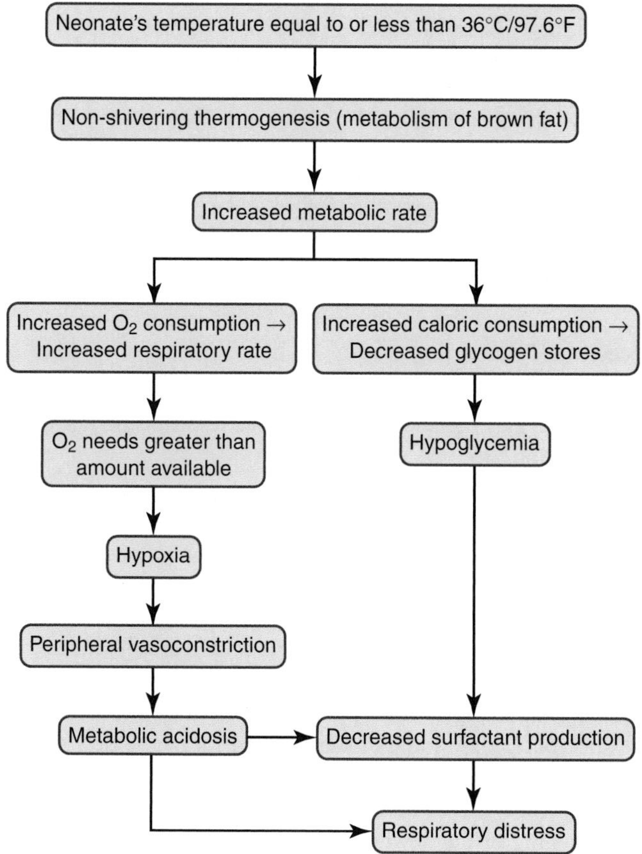

Figure 7–5 Cold stress.

- *Wrap the infant in t-shirt, pajamas, and two blankets to decrease heat loss from convection and radiation.*
- *If these measures are not effective, place the naked infant on a radiant warmer, place the servo-control probe on the infant's abdomen (avoiding bony prominences, liver, and brown fat areas), and set the temperature at least to 36.5°C.*
- *A radiant warmer only heats the outer surfaces, so do not clothe or cover the infant.*
- *Do not attempt to rewarm the infant by microwaving or artificially heating an IV bag or K-pad device and applying it to the infant. Extensive burns may result owing to overheating or uneven heat dispersion.*
- *Closely monitor temperature fluctuations when using a radiant warmer, which may mask the signs and symptoms of temperature instability in the neonate, an indication of sepsis.*
- *Monitor fluid status to determine insensible water losses if using a radiant warmer.*
- *Closely monitor the neonate's temperature, respiratory rate, and glucose levels per institution guidelines.*
- *Recognize that alterations in temperature are directly proportional to gestational age and may indicate the need for physician intervention and notification.*

Evidence-Based Practice: Kangaroo Care

Kangaroo care (or skin-to-skin contact) care has been used in developing countries throughout the world for the past 25 years as an alternative to conventional methods of neonatal care, with the aim to improve the health and survival of low-birth-weight infants and stabilize thermoregulation (Mercer, Erickson-Owens, Graves, & Mumford Haley, 2007). The neonatal mortality rate of high-risk babies is high, with more than 30% of babies dying before stabilization. Evidence to date seems to suggest that that the outcomes for these babies improve if kangaroo mother care is started early to allow for earlier stabilization (Blackwell & Cattaneo, 2007).

Metabolic System Transition and Assessment

- In the last 2 months of fetal life, glucose is stored as glycogen in the liver and is used after birth for:
  - *Coping with the stress of birth*
  - *Breathing*
  - *Heat production*
  - *Muscular activity*
- Glucose is the main source of energy for the brain (Acute Care of at-Risk Newborns Neonatal Society, 2009).
  - *The newborn brain depends on glucose metabolism for 90% of its needs.*
  - *The liver converts glycogen to glucose, which is essential to the newborn's brain and other vital organs.*
  - ***Gluconeogenesis** is the breakdown of glycogen into glucose.*
  - *Clamping of the cord results in a decrease in the level of circulating glucose.*
  - *Glucose levels at birth are 80% of maternal blood glucose levels.*
  - *A decrease in glucose results in an increase in epinephrine, norepinephrine, and glucagon, as well as decreased insulin levels (Polin & Yoder, 2007).*
  - *Hypoglycemia occurs with levels <45 mg/dL (American Academy of Pediatrics [AAP], 2011a).*
    - Increased glucose utilization demands can be due to hypothermia, hypoxia, or sepsis.
    - Prematurity, intrauterine growth restriction, and inborn errors of metabolism can result from a decrease in glycogen stores.
    - A decrease in postmaturity can be due to deterioration of the placenta, which provides nutrition.
    - Large-for-gestational-age babies, infants of diabetic mothers (IDMs), erythroblastosis fetalis, and Beckwith-Wiedemann syndrome can result from overproduction of insulin in the neonate as a result of high intrauterine glucose levels.
    - A hyperglycemic state in diabetic mothers results in beta cell hypertrophy, increased fetal oxygen consumption, and inhibited surfactant and insulin production (Polin & Yoder, 2007).
    - Decreases can also result from maternal intake of certain medications, such as terbutaline.

- *Alterations in glucose levels can predispose an infant to the development of metabolic acidosis.*
- *Monitor glucose levels especially closely with evidence of risk factors, congenital metabolic conditions, birth defects, stress, jitteriness, or neonatal depression.*
- *Normal glucose levels vary from institution to institution.*

CRITICAL COMPONENT

Recognizing Hypoglycemia in the Neonate

- Irritability
- Jitteriness
- Hypotonia
- Temperature instability
- Apnea
- Poor feeding
- Lethargy
- Seizures
- Lack of symptoms does not always indicate absence of alteration

Nursing Interventions

- Monitor for signs and symptoms of hypoglycemia.
- Recognize risk factors for hypoglycemia.
- Assess blood glucose with glucometer, i-STAT.
- Assist with breastfeeding.
- Per institutional protocol, feed full-term neonate with glucose levels between 20 and 40 mg/dL with formula or dextrose water if capable, usually 5 mL/kg (Ward & Hisley, 2009).
- If infant is symptomatic and unable to feed, administer glucose intravenously as per institution's guidelines, usually 2 to 3 mL/kg of 10% dextrose.
- Begin intravenous glucose maintenance, and rigorously follow guidelines on repeat blood serum glucose levels.
- Maintain NTE to prevent cold stress, which increases utilization of glucose.

Evidence-Based Practice: Glucose Levels

Critical glucose levels less than 45 mg/dL obtained with point-of-care devices such as glucometers must be confirmed by serum levels sent STAT to the laboratory. Target glucose levels are >45 mg/dL before feedings. At-risk infants should be fed at 1 hour of age and glucose levels checked 30 minutes after feedings. In infants who are poor feeders, tube feedings should be considered (AAP, 2011).

Newborn Screening

- Every year, 3000 infants in the United States are diagnosed with serious metabolic disorders as a result of the newborn screening process.

Inborn Errors of Metabolism

- Absence or abnormality of an enzyme or cofactor leads to excessive accumulation or deficiency of a specific metabolite (Sutton, 2008).
- Disorders of amino acids, organic acids, carbohydrates, and the urea cycle as well as of mitochondrial, fatty acid, peroxisomal, lysosomal, purine, pyrimidine, and metal metabolism are some of those tested for in the newborn period.
- Each state has its own statutes or regulations regarding screening of the newborn based on state requirements, family history, or diagnosis of a symptomatic infant.
- Most tests are performed within the first 24 to 48 hours owing to early discharges or at follow-up newborn wellness checks.
- Some states require parental written consent.
- Tests utilize capillary blood drawn by nursing or lab personnel and placed on filter paper cards (**Figure 7-6**).
- Tests can detect up to 100 different inborn errors of metabolism or deviations.
- See the National Genetics website at http://genes-r-us.uthscsa.edu/nbsdisorders.pdf

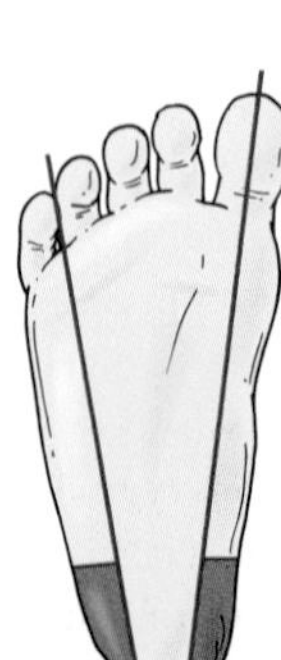

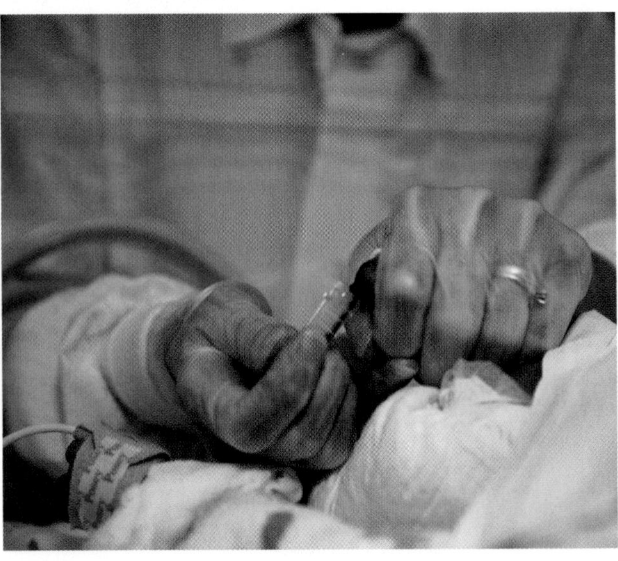

Figure 7-6 Heel stick of foot.

- Phenylketonuria (PKU) is an autosomal recessive deficiency of the enzyme phenylalanine.
  - *Deficiency prevents the conversion of the essential amino acid phenylalanine to tyrosine.*
  - *The elevated levels of phenylalanine can result in mental retardation owing to defective myelinization and degeneration of the white and gray matter of the brain (Taeucsh, Ballard, & Gleason, 2005).*
  - *This metabolic disorder is tested for in all 50 states, including the District of Columbia.*
  - *Infant must be on feedings for 3 full days, so that the liver enzyme that converts phenylalanine to tyrosine will be secreted.*
  - *Guthrie blood test is performed.*
  - *A low-phenylalanine diet must be implemented for the rest of the child's life.*
- Congenital hypothyroidism can lead to mental retardation and is tested for in all 50 states, including the District of Columbia (National Newborn Screening & Genetics Resource Center, 2009).
  - *Underactive or absent thyroid gland*
  - *Hypotonia, lethargy, poor temperature control, respiratory distress*
  - *Replacement hormone necessary throughout life*
  - *Parental education regarding the need for replacement hormone and close follow-up*
- Congenital adrenal hyperplasia
  - *Inability to produce cortisol in the adrenal glands is due to a defect in the enzyme 21-hydroxylase.*
  - *Autosomal recessive: affects 1 in 12,000 to 1 in 680 Eskimos (Taeusch et al., 2005).*
  - *Hyperplasia of the adrenal gland develops.*
  - *End result is excessive androgen production from the adrenal glands (Riepe & Sippell, 2007).*
- Galactosemia is a common enzyme deficiency.
  - *Prevents the breakdown of galactose to glucose*
  - *Can lead to mental retardation, failure to thrive*
  - *Tested for in all 50 states, including the District of Columbia*
- Maple syrup disease
  - *Rare autosomal recessive disorder common in those of Amish and Mennonite descent*
  - *Buildup of metabolic enzyme leads to severe ketoacidosis and encephalopathy*
  - *Protein-free diet implemented for the rest of the infant's life (Rathnau-Minnella, 2008)*

Hepatic System and Assessment

- The full-term neonatal liver is responsible for carbohydrate metabolism, iron storage, bilirubin conjugation, and blood coagulation. The stressed or immature infant is susceptible to alterations in these critical homeostasis maintenance mechanisms (Chapman & Durham, 2010).
  - *Iron stores in fetal liver are put down in the last weeks of pregnancy; as RBCs are broken down, they are added to the liver stores until future RBCs are produced.*
    - Term infants who are breastfed do not need supplemental iron until 6 months of age.
    - Term infants who are bottle feeding require iron-fortified formula.
    - All infants at 6 months of age require iron supplementation through supplements or iron-rich foods.
- *Coagulation*
  - Activation of clotting factors II, VII, IX, and X and prothrombin is influenced by vitamin K.
  - At birth, maternal sources of vitamin K are removed.
  - Intestinal flora are absent in the newborn until after the first feeding, which puts neonates at higher risk for coagulation issues.
  - It is recommended that infants receive a 1-mg intramuscular (IM) injection of vitamin K within 1 hour after birth (AAP, 2009).
  - Infants who are breastfed or asphyxiated or who have mothers who are treated with anticoagulants are at risk for decreased vitamin K levels (Chapman & Durham, 2010).
  - Infants can be at risk for clotting delays and potential hemorrhage, called hemorrhagic disease of the newborn.
- *Newborns have a higher hematocrit, slower bilirubin clearance, shorter RBC life span, and more immature liver conjugation processing.*
- ***Conjugation** is the process of converting lipid-soluble (nonexcreted or indirect) bilirubin into a water-soluble (excreted or direct) form (Ward & Hisley, 2009).*
  - Bilirubin pigment discolors the skin, sclera, and oral mucus membranes and is known as **jaundice** when it discolors these areas.
  - Bilirubin is released from the breakdown of hemoglobin.
  - Elevated levels are mainly due to the infant's immature liver.
  - Hyperbilirubinemia is an excessive amount of bilirubin in the blood.
  - Unconjugated bilirubin (indirect bilirubin) is fat soluble and nonexcretable. Unconjugated bilirubin binds to albumin.
    - *The liver must conjugate, or change, this form of bilirubin via liver enzymes into conjugated (direct) bilirubin so that it can be eliminated in the urine and stool (**Figure 7-7**).*
    - *Increased levels of unconjugated bilirubin (indirect bilirubin) that saturate the albumin-binding sites cross the blood–brain barrier and at this point can result in **kernicterus**, a life-threatening buildup of bilirubin in the brain and spinal cord.*
    - *The total serum bilirubin (TSB) is the combination of direct bilirubin and indirect bilirubin.*
- *Risk factors for hyperbilirubinemia*
  - Infant of diabetic mother
  - ABO incompatibility: When mother and baby have different blood types—specifically, the mother has type O and the baby has type A or B—an immune system reaction occurs that results in excessive breakdown of RBCs and the release of bilirubin.

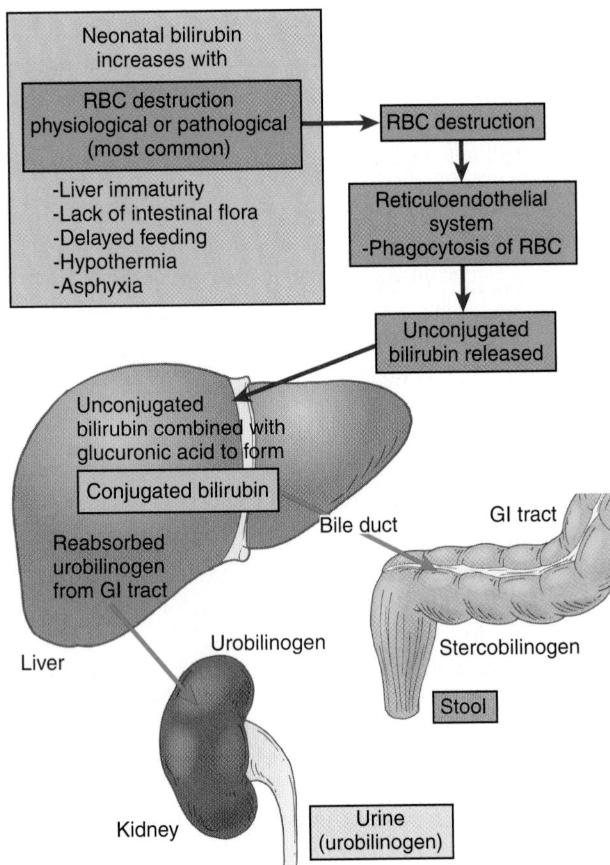

Figure 7–7 Physiological pathway for excretion of bilirubin.

- Rh incompatibility: When the mother is Rh negative and the baby is Rh positive, the mother will produce antibodies against the baby's blood, and hemolysis of the neonate's blood will occur. Bilirubin levels will rise dramatically, and the infant is at risk for kernicterus and erythroblastosis fetalis as well as severe hemolytic anemia and jaundice. This condition is preventable with the administration of RhoGam.
- Prematurity
- Delayed feeding, which delays the passage of bilirubin-rich meconium
- Birth trauma due to accelerated breakdown of RBCs in bruising, asphyxia
- Liver immaturity
- Stress in the neonate (cold stress, asphyxia, hypoglycemia)
- Use of Pitocin in labor
- Cultural background such as Asian, American Indian
- Sibling history of jaundice
- Breastfeeding

- *Monitoring for hyperbilirubinemia*
  - Observe the skin of the neonate; the progression of jaundice begins on the face and nose, and then progresses down the trunk to the extremities (El-Beshbishi, Shattuck, Mohammad, & Peterson, 2009). This is not an accurate method of assessment, especially in darker-skinned infants.

Evidence-Based Practice: Delayed Clamping of the Cord

Dewey, K., & Chaparro, C. (2006). Delayed umbilical cord clamping boosts iron in infants. Retrieved from http://www.sciencedaily.com/releases/2006/06/060618224104.htm

Ceriani Cernadas, J. M., Carroli, G., Pellegrini, L., Otano, L., Ferreira, M. Ricci, C., Lardizabal, J. (2006). The effect of timing of cord clamping on neonatal venous hematocrit values and clinical outcome at term: A randomized controlled trial. *Pediatrics, 117*, 779–786. doi: 10.1542/peds.2005-1156

The delay of cord clamping in the past has been associated with an increased incidence of hyperbilirubinemia in the neonate. Recent studies published by Dewey and Chaparro in 2006 and Ceriani Cernadas et al. in 2006 showed that the benefits of delay of cord clamping for 1 to 3 minutes or until the cord stops pulsating resulted in increased levels of iron, decreased risk of anemia, decreased risk for intraventricular hemorrhage, and no effects on bilirubin levels.

  - All neonates should be screened prior to discharge with a measurement of bilirubin levels and the assessment of clinical risk factors. Bilirubin levels are then plotted on the Bhutani nomogram.
  - The Bhutani nomogram is an hour-specific tool used for prediction in those at-risk neonates who are >36 weeks' gestation, >2000 gm, and otherwise well who do not have ABO incompatibilities (Bhutani, Johnson, & Sivieri, 1999; Keren et al., 2006).
    - *Infants are rated as low, intermediate, or high risk for developing clinically significant hyperbilirubinemia.*
    - *Severely at-risk infants are those with total serum bilirubin levels ≥95 percentile for age in hours (Bhutani et al., 1999).*
  - The **Coombs' test** is also utilized in monitoring.

CLINICAL PEARL

Coombs' Test

The Coombs' test is a measurement of antibodies that are attached to the newborn's RBCs that occur with Rh-negative mothers. Rh-negative mothers produce antibodies against the Rh-positive baby, or in ABO incompatibilities. If there is an abnormal coating of the neonate's RBCs with an antibody globulin from the mother, it is considered a positive Coombs' test, and the neonate is at a higher risk of hemolytic disease of the newborn (Chapman & Durham, 2010).

- *A heel stick is performed with a sharp lancet to remove small drops of capillary blood to test for total, direct, and indirect serum bilirubin levels.*
  - Transcutaneous bilirubin (TcB) measurement—noninvasive multiwavelength spectral skin monitoring of bilirubin levels via the forehead or upper part of the sternum. Up to 15 mg/dL, the TcB correlates with serum blood levels (Keren et al., 2006).
- *Physiological jaundice*
  - Transient rise within the first 24 to 48 hours of life
  - Affects 60% of term newborns, 80% of preterms (Ward & Hisley, 2009)

    - Peaks at 3 to 7 days of life
    - Bilirubin levels are benign and usually do not exceed 15 mg/dL. Levels from 17 to 18 mg/dL may be accepted as normal in term infants (AAP, 2004).
- *Pathological jaundice*
    - Occurs within the first 24 hours of life
    - Results from excessive destruction of RBCs, infection, incompatibilities, or metabolic disorders
    - Consider if bilirubin levels are levels >12.9 mgm/dL in term infant, >15 mgm/dL in preterm infants within a day of birth (AAP, 2004)
    - Consider with bilirubin levels that increase by more than 5 mg/dL/day (AAP, 2004)
    - Diagnosed with jaundice lasting longer than 1 week in a term newborn, or more than 2 weeks in a premature infant (AAP, 2004)
- *Breast milk jaundice*
    - Affects 1% to 2% of breastfed babies
    - Early onset—poor feeding patterns; bilirubin levels may spike to 19mg/dL (Ward & Hisley, 2009).
    - Late onset-peaks 2 to 3 weeks after birth; there is an increased absorption of bilirubin as a result of a factor in breast milk that increases the absorption of bilirubin from the intestines (**Table 7-3**; Ward & Hisley, 2009).

Nursing Interventions

- Identify infants at risk.
- Monitor bilirubin levels through close skin monitoring; digitally compress the skin.
- Monitor point-of-care heel sticks, transcutaneous bilirubin levels, and serum bilirubin levels.
- Support early and frequent feedings.
- Support and work with lactating mothers.
- Consult with lactation consultants.
- Monitor stooling and voiding patterns.
- Monitor and screen for lethargic or sleepy infants.
- Monitor for high-pitched cry and arching of the body.
- Maintain phototherapy.

Phototherapy

- In phototherapy, blue-green fluorescent light is absorbed into the skin, mixes with the bilirubin, and converts bilirubin into lumirubin, which is water soluble and thereby allows the infant to excrete bilirubin in the stool and urine.
- Fluorescent lights should be calibrated periodically according to the manufacturer's guidelines.
- Cover the infant's eyes to prevent cataracts.
- Infants should be fully exposed, except for the diaper, and placed in a low-heat-setting isolette. Place lamp 45 to 50 cm away from infant, or 2 inches from the top of the isolette (Chapman & Durham, 2010).
- Remove eye patches and hold infant only during feedings.
- Closely monitor temperature during phototherapy.
- Single phototherapy is the use of one light, double phototherapy the use of two, and triple phototherapy the use of three—choice of method depends on the bilirubin levels and the rate of the rise of the levels (**Figure 7-8**).
- A fiberoptic blanket or band can be used at home and provides light similar to that found in sunlight.
- Fluid requirements increase during therapy owing to insensible water loss.
- Partial-, single-, or double-volume-exchange blood transfusion may be necessary in a neonatal intensive care unit.

CULTURAL AWARENESS: Communication and Client Teaching

Routine discharge teaching needs to be completed in the language spoken in the home. Teaching needs to be in both written and oral formats with patient-friendly information, including signs and symptoms of an infant's deteriorating status, follow-up monitoring instructions, and office contacts for questions (Moerschel, Cianciaruso, & Tracy, 2008).

TABLE 7–3 HYPERBILIRUBINEMIA IN BREASTFEEDING JAUNDICE VS. BREAST-MILK JAUNDICE

Breastfeeding Jaundice	Breast-Milk Jaundice
Early onset of jaundice (within the first few days of life) Associated with ineffective breastfeeding Dehydration can occur Delayed passage of meconium stool promotes reabsorption of bilirubin in the gut **Treatment:** Encourage early, effective breastfeeding without supplementation of glucose water or other fluids	Late onset (after 3–5 days) Gradual increase in bilirubin that peaks at 2 weeks of age Associated with breast-milk composition in some women that increases the enterohepatic circulation of bilirubin **Treatment:** Continued breastfeeding in most infants. In some cases where bilirubin levels are excessively high, breastfeeding may be interrupted and formula feedings can be given for several days. This typically results in a decline of the bilirubin level. Breastfeeding is resumed when bilirubin levels decline

From Chapman, L., & Durham, R. (2010). *Maternal-newborn nursing: Critical components of nursing care.* Philadelphia: F.A. Davis.

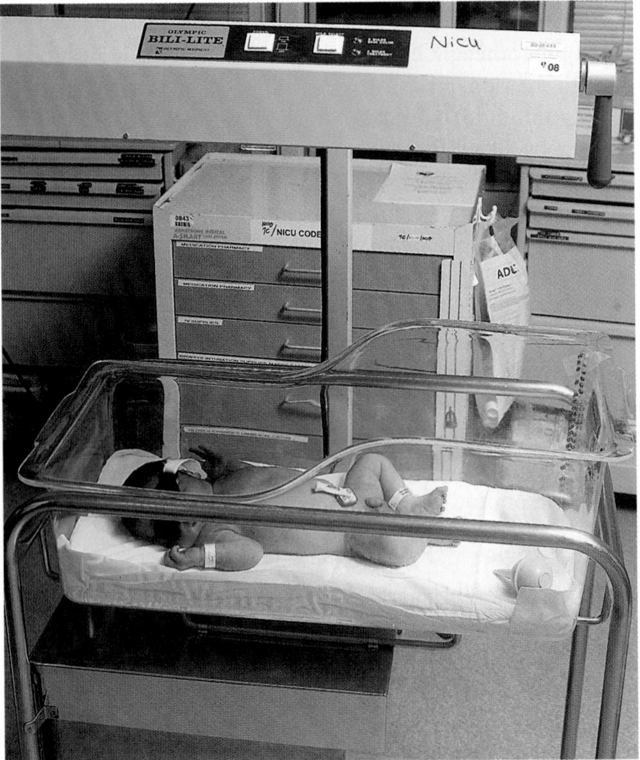

Figure 7–8 Phototherapy.

Gastrointestinal System Transition and Assessment

See Chapter 15 for further details.

- The abdomen should be cylindrical; a sunken abdomen should be reported.
- The stomach is immature but rapidly adjusts.
- Stomach capacity is 30 to 60 mL at birth and then rapidly increases.
- The infant may be uninterested in feeding owing to a quiet sleep state.
- Both the desire for feeding and stomach size increase rapidly during infancy.
- Enzymes are present at birth to digest proteins, moderate fats, and simple sugars.
- Decreased esophageal sphincter pressure is present at birth but increases with age.
- The first stool is black and tarry and is known as **meconium**. Meconium is formed starting around 16 weeks of gestation and usually is passed within 24 to 48 hours of age.
- Stool then becomes transitional around day 3 of life, with color and consistency dependent on feeding.
  - *Breastfeeding stool beyond transitional is golden and semiformed.*
  - *Bottle-fed stool beyond transitional is drier and pale yellow or greenish-black to brownish.*
  - *A loose or green stool is considered diarrhea (Chapman & Durham, 2010).*
- Breastfed babies eat more frequently owing to the increased digestibility of breast milk. Breast milk is composed of 60% whey and 40% casein, whereas cow's milk has 20% whey and 80% casein. Casein forms a hard curd that is difficult to digest.
- Constipation does not occur in breastfed newborns.
- Breastfed babies often produce stool with every feeding, and by 1 month of age may progress to one stool every day or every other day.
- Bottle-fed babies may become constipated owing to improper formula mixing. Normal elimination patterns for bottle-fed infants are one or two stools a day.
- After the second month of life, stool increases in volume and decreases in frequency.
- Feeding should be at least every 4 hours but may need to be more frequent owing to stomach emptying time.
- Infants progress from being able to only suck, drink liquids, and be fed by a caregiver to children who are able to feed themselves and digest solids.
- As the infant is weaned from the breast or bottle to solid foods, the consistency of the stool will change. It is not uncommon to see pieces of food in the stool.

Genitourinary System Transition and Assessment

See Chapter 16 for further details.

- Nephrons are fully functional at 34 to 36 weeks of gestation.
- The fetus produces urine within the first 3 months of gestation.
- The first urine output should occur within 24 hours after birth.
- In the first 1 or 2 days, urine may be stained orange or pink owing to urate crystals.
- Newborns do not have the ability to concentrate or dilute urine in response to changes in intravascular fluid status and therefore are at risk for dehydration or fluid overload.
- Infants are more prone to extracellular fluid (ECF) loss than intracellular fluid (ICF) loss.
- The term neonate is composed of 75% water (40% ECF, 35% ICF), and term neonates usually lose 5% to 10% of their weight in the first week of life, almost all of which is water loss.
- Fluid requirements during the first 2 days of life are 80 to 100 mL/kg/day, then increase to 100 to 150 mL/kg/day.
- The glomerular filtration rate decreases at birth.
- Specific gravity averages 1.001 to 1.010 during infancy.
- Infants do not have the ability to correct acid–base balance through bicarbonate and hydrogen ion concentration.
- Urine output should be 1 to 3 mL/kg/hour if monitored in the hospital to maintain adequate fluid maintenance.
- Strict input and output (I&O) is essential in the nursing care of any infant in the hospital.
- By 3 months of age, infants are able to concentrate urine.
- Normal urine output is calculated based on weight.
- Six to 10 wet diapers/day is considered normal urine output (**Table 7-4**).

TABLE 7-4 TABLE OF FLUID INTAKE

General Guidelines for a 24-Hour Period	Fluid Intake	Based on Increments of 10 kg per Body Weight
<10 kg	100 mL/kg	
>10 and <20 kg	1000 mL for 1st 10 kg	+50 mL/kg for each kg >10 and <20
>20 kg	1500 mL for 1st kg	+20 mL/kg for each kg >20

Genitalia

See Chapter 18 for further details.

- The normal male has descended testes, and the urethral opening in the center of the penis.
- The scrotum at first appears edematous and disproportionately large.
- **Hypospadias** is when the urethral opening is on the underside (ventrum) of the penis. **Epispadias** is when the urethral opening is on the upper portion (dorsum) of the penis. In both of these conditions, there will be a delay in circumcision so that the prepuce can be used for surgical correction.
- **Circumcision** is the surgical removal of the foreskin of the penis.
- In the normal female, the labia majora are larger than the labia minora.
- Observe for vaginal tags.
- Observe for ambiguous genitalia, a genetic defect in which the outward appearance of the genitalia does not resemble either a boy or a girl. The penis may be very small, the clitoris may be very large, or the labia may be fused, resembling a scrotum.
- **Pseudomenstruation**—a thin white or blood-tinged mucus may be present due to withdrawal of maternal hormones.
- The breasts may be enlarged in both male and female infants at birth.

Skin System Transition and Assessment

- Provide adequate lighting for assessment.
- Color is influenced by ethnicity.
- Skin should be pink. Pale or dusky skin may indicate congenital heart disease (see Chapter 12).
- Observe for jaundice; apply pressure and remove with your fingertip over bony prominences such as the nose, sternum, or sacrum.
- Observe for the presence of body hair, fine downy **lanugo**.
- Observe for acrocyanosis (normal and disappears with crying).
- Observe for petechiae, skin tags, breaks in the skin, forceps marks on the face or scalp, and electronic fetal monitoring marks on the scalp.
- Observe for **milia** (small white sebaceous cysts), usually present on the face.
- **Vernix caseosa**—cheesy substance found mainly in the creases of the armpits and groin but may cover the entire body. This protective covering should not be removed, as it provides an emollient effect to the skin.
- **Erythema toxicum** (newborn rash)—tiny pimples that disappear within the first few weeks
- **Mongolian spots**—areas located over sacral region that are grayish, dark blue, or black; prominent in certain ethnic cultures from Asia, Africa, and Mediterranean areas (**Figure 7-9**).
- Observe for birthmarks, nevi, or stork bites (**Figure 7-10**).
- Cord begins to dry following the cutting of the cord. The cord clamp should be removed 24 to 48 hours after birth. Cord care includes keeping it dry. Some institutions leave the cord open to air, apply methylene blue to the cord as a drying agent, or apply alcohol to the cord. Keep the

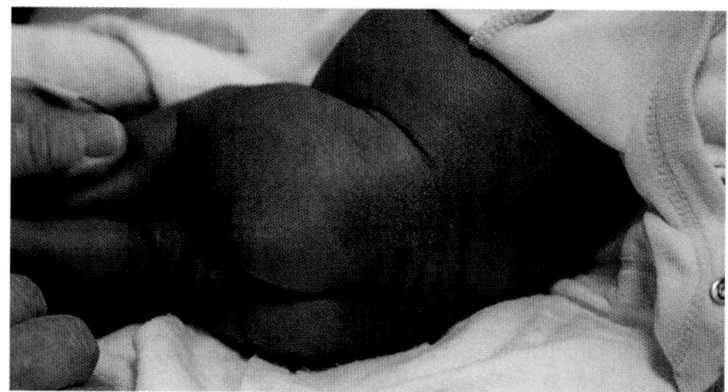

Figure 7-9 Mongolian spots.

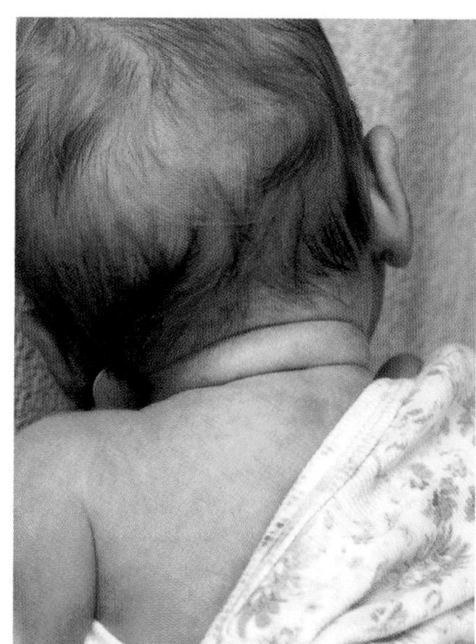

Figure 7-10 Stork bite.

diaper below the cord. As it dries, the cord becomes black and hard, and it falls off within 2 weeks. Be aware that some cultures save the cord detachment (see Chapter 4).

- Diapering can be with disposable or cloth diapers. Most parents choose disposable. The newborn infant should have between 6 and 10 wet diapers per day. Water should be used to clean the genital and rectal area, wiping in girls from front to back. Nurses need to instruct caregivers to wash their hands following every diaper change.
- Diaper rash—red and sore areas in the diaper region from urine and stool, often a result of *Candidiasis.*
- Heat rash or prickly heat is due to overdressing in warm weather.
- Cradle cap—scaly or crusty skin on the scalp due to buildup of oils, scales, and dead skin
- See **Table 7-5** for common newborn characteristics.

Evidence-Based Practice: Care of Neonatal Skin

Association of Women's Health, Obstetric, and Neonatal Nurses. (2007). Quick care guide for neonatal skin care (2nd ed.). Retrieved from http://www.awhonn.org/awhonn/content.do?name=07_PressRoom/7-07Nov14_SkinCareEBG.htm

The American Association of Women's Health, Obstetric, and Neonatal Nurses (AWHONN) developed the *Neonatal Skin Care Evidence-Based Clinical Practice Guideline,* an evidence-based practice guideline for the care of neonatal skin related to bathing, cord care, disinfectants, wound care, and the relationship between term infant and preterm infant skin care in the first 28 days of life.

Immune System Transition and Assessment

- The infant in utero is considered to be in a sterile environment.

TABLE 7–5 COMMON NEWBORN CHARACTERISTICS

Characteristic	Appearance	Significance
ACROCYANOSIS	Hands and/or feet are blue	Response to cold environment Immature peripheral circulation
CIRCUMORAL CYANOSIS	A benign localized transient cyanosis around the mouth	Observed during the transitional period; if it persists it may be related to a cardiac anomaly
MOTTLING	A benign transient pattern of pink and white blotches on the skin	Response to cold environment
HARLEQUIN SIGN	One side of the body is pink, and the other side is white	Related to vasomotor instability
MONGOLIAN SPOTS	Flat bluish discolored area on the lower back and/or buttocks Seen more often in African American, Asian, Latin, and Native American infants	Might be mistaken for bruising Need to document size and location Resolves on own by school age
ERYTHEMA TOXICUM	A rash with red macules and papules (white to yellowish-white papule in center surrounded by reddened skin) that appears on different areas of the body, usually the trunk area Can appear within 24 hours of birth and up to 2 weeks after birth	Benign Disappears without treatment

TABLE 7–5 COMMON NEWBORN CHARACTERISTICS—cont'd

Characteristic	Appearance	Significance
MILIA 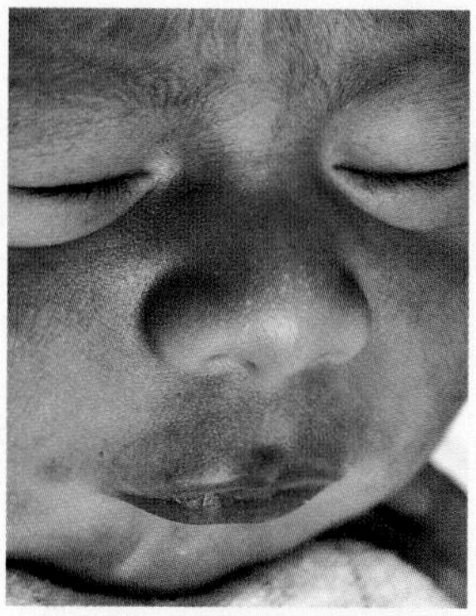	White papules on the face; more frequently seen on the bridge of the nose and chin	Exposed sebaceous glands that resolve without treatment Parents might mistake these for "whiteheads" Inform parents to leave them alone and let them resolve on their own
LANUGO 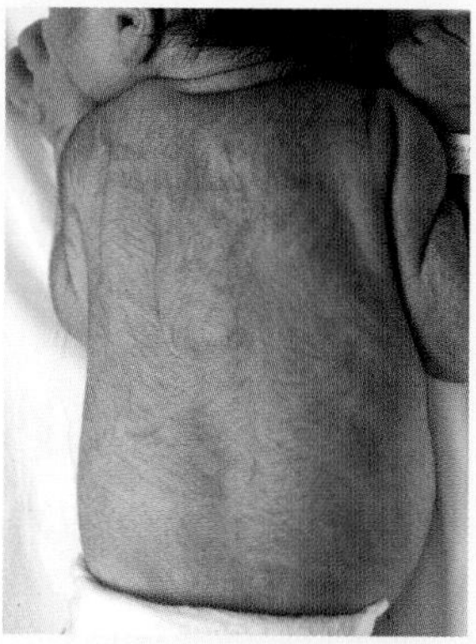	Fine, downy hair that develops after 16 weeks of gestation The amount of lanugo decreases as the fetus ages Often seen on the neonate's back, shoulders, and forehead	Gradually falls out The presence and amount of lanugo assist in estimating gestational age Abundant lanugo may be a sign of prematurity or a genetic disorder
VERNIX CASEOSA 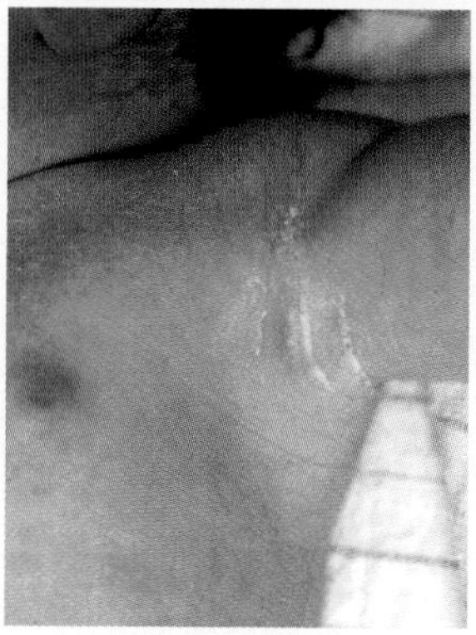	A protective substance secreted from sebaceous glands that covered the fetus during pregnancy It looks like a whitish, cheesy substance May be noted in the axillary and genital areas of full-term neonates	The presence and amount of vernix assist in estimating gestational age Full-term neonates usually have no vernix or only small amounts

Continued

TABLE 7–5 COMMON NEWBORN CHARACTERISTICS—cont'd

Characteristic	Appearance	Significance
JAUNDICE	Yellow coloring of the skin First appears on the face and extends to the trunk and eventually the entire body Best assessed in natural lighting When jaundice is suspected, the nurse can apply gentle pressure to the skin over a firm surface such as the nose, forehead, or sternum; the skin blanches to a yellowish hue	Jaundice within the first 24 hours is pathological; it is usually related to a problem of the liver (see Chapter 17) Jaundice occurring after 24 hours is referred to as physiological jaundice and is related to an increased amount of unconjugated bilirubin in the system (see Chapter 17)
EPSTEIN PEARLS	White, pearl-like epithelial cysts on gum margins and palate	Benign and usually disappear within a few weeks
NATAL TEETH	Immature caps of enamel and dentin with poorly developed roots Usually only one or two teeth are present	They are usually benign, but can be associated with congenital defects Natal teeth are often loose and need to be removed to decrease the risk of aspiration

Modified from Chapman, L., & Durham, R. (2010). *Maternal-newborn nursing: Critical components of nursing care* (pp. 294–297). Philadelphia: F.A. Davis; and Dillon, P. (2007). *Nursing assessment* (pp. 855–867). Philadelphia: F.A. Davis.

- The infant is provided with maternal immunity through antibodies that bind to bacteria, viruses, and fungi that enter the body.
- Following birth
  - *Active humoral immunity is provided through acquired immunity from vaccination, or natural immunity from one's own production of antibodies in response to exposure to antigens.*
  - *Passive immunity is temporary and is provided by those maternal antibodies that cross the placenta; the lymphocytes are T and B cells. Passive immunity is provided by breast milk, which contains all five immunoglobulins: IgG, IgA, IgD, IgM, and IgE.*
- *Immunoglobulins are maternal antibodies that cross the placenta and provide passive immunity—IgG, IgM, IgE, IgD, and IgA (**Table 7-6**).*
  - IgG is the only immunoglobulin that crosses the placenta during pregnancy and makes up 75% to 85% of all antibodies in the infant.
  - IgA is primarily found in breast milk.

TABLE 7–6 CLASSES OF IMMUNOGLOBULINS

NAME	LOCATION	FUNCTION
IgG	Blood Extracellular fluid	Crosses the placenta to provide passive immunity for newborns Provides long-term immunity after recovery or a vaccine
IgA	External secretions (tears, salvia, etc.)	Present in breast milk to provide passive immunity for breast-fed infants Found in secretions of all mucous membranes
IgM	Blood	Produced first by the maturing immune system of infants Produced first during an infection (IgG production follows) Part of the ABO blood group
IgD	B lymphocytes	Receptors on B lymphocytes
IgE	Mast cells or basophils	Important in allergic reaction (mast cells release histamine)

From Chapman, L., & Durham, R. (2010). *Maternal-newborn nursing: Critical components of nursing care* (p. 286). Philadelphia: F.A. Davis; original source Scanlon, V., & Sanders, T. (2007). *Essentials of anatomy and physiology* (5th ed.). Philadelphia: F.A. Davis.

- IgM is primarily found in the lymph and bloodstream.
- IgD is primarily found in the abdomen and chest areas of the body.
- IgE is found in the lungs, skin, and mucous membranes.

- *The infant's immune system is not fully developed until 6 months of age, and begins to produce antibodies around 2 to 3 months of age.*
- *Infants who are fed early have a higher incidence of developing food allergies as a result of exposure to proteins in the food (Greer, Sicherer, & Burks, 2008).*
- *Infants are at risk for infection because of immature immune responses, lack of maternal antibodies, stress that depletes the immune system, and breaks in the skin due to invasive procedures that introduce bacteria or viruses.*

Head and Neck Assessment

- The anterior and posterior fontanels (soft spots) should be assessed with the infant in an upright position.
  - *The anterior fontanel is diamond shaped, averages 2 to 3 cm wide by 3 to 4 cm long, and closes at 12 to 18 months. You should be able to feel slight pulsations in this area. Abnormal findings are full or bulging fontanels, sunken fontanels, or closed suture lines.*
  - *The posterior fontanel is triangular, averages 1 to 2 cm wide, and closes in the second month of life.*
  - *Bulging fontanels may occur with crying or increased intracranial pressure.*
  - *Sunken fontanels indicate dehydration.*
  - *Average head circumference is 35 centimeters but can range from 33 to 37 cm.*
  - ***Molding** of the head occurs with normal vaginal deliveries, causing misshapen or elongated scalp.*
  - *Bruising or swelling of the scalp may occur as the result of a difficult delivery or use of a vacuum or forceps.*
  - *Bleeding of the skull bone and its outer covering may cause a small bump, which will reabsorb in a few weeks.*
    - **Caput succedaneum** is the cone shape to the back of the head that crosses suture lines (**Figure 7-11A**). This shape occurs when blood and tissue become edematous as a result of pushing against the mother's cervix.
    - **Cephalhematoma** is a swelling on one or both sides of the scalp that does not cross suture lines (**Figure 7-11B**). It is a result of bleeding over the skull bone or within

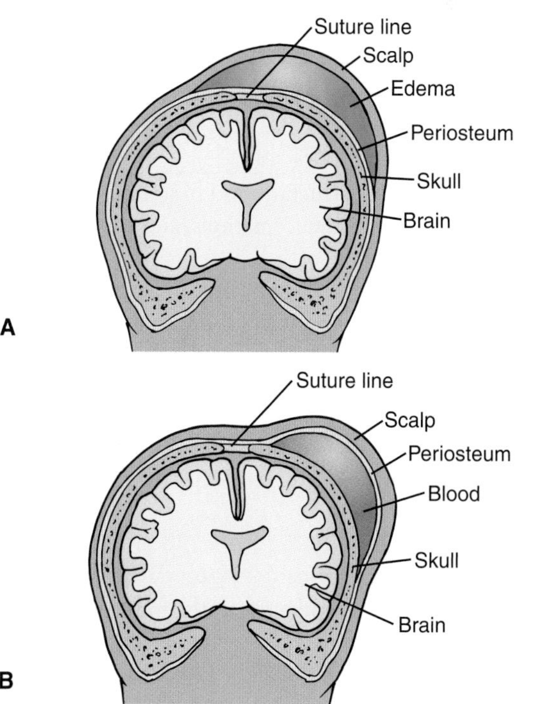

Figure 7–11 **A,** Caput succedaneum; **B,** cephalhematoma.

the periosteum due to pressure against the pelvic bone. It can be life threatening as a result of blood loss.
  - **Craniosynostosis** is the premature closure of one or more of the cranial sutures.

Eyes

- The eyelids may be edematous from the birthing process; resolves spontaneously.
- The iris should be grayish-blue or gray-brown. The sclera should be blue or white. Jaundiced sclera is an abnormal finding.
- Pupils should be equal, round, and reactive to light activity. The cornea should be clear, and the red reflex should be present.

> **Evidence-Based Practice: Red Reflex**
>
> American Academy of Pediatrics. (2008). Red reflex examination in neonates, infants, and children. *Pediatrics, 122,* 1401–1404. doi:10.1542/peds.2008-2624
>
> The red reflex is an important test in determining life-altering abnormalities such as cataracts, glaucoma, retinoblastoma, retinal abnormalities, and systemic abnormalities that may show signs or symptoms in the eye. A light is used to reflect off the ocular fundus of the eye. Obstructions can occur with mucus or abnormalities, and there are differences in the red reflex depending upon race, ethnicity, and pigmentation of the fundus. A position statement by the AAP (2008) indicates the need for a red reflex examination to be completed by a pediatrician or other trained primary care provider prior to discharge from the newborn nursery.

- The line from the inner epicanthal fold, to the outer canthus, to the top notch of the ear where it connects with the scalp should be symmetrical.
- Tears are not produced until the second month of life.
- Strabismus is an imbalance in ocular motor capacity.
- The visual acuity of a newborn is 20/400, improving in the first 2 years of life to 20/30.

Ears

- Examine for position, structure, and function.
- Note absence of clefts, malformations, and cartilage or abnormalities.
- The infant should startle to noise and move eyes to sound.
- The infant should respond to soothing sounds.
- Unresponsiveness to noises should be investigated.

Nose

- Check the patency of the nares.
- Infants are obligatory nose breathers.
- Monitor for nasal flaring.

Mouth

- The mouth should be symmetrical; the tongue should not protrude between the lips.
- The hard and soft palates should be intact and high arched.
- **Epstein pearls**—yellow or white fluid-filled papules on the palate of the mouth that spontaneously resolve.

Dental Development and Assessment

- Tooth buds are present during the third month of pregnancy.
- Natal teeth can be present at birth (usually lower central incisors without a root) and can interfere with breastfeeding.
- Teething is the eruption of the teeth through the gums.
- Teeth erupt at 4 to 10 months of age (usually around 6 months), starting with the two lower center teeth; the upper center teeth come in at about 8 to 12 months old. At the end of the first year, the child will have six to eight teeth.
- The primary teeth are calcifying.
- The American Dental Association (ADA) recommends that the first dental visit occur by 1 year of age (ADA, 2009).
- A soft clean cloth should be used to clean the teeth as they erupt or to bite down on to decrease the pain of teething.
- Signs and symptoms of teething including drooling, restlessness or difficulty falling asleep, sucking on the hands, and mild rash around the mouth due to drooling.
- Teething is not associated with generalized rash, fever, diarrhea, or prolonged fussiness. Numbing over-the-counter medications are brief in action and may also numb the throat and have a taste that is not pleasant for infants. Infants should never be given any medication with alcohol in the ingredients.

> CLINICAL PEARL
>
> **Dental Care for the Infant**
>
> - Feed only formula, breast milk, or water in a bottle.
> - Serve juice only in a cup.
> - Do not put infants to bed at night or for a nap with a bottle.
> - Brush teeth with a soft cloth once they erupt.
> - Do not use cold juice to soothe an infant's gums.
> - Begin regular dental appointments by the first birthday.

Neck

- The head should move freely from side to side.
- The infant should not move the head past the shoulder.
- The neck is short and thick; skin folds are present.
- No masses should be felt or observed.

Neurological Transition and Assessment and Development

See Chapter 13 for further details.

- The brain reaches 90% of its total size during infancy.
  - *All neurons are present by the end of the first year of life.*
  - *Maturation follows **cephalocaudal** (head-to-toe) and **proximodistal** (center-to-extremity) progression.*
  - *Uncoordinated movements*
  - *Tremors in the extremities*
  - *Poor muscle control*

- Abnormalities are determined by testing the baby's reflexes; they need to be symmetrical on each side of the body. Asymmetry suggests abnormality or weakness.
  - *Moro reflex or startle reflex—occurs when the infant is startled with noise or rapid change in position; the infant throws the arms and legs out, cries, and then recoils the arms and legs. The neonate makes a "C" with the thumb and forefinger. This reflex disappears around 5 to 6 months of age.*
  - *Rooting reflex—when the side of mouth is touched or stroked, the infant will turn its head and seek to suck. Disappears between 3 and 6 months of age.*
  - *Sucking reflex—present at birth; disappears at 10 to 12 months of age.*
  - *Palmar grasp reflex—grasping of a person's finger in the infant's hand; disappears around 3 months and is replaced by the voluntary grasp.*
  - *Plantar reflex—the infant's toes flex in a grasping motion in response to a thumb pressed against the ball of the foot; disappears around 9 to 12 months of age.*
  - *Tonic neck or fencing position reflex—the arm and leg are extended while the opposite side of the body is flexed; disappears around 4 to 6 months of age.*
  - *Babinski reflex—the infant's toes flare when the foot is stroked in an upward motion; normal in children up to 2 years old, but disappears as the child ages and the nervous system becomes more developed. It may disappear as early as 12 months.*
  - *Stepping or dancing reflex—the neonate steps up and down in place when held upright; disappears at 3 to 4 weeks of age. See **Table 7-7**.*

PHYSICAL DEVELOPMENT

Gestation

- Gestational age is based on mother's menstrual history, prenatal ultrasound, or neonatal maturation examination.

TABLE 7–7 NEWBORN REFLEXES

Reflex	How Elicited	Expected Response	Abnormal Response
MORO Present at birth; disappears by 6 months	Jar the crib or hold the baby in a semisitting position and let the head slightly drop back	Symmetrical abduction and extension of arms and legs, and legs flex up against trunk The neonate makes a "C" shape with the thumb and index finger	A slow response might occur with preterm infants or sleepy neonates An asymmetrical response may be related to temporary or permanent birth injury to clavicle, humerus, or brachial plexus
STARTLE Present at birth; disappears by 4 months	Make a loud sound near the neonate	Same as Moro response	Slow response when sleeping Possible deafness Possible neurological deficit
TONIC NECK Present between birth and 6 weeks; disappears by 4 to 6 months	With the neonate in a supine position, turn the head to the side so that the chin is over the shoulder	The neonate assumes a "fencing" position with arms and legs extended in the direction in which the head was turned	Response after 6 months may indicate cerebral palsy
ROOTING Present at birth; disappears between 3 and 6 months	Brush the side of a cheek near the corner of the mouth	The neonate turns his or her head toward the direction of the stimulus and opens the mouth Instruct mothers who are lactating to touch the corner of the neonate's mouth with a nipple and the infant will turn toward the nipple for feeding	May not respond if recently fed. Prematurity or neurological defects may cause weak or absent response
SUCKING Present at birth; disappears at 10–12 months	Place a gloved finger or nipple of a bottle in the neonate's mouth	Sucking motion occurs	May not respond if recently fed Prematurity or neurological defects may cause weak or absent response

Continued

TABLE 7–7 NEWBORN REFLEXES—cont'd

Reflex	How Elicited	Expected Response	Abnormal Response
PALMAR GRASP Present at birth; disappears at 3–4 months	The examiner places a finger in the palm of the neonate's hand	The neonate grasps the finger tightly; if the neonate grasps the examiner's finger with both hands, the neonate can be pulled to a sitting position	Absent or weak response indicates a possible central nervous system defect, or nerve or muscle injury
PLANTAR GRASP Present at birth; disappears at 3–4 months	Place a thumb firmly against the ball of the infant's foot	Toes flex tightly down in a grasping motion	Weak or absent response may indicate possible spinal cord injury
BABINSKI Present at birth; disappears at 1 year	Stroke the lateral surface of the sole in an upward motion	Hyperextension and fanning of toes	Absent or weak response may indicate a possible neurological defect
STEPPING OR DANCING Present at birth; disappears at 3–4 weeks	Hold the neonate upright with feet touching a flat surface	The neonate steps up and down in place	Diminished response may indicate hypotonia

From Chapman, L., & Durham, R. (2010). *Maternal-newborn nursing: Critical components of nursing care* (pp. 297–299). Philadelphia: F.A. Davis; originally adapted from Dillon, P. (2007). *Nursing assessment* (pp. 868–873). Philadelphia: F.A. Davis.

- Gestational age can be calculated using the Dubowitz neurological examination or the Ballard scoring method.
- The Dubowitz neurological exam for infants in a neonatal intensive care unit (NICU) measures habituation, movement and muscle tone, reflexes, and neurobehavioral areas.
- Ballard Maturational Scoring consists of six areas of neuromuscular maturity and six areas of observed physical maturity (**Table 7-8**). A score is assigned to each area. The physical maturity scoring should be completed within the first 2 hours of birth, and the neuromuscular scoring should be completed within the first 24 hours.
- *Neuromuscular activity*
  - Posture—the position of the infant at rest, flaccid or flexed
  - Square window—how far the infant's hand can be flexed toward the wrist
  - Arm recoil—how well the arms recoil back when flexed
  - Popliteal angle—how far the infant's knees can be flexed
  - Scarf sign—how far the infant's arm can be moved across the chest

TABLE 7–8 BALLARD MATURATIONAL ASSESSMENT TOOL

Neuromuscular Maturity	Physical Maturity
POSTURE Assess the position the neonate assumes while lying quietly on his or her back The more mature, the greater degree of flexion in the legs and arms	SKIN The examiner inspects the neonate's chest and abdominal skin areas for texture, transparency, thickness, and peeling and/or cracking A preterm neonate's skin is smooth, thin, and translucent (numerous veins visible) A full-term neonate's skin is thicker and more opaque, with some degree of peeling
SQUARE WINDOW Assess the degree of the angle created when the examiner flexes the neonate's hand toward the forearm The more mature, the greater the flexion	LANUGO The examiner assesses the amount of lanugo on the neonate's back Lanugo begins to form around the 24th week of gestation; it is abundant in preterm neonates and decreases in amount as the neonate matures

TABLE 7–8 BALLARD MATURATIONAL ASSESSMENT TOOL—cont'd

Neuromuscular Maturity	Physical Maturity
ARM RECOIL With the neonate in a supine position, the examiner fully flexes the forearm against the neonate's chest for 5 seconds The examiner extends the arms and releases them The more mature, the faster the arms return to the flexed position (recoil)	PLANTAR CREASES The examiner inspects the bottom of the feet for location of creases The more mature, the more creases over the greater proportion of the foot
POPLITEAL ANGLE With the neonate in a supine position and the pelvis flat, the examiner flexes the neonate's thigh to the abdomen; the leg is extended; the angle at the knee is estimated The more mature, the lesser the angle	BREAST TISSUE The examiner assesses the degree of nipple formation The size of the breast bud is measured by gently grasping the tissue with the thumb and forefinger and measuring the distance between the thumb and forefinger The more mature, the greater the degree of nipple formation and the size of the breast bud
SCARF SIGN With the neonate in a supine position, the examiner takes the neonate's hand and moves the arm across the chest toward the opposite shoulder The examiner notes where the elbow is in relationship to the midline of the chest The more preterm, the more the elbow crosses the midline	EAR FORMATION The examiner assesses the ear for form and firmness The more mature, the more defined and firmer the ear is
HEEL TO EAR With the neonate in a supine position, the examiner takes the neonate's foot and moves it toward the ear The more mature, the lesser the flexion (the further the heel is from the ear)	GENITALIA **Male:** The examiner palpates the scrotum for the presence of testis and inspects the scrotum for appearance The more mature, the greater the descent of the testis and the greater the degree of rugae (creases) **Female:** The examiner moves the neonate's hip one-half abduction and visually inspects the genitalia The more mature, the more the labia majora cover the labia minora and clitoris

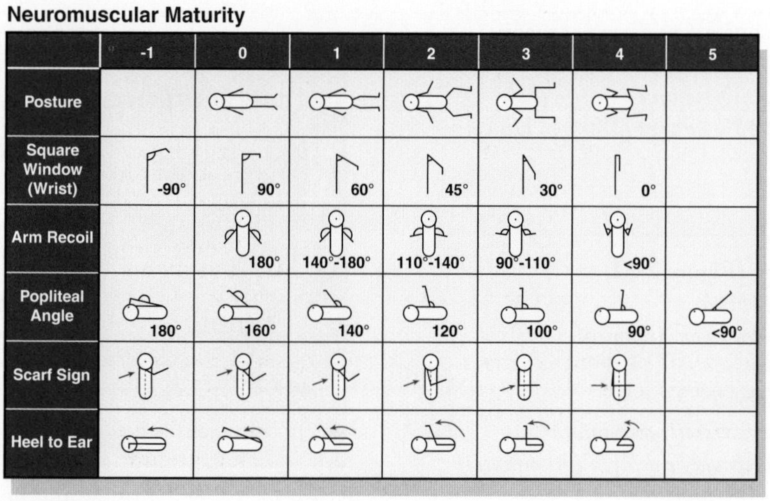

Neuromuscular Maturity

	-1	0	1	2	3	4	5
Posture							
Square Window (Wrist)	-90°	90°	60°	45°	30°	0°	
Arm Recoil		180°	140°-180°	110°-140°	90°-110°	<90°	
Popliteal Angle	180°	160°	140°	120°	100°	90°	<90°
Scarf Sign							
Heel to Ear							

Continued

TABLE 7–8 BALLARD MATURATIONAL ASSESSMENT TOOL—cont'd

Physical Maturity

Skin	sticky friable transparent	gelatinous red translucent	smooth pink visible veins	superficial peeling or rash, few veins	cracking pale areas rare veins	parchment deep cracking no vessels	leathery cracked wrinkled
Lanugo	none	sparse	abundant	thinning	bald areas	mostly bald	
Plantar Surface	heel-toe 40–50 mm:-1 <40 mm:-2	>50 mm no crease	faint red marks	anterior transverse crease only	creases ant. 2/3	creases over entire sole	
Breast	imperceptible	barely perceptible	flat areola no bud	stippled areola 1–2 mm bud	raised areola 3–4 mm bud	full areola 5–10 mm bud	
Eye/ear	lids fused loosely:-1 tightly:-2	lids open pinna flat stays folded	sl. curved pinna; soft; slow recoil	well-curved pinna; soft but ready recoil	formed and firm instant recoil	thick cartilage ear stiff	
Genitals (Male)	scrotum flat, smooth	scrotum empty faint rugae	testes in upper canal rare rugae	testes descending few rugae	testes down good rugae	testes pendulous deep rugae	
Genitals (Female)	clitoris prominent labia flat	prominent clitoris small labia minora	prominent clitoris enlarging minora	majora and minora equally prominent	majora large minora small	majora cover clitoris and minora	

Maturity Rating

Score	Weeks
−10	20
−5	22
0	24
5	26
10	28
15	30
20	32
25	34
30	36
35	38
40	40
45	42
50	44

From Chapman, L., & Durham, R. (2010). *Maternal-newborn nursing: Critical components of nursing care* (p. 300). Philadelphia: F.A. Davis.

    - Heel to ear—with the hips on the bed, how far the baby's feet can be moved toward the ear
  - *Physical maturity*
    - Skin—dryness, peeling, moisture
    - Lanugo—presence or absence
    - Plantar surfaces—presence or absence and their depth
    - Breasts (normal 3 to 10 mm, nipples prominent)
    - Ear/eyes—open or fused, amount of cartilage in the pinna
    - Genitalia—size of clitoris, labia minor, and labia majora
  - *Scores for these provide a gestational age based on weight, length, and head circumference. Term infants have higher scores than premature infants.*
- *Viability* is a term used to determine the rate of survival.
  - *Less than 22 weeks' gestation considered not viable*
  - *At 23 weeks' gestation, only 10% survive*
  - *At 24 weeks' gestation, 33% survive*
  - *At 25 weeks' gestation, 58% survive (Ward & Hisley, 2009)*

Periods of Reactivity

- Initial period of reactivity (**Figure 7-12**)
  - *Initial 30 minutes after birth*
  - *Active and very interested in environment*
  - *Bursts of eye movements*
  - *Responds to external stimuli*
  - *Excellent bonding time for family and infant*
  - *Eyedrops and ointment should be delayed (30 minutes) until family has made eye contact*
  - *Excellent time for breastfeeding*
  - *Heart rate, respiratory rate, and mucous production increase*
  - *Brief periods of tachypnea, tachycardia, apnea, cyanosis*
- Period of relative inactivity
  - *Begins 30 minutes to 2 hours after birth*
  - *Infant very sleepy and unresponsive to stimuli in the environment*
  - *Difficult periods for feeding*
  - *Heart rate, respiratory rate, and mucous production decrease*
- Second period of reactivity
  - *Begins 2 to 8 hours after birth*
  - *Alert and responsive*
  - *Heart rate and respiratory rate increase*
  - *Increased stooling*
  - *Increased muscle tone*

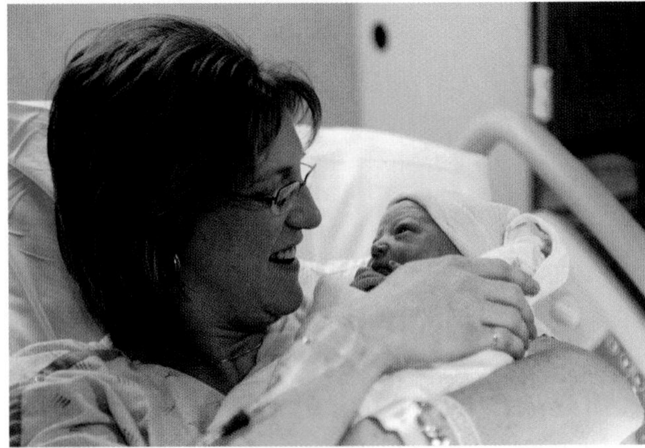

Figure 7–12 The mother and her newborn become acquainted during the first period of reactivity.

Weight

- Average birth weight: 7.5 pounds
- Appropriate for gestational age (AGA): between the 10th and 90th percentiles
- Small for gestational age (SGA): below the 10th percentile
- Large for gestational age (LGA): above the 90th percentile
- Low birth weight (LBW): 2500 grams or less (6 lb)
- Very low birth weight (VLBW): 1500 grams or less (3.5lb)
- Intrauterine growth restriction (IUGR)—growth of the fetus does not meet expected norms for gestational age.
- Large body surface area in comparison to total weight for infants

Height

- The National Center for Health Statistics has developed growth charts that are used to compare a child's measurements with those of other children the same age (**Figures 7-13** and **7-14**; Centers for Disease Control and Prevention [CDC], 2009).
- Average length is 20 inches long.
- The best predictor of adult height is family history.

Head Circumference

- Head and chest circumference are usually equal, with chest slightly smaller, usually 1 to 2 cm less than head (**Figures 7-15** and **7-16**).
- If the head is smaller than the chest, consider **microcephaly**, or small head.

ANTICIPATORY GUIDANCE

- Psychological preparation of a caregiver is necessary to alleviate fears and anxiety in the care of the infant.
  - *Caregivers must first understand the developmental milestones.*
  - *Educate caregivers on healthy and safe habits related to injury and illness prevention and childproofing their home.*
  - *Explain nutrition.*
  - *Explain oral health.*
  - *Discuss family relationships and the understanding that all relationships will change.*
  - *Explain infant care.*
  - *Discuss parent–infant interactions, including playing, cuddling, and separation anxiety.*

DEVELOPMENTAL MILESTONES

- Birth to 3 months
  - *Weight—gains 5 to 7 ounces weekly during the first month and then 1 to 2 pounds per month*
  - *Feeding—breastfed every 2 to 3 hours, formula fed every 4 hours*
  - *Height—grows 1 inch per month for first 6 months of life*
  - *Head circumference—grows ½ inch per month for first 6 months of life*
  - *Motor skills—wobbly at first, but begins to be able to lift head when on his or her abdomen. Grasps an object, kicks vigorously, and turns head from side to side. Infants need to have the head and neck supported. They can get their hands and thumbs to their mouths.*
  - *Reflexes—primitive reflexes remain.*
  - *Hearing—should respond to parent's voice and respond to loud noises by blinking, startling, frowning, or waking from light sleep*
  - *Vision—most newborns focus best on objects about 8 to 10 inches away, or the distance to your face during a feeding; acuity is 20/100; they begin to recognize mother visually. Are able to track objects visually with more accuracy*
  - *Communication—sensitive to the way they are held, rocked, and fed. By age 2 months, the infant may smile on purpose, blow bubbles, and coo when talked to. At 3 months the infant may laugh out loud, express moods.*

Clinical Reasoning

Anticipatory Guidance Regarding Breastfeeding

The Jones family had a baby girl 3 months ago. Mrs. Jones has been breastfeeding her little girl exclusively since birth, and both are satisfied with the breastfeeding process. Mrs. Jones, however, feels trapped in her home, and her little girl cries and will not eat for anyone else in the family. Mr. and Mrs. Jones want to be able to go out together for dinner and a movie, and the baby's grandma is a willing babysitter, but Mrs. Jones is feeling guilty because her baby will not eat for anyone else.

1. What anticipatory guidance can the nurse provide to the Jones family regarding the developmental stage of their baby daughter?
2. What information can the nurse provide to the Jones family in regard to making the transition to being able to go out for dinner and a movie?
3. What anticipatory guidance can the nurse provide to Mrs. Jones about her relationship with her daughter and her husband?

- Three to 6 months
  - *Birth weight doubles by 6 months of age.*
  - *Height increases 1 inch per month for first 6 months.*
  - *Can raise head (see **Figure 7-17**)*
  - *Reaches and grasps objects, plays with hands, moves objects to mouth, plays with toes*
  - *Rolls from abdomen to back*
  - *More stabilized sleeping patterns at 3 months*
  - *Opens mouth for spoon*
  - *Binocular vision—ability to see with both eyes coordinated*
  - *Primitive reflexes begin to disappear, such as Moro, grasp, and tonic neck reflexes.*
  - *Begins to drool, chew on toys as teething begins (6 months)*
  - *Can sit when propped at 6 months (see **Figure 7-18**)*
  - *Can support some weight when held in a standing position*

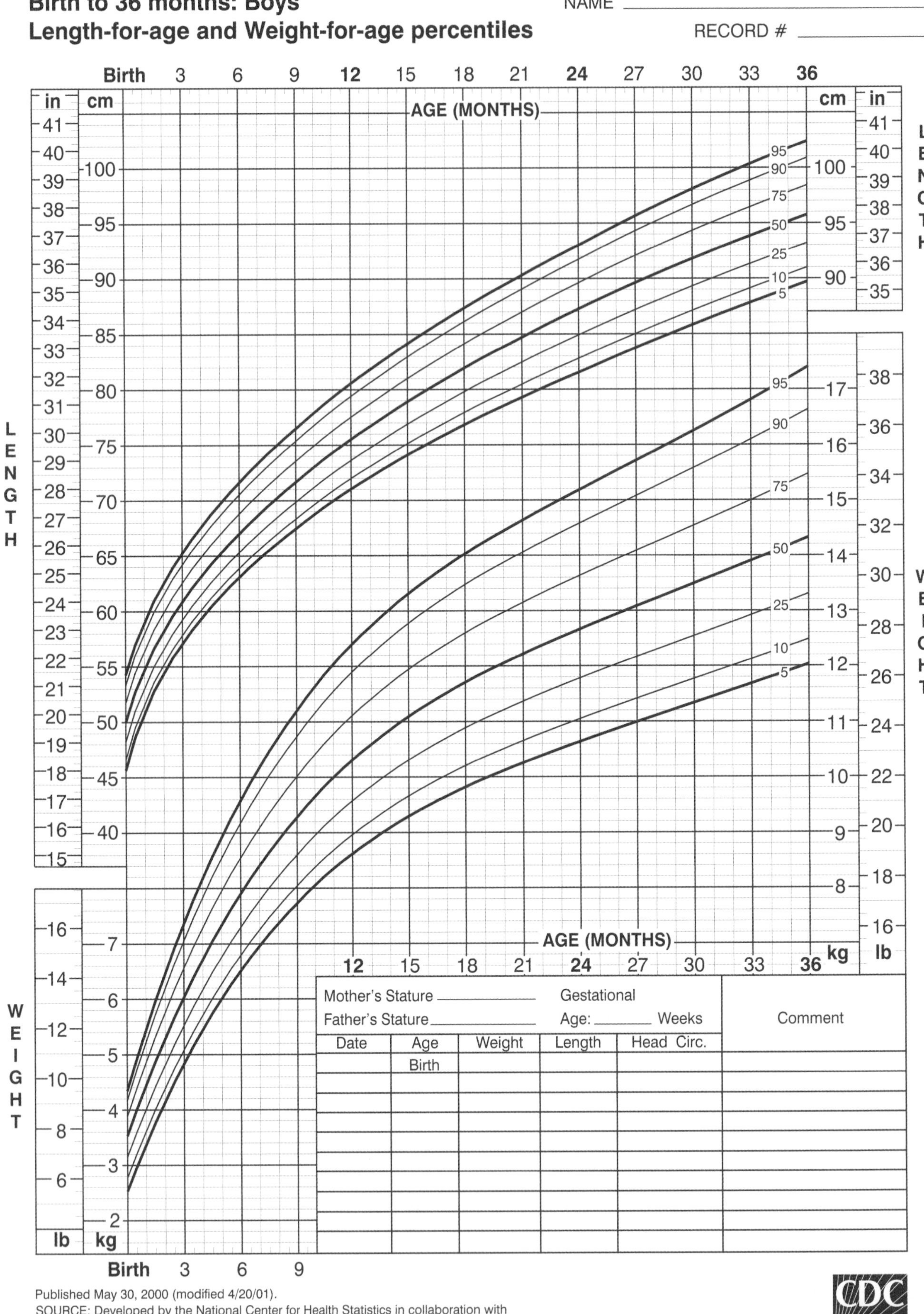

Figure 7–13 Chart of height/weight growth for boys, birth to 36 months. *(From the Centers for Disease Control and Prevention. Developed by the National Center for Health Statistics in collaboration with the National Center for Chronic Disease Prevention and Health Promotion, published May 30, 2000, modified April 20, 2001, http://www.cdc.gov/growthcharts.)*

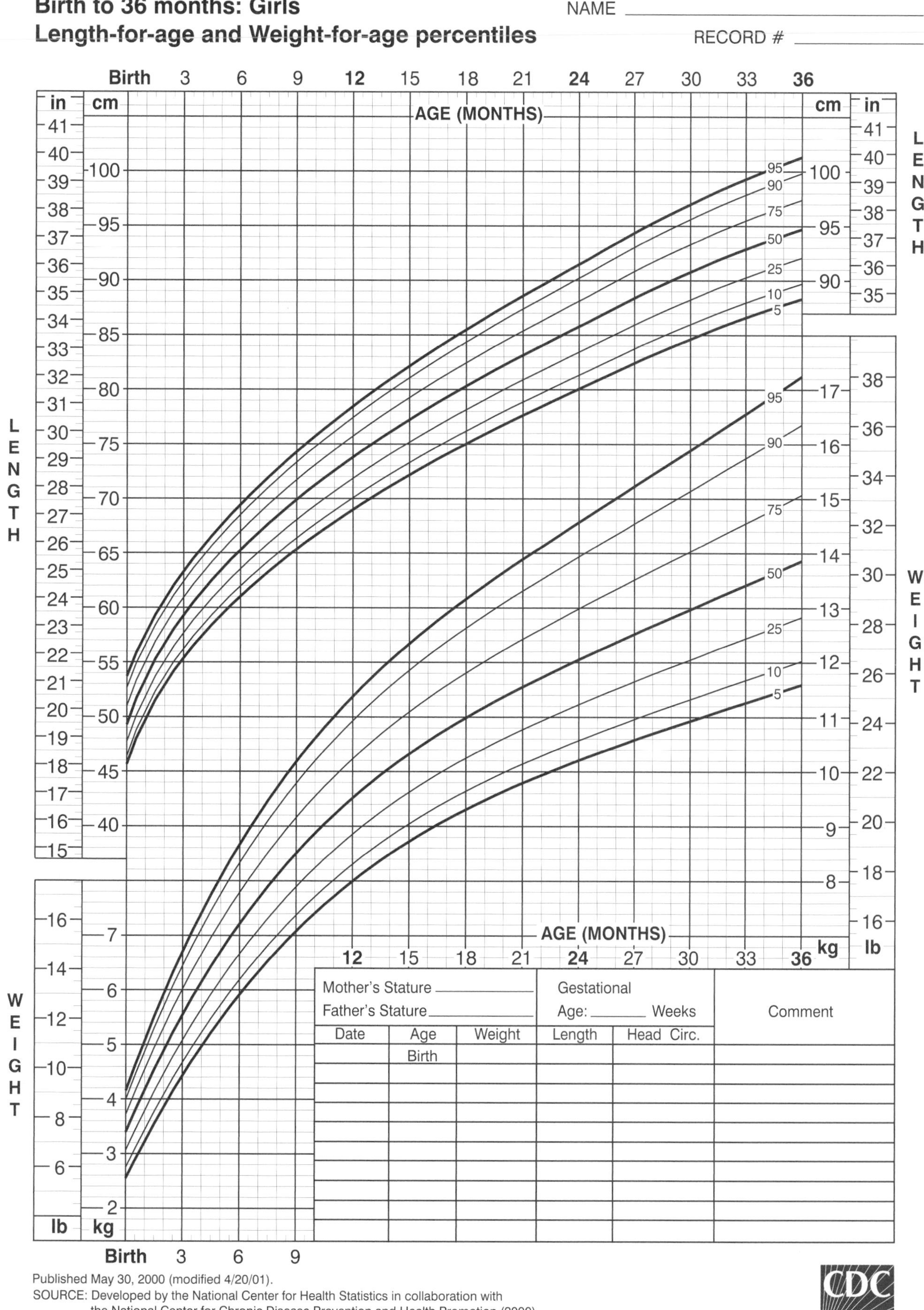

Figure 7–14 Chart of height/weight growth for girls, birth to 36 months. *(From the Centers for Disease Control and Prevention. Developed by the National Center for Health Statistics in collaboration with the National Center for Chronic Disease Prevention and Health Promotion, published May 30, 2000, modified April 20, 2001, http://www.cdc.gov/growthcharts.)*

Birth to 36 months: Girls
Head circumference-for-age and Weight-for-length percentiles

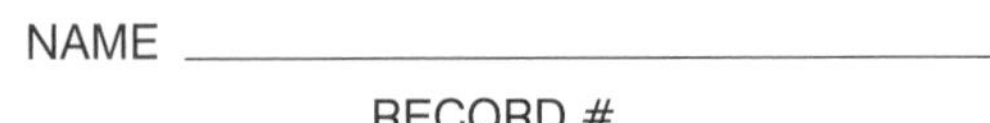

Date	Age	Weight	Length	Head Circ.	Comment

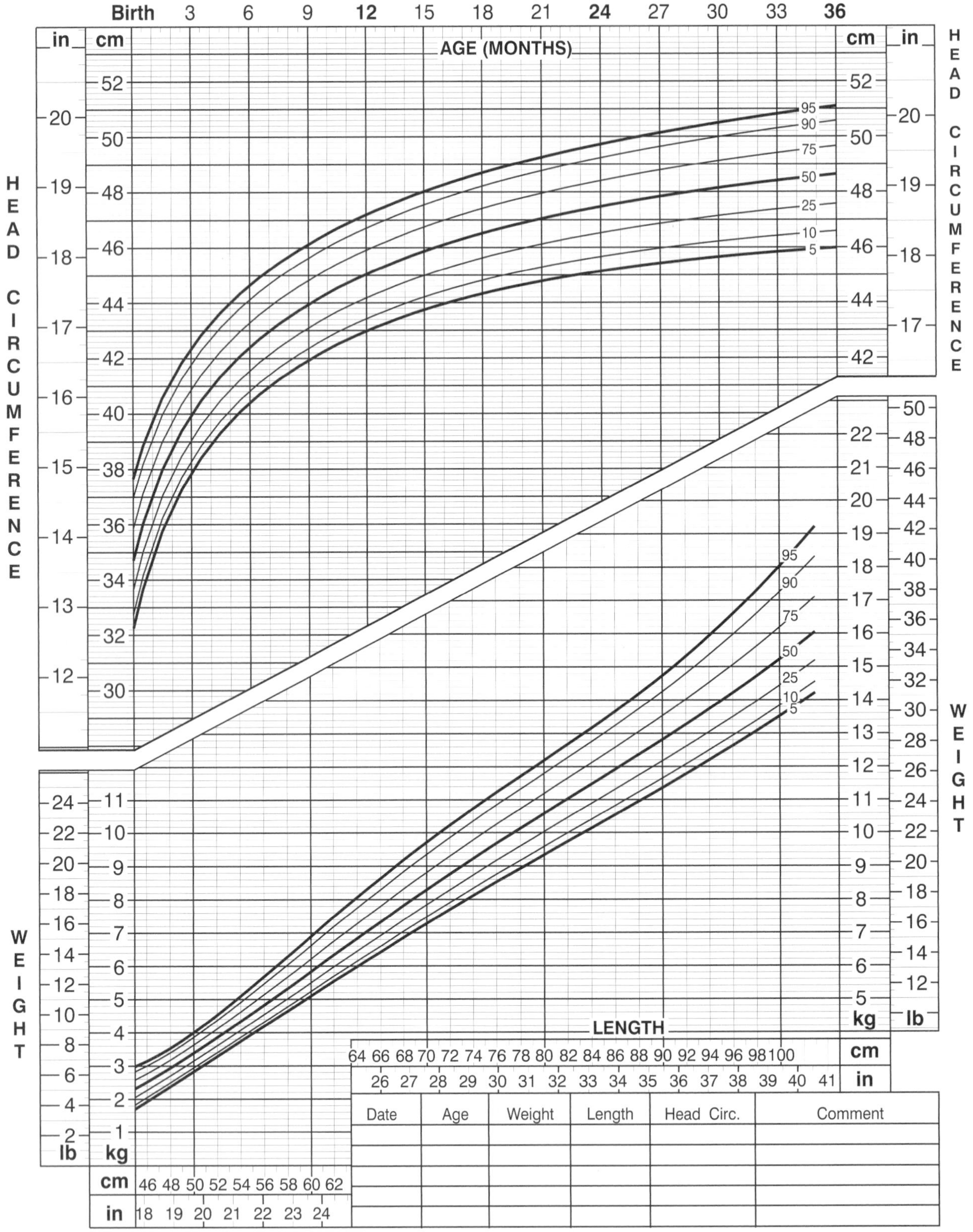

Published May 30, 2000 (modified 10/16/00).
SOURCE: Developed by the National Center for Health Statistics in collaboration with the National Center for Chronic Disease Prevention and Health Promotion (2000).
http://www.cdc.gov/growthcharts

CDC
SAFER • HEALTHIER • PEOPLE™

Figure 7–15 Chart of head circumference for girls, birth to 36 months. *(From the Centers for Disease Control and Prevention. Developed by the National Center for Health Statistics in collaboration with the National Center for Chronic Disease Prevention and Health Promotion, published May 30, 2000, modified October 16, 2000, http://www.cdc.gov/growthcharts.)*

Birth to 36 months: Boys
Head circumference-for-age and Weight-for-length percentiles

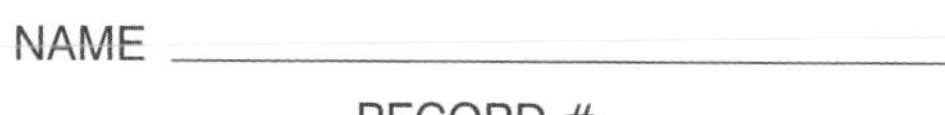

Date	Age	Weight	Length	Head Circ.	Comment

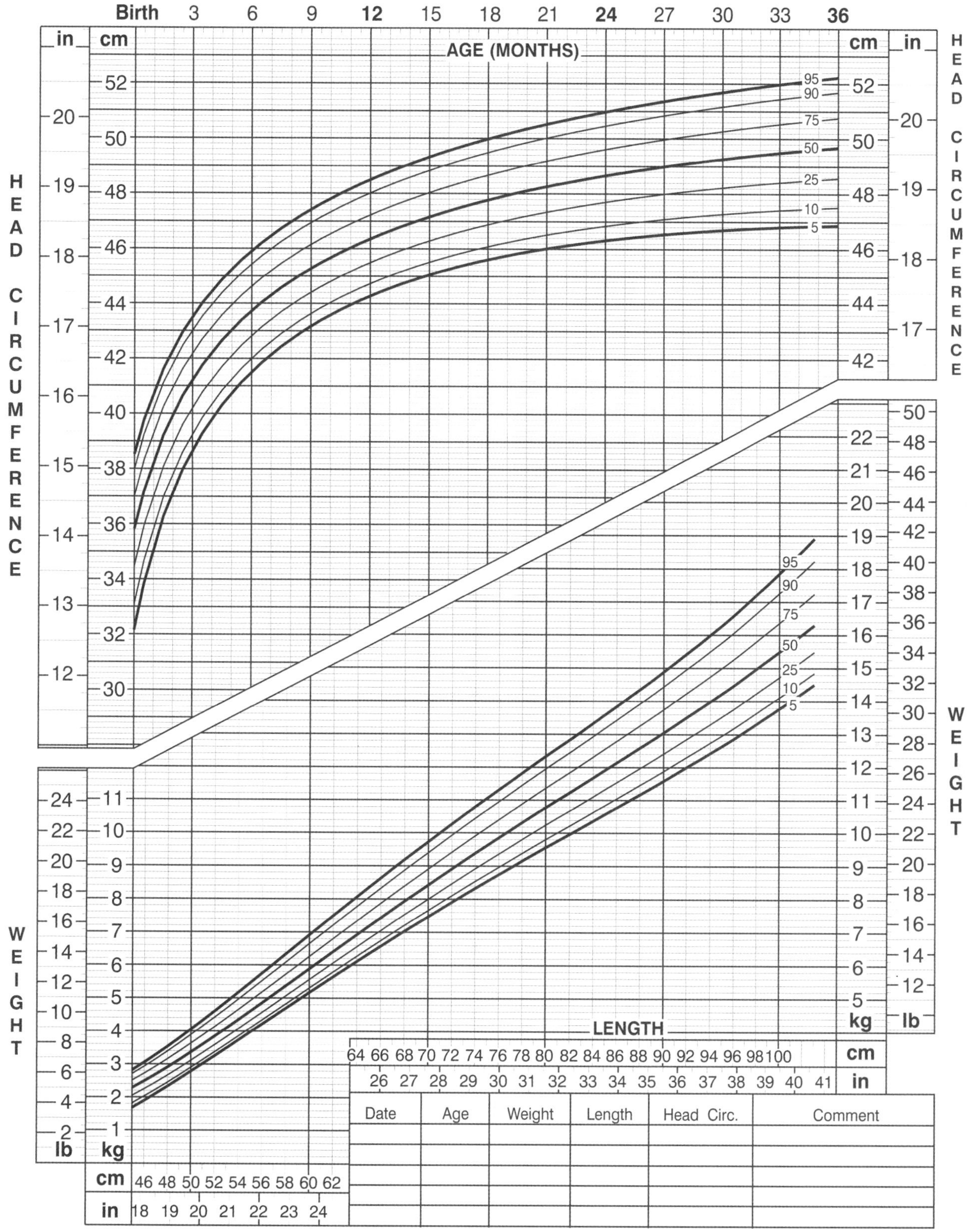

Published May 30, 2000 (modified 10/16/00).
SOURCE: Developed by the National Center for Health Statistics in collaboration with the National Center for Chronic Disease Prevention and Health Promotion (2000).
http://www.cdc.gov/growthcharts

CDC
SAFER • HEALTHIER • PEOPLE™

Figure 7–16 Chart of head circumference for boys, birth to 36 months. *(From the Centers for Disease Control and Prevention. Developed by the National Center for Health Statistics in collaboration with the National Center for Chronic Disease Prevention and Health Promotion, published May 30, 2000, modified October 16, 2000, http://www.cdc.gov/growthcharts.)*

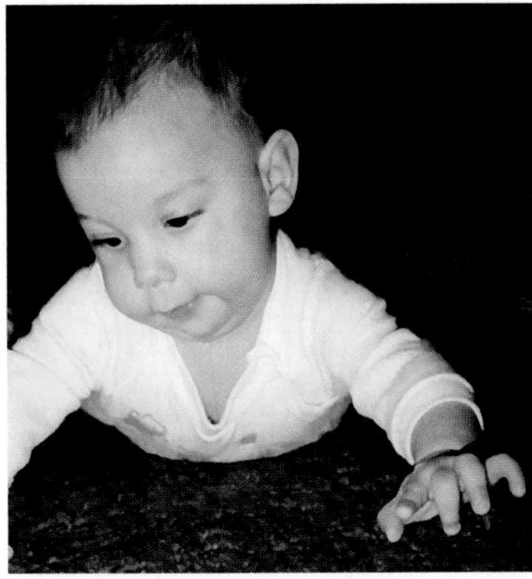

Figure 7-17 Infant lifting head up.

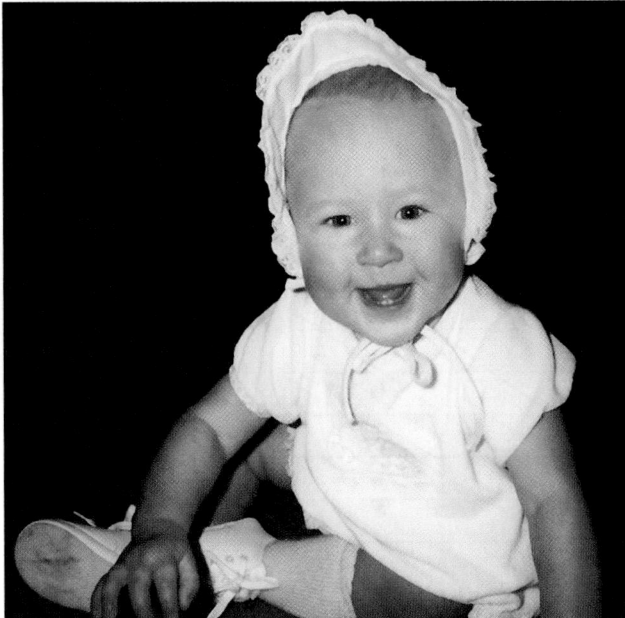

Figure 7-18 Infant sitting up.

- *Coordinated eye movements*
- *Recognizes familiar objects and people, expresses displeasure when those objects or people are removed, babbles to self*

- Six to 9 Months
  - *All infants should be screened for developmental delays and disabilities at 9 months at the well-child visit (AAP, 2006c).*
  - *Rolls from back to stomach and stomach to back*
  - *Transfers objects from hand to hand, points at objects, and picks them up at 9 months*
  - *Fine motor skills*
  - *Puts feet in mouth, plays pat-a-cake, loves to see own image in a mirror*
  - *Taste preferences*
  - *Begins to understand differences between inanimate and animate objects*
  - *Stranger anxiety*
  - *Vocalizes with many-syllable vowel sounds and m-m with crying*
  - *Around 9 months, says Dada and Mama and understands bye-bye and no*
  - *Around 8 to 9 months begins to pull to stand, develops pincer grasp, crawls backward and then forward, and responds to own name (see* ***Figure 7-19****).*
  - *Understands where to look for an object that has been dropped; practices grasp–release movements*
  - *Begins to test parent's responses, such as watching the parent while dropping food on the floor*
  - *Distinguishes colors*
  - *Distance vision*
  - *Expresses emotions—frustration and anger*
- Nine to 12 Months
  - *Birth weight triples.*
  - *Birth length increases by 50%.*
  - *Head and chest circumference are equal.*
  - *Total of 6 to 8 teeth*
  - *Knows name*
  - *Creeps along furniture*
  - *Drinks from a cup; should be weaned from a bottle*
  - *Stands alone for brief periods of time; raises arms when wants to be picked up*
  - *May take first steps or walk alone*
  - *Eats with spoon and cup but prefers fingers*
  - *Enjoys familiar surroundings and people, expresses dissatisfaction with strangers or strange surroundings (stranger anxiety)*
  - *May develop security objects such as favorite toys, blankets*
  - *Enjoys books, especially board books*

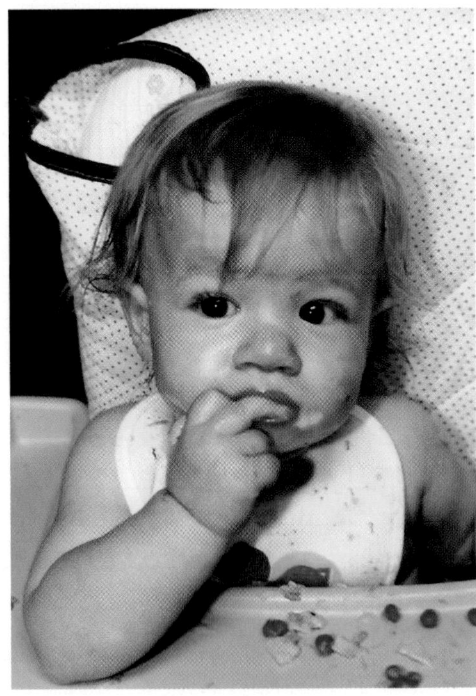

Figure 7-19 Infant with pincer grasp.

- *Can understand simple communication or direction; says two or three words beyond Dada and Mama*
- *One or both feet may slightly turn in; the infant's lower legs are normally bowed.*
- *At around 12 months of age can transition to whole cow's milk; do not use 1% or 2%, as the infant needs the fat content for continuing brain development*

COGNITIVE DEVELOPMENT

- Primitive reflexes are controlled by lower brain functions at birth, which quickly disappear.
- Intellectual growth begins at birth and focuses on memory, problem solving, exploration of the environment, and understanding concepts.
- Cognitive development involves the infant's processing of information, conceptual processes, intelligence, language development, memory, and perceptual skills.
- Cognitive development varies greatly from month to month and develops at a fast rate.
- Infants learn through a cultural context in their development.
- Infants develop on all levels and are influenced by neurological development and experience with others.
- The Brazelton Neonatal Behavioral Assessment Scale tests an infant's neurological development, behavior, and responsiveness. It is utilized only in the neonatal period.
- The Gesell Developmental Schedules test for fine and gross motor skills, language, eye–hand coordination, imitation, object recovery, personal-social behavior, and play response.
- The Denver Developmental Screening Test is used to identify problems or delays. It measures personal/social, fine and gross motor, language, and social skills.
- The Bayley Scales of Infant Development (BSID) test the cognitive, behavioral, and motor domains of the infant. The assessment is used to assist in identifying infants with developmental disabilities. It is a highly reliable tool that utilizes mental, motor, and behavioral scales to rate an infant's functioning. The mental test screens for such items as whether the infant turns to a sound or looks for a fallen object. The motor test screens for gross and fine motor skill development.

Developmental Theorists

- Piaget (theory of cognitive development): in sensorimotor stage, infants use five senses to explore their world; theory includes six substages that describe the infant's mental representation (see Chapter 6). Infants learn about their environment through their senses and begin to engage in goal-directed behaviors (Ward & Hisley, 2009).
- Vygotsky (social context of cognitive development): describes how complex mental functioning originates in infants through social interactions. Cultural factors influence attainment. There is a close correlation between language acquisition and the development of thinking (see Chapter 6).
- Erikson (social development): highlights trust versus mistrust as the first psychosocial stage during the first year of life. This theory explains how the infant's personality develops.
    - *Trust requires a feeling of physical comfort and a minimal amount of fear and apprehension about the future. It is a time where the infant has certain expectations about the predictability of the environment. If this stage is not attained, the infant feels insecure and learns mistrust (see Chapter 6).*
    - *Trust in infancy provides lifelong expectation that the world will be a good and pleasant place to live.*
- Mahler (social development): describes how an infant develops a sense of self through symbiosis and separation, or individualism (see Chapter 6).
- Kohlberg (moral development): describes that moral reasoning aids in the development of ethical behavior and proceeds through six stages (see Chapter 6).

Sensory Development

- Vision—least developed sense; attracted to bright colors, black and white because of limited vision; objects are seen as two-dimensional with poor peripheral vision until 2 to 3 months of age
- Smell—well-developed sense; especially recognizes smell of own mother (Schaal, Hummel & Soussignan, 2004)

Evidence-Based Practice: Soothing Odors

Laudert, S., Liu, W. F., Blackington, S., Perkins, S., Martin, S., MacMillan-York, E., Handyside, J. (2007). Implementing potentially better practices to support the neurodevelopment of infants in the NICU. *Journal of Perinatology, 27,* S75–S93. doi: 10.1038/sj.jp.7211843

Studies have shown that biologically meaningful odors such as amniotic fluid, colostrum, and breast milk are soothing to infants, particularly when obtained from the infant's own mother (Laudert et al., 2007).

- Taste—well-developed sense; sweet tastes are preferred
- Hearing—can hear inside womb and can identify mother's voice
- Hearing—differentiates between male and female voices, recognizes mom's voice, important for language development
- Hearing test is administered prior to discharge, either through otoacoustic (OAC) emissions or auditory brainstem response (ABR) (**Figure 7-20**).
    - *Thirty-six states, including Puerto Rico, Guam, and the District of Columbia, require hearing screening for newborns.*
    - *Tests are noninvasive, conducted prior to discharge by a trained professional, and performed in a quiet environment. Vernix, other fluids, and a withdrawing infant may affect the test.*

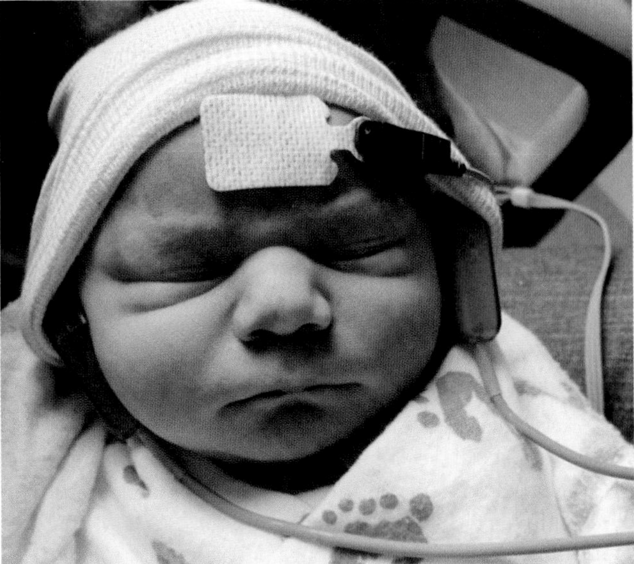

Figure 7–20 Neonatal hearing screening.

CLINICAL PEARL

Hearing Screening at Birth

The U.S. Preventative Task Force, the Centers for Disease Control and Prevention, and the American Academy of Pediatrics recommend that all newborn infants undergo screening at birth (Harlor & Bower, 2009). Some degree of hearing loss occurs in 1 to 6 out of 1000 infants (Bachmann & Arvedson, 1998).

- *ABR is a physiological measurement of the brainstem's response to sound. A clicking sound is produced, and the electrical activity response from the nerve is recorded as waveforms on a computer. This noninvasive test requires electrodes to be placed on the infant's scalp with adhesive and is conducted while the infant is sleeping.(Chapman & Durham, 2010)*
- *The OAC emissions method utilizes an earplug that tests and measures the responses of the cochlea to clicking sounds produced by a microphone. The infant is sleeping during the test. It is a noninvasive procedure.*

- Examination of the ears of an infant: pull the pinnae straight back and down.
- Communications have been found to be similar in different cultures, with a higher-pitched voice being used when attempting to get the infant's attention; deaf mothers utilize a slower pattern and sign more often.
- Touch—gentle touch or massage is calming and pleasurable.
- Touch is extremely important.
- Pain is a protective device; the infant responds by extending and retracting the extremities and crying.

Language Acquisition

- Language acquisition is a partly innate and partly learned process.
- Early speech is evidenced by crying, babbling, and mimicking of repetitive vowel sounds such as *ma-ma-ma* and *da-da-da*.
- Single words are then used and accumulated into the infant's vocabulary.
- Children interact with other people and the environment.
- Favorable responses to speech encourage the infant to communicate.
- Linguist Norm Chomsky (nativist theory) describes the infant's acquisition of language as complex and not well understood; he coined the term *language acquisition device*.
- Vygotsky proposed the interactionist theory of language acquisition, which states that language is learned through socialization within the family context.

Discipline

- You cannot spoil an infant.
- At 6 months of age, when the child is more mobile, use distraction to keep the child away from dangerous areas.
- Set limits.
- Temper tantrums are the infant's way of expressing frustration, hunger, anger, illness, or fatigue.
- Reward good behavior.
- Remain calm, firm, and consistent.
- Maintain a set routine.

Promoting Safety

Corporal punishment, such as spanking or hitting, of children has been found to have negative consequences and to be no more effective than other forms of discipline, such as the withdrawal of positive reinforcement (withdrawal of privileges, time outs). Spanking has been associated with a higher incidence of aggressive behavior in children, increased substance abuse, and higher rates of crime and violence in older children (American Academy of Pediatrics, Committee on Psychosocial Aspects of Child and Family Health, 1998; Straus, 2005).

Clinical Reasoning

Anticipatory Guidance for Temper Tantrums

At a well-child appointment, the nurse is taking a history of 9-month-old Johnny, who is accompanied by his mother and one older sibling. During data collection, Johnny is trying to get down from his mother's lap and begins to throw a temper tantrum. Johnny's mother becomes very frustrated and embarrassed. She lets Johnny first sit on the floor, then yanks him up on her lap, cursing under her breath and saying, "Why are you doing this to me?" As a nurse, you understand that you have some caregiver education to perform.

1. What anticipatory guidance can the nurse provide to Johnny's mother in regard to Johnny's development?
2. What anticipatory guidance can the nurse provide in regard to discipline for a 9-month-old?
3. What anticipatory guidance can the nurse provide to Johnny's mother related to her frustration in caring for Johnny and his sibling?

Colic

> **CLINICAL PEARL**
>
> **Diagnostic Criteria for Infant Colic**
>
> - Paroxysms of irritability, fussing, or crying that start or stop without obvious cause
> - Episodes lasting 3 hours or more, occurring 3 days a week, lasting longer than a week
> - Infant thriving (Hyman et al., 2006)

- Make sure the infant is burped frequently.
- Usually no medical problem is present, but the infant should be assessed by a pediatrician if it continues.
- Some infants experience a great deal of intestinal gas.
- Colic usually happens at the end of the day.
- Infants tend to be sensitive to stimulation.
- A car ride and movement can soothe an infant.
- Infant massage may help.
- Infant carriers that are positioned on the parent's chest, back, or side can soothe a colicky baby (Garrison & Christakis, 2000)
- Create a white noise environment—turn on a fan in the room (not blowing on the infant).
- If a pacifier is used, it can help calm the infant; pacifiers have been shown to decrease the incidence of sudden infant death syndrome.
- Colic usually disappears by about 6 to 12 weeks of age.

> **CLINICAL PEARL**
>
> **Care of the Infant with Colic**
>
> - Swaddle infant.
> - Place in a safe area.
> - Remove yourself from the infant for a 10-minute break once the child is secured in a safe place.
> - Educate caregivers that colic is not a reflection of their caregiving skills.
> - Realize that it is a heightened time of stress for caregivers.
> - Simethicone drops have been prescribed to ease intestinal gas, but never give an infant an over-the-counter medication without consulting the child's pediatrician.

Play

- Play is how infants learn about the world and themselves.
- Safety is the number one consideration.
- Infants are primarily sensorimotor-focused, so play involves sensory stimulation.
- Simple toys should be used because attention span is short. These include unbreakable mirrors, rattles, soft (nonremovable pieces) stuffed animals, large snap toys, and musical pull toys.
- Place infants on their stomachs for supervised tummy time.
- Engage the infant with soothing tones and use of facial expressions.
- Use soothing music.
- Avoid detachable or removable pieces or parts.
- Infants explore and imitate.
- Infants explore the world with their mouths; everything goes into their mouths.
- If other siblings' toys are lying around, safety for the infant requires the caregiver to be aware of small pieces.
- Toys should help the infant in physical and fine motor development.
- Infants enjoy looking at themselves in mirrors.
- Infants enjoy toys with bright colors, simple designs, dangling objects, and human faces, as well as manipulative toys such as discs, keys on a ring, squeeze toys, and rattles.
- Play is essential in a hospitalized environment.
- The theorist Watson described the importance of positive play in fostering attachment between the infant and the caregiver. See Chapter 6 for further details.

NUTRITION

- Physical and psychosocial needs change rapidly.
- Two choices for newborns to infants 6 months of age: breastfeeding or bottle-feeding a commercially prepared formula. Because of the infant's developmental stage, he or she will push solids forward and out of the mouth.
- Decision to breastfeed versus bottle feed is dependent on maternal knowledge, past exposure to breastfeeding, educational level, perceptions of the benefits of breastfeeding, cultural factors, family and friend support, career barriers, husband or partner support, and support from health-care providers.
- The World Health Organization recommends exclusive breastfeeding until the age of 6 months, with no supplementation of water, formula, or solids prior to this point (World Health Organization Position Statement, 2011).
- Sufficient protein is needed to support growth and development.
- Fats are needed to provide calories and support brain development.
- Carbohydrates are needed to provide energy.
- Infants need 100 to 116 kcal/kg/day for basic growth and development.
- Adequate fluid and electrolyte intake is necessary.
- Fluids, mainly water, should total 140 to 160 mL/kg/day for infants.
- Supplemental iron is not necessary for breastfed infants prior to 6 months of age.
- All infants 6 months or older require iron supplementation. Iron can be supplied through lean red meats, fortified infant cereals, dried fruit, and tofu.
- Do not feed cow's milk until after 1 year of age.
- Soy formula is utilized for galactosemia, lactose intolerance, and allergies to cow's milk.

CLINICAL PEARL

Soy Protein–Based Formula

Isolated soy protein-based formulas are safe and effective for normal growth and development of infants but are not to be used for preterm infants. Soy protein-based formulas have no advantage in the prevention of colic or as a supplement for breastfed infants (American Academy of Pediatrics, Committee on Nutrition, 1998).

Nonnutritive Sucking

- The infant's sucking ability is necessary for neurological development and survival.
- Nonnutritive sucking is a self-soothing or comforting measure utilized by infants.
- Pacifiers, fingers, or fists are used in self-sucking.
- Suckling, which the infant does at the breast, requires a different set of mouth movements than does bottle feeding or the use of fingers, fists, or a pacifier.
- Avoid using pacifiers in the early days of breastfeeding.
- Educate caregivers on the use of a pacifier, such as not using it as a substitute for feeding or holding.
- Never tie or clip the pacifier to the child's clothing, becausae this can be a source of strangulation, even in older infants.
- Limit the use of the pacifier as the infant gets older to prevent prolongation of a habit that will be difficult to break; distract the infant with an alternative.

Breastfeeding

- This is the optimal method of feeding because it provides all necessary nutrients, minerals, and vitamin (**Table 7-9**).
- Should be begun within the first hour after birth during the initial period of reactivity
- Should be on demand throughout the day and night
- Reduces costs and preparation time
- Promotes positive bonding between infant and mother
- Decreases risk of obesity

Composition of Breast Milk

- Breast milk development begins early in pregnancy through the hormones of estrogen, progesterone, and prolactin.
- It is high in immunoglobulins A and G and contains higher levels of a protein with a laxative effect that aids in the passage of meconium. No immunoglobulins are found in formulas.
- Concentration of nutrients differ between women.
- Rare to have an infant have an allergic response to breast milk
- Components of breast milk
- Large water content; fat content accounts for 52% (Chapman & Durham, 2010)
- Carbohydrates (lactose, 37%)
- Protein, specifically whey (60% to 80%) and casein (20% to 40%)(Chapman & Durham, 2010)
- Antibodies, bifidus factor (which stimulates the growth of lactobacillus)

TABLE 7–9 SELECTED BENEFITS OF BREASTFEEDING

FOR MOTHERS
• Decreased risk of breast cancer
• Lactational amenorrhea (LAM) (although breastfeeding is not considered an effective form of contraception)
• Enhanced involution (due to uterine contractions triggered by the release of oxytocin) and decreased risk of postpartum hemorrhage
• Enhanced postpartum weight loss
• Increased bone density
• Enhanced bonding with infant
FOR INFANTS
• Enhanced immunity through the transfer of maternal antibodies; decreased incidence of infections, including otitis media, pneumonia, urinary tract infections, bacteremia, and bacterial meningitis
• Enhanced maturation of the gastrointestinal tract
• Decreased likelihood of developing insulin-dependent (type 1) diabetes
• Decreased risk of childhood obesity
• Enhanced jaw development
• Protective effects against certain childhood cancers

From Ward, S. L., & Hisley, S. M. (2009). *Maternal-child nursing care: Optimizing outcomes for mothers, children, & families* (p. 489). Philadelphia: F.A. Davis.

- Lipase, amylase, and other enzymes
- Also includes epidermal growth factor, nerve growth factor, other growth factors, and interleukins (Wagner, 2010)

Stages of Breast Milk

- Stage one—**colostrum**, a yellowish fluid that is the first fluid from the breast, is present in the first 2 to 3 days after birth.
- Stage two—the milk becomes transitional from 3 to 10 days after birth.
- Stage three—the mature milk begins after 10 days of birth. This mature milk has approximately 23 calories per ounce and is composed of foremilk and hind milk.
  - *Foremilk is the milk that is produced and released at the beginning of the feeding and has a higher water and lactose content and a lower fat content.*
  - *The hind milk is released at the end of the feeding and has a higher fat content.*

Lactation, the Production of Breast Milk

- Lactation is the process of milk production (**Figure 7-21**).
- Once the baby is born, the levels of estrogen and progesterone are eliminated and prolactin becomes the predominant hormone.

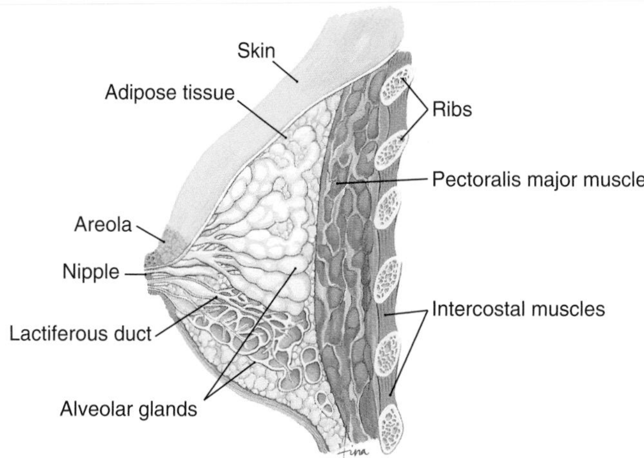

Figure 7-21 Mammary gland shown in midsagittal section.

- Infant stimulation influences supply and demand—as the infant demands, the woman's body supplies.
- Oxytocin is released from the posterior pituitary, which affects the breasts and the uterus. Oxytocin produces the **let-down reflex**, which forces milk into the lacteriferous ducts of the breast. The let-down reflex is responsible for milk ejection. This reflex can occur during sexual stimulation, when hearing a baby cry, or when thinking of the infant. It can be inhibited by stress, fatigue, and pain. (Chapman & Durham, 2010)
- Infant cues and readiness to breastfeed are important adaptations that mom and infant need to make to facilitate the supply and demand.
- Early clues
  - *Rooting*
  - *Head bobbing up and down*
  - *Stirring and increased arm and leg movement*
  - *Burying head in mattress or mom's chest*
- Late cues
  - *Crying—extended crying can inhibit latching onto the breast.*
  - *Agitation*
- See Figure 7-22 for breastfeeding positions
- Latching on
  - *If placed on the mom's abdomen, the infant at birth will make crawling movements to reach the breast (**Figure 7-22**).*
  - *Process of infant attaching to the breast for feeding—hold the breast like a sandwich with the thumb on the top and the other fingers underneath. The baby should be held close; as the baby's mouth is opened wide, place the breast fully (including the nipple and areola) into the baby's mouth (**Figure 7-23**).*
  - *Encourage the infant's mouth to open by stimulating the rooting reflex.*
  - *A successful latch is when the infant's mouth is around the areola with the nipple at the back of its mouth.*
  - *The infant draws the milk forward in the breast.*
  - *The tip of nose, cheeks, and chin should be touching the breast. Align the breast with the infant's nose.*

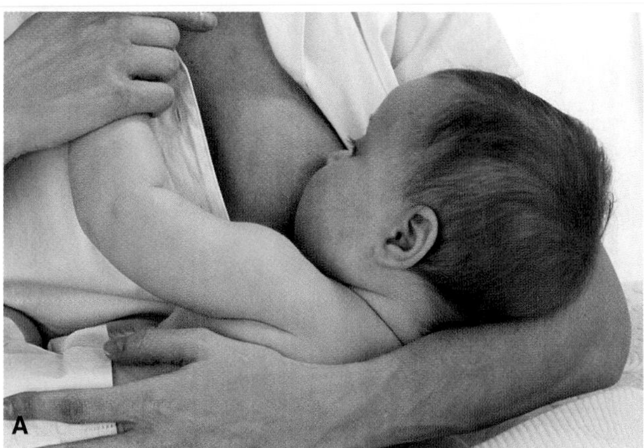

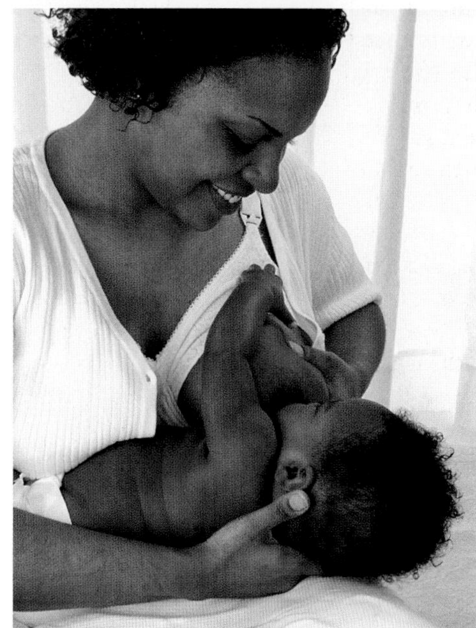

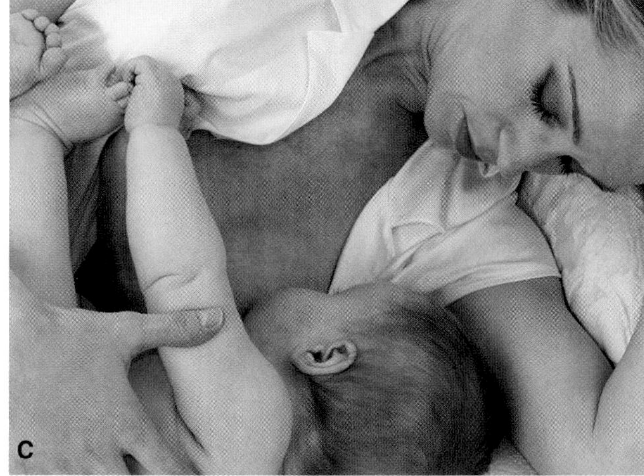

Figure 7-22 Common positions for breastfeeding. **A,** Cradle hold; **B,** football hold; **C,** side-lying position. *(Courtesy of Medela Corporation, McHenry, Illinois. © 2011)*

  - *Suck and swallow should follow.*
  - *Often infants will feed from only one breast at a time for each feeding.*
  - *Latch Scoring System (**Table 7-10**)*

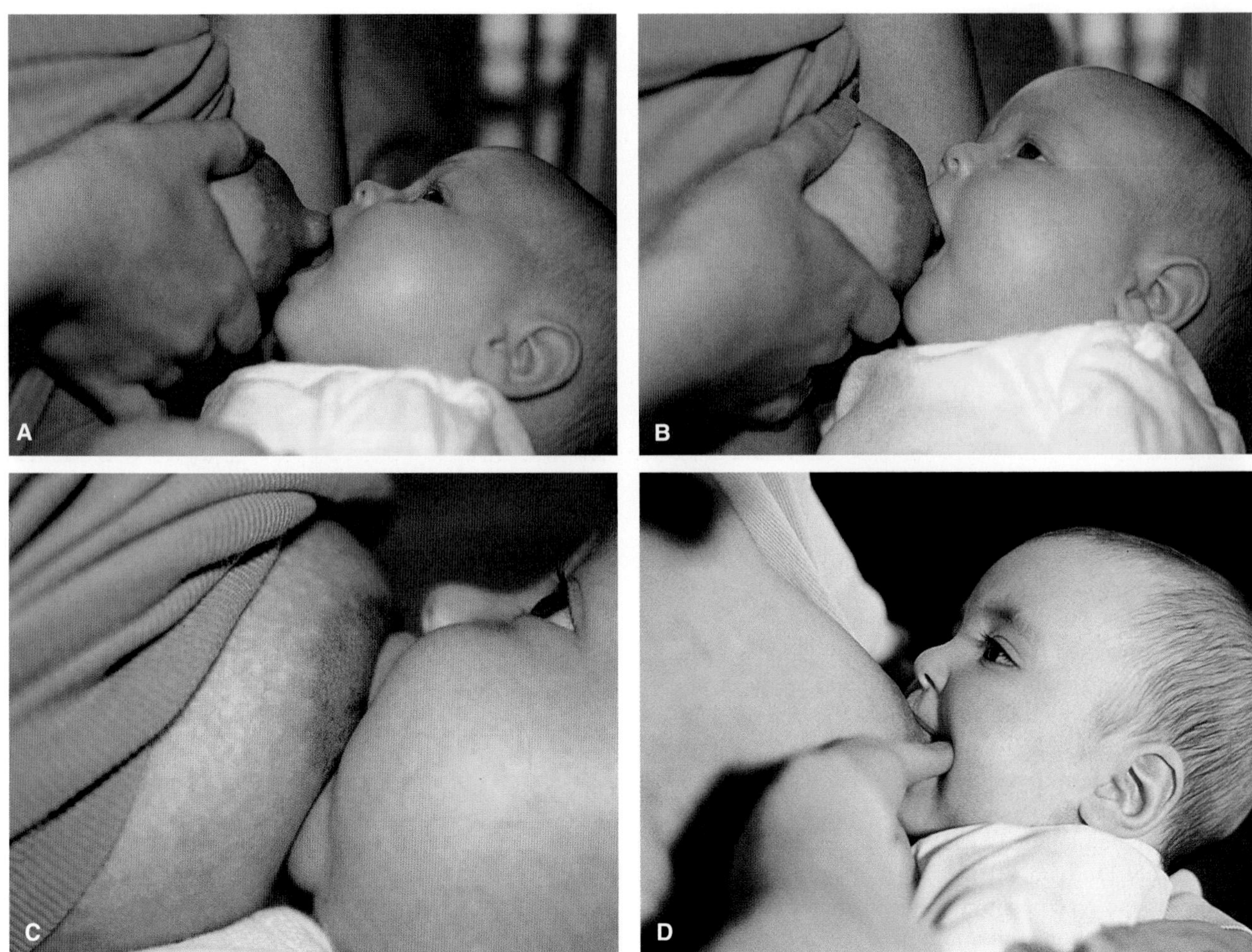

Figure 7–23 Infant latching on. *(Courtesy of Medela Corporation, McHenry, Illinois. © 2011)*

TABLE 7–10 LATCH SCORING SYSTEM

	0	1	2
L Latch	Too sleepy or reluctant No latch achieved	Repeated attempts Hold nipple in mouth Stimulate to suck	Grasps breast Tongue down Lips flanged Rhythmic sucking
A Audible swallowing	None	A few with stimulation	Spontaneous and intermittent <24 hours old Spontaneous and frequent >24 hours old
T Type of nipple	Inverted	Flat	Everted (after stimulation)
C Comfort (breast/nipple)	Engorged Cracked, bleeding, large blisters, or bruises Severe discomfort	Filling Reddened/small blisters or bruises Mild/moderate pain	Soft Tender

TABLE 7–10 LATCH SCORING SYSTEM—cont'd

	0	1	2
H Hold (positioning)	Full assist (staff holds infant at breast)	Minimal assist (i.e., elevate head of bed; place pillow for support) Teach one side; mother does the other side Staff holds and then mother takes over	No assist from staff Mother able to position/hold infant

From Chapman, L., & Durham, R. (2010). *Maternal-newborn nursing: Critical components of nursing care* (p. 320). Philadelphia: F.A. Davis, p. 320; original source from Jensen, D., Wallace, S., & Kelsay, P. (1994, January). LATCH: A breastfeeding charting system and documentation tool. *Journal of Obstetric, Gynecologic, and Neonatal Nursing, 23*(1), 27–32.

- Breastfeeding success
  - *Feedings should last between 10 and 30 minutes—shorter times may indicate poor positioning or a sleepy infant; longer times can indicate nonnutritive sucking.*
  - *Removing an infant from the breast is accomplished by inserting a clean finger into the corner of the infant's mouth to break the suction.*
  - *Successful breastfeeding results in the infant gaining ½ to 1 ounce per day (AAP, 2004).*
  - *Expressed breast milk may be kept for 4 hours at room temperature, for 5 to 7 days in the refrigerator, and for 6 to 12 months in a deep freezer.*
  - *Never reheat breast milk in a microwave or leave it on the counter to thaw or warm up.*
  - *Thaw in the refrigerator.*
  - *The AAP recommends breastfeeding for a full year.*

CLINICAL PEARL

Lactation Consultant

A lactation consultant is a trained provider who is an expert in the field of lactation and breastfeeding. The AAP recognizes these consultants as being responsible for maintaining a higher percentage of breastfeeding in the short and long term if their guidance is followed for 12 months.

Weaning an Infant

- Eliminate one feeding at a time.
- Observe for signs that the infant is having emotional or physical issues.
- Usually the last feeding to be eliminated is the nighttime feeding.

Bottle Feeding

- Read the manufacturer's mixing instructions; carefully dilute.
- Some preparations are ready to feed.
- Bottles and nipples must be washed thoroughly; use a dishwasher or boil all bottles, rings, and nipples.
- If formula needs to be heated, put it in a pan of hot water (not boiling) or use an electric warmer. Never microwave owing to uneven heat distribution.
- Burp the infant frequently to prevent emesis.
- Facilitate parent bonding by holding the infant close. Never prop a bottle.
- Liquid formulas are sterile due to the manufacturing process.
- Powdered formulas are not sterile, thereby increasing incidence of infections.
- Parents should be provided detailed instructions on hand hygiene, preparation, and equipment sterilization to prevent disease.

Advancing Feeding in Infants

- An infant's requirement for calories is determined by size, rate of growth, activity, and energy needed for metabolic activities. Calorie needs per pound of body weight are higher during the first year of life than at any other time. (Chapman & Durham, 2010)
- An infant is ready for solid foods around 6 months of age. At this time, babies are able to move food around in their mouths. Breastfeeding should be on demand and average four to seven feedings per day; bottle feeding should average 24 to 40 ounces of formula; and no fruit juices should be given at this time.
- Advance to a double-handled cup with a snap-on lid.
- The nighttime feeding is the last feeding to be removed, as it is a source of comfort for the infant.
- All foods should be placed on a spoon, not put in a bottle.
- Baby rice cereal is usually indicated for the first solid food (2 to 3 teaspoons) because it is iron fortified and is associated with a decreased incidence of allergic reactions.
- Around 8 months, the next foods to be tried are strained fruit, vegetables, and strained meats. The caregiver should be taught to introduce each type of food for 2 to 3 days to observe for reactions such as rashes, diarrhea, abdominal cramping, or vomiting.
- Use single-ingredient foods.
- Do not add sugar, sweeteners, or corn syrup to any foods.

- Self-feeding should begin when infants can sit up alone, hold their necks steady, draw in their lips when food is introduced into the mouth, and keep the food in their mouths and not push it back out. Offer soft, mashed table food.
- The infant should receive only home-cooked food.
- Always cut up the infant's food into small pieces to prevent choking. The first teeth are biting teeth, not grinding teeth.

Promoting Safety

Foods and food preparation practices that result in a decreased risk of choking in the infant:

- Cooked macaroni
- Small pieces of cheese
- Soft cooked vegetables such as potatoes
- Small pieces of fruit such as bananas, peaches, or pears
- Small pieces of toast
- Grapes cut into fourths
- Thoroughly cook and cut all foods into small pieces.
- Remove pits or seeds from fruit.
- Grind, mash, and add liquid to foods for younger infants.

- Juice should be placed in a cup, not a bottle, to decrease the incidence of dental decay.
- Between 10 and 12 months, the infant will mimic the feeding habits of other family members.
- Do not feed an infant cow's milk until after 12 months of age. Cow's milk is deficient in iron, and the infant will develop anemia (see http://www.mypyramid.gov/kids/index.html).

Promoting Safety

Infants less than 1 year of age should never be given honey or corn syrup because this may result in the ingestion of *Clostridium botulinum* bacteria, which is a spore-producing organism. The spores are found in improperly stored foods, home-canned foods, processed foods such as potato salad, restaurant-prepared foods, and bottled garlic (AAP, 2006b).

SLEEP

- "Back to Sleep" program to prevent sudden infant death syndrome (SIDS)
  - *SIDS is the leading cause of death from 1 month to 1 year, with peaks between 2 and 4 months.*
  - *Occurs more often with males than with females, in winter months, and in African Americans and American Indians*
  - *Occurs more often in babies of mothers who did not have prenatal care and those who smoke*
  - *Unknown causes, but is not due to infections, choking, vomiting, or abuse*

Evidence-Based Practice: Healthy Child Care America "Back to Sleep" Campaign

- Always place babies to sleep on their backs during naps and at nighttime. Babies sleeping on their sides are more likely to accidentally roll onto their stomachs; the side position is not as safe as the back and is not recommended.
- Do not cover the heads of babies with a blanket or overbundle them in clothing and blankets.
- Avoid letting the baby get too hot. The baby could be too hot if you notice sweating, damp hair, flushed cheeks, heat rash, and rapid breathing. Dress the baby lightly for sleep.
- Place your baby in a safety-approved crib with a firm mattress and a well-fitting sheet. (Cradles and bassinets may be used, but choose those that are certified for safety by the Juvenile Products Manufacturers Association [JPMA].)
- Place the crib in an area that is always smoke free.
- Do not allow babies to sleep on adult beds, chairs, sofas, waterbeds, or cushions.
- Toys and other soft bedding, including fluffy blankets, comforters, pillows, stuffed animals, and wedges, should not be placed in the crib with the baby. These items can impair the infant's ability to breathe if they cover the infant's face.
- Breastfeed your baby. Experts recommend that mothers feed their children human milk at least through the first year of life (AAP, 2008, retrieved from http://www.nichd.nih.gov/publications/pubs/upload/090458_BTS_general.pdf).

Promoting Safety

In 2011, the AAP recommended that bumper pads never be used in the cribs of infants. This organization states that there is no clinical evidence that bumper pads prevent injuries, but they do pose a significant risk of suffocation or entrapment because infants do not have the motor skills to turn their heads.

- Newborns sleep from feeding to feeding; with age, the amount and length of wakeful periods increase.
- Newborns can sleep up to 16 hours a day in 3- to 4-hour intervals. Sleep deprivation is a factor for caregivers of newborns.
- By 3 months of age, the infant begins to sleep 6 to 8 hours a night.
- At 6 months, an infant takes two naps a day.
- At 1 year of age, the infant sleeps 14 hours a day—3 hours during the day and 11 hours at night.
- Infants, like adults, progress through REM and non-REM sleep cycles.
- Infants' increase in sleep patterns is tied to growth spurts (Mann, 2011).
- The AAP and the U.S. Product Safety Commission recommend against co-bedding, or allowing the infant to sleep with parents/caregivers or siblings. Co-bedding is practiced in many cultures (AAP, 2011b)

Evidence-Based Practice: Infant Sleep and Parental Behavior

Sadeh, A., Tikotzky, L., & Scher, A. (2009). Parenting and infant sleep. *Sleep Medical Review, 14,* 89–96. doi: 10.1016/j.smrv.2009.05.003

Infant sleep patterns undergo dramatic evolution during the first year of life. This process is driven by underlying biological forces but is highly dependent on environmental cues, including parental influences. There are links between infant sleep and parental behaviors, cognitions, emotions, and relationships, as well as psychopathology. "Parental behaviors, particularly those related to bedtime interactions and soothing routines, are closely related to infant sleep" (Sadeh, Tikotzky, & Scher, 2009).

Evidence-Based Practice: Bedtime Routines

American Academy of Sleep Medicine. (2009). Bedtime routine improves sleep in infants and toddlers, maternal mood. Retrieved from http://www.sciencedaily.com/releases/2009/05/090501090916.htm

A study conducted in 2009, entitled *A Nightly Bedtime Routine: Impact on Sleep in Young Children and Maternal Mood,* indicates that the establishment of a nightly bedtime routine produces significant reductions in problem sleep behaviors in infants. Sleep onset and the number and duration of night awakenings improve with the institution of a sleep routine for infants. According to the study, sleep problems are one of the most common concerns of parents of young children, with as many as 20% to 30% of infants experiencing sleep difficulties, causing disruptions in the family routines. Previous studies have demonstrated that improvement in sleep patterns can significantly improve the family's overall feelings of well-being.

Data were collected from 405 mothers and their infants or toddlers (206 infants between the ages of 7 and 18 months and 199 toddlers between the ages of 18 and 36 months), in 3-week study frames. Families were randomly assigned to a routine or control group. During the first week of the study, the families followed the normal sleep behaviors and patterns as a baseline. During the next 2 weeks, mothers in the study group were instructed to conduct a specific bedtime routine, while the control group continued with their child's normal bedtime patterns. Parents in the infant study group were instructed to follow a three-step bedtime procedure that included a bath, a massage, and quiet activities (such as cuddling and singing); lights were to be turned out within 30 minutes of the end of the sleep routine. Mothers then put their children to bed. The control group members continued with their normal sleep routines. The research indicated that daily routines led to predictable and less stressful environments for infants and were related to parenting competence, improved behaviors, and lower maternal distress (American Academy of Sleep Medicine, 2009).

NURSING PROCEDURES SPECIFIC TO INFANTS AND NEWBORNS

Assisting with Circumcisions

- Circumcision is the removal of the prepuce of the penis.
- It is performed for religious, cultural, hygienic, or social reasons.
- There is no identified medical reason for circumcision.
- Infants with hypospadias or epispadias are not circumcised until after correction of the condition.
- Administer acetaminophen 1 hour prior to the procedure.
- Provide pain relief with a topical prilocaine-lidocaine (EMLA) cream applied to the distal half of the penis 60 to 90 minutes prior to the procedure.
- The infant is positioned on a circumcision board, which positions the arms and legs in a straddled position. The upper body should be covered to minimize heat loss.
- Suction should be available in case of emesis.
- Dorsal penile blocks are used.
- Small needles are used.
- Swaddling aids in increasing comfort.
- Sucrose (24% sugar water) solution can help to relieve pain.
- Nonnutritive sucking can also help to relieve pain.
- Decrease environmental stimuli (Anand et al., 2005).
- Infant must be hospitalized for procedure if more than 1 month of age.

Medication

Sucrose Solution

- Sucrose solution, which is 24% sucrose and water, induces endogenous opioids that provide analgesia for minor procedures.
- A pacifier, or a gloved finger if breastfeeding, used in conjunction with sucrose water enhances the analgesic effect.
- Do not use more than three doses during a single procedure.
- Do not use for infants requiring ongoing pain relief; these infants will require acetaminophen or an opioid such as fentanyl or morphine.
- Although an infant may cry and show signs of pain when 24% sucrose water is used, studies have consistently shown that the sensation of pain and its negative effects will be diminished (Schechter et al., 2007).
- The analgesic effect of 24% sucrose water appears to be reduced after 46 weeks post-conceptual age.
- Sucrose water needs to be ordered by a practitioner and documented as an administered medication.

Evidence-Based Practice: The Brain's Natural Pain Relievers

Gibbins, S., & Stevens, B. (2001). Mechanisms of sucrose and non-nutritive sucking in procedural pain management in infants. *Pain Research and Management, 6,* 21–28. Retrieved from http://www.ncbi.nlm.nih.gov/pubmed/11854758

Stevens, B., Yamada, J., & Ohlsson, A. (2010). Sucrose for analgesia in newborn infants undergoing painful procedures. Retrieved from http://www.ncbi.nlm.nih.gov/pubmed/15266438

The administration of sucrose and the application of nonnutritive sucking are theorized to activate endogenous opioid pathways (natural pain relievers produced in the brain), with resulting calming and pain-relieving effects. The analgesic effects of nonnutritive sucking are thought to be activated through nonopioid pathways by stimulation of orotactile and mechanoreceptor mechanisms.

- Two main types of procedures: Gomco and plastibell (**Figure 7-24**). After the procedure, a petroleum gauze should be applied to the head of the penis to prevent irritation from the diaper.
- The penis is assessed every 15 minutes for the first hour and then every 2 to 3 hours depending on institution policy.
- The neonate should void within 24 hours of the procedure or prior to discharge.
- Instruct parents not to remove the gauze but to allow it to fall off, fasten diapers loosely, observe for bleeding every 4 hours during the first day, and observe for signs and symptoms of infection.
- Acetaminophen orally may be ordered every 4 to 6 hours for 24 hours after the procedure for pain (**Figure 7-25**).
- Educate caregivers that the healing penis develops a yellowish eschar, which should not be wiped off or removed because doing so will start the healing process all over again.

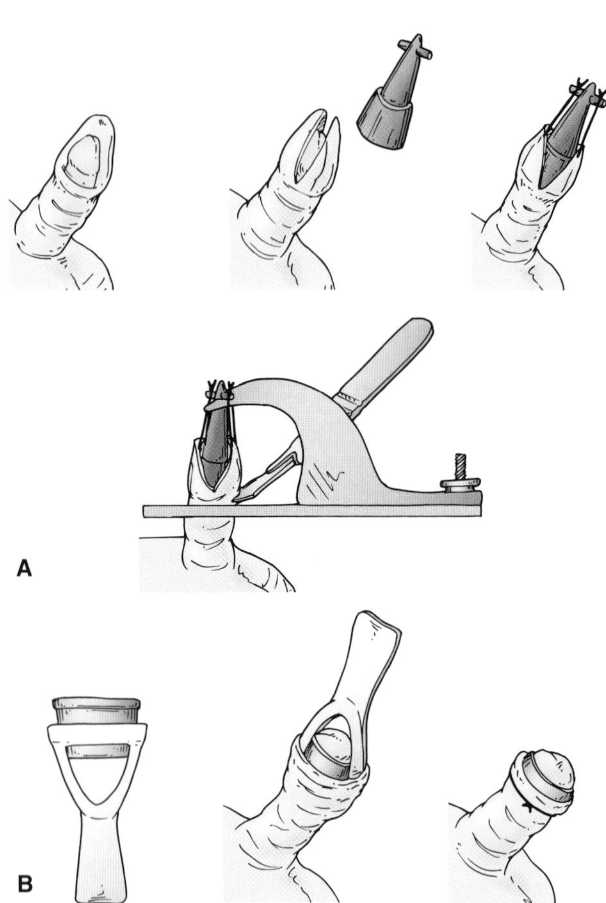

Figure 7-24 Removal of the prepuce during circumcision. **A,** Gomco clamp; **B,** plastibell.

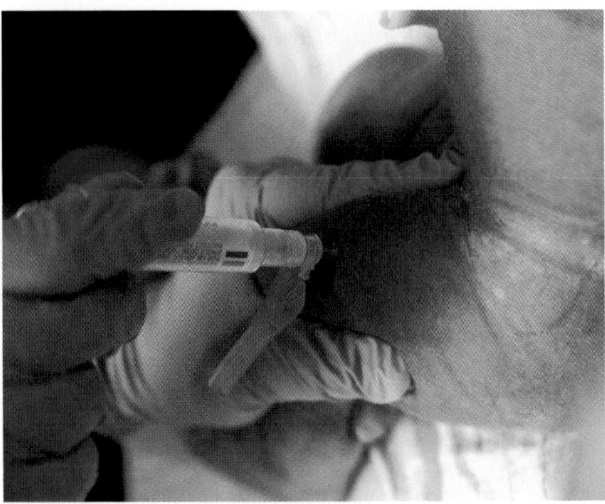

Figure 7-25 Medication administration.

Evidence-Based Practice: Neonatal Circumcision

American Academy of Pediatrics. (1989). Report of the Task Force on Circumcision. *Pediatrics, 3,* 388-391. Retrieved from http://www.cirp.org/library/statements/aap/#a1989

American Academy of Pediatrics, Task Force on Circumcision. (1999). Circumcision policy statement. *Pediatrics, 103,* 686-693. Retrieved from http://www.cirp.org/library/ statements/aap1999/

A 1989 supplement to the 1971 hospital care manual issued a statement that for the first time recognized neonatal pain, in addition to reaffirming a previous position that there is no medical indication for neonatal circumcision (AAP, 1989). The current position statement issued in 1999 does not recommend routine circumcision of the newborn and stresses the importance of obtaining the well-informed consent of both parents (American Academy of Pediatrics, Task Force on Circumcision, 1999).

CULTURAL AWARENESS: Circumcision and Culture

The origin of circumcision has religious foundations going back to the time of the Egyptians and was instituted as a religious practice to ensure fertility, as a rite of passage, or for hygiene purposes. In 2009, 55% to 65% of newborn infants in the United States and Canada were circumcised within 48 hours to 10 days following birth. Circumcision is more common in the United States, Canada, and the Middle East and very rare in Asia, South America, Central America, and Europe. Prior to World War II, the male population in the United States was very infrequently circumcised. In recent years, the trend not to circumcise has witnessed a resurgence (American Academy of Pediatrics, Task Force on Circumcision, 1999).

American Academy of Pediatrics, Task Force on Circumcision. (1999). Circumcision policy statement. *Pediatrics, 103,* 686-693. Retrieved from http://www.cirp.org/library/statements/aap1999/

Discharge Care for the Circumcised Infant

- Notify the physician if:
  - *Persistent bleeding or blood on diaper (more than quarter-sized)*
  - *Increasing redness*
  - *Fever*
  - *Other signs of infection, such as increased swelling or discharge, or the presence of pus-filled blisters*
  - *Not urinating normally within 12 hours after the circumcision*

Care of the Uncircumcised Male

- Do not force the foreskin over the penis.
- Make sure that the penis is cleaned meticulously to prevent infection.
- Do not insert any objects under the foreskin to clean it, such as cotton-tip applicators.

Medication Administration

- Pediatric dosing must be precise to ensure adequate therapeutic levels; dosing is based on weight.
- Children are not little adults.
- When possible, caregivers should use syringes to measure and administer liquid medications.
- Caretakers should be discouraged from using household spoons because they may vary in size, which can lead to inaccurate dosing.

CLINICAL PEARL

Neonates and Medication Administration

In neonates there is an absence of hydrochloric acid, which may interfere with absorption of some medications.

- Variable weight and differences in body surface area affect medication administration.
- Infants are at greater risk for toxic levels that produce untoward effects.
- Infants have smaller amounts of pancreatic enzymes.
- Kidney function is immature in infants.
- Approach infant slowly, at eye level.
- Handle infant gently, keep infant on caregiver's lap, and utilize distraction.
- Do not put medications in a bottle of formula or breast milk because the infant must drink the entire amount to receive the appropriate dosage.
- Hold the infant in the nursing position, allowing the infant to swallow in between squirts of the medication in the buccal area of the mouth; do not lay the infant down until he or she swallows.
- Never give an infant over-the-counter medications. Instruct caregivers to call practitioner with concerns.
- For rectal medications, lubricate the blunted end with water-soluble gel, insert approximately ½ inch, and hold the buttocks closed for approximately 10 minutes to allow for dissolution and absorption of the medication.

HEALTH PROMOTION AND THE FAMILY OF A NEWBORN

Umbilical Cord Blood Banking

- Umbilical cord blood banking is a fee-for-service option that stores cord blood obtained at the time of delivery.
- It is a means of providing possible reimplantation through the cryostorage of stem cells from the cord blood.
- Stem cells can produce all blood cells, which can be used in the future to replace bone marrow that has been destroyed by disease, radiation, or chemotherapy.
- A strict protocol must be followed in the recovery of the stem cells.
- Cord blood banking is not compatible with a delay in cord clamping; harvesting of the stem cells prevents them from returning to the infant.

Education on the Need for Immunizations

"Benefits and risks are associated with using all immunobiologics (i.e., an antigenic substance or antibody-containing preparation). No vaccine is completely safe or effective. Benefits of vaccination include partial or complete protection against infection for the vaccinated person and overall benefits to society as a whole" (Kroger, Sumaya, Pickering, & Atkinson, 2011). See **Figure 7-26** for the recommended immunization schedule.

Education of the Caregiver on Taking Temperature

- Instruct caregivers to take the infant's temperature if they suspect a fever.
- Digital thermometers are preferred over mercury-filled thermometers.
- Rectal temperatures are taken for children less than 3 years of age.
- For rectal temperatures, lubricate the end with a water-soluble solution and insert the rectal thermometer no further than ½ inch into the rectum.
- For axillary temperatures, place the nonlubricated end in the armpit and hold the infant's arm at his or her side for approximately 1 minute; use with infants 3 months or older.

Education of the Caregiver on Signs of Illness in the Newborn and Infant

- Notify the health-care practitioner with any of these concerns:
  - *Axillary temperature >99.3°F*
  - *Vomiting*
  - *Decrease in the number of wet diapers*
  - *Sunken fontanels*

Recommended Immunization Schedule for Persons Aged 0 Through 6 Years—United States • 2011

For those who fall behind or start late, see the catch-up schedule

Vaccine ▼ Age ►	Birth	1 month	2 months	4 months	6 months	12 months	15 months	18 months	19–23 months	2–3 years	4–6 years
Hepatitis B[1]	HepB	HepB				HepB					
Rotavirus[2]			RV	RV	RV[2]						
Diphtheria, Tetanus, Pertussis[3]			DTaP	DTaP	DTaP	see footnote[3]	DTaP				DTaP
Haemophilus influenzae type b[4]			Hib	Hib	Hib[4]	Hib					
Pneumococcal[5]			PCV	PCV	PCV	PCV				PPSV	
Inactivated Poliovirus[6]			IPV	IPV		IPV					IPV
Influenza[7]								Influenza (Yearly)			
Measles, Mumps, Rubella[8]						MMR			see footnote [8]		MMR
Varicella[9]						Varicella			see footnote [9]		Varicella
Hepatitis A[10]							HepA (2 doses)			HepA Series	
Meningococcal[11]										MCV4	

Range of recommended ages for all children

Range of recommended ages for certain high-risk groups

This schedule includes recommendations in effect as of December 21, 2010. Any dose not administered at the recommended age should be administered at a subsequent visit, when indicated and feasible. The use of a combination vaccine generally is preferred over separate injections of its equivalent component vaccines. Considerations should include provider assessment, patient preference, and the potential for adverse events. Providers should consult the relevant Advisory Committee on Immunization Practices statement for detailed recommendations: **http://www.cdc.gov/vaccines/pubs/acip-list.htm**. Clinically significant adverse events that follow immunization should be reported to the Vaccine Adverse Event Reporting System (VAERS) at **http://www.vaers.hhs.gov** or by telephone, **800-822-7967**. Use of trade names and commercial sources is for identification only and does not imply endorsement by the U.S. Department of Health and Human Services.

1. **Hepatitis B vaccine (HepB).** (Minimum age: birth)
   At birth:
   - Administer monovalent HepB to all newborns before hospital discharge.
   - If mother is hepatitis B surface antigen (HBsAg)-positive, administer HepB and 0.5 mL of hepatitis B immune globulin (HBIG) within 12 hours of birth.
   - If mother's HBsAg status is unknown, administer HepB within 12 hours of birth. Determine mother's HBsAg status as soon as possible and, if HBsAg-positive, administer HBIG (no later than age 1 week).

   Doses following the birth dose:
   - The second dose should be administered at age 1 or 2 months. Monovalent HepB should be used for doses administered before age 6 weeks.
   - Infants born to HBsAg-positive mothers should be tested for HBsAg and antibody to HBsAg 1 to 2 months after completion of at least 3 doses of the HepB series, at age 9 through 18 months (generally at the next well-child visit).
   - Administration of 4 doses of HepB to infants is permissible when a combination vaccine containing HepB is administered after the birth dose.
   - Infants who did not receive a birth dose should receive 3 doses of HepB on a schedule of 0, 1, and 6 months.
   - The final (3rd or 4th) dose in the HepB series should be administered no earlier than age 24 weeks.
2. **Rotavirus vaccine (RV).** (Minimum age: 6 weeks)
   - Administer the first dose at age 6 through 14 weeks (maximum age: 14 weeks 6 days). Vaccination should not be initiated for infants aged 15 weeks 0 days or older.
   - The maximum age for the final dose in the series is 8 months 0 days
   - If Rotarix is administered at ages 2 and 4 months, a dose at 6 months is not indicated.
3. **Diphtheria and tetanus toxoids and acellular pertussis vaccine (DTaP).** (Minimum age: 6 weeks)
   - The fourth dose may be administered as early as age 12 months, provided at least 6 months have elapsed since the third dose.
4. ***Haemophilus influenzae* type b conjugate vaccine (Hib).** (Minimum age: 6 weeks)
   - If PRP-OMP (PedvaxHIB or Comvax [HepB-Hib]) is administered at ages 2 and 4 months, a dose at age 6 months is not indicated.
   - Hiberix should not be used for doses at ages 2, 4, or 6 months for the primary series but can be used as the final dose in children aged 12 months through 4 years.
5. **Pneumococcal vaccine.** (Minimum age: 6 weeks for pneumococcal conjugate vaccine [PCV]; 2 years for pneumococcal polysaccharide vaccine [PPSV])
   - PCV is recommended for all children aged younger than 5 years. Administer 1 dose of PCV to all healthy children aged 24 through 59 months who are not completely vaccinated for their age.
   - A PCV series begun with 7-valent PCV (PCV7) should be completed with 13-valent PCV (PCV13).
   - A single supplemental dose of PCV13 is recommended for all children aged 14 through 59 months who have received an age-appropriate series of PCV7.
   - A single supplemental dose of PCV13 is recommended for all children aged 60 through 71 months with underlying medical conditions who have received an age-appropriate series of PCV7.
   - The supplemental dose of PCV13 should be administered at least 8 weeks after the previous dose of PCV7. See *MMWR* 2010:59(No. RR-11).
   - Administer PPSV at least 8 weeks after last dose of PCV to children aged 2 years or older with certain underlying medical conditions, including a cochlear implant.
6. **Inactivated poliovirus vaccine (IPV).** (Minimum age: 6 weeks)
   - If 4 or more doses are administered prior to age 4 years an additional dose should be administered at age 4 through 6 years.
   - The final dose in the series should be administered on or after the fourth birthday and at least 6 months following the previous dose.
7. **Influenza vaccine (seasonal).** (Minimum age: 6 months for trivalent inactivated influenza vaccine [TIV]; 2 years for live, attenuated influenza vaccine [LAIV])
   - For healthy children aged 2 years and older (i.e., those who do not have underlying medical conditions that predispose them to influenza complications), either LAIV or TIV may be used, except LAIV should not be given to children aged 2 through 4 years who have had wheezing in the past 12 months.
   - Administer 2 doses (separated by at least 4 weeks) to children aged 6 months through 8 years who are receiving seasonal influenza vaccine for the first time or who were vaccinated for the first time during the previous influenza season but only received 1 dose.
   - Children aged 6 months through 8 years who received no doses of monovalent 2009 H1N1 vaccine should receive 2 doses of 2010–2011 seasonal influenza vaccine. See *MMWR* 2010;59(No. RR-8):33–34.
8. **Measles, mumps, and rubella vaccine (MMR).** (Minimum age: 12 months)
   - The second dose may be administered before age 4 years, provided at least 4 weeks have elapsed since the first dose.
9. **Varicella vaccine.** (Minimum age: 12 months)
   - The second dose may be administered before age 4 years, provided at least 3 months have elapsed since the first dose.
   - For children aged 12 months through 12 years the recommended minimum interval between doses is 3 months. However, if the second dose was administered at least 4 weeks after the first dose, it can be accepted as valid.
10. **Hepatitis A vaccine (HepA).** (Minimum age: 12 months)
    - Administer 2 doses at least 6 months apart.
    - HepA is recommended for children aged older than 23 months who live in areas where vaccination programs target older children, who are at increased risk for infection, or for whom immunity against hepatitis A is desired.
11. **Meningococcal conjugate vaccine, quadrivalent (MCV4).** (Minimum age: 2 years)
    - Administer 2 doses of MCV4 at least 8 weeks apart to children aged 2 through 10 years with persistent complement component deficiency and anatomic or functional asplenia, and 1 dose every 5 years thereafter.
    - Persons with human immunodeficiency virus (HIV) infection who are vaccinated with MCV4 should receive 2 doses at least 8 weeks apart.
    - Administer 1 dose of MCV4 to children aged 2 through 10 years who travel to countries with highly endemic or epidemic disease and during outbreaks caused by a vaccine serogroup.
    - Administer MCV4 to children at continued risk for meningococcal disease who were previously vaccinated with MCV4 or meningococcal polysaccharide vaccine after 3 years if the first dose was administered at age 2 through 6 years.

The Recommended Immunization Schedules for Persons Aged 0 Through 18 Years are approved by the Advisory Committee on Immunization Practices (**http://www.cdc.gov/vaccines/recs/acip**), the American Academy of Pediatrics (**http://www.aap.org**), and the American Academy of Family Physicians (**http://www.aafp.org**).

Department of Health and Human Services • Centers for Disease Control and Prevention

Figure 7–26 Recommended immunization schedule for persons aged 0 through 6 years, United States, 2012. *(From the Centers for Disease Control and Prevention, Department of Health, approved by the Advisory Committee on Immunization Practices, the American Academy of Pediatrics, and the American Academy of Family Physicians.)*

- *Loss of appetite*
- *Foul odor or bleeding from the cord or circumcision*
- *Decreased level of consciousness; lethargy*
- *Increased irritability*
- *Blue or cool hands and feet*
- *Skin rash*

Sibling Rivalry

- May occur because of changes in family structure and routine
- Not indicative of maladjustment or lack of preparation
- Encourage older children to attend sibling classes.
- Preparation for the changes is necessary based on the developmental age of the siblings.
- Instruct caregivers to include siblings in the supervised care of the infant as appropriate.
- Do not leave the young infant alone with unsupervised younger siblings.
- Foster opportunities for siblings to bond with the infant.
- Educate the caregiver on the need to spend alone/quality time with each of the siblings.

Education of the Caregiver on Milestone Concerns or Red Flags

- No attempts by the infant to lift head when lying face down
- No improvement in head control
- Does not respond to loud noises
- Extreme floppiness
- Lack of response to sounds or visual cues, such as loud noises or bright lights
- Inability to focus on a caregiver's eyes
- Poor weight gain
- Does not crawl by 12 months (AAP, 2006c)

Fostering Positive Parenting Skills

- Talk to the infant.
- Respond to infant's sounds by repeating and adding words.
- Read to the infant; this helps to develop and foster understanding of language and sounds.
- Sing to or play music for the infant.
- Praise the infant and give the infant attention.
- Spend time cuddling and holding the infant so that the infant feels cared for and secure.
- Play with the infant when he or she is alert and relaxed. Watch for signs of being tired or fussy so that the infant can take a break (CDC, 2012).

EMERGENCY CARE RELATED TO THE INFANT AND NEWBORN

In Cases of Emergency

- Stay calm—most serious illnesses provide warnings.
- Begin rescue breathing if infant is not breathing.
- Call 911.
- Apply pressure with a clean cloth to an area that is bleeding.
- If the infant is having a seizure, lower the infant to the floor, turn his or her head to the side, and do not put anything in the infant's mouth.
- Do not move a seriously injured infant unless he or she is in an unsafe situation, such as in a burning house, in a car, or underwater.
- Stay with the infant until help arrives.
- Bring all medication and/or poisons to the emergency room.
- Provide an accurate history of the preceding events, including the last time that the child ate and what was eaten.

Accidents Resulting in Serious Emergency Events

- Falls
- Car accidents
- Drownings
- Electrocution
- Suffocation
- Choking
- Burns
- Firearms incidents

HOSPITALIZED INFANT AND NEWBORN

Nursing Care

- Encourage caregivers to room in.
- Educate caregivers on the normal developmental milestones and stages.
- Educate caregivers on the fact that a hospitalized infant may regress in behavior.
- Encourage caregivers to provide security items such as a favorite toy or blanket.
- Educate caregivers on safety risks in the hospital, such as lowered crib rails, the infant's crawling on the floor, or the presence of items that may not be in the infant's home.
- Reinforce the importance of therapeutic play.
- The least invasive and least painful procedures should be performed first.
- At 6 months of age, infants suffer separation anxiety and can be sensitive to caregiver cues.
- Child life specialists are essential in describing developmental aspects related to play.

Evidence-Based Practice: The Child Life Specialist

Child Life Council, Inc., Rockville, MD, http://www.childlife.org

A child life specialist is a trained individual who works in a hospital or outpatient facility and is responsible for assisting in the stabilization of the psychological aspects of the child, the child's parents/caregivers, and the child's siblings in the healthcare environment. The goal of the child life specialist is to reduce stress by explaining procedures, preparing the child for procedures, and comforting the child throughout procedures or hospitalizations. With infant patients, the specialist may focus on the family unit or the siblings. (See Chapter 2 for further details.)

Pain Management

- Infants feel pain.
- Pain is assessed in newborns and infants by observing facial expressions such as bulged brow, eyes squeezed shut, open mouth, and quivering chin.
- Physiological responses are increased heart rate, respiratory rate, and blood pressure and decreased oxygen saturation.
- Pain causes increased fluid and electrolyte losses.
- Pain causes depression of the immune system through the depletion of mature white blood cells (WBCs) as a result of heightened stress responses.
- Gastric acid production increases.
- Dilated pupils and sweating may be observed.
- Newborns and infants are susceptible to the detrimental effects of pain because of their inability to communicate (Cignacco et al., 2007).
- Cultural influences affect responses to pain.
- Pain relief for infants should be intravenous or oral; if administering opioids, closely monitor respiratory rate and pulse oximetry (AAP, 2006a).
- Utilize EMLA cream or similar topical anesthetics when starting IVs.

Pain Scales

- Infants are exposed to a variety of painful stimuli, from blood draws to circumcision.
- Ongoing assessment is essential for type of pain, origin of pain, and behavioral responses to pain.
- Several reliable infant pain scales are used: PIPP, NIPS, CRIES, FLACC (Zanni, 2007).
- CHEOPS—Children's Hospital of Eastern Ontario Pain Scale (**Table 7-11**)
- FLACC—faces, legs, activity, crying, and consolability (**Table 7-12**)

TABLE 7–11 CHILDREN'S HOSPITAL OF EASTERN ONTARIO PAIN SCALE (CHEOPS) IN YOUNG CHILDREN

OVERVIEW

The CHEOPS is a behavioral scale for evaluating postoperative pain in young children. It can be used to monitor the effectiveness of interventions for reducing the pain and discomfort.

PATIENTS

- The initial study was done on children 1 to 5 years of age.
- It has been used in studies with adolescents, but this may not be an appropriate instrument for that age group.
- According to Mitchell (1999), it is intended for ages 0 through 4.

Parameter	Finding	Points	Parameter	Finding	Points
Cry	No cry	1	Touch	Not touching	1
	Moaning	2		Reach	2
	Crying	2		Touch	2
	Screaming	3		Grab	2
Facial	Smiling	0		Restrained	2
	Composed	1	Legs	Neutral	1
	Grimace	2		Squirming kicking	2
Child verbal	Positive	0		Drawn up tensed	2
	None	1		Standing	2
	Complaints other than pain	1		Restrained	2
	Pain complaints	2			
	Both pain and nonpain complaints	2			
Torso	Neutral	1			
	Shifting				
	Tense	2			
	Shivering	2			
	Upright	2			
	Restrained	2			

TABLE 7–11 CHILDREN'S HOSPITAL OF EASTERN ONTARIO PAIN SCALE (CHEOPS) IN YOUNG CHILDREN—cont'd

Definitions:

- No cry: child is not crying.
- Moaning: child is moaning or quietly vocalizing silent cry.
- Crying: child is crying but the cry is gentle or whimpering.
- Screaming: child is in a full-lunged cry; sobbing may be scored with complaint or without complaint.
- Smiling: score only if definite positive facial expression.
- Composed: neutral facial expression.
- Grimace: score only if definite negative facial expression.
- Positive (verbal): child makes any positive statement or talks about other things without complaint.
- None (verbal): child not talking.
- Complaints other than pain: child complains, but not about pain (e.g., "I want to see mommy"; or "I'm thirsty").
- Pain complaints: child complains about pain.
- Both pain and nonpain complaints: child complains about pain and about other things (e.g., "It hurts"; "I want mommy").
- Neutral (torso): body (not limbs) is at rest; torso is inactive.
- Shifting: body is in motion in a shifting or serpentine fashion.
- Tense: body is arched or rigid.
- Shivering: body is shuddering or shaking involuntarily.
- Upright: child is in a vertical or upright position.
- Restrained: body is restrained.
- Not touching: child is not touching or grabbing at wound.
- Reach: child is reaching for but not touching wound.
- Touch: child is gently touching wound or wound area.
- Grab: child is grabbing vigorously at wound.
- Restrained: child's arms are restrained.
- Neutral (legs): legs may be in any position but are relaxed; includes gently swimming.
- Squirming kicking: definitive uneasy or restless movements in the legs and/or striking out with foot or feet.
- Drawn up tensed: legs tensed and/or pulled up tightly to body and kept there.
- Standing: standing, crouching, or kneeling.
- Restrained: child's legs are being held down.

CHEOPS pain score = SUM (points for all 6 parameters)

Interpretation

- Minimum score: 4
- Maximum score: 13

From Beyer, J. E., McGrath, P. J., & Berde, C. B. (1990). Discordance between self-report and behavioral pain measures in children aged 3–7 years after surgery. *Journal of Pain Symptom Management, 5,* 350–356; Jacobson, S. J., Kopecky, E. A., et al. (1997). Randomised trial of oral morphine for painful episodes of sickle-cell disease in children. *Lancet, 350,* 1358–1361; McGrath, P. J., Johnson, G., et al. (1985). CHEOPS: A behavioral scale for rating postoperative pain in children. *Advanced Pain Research Therapy, 9,* 395–402; McGrath, P. J., & McAlpine, L. (1993). Physiologic perspectives on pediatric pain. *The Journal of Pediatrics, 122,* S2–S8; and Mitchell P. (1999). Understanding a young child's pain. *Lancet, 354,* 1708.

TABLE 7–12 FLACC PAIN SCALE

	SCORING		
Categories	0	1	2
Face	No particular expression or smile; disinterested	Occasional grimace or frown; withdrawn	Frequent to constant frown, clenched jaw, quivering chin
Legs	Normal position or relaxed	Uneasy, restless, tense	Kicking, or legs drawn up
Activity	Lying quietly, normal position, moves easily	Squirming, shifting back and forth, tense	Arched, rigid, or jerking
Cry	No cry (awake or asleep)	Moans or whimpers, occasional complaint	Crying steadily, screams or sobs, frequently complains
Consolability	Content, relaxed	Reassured by occasional touching, hugging, or talking to; distractible	Difficult to console or comfort

Each of the five categories—(F) face; (L) legs; (A) activity; (C) cry; (C) consolability—is scored from 0 to 2, which results in a total score between 0 and 10.
With permission from Sandra I. Merkel, MS, RN, Clinical Nurse Specialist. © 2002, The Regents of the University of Michigan. Original source: Merkel, S., Voepel-Lewis, T., Shayevitz, J., & Malviya S. (1997). The FLACC: A behavioral scale for scoring postoperative pain in young children. *Pediatric Nursing, 23*, 293–297.

- Riley Infant Pain Scale—based on similar criteria; used on infants <36 months and those with cerebral palsy
- PIPP—premature infant pain profile mainly geared to premature hospitalized infants
- CRIES (Crying Requires Oxygen Increased Vital Signs Expression Sleep)—a tool for measuring postoperative neonatal pain
  - *Nonpharmacological pain prevention*
    - Breastfeeding
    - Non-nutritive sucking
    - Kangaroo care
    - Swaddling
    - Limiting environmental stimuli
    - Attention to behavioral cues

ALTERNATIVE AND COMPLEMENTARY THERAPIES FOR THE INFANT AND NEWBORN

Infant Massage

- Stimulates organized sleep patterns
- Enhances growth
- May assist with colic in infants
- Promotes bonding with caregiver
- A position statement by the American Massage Therapy Association (AMTA) in 2008 recognizes that newborns benefit from massage therapy, especially premature infants.

Music Therapy

- Promotes sleep patterns and circadian rhythms
- Slows heart rate
- Singing by caregiver has positive emotional and physiological benefits.
- Aids in communication and language acquisition
- Assists in concentration

Evidence-Based Practice: Music Therapy and Infants

Loewy, J., MacGregor, B., Richards, K., & Rodriquez, J. (1997). Music therapy in pediatric pain management: Assessing and attending to the sounds of hurt, fear, and anxiety. In J. Loewy (Ed.), *Music therapy and pediatric pain*. New Jersey: Jeffrey Brooks.

Researchers and studies have shown that music therapy has the potential to improve cognitive development. Singing of lullabies by caregivers has a calming effect on infants, even if caregivers do not know the words to the songs. Playing soft and soothing music improves psychological well-being. Music has been shown to stimulate neurological growth and development, to calm, and to improve sleeping patterns in infants.

CHRONIC CARE AND THE INFANT AND NEWBORN

Premature Infants

- Prematurity is the primary reason for low birth weight.
- High risk of developmental and motor delay
- Ballard scoring is ≤37 weeks.
- The multidisciplinary team focuses on maximizing the infant's long-term outcomes.
- Neonatologists, pediatricians, cardiologists, pulmonologists, social service workers, physical therapists, and pediatric neurologists are some of the specialists who may be involved.
- Developmental and neurological examinations are performed at routine and serial visits.

- **Respiratory syncytial virus (RSV)** is an acute infection limited to the upper respiratory tract and sometimes accompanied by fever in most healthy full-term infants. In 25% to 40% of RSV infections, the lower respiratory tract becomes infected, and the infant may develop bronchiolitis or pneumonia. Very young infants, preterm infants, or high-risk infants with chronic conditions are at increased risk for hospitalization (CDC, 2009).
- Mortality and morbidity are influenced by numerous factors.

Congenital and Acquired Conditions

See Chapters 17 and 18 for information on the endocrine system and genetics.

- Team of physicians, nurses, respiratory therapists, social workers, and other health professionals work together to meet the infant's needs and provide family-centered care.

Gastroesophageal Reflux

See Chapter 15 for further details.

- Gastroesophageal reflux is due to a weakness in the lower esophageal sphincter (LES) that results in stomach contents leaking backward from the stomach into the esophagus.
- Infants should be frequently burped during feedings.
- Infants should be placed upright for 30 minutes following feeding.
- Raise the head of the crib.
- When the infant is taking solids, thicken foods.
- Certain medications may be prescribed by the physician to increase LES pressure, or to decrease the acid content in the stomach.
- Licorice—although this may ease indigestion, many licorice products contain sugar and alcohol and should not be used in infants. Women who are breastfeeding should not consume products containing licorice because it will pass into the breast milk.
- Acupuncture can be used in combination with diet adjustments, such as for overfeeding or feeding too-complex foods.

SAFETY MEASURES RELATED TO INFANT AND NEWBORN

Injury Prevention—Anticipatory Guidance

- Make and keep infant appointments for medical checkups and vaccinations (2 months, 4 months, 6 months, 9 months, and 1 year).
  - *Immunizations are important because children are susceptible to many potentially serious diseases.*
  - *Consult local health-care provider to ensure that childhood immunizations are up to date. Visit the CDC immunization Web site to obtain a copy of the recommended immunization schedule for U.S. children (http://www.cdc.gov/mmwr/preview/mmwrhtml/rr5515a1.htm).*
- Use "back to sleep" positioning.
- Infants spend most of their time in cribs, which must be safe—no bumper pads, slats no more than 2-3/8 inches apart (JPMA approved).
- Prevent diaper rash with frequent diaper changes, and wiping front to back in girls.
- Childproof the home.
- Have doctor, police, fire, and poison control numbers at caregiver's fingertips.
- Use childproof locks, safety gates, and window guards to prevent accidents and falls.
- Keep anyone with a cough, cold, or infectious disease away from the infant.
- Call a physician if the infant seems sick.
- Call a physician if the infant has a fever, refuses to eat, or has vomiting and/or diarrhea.
- Call a physician if the infant is more fussy or quieter than usual or looks jaundiced.
- Call infant's physician or health-care provider if worried or there are questions about the baby's growth or development.
- Keep the infant in a smoke-free area.
- Keep firearms in a locked cabinet.
- Never leave the child home alone or in an enclosed nonrunning car. The temperature inside the car can change dramatically.
- Pay attention to product recalls of both infant equipment and toys.
- Install fire/smoke and carbon monoxide detectors on every level of the home.
- Pets
  - *Acclimate any pets to the new room setup prior to the baby's coming home.*
  - *Make sure that the pet does not attempt to bite or unintentionally suffocate the infant, and never leave the infant alone with a pet.*
- Drowning
  - *Never leave the infant alone in water or near standing water.*
  - *Do not leave the infant to answer the phone or doorbell.*
  - *Keep toilet lids closed.*
  - *Empty buckets immediately.*

CLINICAL PEARL

Safety Precautions Near Water

Parents and caregivers need to be advised that they should never—even for a moment—leave children alone or in the care of another young child while in bathtubs, pools, spas, or wading pools or near irrigation ditches or other open standing water. Infant bath seats or supporting rings are not a substitute for adult supervision (Rauchschwalbe, Brenner, & Smith, 1997). Remove all water from containers, such as pails and 5-gallon buckets, immediately after use. To prevent drowning in toilets, young children should not be left alone in the bathroom, and unsupervised access to the bathroom should be prevented (Rauchschwalbe et al., 1997).

Promoting Safety

Prolonged submersion in water, such as through infant swimming classes, increases the risk of water intoxication as well as exposure to *Escherichia coli* contamination, both of which can be fatal. Many learn-to-swim programs limit an infant's pool time to 30 minutes. Additionally, contamination of the pool from diapers may result in higher incidence of diarrhea (Position Statement on Drownings, 2003).

- *Burns*
  - Do not hold infant when smoking, drinking hot liquids, or cooking.
  - Do not heat formula or breast milk in the microwave as it causes uneven heating and may also inactivate nutrients in breast milk.
  - An infant's skin is very sensitive to the sun.
    - *Keep infants out of direct sunlight to prevent sunburn.*
    - *Use sunscreen for infants over the age of 6 months.*
  - Turn pot handles away from the outside of the stove, where they can be pulled on by infants beginning to creep.
  - Check the water temperature before putting a child in the tub.
  - Reduce the water heater setting to less than 120°F to lessen the chance of an accidental burning.
  - Keep electrical cords out of infant reach; cap electrical outlets.
  - Use flame-retardant sleepwear for the infant.
- *Choking*
  - Do not attach pacifiers or other objects to the crib or body with a string or cord.
  - Keep small objects away from infants, including toys or stuffed animals with small breakaway parts.
  - Never leave plastic bags or wrappings where the infant can reach them.
  - Keep objects that are choking hazards away from the infant, such as batteries (especially watch batteries), magnets, and balloons.
  - Cut or remove pull cords on blinds and drapes.
  - Anything smaller than your pinky finger can cause a choking situation. This includes foods such as hot dogs, whole grapes, whole raw carrots, raw celery, peanuts, popcorn, chips, candy, marshmallows, pretzels, and peanut butter.
  - Cut all foods into small-sized bites.
- *Poisoning*
  - Keep the poison control number at every phone.
  - Keep all medicines, cleaning products, nail-polish remover, alcohol, and other household chemicals locked in their original containers, and out of reach.
  - Take all suspected poisons to the phone when poison control is called in order to be able to read the ingredients to the center.
  - Remove lead paint from older cribs, infant furniture, walls, and window sills.
  - Never leave an infant alone in a yard.
  - Do not apply sunscreen or perfumed creams or lotions, because they will be absorbed in an infant less than 6 months of age.
  - Keep indoor plants out of the infant's reach.
- *Falls*
  - Never leave the infant alone on a changing table, couch, chair, or bed.
  - Always keep a hand on the baby.
  - Use gates at the top of stairwells.
  - Do not use walkers; they have resulted in serious injuries and even death if they cause the infant to fall down stairs.
  - Make sure that heavy furniture is secure and cannot be toppled over on top of an infant.
  - Educate caregivers on how young children should carry an infant.
- *Car seat*
  - Always use a car seat when traveling in a car or airplane.
  - Use approved car seats correctly.
  - Check the age and weight limits for the seat.
  - Put the car seat in the back seat of the car and secure it facing backwards.
  - Never put the infant in a front seat with a safety airbag.
  - Rear-facing infant seats are used from birth up to 2 years of age, until the child has reached the height and weight limits for the car seat per 2010 AAP guidelines (AAP, 2010).
    - *Parents can contact a certified Child Passenger Safety Technician (CPST) to correctly install infant car seats at http://www.seatcheck.org.*
    - *Each state has its own specific laws related to car seats.*
    - *Caregivers should never leave an infant in the car unattended.*

Evidence-Based Practice: Car-Seat Challenge Test

McGuire, P. E. (2006). Pre-discharge "car seat challenge" for preventing morbidity and mortality in preterm infants. *Cochrane Database of Systematic Reviews*, 1(CD005386). doi: 10.1002/14651858.CD005386.pub2

Physiological monitoring studies indicate that some preterm infants experience episodes of oxygen desaturation, apnea, or bradycardia when seated in standard car-safety seats. The AAP recommends that all preterm infants younger than 37 weeks or less than 5 pounds, 8 ounces should be assessed for cardiorespiratory stability in their car seat prior to discharge or the "car seat challenge" (McGuire, 2006).

- *Electrocution*
  - Keep cords unplugged when not needed.
  - Watch for chewing marks on electrical cords.
- *Suffocation*
  - Remove excess bedding from crib.
  - Remove stuffed toys from crib.
  - Keep all plastic garbage bags, shopping bags, and dry cleaning bags out of reach of the infant.
  - Monitor for issues in sling carriers; make sure that infant does not get wrapped up in clothing and that the head does not fall forward, cutting off the airway.

CHILD ABUSE CONSIDERATIONS

- Abuse consists of intentional, improper actions that result in harm or injury.
- Abuse can be physical, sexual, or mental.
- Neglect is failure to provide the infant with his or her basic needs.

Shaken Baby Syndrome

- The anatomy of infants puts them at particular risk for injury from this kind of action.
- The vast majority of victims are infants younger than 1 year old.
- Pay special attention when choosing a babysitter.
- The average age of victims is between 3 and 8 months.
- Research suggests that teenage fathers are more likely to cause shaken baby syndrome.
- Head trauma results from injuries caused by vigorously shaking a child.
- Contrecoup or injuries to the opposite side of the head are common.
- Detached retinas may result.
- Permanent brain damage may result.
- Death may result.

CLINICAL PEARL

Daddy Boot Camp

- Programs that are taught by men for men
- Aim to support dads and foster improved relationships that translate into improved caregiving behaviors
- Programs stress that babies cry and educate fathers about proper responses. For example, if frustrated, the father should place the infant in a safe place and remove himself from the room.
- Instruct fathers-to-be and new fathers on the care and handling of the new infant.
- Explain importance of providing neck support, holding an infant correctly, and monitoring of soft spots.
- Discuss shaken baby syndrome and methods to deal with frustrations of new parenthood.
- Discuss postpartum depression.

Abduction Prevention

Educate the caregiver as follows:

- In the hospital, infants will be banded with electronic tags to prevent abduction.
- Hospital staff should be properly identified with hospital badges to identify that they have access to the postpartum and newborn areas.
- Be suspicious of casual acquaintances or strangers who attempt to befriend the parent.
- Learn hospital procedures for care after discharge if a visiting nurse is to come to your home.
- Demand positive identification before allowing anyone into your home.
- Do not post information about the infant on social media.
- Under no circumstances should the caregiver give the baby to a stranger.
- Do not allow casual acquaintances or strangers to babysit the infant.
- Never leave the infant alone at home.
- Do not place birth announcements in the newspaper.
- In shopping areas, do not turn your back on the infant. Make sure infant is secured in a car seat that is buckled into a shopping cart.
- Place the infant in the car seat in the car, lock the doors, and then load your groceries or items from the store.
- Educate family members and friends who babysit the infant about infant security.
- Call police anytime you are suspicious or concerned about the infant's safety.

Sexual Abuse

- Stained or bloody diapers
- Genital or rectal pain, swelling, redness, or discharge
- Bruises or other injuries in the genital or rectal area
- Child has behavioral and emotional signs such as:
  - *Difficulty eating or sleeping*
  - *Excessive crying*
  - *Withdrawing from others*
  - *Failure to thrive*

Physical Abuse

- Unexplained or repeated injuries such as welts, bruises, burns, fractured scalp, and broken bones
- Injuries that are in the shape of an object (e.g., belt buckle, electrical cord, cigarette)
- Injuries that are not likely to have happened given the age or ability of the child, such as broken bones in a child too young to walk or climb
- Disagreement or inconsistency in parent/caregiver explanation of the injury
- Unreasonable explanation of the injury
- Fearful or detached behavior by the infant

Emotional Abuse

- Aggressive or withdrawn behavior
- Shying away from physical contact with parents or adults
- Not meeting the infant's basic needs of food, warmth, and cuddling

Neglect

- Consistent failure to respond to the child's need for stimulation, nurturing, encouragement, and protection, or failure to acknowledge the child's presence
- Actively refusing to respond to the child's needs, such as refusing to show affection

- Parents/caregivers expressing the fact that they are not going to spoil the baby or referring to the baby as evil
- Infant with malnourished appearance
- Obvious neglect of the child (e.g., dirty, undernourished, inappropriate clothes for the weather, lack of medical or dental care)
- Failure to provide necessary medications for chronic conditions, such as inhalers for asthmatics
- Delays in calling for help or taking infant to the doctor

Review Questions

1. The caregiver brings her 7-month-old infant to the clinic for a regular checkup. When assessing this infant, the nurse would expect to see which developmental functions?
   A. Sits up without support
   B. Pulls oneself to a stand
   C. Rolls over front to back only
   D. Reaches for toys
2. By what age does attainment of developmental milestones or lack thereof become very apparent to both caregivers and health providers?
   A. 2 weeks of age
   B. 2 months of age
   C. 9 months of age
   D. 2 years of age
3. The mother of a 4-month-old tells the nurse that her baby is taking juice in the afternoon and whole milk at all other feedings. Which of the following is the best response by the nurse?
   A. "That should be fine."
   B. "Juice should not be given until 1 year of age, but the milk is fine."
   C. "The infant should be kept on formula only until after the first birthday."
   D. "The juice is fine, but switch the baby to 2% milk."
4. When are infants at risk for sudden infant death syndrome (SIDS)?
   A. 2 weeks to 2 months of age
   B. 6 months to 8 months of age
   C. 4 months to 6 months of age
   D. 2 months to 4 months of age
5. The research on shaken baby syndrome describes the primary offenders as being
   A. young unmarried mothers.
   B. older mothers >35 years of age.
   C. young fathers.
   D. siblings.
6. Vitamin K is given at birth because it
   A. assists in promoting brain growth.
   B. is essential for myelinization in the brain.
   C. is synthesized by bacteria in the colon, so that the infant is born with a sterile colon.
   D. is responsible for aiding in digestion of simple sugars.
7. At birth, the nurse should suction the infant using which method?
   A. Nose first, then mouth
   B. Mouth first, then nose
   C. Mouth only
   D. Either order
8. Separation anxiety is a normal occurrence in infants beginning primarily around the age of
   A. 1 month.
   B. 2 months.
   C. 4 months.
   D. 8 months.
9. According to Piaget's theory of cognitive development, an infant less than 1 year of age is in which stage?
   A. Preoperational
   B. Sensorimotor
   C. Concrete
   D. Sensual
10. By 6 months of age, infants should
    A. triple the birth weight.
    B. gain 4 pounds per month.
    C. double the birth weight.
    D. lose weight if not eating table food.

References

Acute Care of at-Risk Newborns Neonatal Society (ACoRN). (2009). *Acute care of at risk newborns, 2010 update.* Vancouver, CA: Author.

American Academy of Pediatrics (AAP). (1989). Report of the Task Force on Circumcision. *Pediatrics, 3,* 388–391. Retrieved from http://www.cirp.org/library/statements/aap/#a1989

American Academy of Pediatrics (AAP). (2004). Management of hyperbilirubinemia in the newborn infant 35 or more weeks of gestation. *Pediatrics, 114,* 297–316. doi: 10.1542/peds.114.1.297

American Academy of Pediatrics (AAP). (2006a). Prevention and management of pain in the neonate: An update. *American Academy of Pediatrics, 118,* 2231–2241. Retrieved from http://www.cps.ca/english/statements/fn/fn07-01.htm

American Academy of Pediatrics (AAP). (2006b). Immunizations and infectious diseases: An informed parent's guide. Retrieved from http://www.healthychildren.org/English/health-issues/conditions/infections/Pages/Botulism.aspx?nfstatus=401&nftoken=00000000-0000-0000-0000-000000000000&nfstatus-description=ERROR%3a+No+local+token

American Academy of Pediatrics (AAP). (2006c). Identifying infants and young children in the medical home: An algorithm for developmental surveillance and screening. *Pediatrics, 118,* 405-420. doi: 10.1542/peds.2006-1231

American Academy of Pediatrics (AAP). (2008). Red reflex examination in neonates, infants, and children. *Pediatrics, 122,* 1401–1404. doi:10.1542/peds.2008-2624

American Academy of Pediatrics (AAP). (2009). Policy Statement-AAP Publications Retired and Reaffirmed. *Pediatrics.* doi: 10.1542/peds.2009-1415

American Academy of Pediatrics (AAP). (2010). Child passenger safety. *Pediatrics.* doi: 10.1542/ peds.2011-0213

American Academy of Pediatrics (AAP). (2011a). Clinical report—Postnatal glucose homeostasis in late-preterm and term infants. *Pediatrics*, *107*, 575–579. doi: 10.1542/peds.2010-3851

American Academy of Pediatrics (2011b). Technical Report: SIDS and Other Sleep-Related Infant Deaths: Expansion of Recommendations for the Safe Infant Sleeping Environment Task Force on Sudden Infant Death Syndrom. *Pediatrics, 128(5)*, e1341-e1367; doi:10.1542/peds.2011-2285

American Academy of Pediatrics, Committee on Nutrition. (1998). Soy protein-based formulas: Recommendations for use in infant feedings. *Pediatrics, 101*, 148–153. Retrieved from http://www.ncbi.nlm.nih.gov/pubmed/11345979

American Academy of Pediatrics, Committee on Psychosocial Aspects of Child and Family Health. (1998). Guidance for effective discipline. Retrieved from http://aappolicy.aappublications.org/cgi/content/full/pediatrics;101/4/723

American Academy of Pediatrics, Task Force on Circumcision. (1999). Circumcision policy statement. *Pediatrics, 103*, 686–693. Retrieved from http://www.cirp.org/library/statements/aap1999/

American Academy of Sleep Medicine. (2009). Bedtime routine improves sleep in infants and toddlers, maternal mood. Retrieved from http://www.sciencedaily.com/releases/2009/05/090501090916.htm

American Dental Association (ADA). (2009). Position statement on dental caries. Retrieved from http://www.ada.org

American Hospital Association. (2005). Resource guide: More information about the concepts of patient- and family-centered care. Retrieved from www.aha.org/aha/content/2005/pdf/resourceguide.pdf

American Massage Therapy Association. (2008). Massage therapy may benefit newborns. Retreived from http://www.amtamassage.org/statement4.html

Anand, I. K., Johnston, C., Oberlander, R., Taddio, A., Lehr, V., & Walco, G. (2005). Prevention and management of pain and stress in the neonate. *Pediatrics, 27*, 884–876. Retrieved from http://aappolicy.aappublications.org/cgi/content/full/pediatrics;105/2/454

Association of Women's Health, Obstetric, and Neonatal Nurses (AWHONN). (2007). Quick care guide for neonatal skin care (2nd ed.). Retrieved from http://www.awhonn.org/awhonn/content.do?name=07_PressRoom/7-07Nov14_SkinCare EBG.htm

Bachmann, K. R., & Arvedson, J. C. (1998). Early identification and intervention for children who are hearing impaired. *Pediatrics in Review, 19*, 155–165. doi: 10.1542/pir.19-5-155

Bhutani, V. K., Johnson, L., & Sivieri, E. M. (1999). Predictive ability of a predischarge hour-specific serum bilirubin for subsequent significant hyperbilirubinemia in term and near term newborns. *Pediatrics, 103*, 6–14. doi: 10.1542/peds.103.1.6

Blackwell, K., & Cattaneo, A. (2007). What is the evidence for kangaroo mother care of the very low birth weight baby? *Problems of the Neonate and Young Infant.* Retrieved from http://www.ichrc.org/pdf/kangaroo.pdf

Centers for Disease Control and Prevention (CDC). (2009). Length, height, and head circumference for age. Retrieved from http://www.cdc.gov/growthcharts/clinical_charts.htm

Centers for Disease Control and Prevention (CDC). (2012). Child development. Retrieved from http://www.cdc.gov/ncbddd/childdevelopment/positiveparenting/infants.html

Ceriani Cernadas, J. M., Carroli, G., Pellegrini, L., Otano, L., Ferreira, M. Ricci, C., . . . Lardizabal, J. (2006). The effect of timing of cord clamping on neonatal venous hematocrit values and clinical outcome at term: A randomized controlled trial. *Pediatrics, 117*, 779–786. doi: 10.1542/peds.2005-1156

Chapman, L., & Durham, R. (2010). *Maternal-newborn nursing: Critical components of nursing care.* Philadelphia, PA: F.A. Davis.

Cignacco, E., Hamers, J. P. H., Stoffel, L., van Lingen, R. A., Gessler, P., & McDougall, J. (2007). The efficacy of nonpharmacologic interventions in the management of procedural pain in preterm and term neonates: A systematic literature review. *European Journal of Pain, 11*, 139–152.

Deglan, J. H., Vallerand, A. H., & Sanoski, C. A. (2011). *Davis's drug guide for nurses* (12th ed.). Philadelphia: F.A. Davis.

Dewey, K., & Chaparro, C. (2006). Delayed umbilical cord clamping boosts iron in infants. Retrieved from http://www.sciencedaily.com/releases/2006/06/060618224104.htm

El-Beshbishi, S. N., Shattuck, K .E., Mohammad, A. A., & Peterson, J. R. (2009). Hyperbilirubinemia and transcutaneous bilirubinometry. *Clinical Chemistry, 55*, 1280–1287. doi: 10.1373/clinchem.2008.121889

Garrison, M., & Christakis, D. (2000). A systematic review of treatments for infant colic. *Pediatrics,* 106, 184–190. Retrieved from http://www.ncbi.nlm.nih.gov/pubmed/10888690

Gibbins, S., & Stevens, B. (2001). Mechanisms of sucrose and non-nutritive sucking in procedural pain management in infants. *Pain Research and Management, 6*, 21–28. Retrieved from http://www.ncbi.nlm.nih.gov/pubmed/11854758

Greer, F. R., Sicherer, S. H., & Burks, W. A. (2008). Effects of early nutritional interventions on the development of atropic disease in infants and children: The role of breastfeeding, timing of complementary foods, and hydrolyzed formulas. *Pediatrics, 121*, 183–191. doi: 10.1542/ peds.2007-3022

Harlor, A. D., & Bower, C. (2009). Hearing assessment in infants and children: Recommendations beyond neonatal screening. *Pediatrics, 124*, 1252–1263. doi: 10.1542/peds.2009-1997

Hyman, P. E., Milla, P. J., Benninga, M. A., Davidson, G. P., Fleisher, D. F., & Taminiau, J. (2006). Childhood functional disorders: Neonate/toddler. *Gastroenterology, 130*, 1519–1526. Retrieved from http://www.romecriteria.org/pdfs/p1519Childhood_Neonate.pdf

Keren, R., Luan, X., Friedman, S., Saddlemire, S., Cnaan, A., & Bhutani, V. K. (2006). A comparison of alternative risk-assessment strategies for predicting significant neonatal hyperbilirubinemia in term and near term infants. *Pediatrics, 121*, e170–e179. Retrieved from doi: 10.1542/peds.2006-3499

Kroger, A. T., Sumaya, C. V., Pickering, L. K., & Atkinson, W. L. (2011). General recommendations on immunization. Retrieved from http://www.cdc.gov/mmwr/ preview/mmwrhtml/rr6002a1.htm

Laudert, S., Liu, W. F., Blackington, S., Perkins, S., Martin, S., MacMillan-York, E., . . . Handyside, J. (2007). *Journal of Perinatology, 27*, S75–S93. doi: 10.1038/sj.jp.7211843

Loewy, J., MacGregor, B., Richards, K., & Rodriquez, J. (1997). Music therapy in pediatric pain management: Assessing and attending to the sounds of hurt, fear, and anxiety. In J. Loewy (Ed.), *Music therapy and pediatric pain.* New Jersey: Jeffrey Brooks.

Mann, D. (2011). Infant growth spurts tied to more sleep. Retrieved from http://www.webmd.com/ parenting/baby/news/20110502/infant-growth-spurts-tied-to-more- sleep

McGuire, P. E. (2006). Pre-discharge "car seat challenge" for preventing morbidity and mortality in preterm infants. *Cochrane Database of Systematic Reviews, 1*(CD005386). doi: 10.1002/14651858.CD005386.pub2

Mercer, J. S., Erickson-Owens, D. A., Graves, B., & Mumford Haley, M. (2007). Evidence-based practices for the fetal to newborn transition. *Journal of Midwifery and Women's Health, 52*, 262–272. doi: 10.1016/j.jmwh.2007.01.005

Merkel, S. I., Voepel-Lewis, T., Shayevitz, J. R., & Malviya, S. (1997). The FLACC: A behavioral scale for scoring postoperative pain in young children. *Pediatric Nurse, 23*, 293–297.

Moerschel, S. K., Cianciaruso, L. B., & Tracy, L. R. (2008). A practical approach to neonatal jaundice. *American Family Physician, 77*, 1255–1262. Retrieved from http://www.aafp.org/afp/2008/0501/p1255.html

National Newborn Screening and Genetics Resource Center. (2009). National newborn screening status report. Retrieved from http://genes-r-us.uthscsa.edu/nbsdisorders.pdf

Polin, R. A., & Yoder, M. C. (2007). *Workbook in practical neonatology* (4th ed.). Philadelphia: Saunders.

Position statement on drownings. (2003). Prevention of drowning in infants, children, and adolescents. *American Academy of Pediatrics Committee on Injury, Violence, and Poison Prevention, 112*, 437–439. Retrieved from http://aappolicy.aappublications.org/cgi/content/full/pediatrics;112/2/437

Rathnau-Minnella, C. H. (2008). *The ABCs of genetics* (2nd ed.). Glenview, IL: National Association of Neonatal Nurses.

Rauchschwalbe, R., Brenner, R. A., & Smith, G. S. (1997). The role of bathtub seats and rings in infant drowning deaths. *Pediatrics, 100*, E1. Retrieved from http://www.ncbi.nlm.nih.gov/pubmed/9310534

Riepe, F. G., & Sippell, W. G. (2007). Recent advances in diagnosis, treatment, and outcome of congenital adrenal hyperplasia due to 21-hydroxylase deficiency. *Reviews in Endocrine and Metabolic Disorders, 8*, 349–363. doi: 10.1007/s11154-007-9053-1

Sadeh, A., Tikotzky, L., & Scher, A. (2009). Parenting and infant sleep. *Sleep Medical Review, 14*, 89–96. doi: 10.1016/j.smrv.2009.05.003

Schaal, B., Hummel, T., & Soussignan, R. (2004). Olfaction in the fetal and premature infant: Functional status and clinical implications. *Clinics in Perinatology, 31*, 261–285. doi: 10.1016/j.clp.2004.04.003

Schechter, N. L., Zempsky, W. T., Cohen, L. L., McGrath, P. J., McMurtry, M., & Bright, N. S. (2007). Pain reduction during pediatric immunizations: Evidence-based review and recommendations. *Pediatrics, 119*, e1184–e1198. doi:10.1542/peds.2006-1107

Stevens, B., Yamada, J., & Ohlsson, A. (2010). Sucrose for analgesia in newborn infants undergoing painful procedures. Retrieved from http://www.ncbi.nlm.nih.gov/pubmed/15266438

Straus, M. A. (2005). Children should never, ever be spanked no matter what the circumstances. In D. R. Loseke, R. J. Gelles, & M. M. Cavanaugh (Eds.), *Current controversies about family violence* (2nd ed., pp. 137–157). Retrieved from http://pubpages.unh.edu/~mas2/ CP67%20Children%20Should%20Never%20be%20Spanked.pdf

Sutton, V. R. (2008). Overview of the classification of inborn errors of metabolism. Retrieved from www.uptodate.com/contents/overview-of-the-classification-of-inborn-errors-of-metabolism?source=search_result&selectedTitle=1~150

Taeusch, H. W., Ballard, R. A., & Gleason, C. A. (2005). *Avery's diseases of the newborn* (8th ed.). Philadelphia: Elsevier.

Wagner, C. L. (2010). Human milk and lactation. Retrieved from http://emedicine.medscape.com/ article/1835675-overview#a0101

Ward, S. L., & Hisley, S. M. (2009). *Maternal-child nursing care: Optimizing outcomes for mothers, children, & families.* Philadelphia: F.A. Davis.

World Health Organization Position Statement. (2011). Exclusive breastfeeding for six months best for babies everywhere. Retrieved from http://www.who.int/mediacentre/news/statements/2011/breastfeeding_20110115/en/index.html

Zanni, G. R. (2007). Joint Commission on Accreditation of Healthcare Organizations 2007 national patient safety goals. Retrieved from http://www.pharmacytimes.com/publications/issue/2007/2007-02/2007-02-6294

From Toddlers to Preschoolers

8

Ludy Caballero, BSN, RN, EMTP
Diane M. Kocisko, MSN, RN, CPN

OBJECTIVES

- ☐ Define key terms.
- ☐ Identify normal growth and development for toddlers and preschoolers.
- ☐ Discuss the nursing assessment of toddlers and preschoolers.
- ☐ Identify safety risks for toddlers and preschoolers.
- ☐ Discuss safety interventions to minimize risks.
- ☐ Identify and discuss pain scales used with toddlers and preschoolers.
- ☐ Identify appropriate nursing interventions and education regarding pain and safety for toddlers and preschoolers and their caregivers.
- ☐ Identify and discuss different challenges faced by toddlers and preschoolers.

KEY TERMS

- Toddler
- Separation anxiety
- Preschooler
- Chief complaint
- Normal vital signs
- Unintentional injury
- Pain scales
- Sibling rivalry
- Appropriate serving size

TODDLER GROWTH AND DEVELOPMENT (AGES 1–3)

Theorists

- Erikson—autonomy vs. shame and doubt. In Erikson's theory of psychosocial development, **toddlers** in this stage seek to attain autonomy by gaining more control over self, in such areas as toileting and food and toy preferences. Success leads to self-confidence and self-control, whereas feelings of shame and doubt in these areas may lead to a sense of inadequacy.
- Piaget—preoperational. In Piaget's cognitive developmental theory, 2- to 7-year-olds are in the preoperational stage, which is characterized by magical thinking and egocentrism, the inability to see things from another's perspective.
- Freud—anal stage. In Freud's psychosexual theory, toddlers are in the anal stage, which focuses on pleasure derived from the toddler's enjoyment of holding and releasing bowel movements.
- Kohlberg—preconventional. In Kohlberg's theory of moral development, 2- to 7-year-olds are in the stage of preconventional moral reasoning, and tend to follow set rules in fear of punishment.

Movements

- Walks alone
- Begins to run
- Stands on tiptoes
- Climbs on furniture
- Builds towers of blocks
- Kicks a ball
- Climbs stairs while holding onto support
- Pulls or carries toys while walking

Language

- Points to objects when named by others
- Recognizes the names of well-known people and things
- Learns own name
- Repeats words that are overheard
- Is able to say 10 words (young toddler) to 250 words (older toddler)
- Later is able to speak in two- to four-word sentences

Cognitive Skills

- Finds objects that are hidden
- Begins to identify and sort colors and shapes
- Begins to play make-believe

Don't have time to read this chapter? Want to reinforce your reading? Need to review for a test? Listen to this chapter on DavisPlus at **davispl.us/rudd1.**

- Begins to scribble and show preference for one hand versus the other
- Asks "why" questions

> **CLINICAL PEARL**
> By 2 years of age, a child can follow simple instructions. A child can and should be encouraged to participate in self-care and the education process to some extent. Providing limited, appropriate choices for the child will allow for a sense of control.

Social and Emotional Milestones

- Imitates others
- Gains awareness of self as separate from others
- Begins to enjoy spending time with other children
- Engages in parallel play, playing near other toddlers but not consistently interacting or playing together
- Shows affection openly
- Begins to display defiance
- Displays **separation anxiety** until approximately the end of the second year

PRESCHOOLER GROWTH AND DEVELOPMENT (AGES 3–5)

Theorists

- Erikson—initiative vs. guilt. Success in this stage involves initiative, wherein **preschoolers** begin to assert power and control over their environment; the opposite result is feelings of guilt and a dependence on others.
- Piaget—preoperational. As described for toddlers, this stage of cognitive development (ages 2 to 7) is characterized by magical thinking and egocentrism.
- Freud—phallic stage. The focus of this stage is pleasure derived from the genitals; childhood masturbation is common, and toddlers may view the opposite-sex parent as a sexual object.
- Kohlberg—preconventional. As described for toddlers, this level of moral reasoning (ages 2 to 7) involves an obedience/punishment mentality.

> **CLINICAL PEARL**
> A child should be given feedback in relationship to his or her behavior. The child should be told "good job" instead of "good boy/girl." Preschoolers cannot understand the process of disease transmission. The child may feel that an illness is a punishment for "being bad."

Movements

- Hops and stands on one foot for 5 to 10 seconds
- Throws objects overhand
- Catches a bounced ball
- Uses scissors
- Dresses and undresses self with assistance (later without assistance)
- Goes up and down the stairs without assistance
- Draws squares, circles, and later triangles
- Draws stick figures with more than two body parts (later draws people with bodies)
- Brushes own teeth and goes to the toilet without assistance (later in stage)
- May learn to skip, ride a bicycle, and swim
- Uses utensils when eating

Language

- Speaks clearly enough for strangers to understand
- Able to say upward of 900 words
- Speaks in sentences of five or more words
- Tells stories
- Uses future tense
- Comprehends rhyming
- States full name and address (later in stage)

Cognitive Skills

- Recalls parts of a story
- Counts to ten
- Correctly identifies at least four colors
- Begins to understand the concept of time
- Knows the meaning of *same* and *different*
- Begins to use imagination and creativity

Social and Emotional Milestones

- Are more independent
- Show interest in new things
- May want to do things by themselves
- Obey rules
- Role play
- Play well with others
- Want to please and be like friends
- Try to negotiate problem solving
- Have trouble in differentiating between reality and fantasy (later preschoolers are able to tell the difference)
- May believe in monsters or be afraid of the dark
- Begin to understand gender differences
- May sometimes be demanding or eager to help

> **CLINICAL PEARL**
> Many preschoolers are afraid of the dark and may be afraid to sleep in a dark room. It is helpful to have a nightlight that sheds minimal light to reduce fear. Providing a bedtime routine will decrease anxiety and provide a relaxing environment.

NURSING ASSESSMENT

Obtain Health History

- **Chief complaint**, current signs/symptoms, or events leading to visit
- Past medical history

- Medications
- Allergies
- Appetite and time of last meal
- Height and weight

> **CLINICAL PEARL**
>
> **Head-to-Toe Assessment**
>
> Conduct head-to-toe assessment from least to most invasive/intrusive, leaving painful areas for last.

Assess Head

- Ears, eyes, nose, mouth, teeth, and throat for symmetry, drainage, enlarged lymph nodes, and pain and/or abnormalities

> **CRITICAL COMPONENT**
>
> Children are anatomically and physiologically different than adults:
>
> - Proportionately larger heads as compared to bodies
> - Greater ratio of body surface area to total weight
> - Larger tongues and greater proportion of soft tissue in and around the airway
> - Shorter, more narrow airway that is more elastic and collapsible
> - More pliable chest
> - Weaker abdominal muscles, creating the look of distention
> - Belly breathers
> - Higher metabolic rates
> - Higher fluid requirements
> - Higher total blood volumes

Assess Torso

- Neck, chest, back, and abdomen for variations of the skin, enlarged lymph nodes, rashes, and pain and/or abnormalities

Assess Extremities

- Movement
- Symmetry
- Variations of the skin
- Pain and/or abnormalities

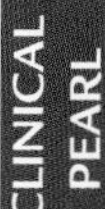

> Assess toddlers in their comfort zone, usually in a parent's lap, remember to protect a preschooler's modesty, and approach children down at their level.

Growth and Development

- See the Centers for Disease Control and Prevention (2009) growth charts (**Figure 8-1**) for typical heights and weights. (Also available at http://www.cdc.gov/growthcharts/clinical_charts.htm.)
- At birth to 36 months, assess:
  - *Length for age and weight for age*
  - *Head circumference for age and weight for length (done with preschoolers, 2 to 5 years)*
  - *Weight for stature*

Nutritional Status

- Hair is evenly dispersed.
- Appearance is not of overweight or underweight.
- Skin is not overly dry.

General Physical Appearance

- Appears to be clean.
- Is dressed appropriately for current weather.
- Is awake and alert.

Hearing

Assess for signs of hearing problems, such as the following:

- Child appears to not be listening.
- Child frequently asks for requests to be repeated.
- Child asks for volume of television to be turned up.

Speech

- Uses words appropriate for age level
- Sentence structure appropriate for age
- Uses eye contact during communication

Vision

- Sits close to television screen or computer monitor (could indicate vision problem)
- Reaches for toys or objects near and far

Measurements

Height

- Standing when able to stand
- Lying down for young toddler, as lordosis is common in this age group

Weight

- Undress young toddlers when dehydration is of concern to obtain accurate weight.

Head Circumference

- Measured for all children under 2 years of age
- May be assessed after 2 years of age if difficulty with bone growth or issues identified that impact the growth of the head

Abdominal Circumference

- Primarily assessed for those under 2 years of age

Birth to 36 months: Girls
Length-for-age and Weight-for-age percentiles

NAME ______________________

RECORD # ____________

Mother's Stature			Gestational Age: ____ Weeks		Comment
Father's Stature					
Date	Age	Weight	Length	Head Circ.	
	Birth				

Published May 30, 2000 (modified 4/20/01).
SOURCE: Developed by the National Center for Health Statistics in collaboration with the National Center for Chronic Disease Prevention and Health Promotion (2000).
http://www.cdc.gov/growthcharts

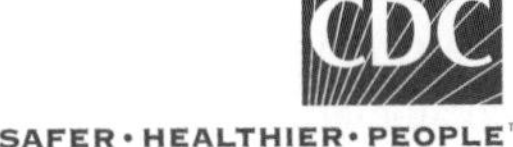

Figure 8–1 Growth charts. *(From the Centers for Disease Control and Prevention. Developed by the National Center for Health Statistics in collaboration with the National Center for Chronic Disease Prevention and Health Promotion, published May 30, 2000, modified April 20, 2001, http://www.cdc.gov/growthcharts.)*

Birth to 36 months: Girls
Head circumference-for-age and Weight-for-length percentiles

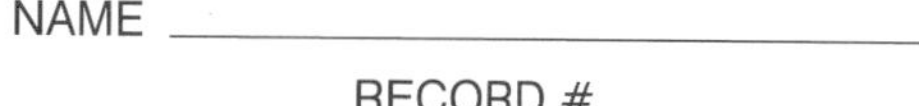

NAME ____________________

RECORD # ____________

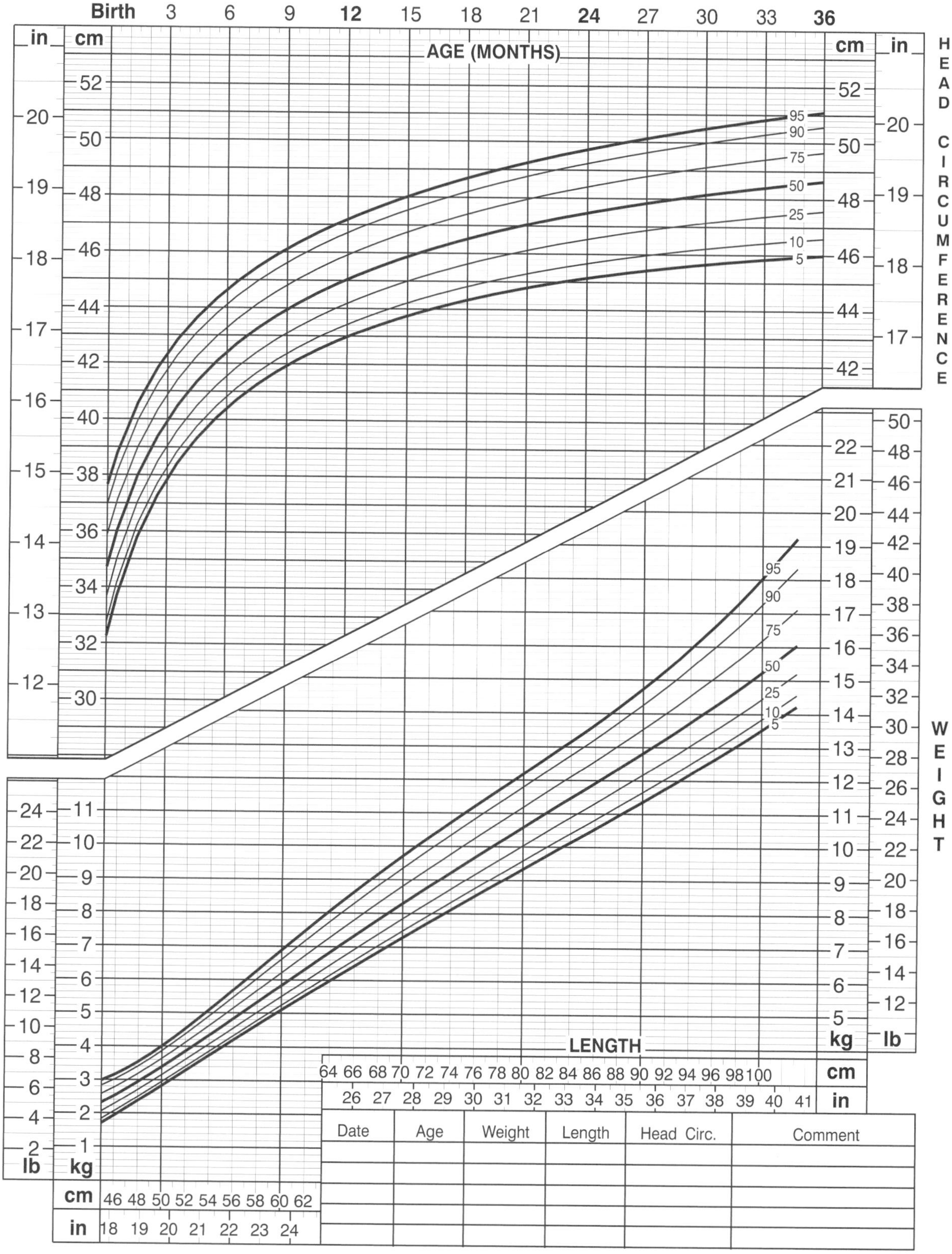

Date	Age	Weight	Length	Head Circ.	Comment

Published May 30, 2000 (modified 10/16/00).
SOURCE: Developed by the National Center for Health Statistics in collaboration with the National Center for Chronic Disease Prevention and Health Promotion (2000).
http://www.cdc.gov/growthcharts

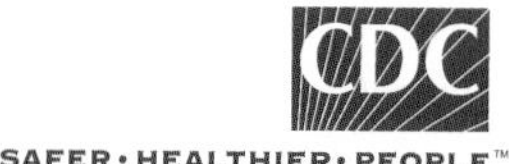

SAFER • HEALTHIER • PEOPLE™

Figure 8-1—cont'd

Continued

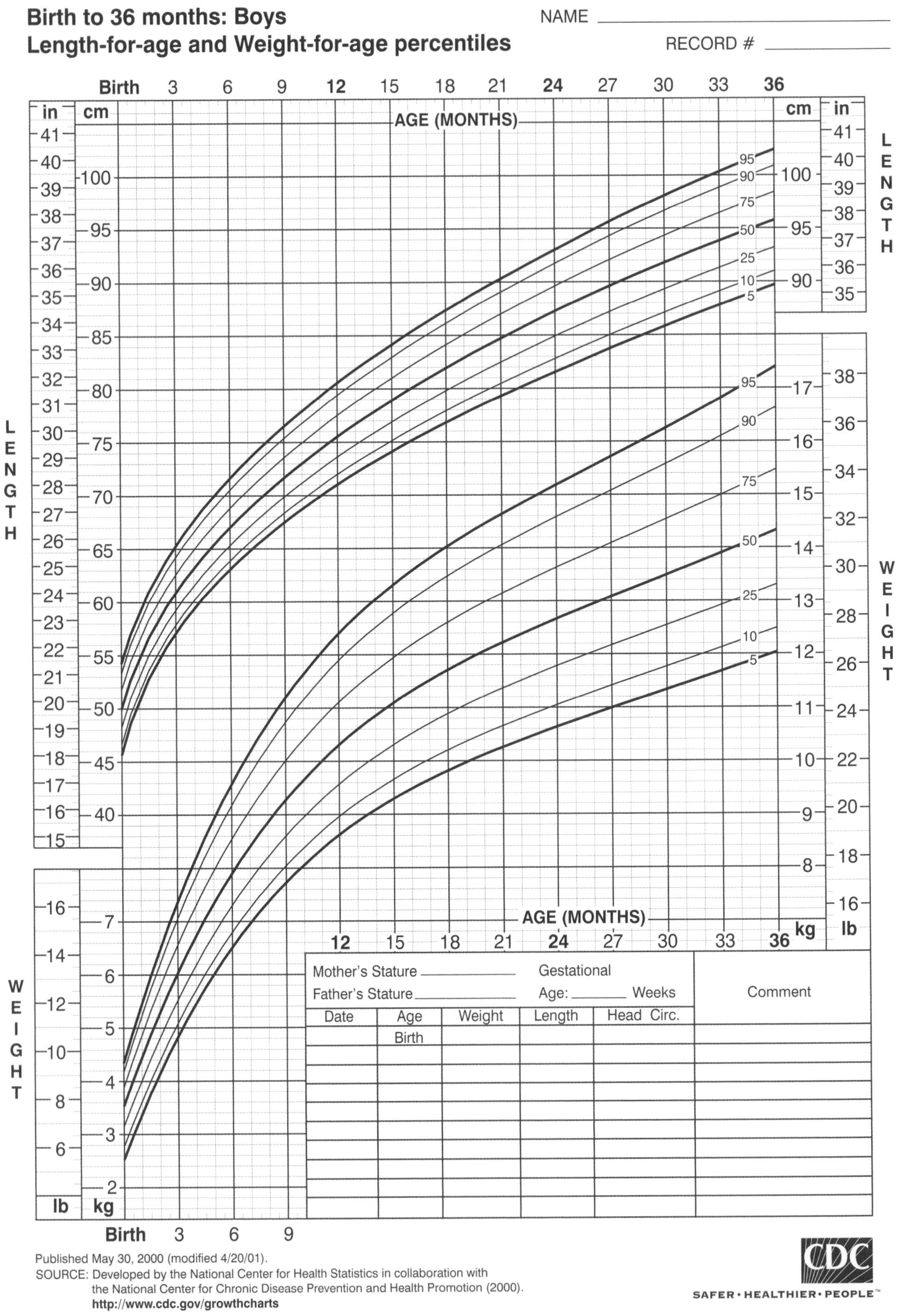

Birth to 36 months: Boys
Length-for-age and Weight-for-age percentiles

NAME ______________________

RECORD # ______________

Mother's Stature		Gestational Age: ____ Weeks			Comment
Father's Stature					
Date	Age	Weight	Length	Head Circ.	
	Birth				

Published May 30, 2000 (modified 4/20/01).
SOURCE: Developed by the National Center for Health Statistics in collaboration with the National Center for Chronic Disease Prevention and Health Promotion (2000).
http://www.cdc.gov/growthcharts

CDC
SAFER • HEALTHIER • PEOPLE™

Figure 8-1—cont'd

Birth to 36 months: Boys
Head circumference-for-age and Weight-for-length percentiles

NAME ______________________

RECORD # ______________

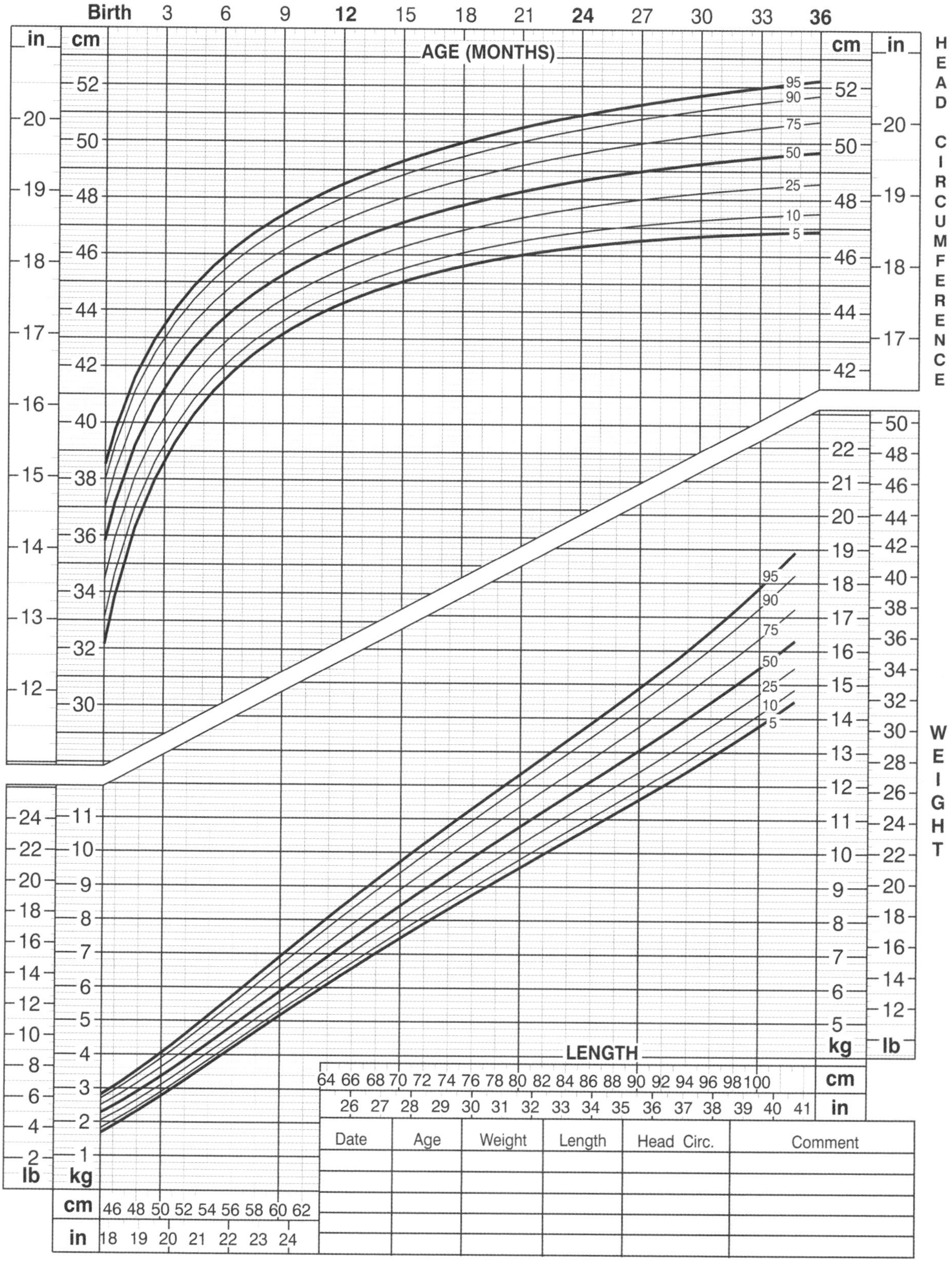

AGE (MONTHS): Birth 3 6 9 12 15 18 21 24 27 30 33 36

HEAD CIRCUMFERENCE (cm): 30 32 34 36 38 40 42 44 46 48 50 52

HEAD CIRCUMFERENCE (in): 12 13 14 15 16 17 18 19 20

Percentiles: 95 90 75 50 25 10 5

WEIGHT (kg): 1 2 3 4 5 6 7 8 9 10 11 12 13 14 15 16 17 18 19 20 21 22

WEIGHT (lb): 2 4 6 8 10 12 14 16 18 20 22 24 26 28 30 32 34 36 38 40 42 44 46 48 50

LENGTH (cm): 46 48 50 52 54 56 58 60 62 64 66 68 70 72 74 76 78 80 82 84 86 88 90 92 94 96 98 100

LENGTH (in): 18 19 20 21 22 23 24 26 27 28 29 30 31 32 33 34 35 36 37 38 39 40 41

Date	Age	Weight	Length	Head Circ.	Comment

Published May 30, 2000 (modified 10/16/00).
SOURCE: Developed by the National Center for Health Statistics in collaboration with the National Center for Chronic Disease Prevention and Health Promotion (2000).
http://www.cdc.gov/growthcharts

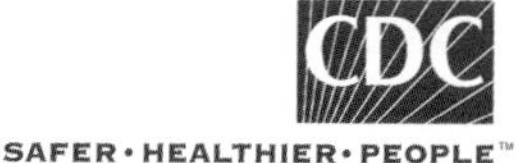

Figure 8-1—cont'd

Vital Signs

Assess for **normal vital signs** in the following areas:

- Temperature (**Figure 8-2**)
  - *Axillary*
- Pulse/heart rate
  - *Listen to apical for a full minute to assess for regular rhythm.*
  - *Pulse quality should be equal bilaterally and equal in upper and lower extremities.*
- Respiration rate
  - *Assess for distress and irregularity.*
  - *Allow child to stay with caregiver so that respiratory rate will not be falsely increased due to anxiety.*
- Blood pressure (**Figure 8-3**)
  - *Allow child to select which arm to use for blood pressure check when appropriate.*
  - *Talk to the child and tell of the tight "hug" feeling to expect on the arm.*
  - ***Table 8-1** shows average ranges for vitals.*
- Pulse oximetry
  - *Allow the child to select which digit to put the pulse oximeter on.*
  - *You may demonstrate use on the caregiver's finger to show that it is a painless procedure.*

Auscultate

- Lung sounds for clarity, wheezing, rhonchi, or crackles
- Neck sounds for stridor or snoring
- Heart sounds for regularity and murmur
- Bowel sounds for abnormalities (absent, hypoactive, or hyperactive)

CLINICAL PEARL

The nurse may hold up an index finger and tell the child to pretend it is a candle. The child is then prompted to blow out the candle. After the child exhales and "blows," the nurse will lower the finger and tell the child that the candle was blown out. This brings fun and a game-like atmosphere to the assessment. The child is then taking in deep breaths to adequately assess breath sounds.

Palpate

- Scalp for suture lines and fontanels
- Abdomen for tenderness and swelling
- Assess for enlarged liver or spleen

CRITICAL COMPONENT

Formula for calculating a child's blood pressure: 70 + 2 × age in years = lower end of systolic blood pressure; 90 + 2 × age in years = upper end of systolic blood pressure (U.S. Department of Health and Human Services, National Institutes of Health, & National Heart, Lung, and Blood Institute, 2005). (See Table 8-1.)

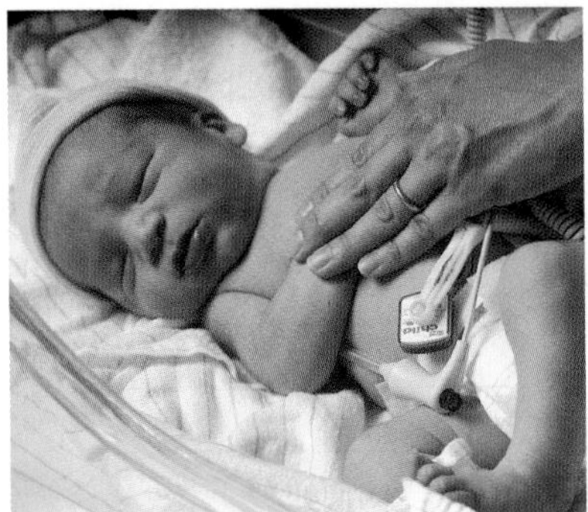

Figure 8–2 Taking vital signs: Temperature.

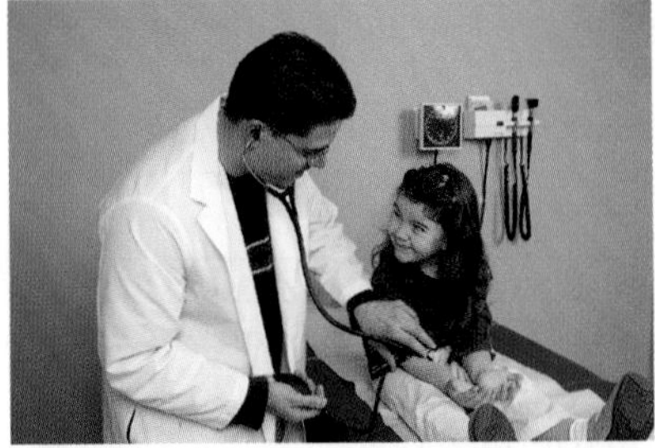

Figure 8–3 Taking vital signs: Blood Pressure.

SAFETY

According to Safe Kids USA (2009), among children under 14 years of age, children ages 4 and under are at greater risk of death as a result of **unintentional injury**. Children less than 4 years of age account for approximately half of all unintentional injury deaths. Each year more children ages 1 to 4 die from unintentional injuries than from all childhood diseases combined (Safe Kids USA, 2009).

- The leading causes of injury deaths in children are motor vehicle crashes, drowning, suffocation, fires and/or burns, and pedestrian-related incidents (Safe Kids USA, 2009).
- Younger children, males, minorities, and poor children tend to suffer disproportionately; poverty is often a predictor of injury (Safe Kids USA, 2009).
- Drowning was the leading cause of injury death for those 1 to 4 years of age (Centers for Disease Control and Prevention [CDC], National Vital Statistics Systems [NVSS], & National Electronic Injury Surveillance System [NEISS], 2006).
- Falls and poisonings were the leading cause of nonfatal injuries of children between 1 and 4 years of age (CDC, NVSS, & NEISS, 2006).

TABLE 8–1 AVERAGE RANGE FOR TODDLER AND PRESCHOOL VITAL SIGNS

Age Group	Pulse/Heart Rate (Beats/Min)	Respiration Rate (Breaths/Min)	Systolic Blood Pressure (mm Hg)	Diastolic Blood Pressure (mm Hg)
Toddlers	70–110	20–30	90–105	55–70
Preschoolers	65–110	20–25	95–110	60–75

From Ward, S. L., & Hisley, S. M. (2010). *Maternal-child nursing care*. Philadelphia: F.A. Davis.

CLINICAL PEARL

In 2011, drop-side cribs were banned for sale and distribution in the United States due to multiple injuries. This style of crib may be passed down through friends and family and thus still be used in homes. Discourage the use of this style of crib to promote injury prevention (Healthy Child Care America, 2011).

Nursing Interventions

- Minimize falls risk by keeping the side rails on beds/cribs up.
- Check equipment regularly—wire and cord placement to minimize entanglement, suction availability at cribside when necessary, and the least amount of equipment and crib attachments to decrease choking and suffocation hazards.
- Check temperature of water, food, and drinks to prevent burns.
- Explore any signs or symptoms that potentially may require a referral to child protective services. This is a legal requirement in most states and provides assistance for children and families of abuse. A child may experience abuse at any age.
- Educate caregiver on basic home, outdoor play, and car safety measures to ensure environmental safety for children.
- Install smoke detectors and ensure they are operational by changing the batteries every six months.

Promoting Safety

A child may become scared and hide in fear during an emergency. Urge families to have an evacuation plan in case of fire or other emergency; the plan should include alternative exits and a meeting place outside of the home.

Safety Education for Caregiver

- Do not carry hot liquids around children or while holding a child.
- Do not allow young children around stoves and fireplaces.
- Use the back burners on the stove and turn pot handles in toward back.
- Do not allow children around smaller hot appliances, such as irons, curling irons, and toasters.
- Set the temperature of hot water tanks to 120 degrees Fahrenheit or lower to prevent scalds (Christopherson, 2011).
- Always check the temperature of water, food, and formula prior to use.
- Use safety gates to block stairs. If placed at top of staircase, secure to wall.
- Keep windows closed. Screens will not hold children in and prevent falls.
- Do not leave young children alone on porches or balconies.
- Use nightlights.
- Keep all medications and poisonous products (e.g., household cleaners and chemicals) in high places out of reach or in a locked cabinet.

Medication

Medication Is Not Candy

Never tell a child medication is candy. Medication should be administered by an adult and kept in a place that is out of a child's reach. Child safety caps are not meant to be the primary prevention for accidental ingestion. Child safety caps are the last means of defense between the child and the medication.

- Have the number to your local poison control center available and keep poisonous materials in original containers so that the information on the labels can be accessed.
- Buy products with childproof tops.
- Clean up any old, chipping paint around the house.
- Look for and take away small toys that could present a choking hazard.
- Buy age-appropriate toys.
- Throw away anything broken.
- Secure any loose cords from blinds, curtains, and clothing out of reach to minimize strangulation hazard.
- Keep up to date on recalled toys and furniture.
- Do not allow children to eat and play at the same time.

- Cut food into bite-size pieces and avoid foods such as nuts, hot dogs, hard candy, and grapes that could cause choking.
- Do not allow children to play with coin money or latex balloons.
- Lock rooms that are not childproofed.
- Supervise children closely around all animals, including family pets.
- Do not leave water in the bathtub or cleaning buckets.
- Close bathroom doors.
- Never leave children alone near any basin of water.

Outdoor Safety

- Childproof swimming areas, including access to pools, ponds, and lakes.
  - *Never leave children unattended near swimming areas, even if they are able to swim.*
  - *Use floatation devices (**Figure 8-4**).*
  - *Never leave toys in a pool, as children may be tempted to retrieve them.*
- Playgrounds and unfamiliar play areas post an increased risk of danger due to the unfamiliarity of the environment.
  - *Teach playground and play area safety rules, such as no running near roped areas, no putting head through bars, and no trampoline use. Trampolines are a safety risk for children of all ages.*

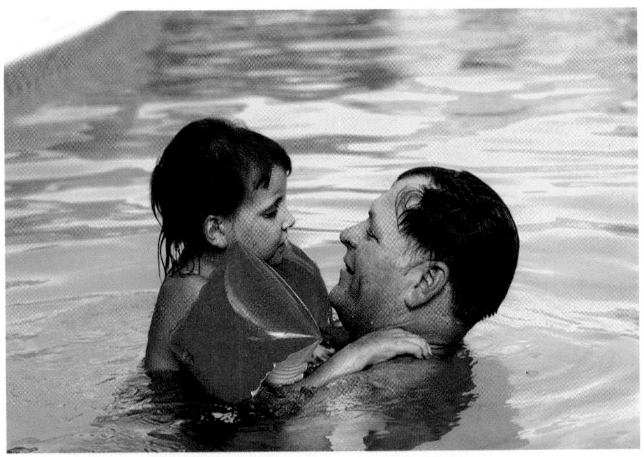

Figure 8-4 Flotation devices can prevent drowning.

  - *Teach crosswalk safety, such as how to cross correctly; running into the street for toys is not allowed; playing in the street is not allowed.*
  - *Children should always wear a bicycle helmet and never ride bicycles in the street.*
  - *Use child safety/booster seats and seat children in the back seat at all times.*
  - ***Table 8-2** shows required U.S. child restraint laws by state.*

TABLE 8-2 CHILD RESTRAINTS REQUIRED BY LAW

State	Child Restraint Required	Adult Safety Belt Permissible	Maximum Fine for First Offense
Alabama	<1 (or <20) in rear-facing infant seat; 1-4 (or 20-40) in forward-facing child safety seat; 5 (but not yet 6) in booster seat	6-14	$25 + points
Alaska	≤1 (or <20) in rear-facing infant seat; 1-4 (and >20) in child safety seat; 4-7 (and 20-64 or <57″) in booster seat	>4 (and ≥65 or ≥57″); 8-16 (and <65 or <57″)	$15 + points
American Samoa	<4	≥4	No data
Arizona	<5	Not permissible	$50
Arkansas	≤5 (and <60)	6-14 (or ≥60)	$100
California	≤5 (or <60) in a rear seat if available	6-15 (or ≥60)	$100 + points
Colorado	<1 (and <20) in rear-facing infant seat in rear seat if available; 1-3 (and 20-40) in forward-facing child safety seat; 4-7 (and <55″) in booster seat	8-15 (or ≥55″)	$82
Connecticut	<1 (or <20) in rear-facing restraint system; 1-6 (and <60) in child restraint system; booster seats only with a lap and shoulder belt	7-15 (and ≥60)	$60 ($15 for 4-16 and ≥40 lbs)
Delaware	≤7 (and <66)	8-15 (or ≥66)	$25
D.C.	≤7	8-15	$75 + points
Florida	≤3	4-5	$60 + points

TABLE 8–2 CHILD RESTRAINTS REQUIRED BY LAW—cont'd

State	Child Restraint Required	Adult Safety Belt Permissible	Maximum Fine for First Offense
Georgia	≤7 (and ≤57″) in rear seat if available (*eff. 7/1/11*)	>57″; ≥40 lbs can use lap belt if lap/shoulder belt unavailable	$50 + points
Guam	<12 in child restraint or booster seat	>12	$100
Hawaii	≤3 in child safety seat; 4–7 in booster seat or child restraint	4–7 (and >4′9″); 4–7 (and ≥40 lbs) in rear seat can use lap belt if lap/shoulder belt unavailable	$100
Idaho	<7	Not permissible	$69
Illinois	≤7	8–15; >40 lbs in rear seat if only lap belt available	$50
Indiana	≤7	8–15; ≥40 lbs can use lap belt if lap/shoulder belt unavailable	$25 + points
Iowa	<1 (and <20) in a rear-facing child seat; 1–5 in child restraint	6–17	$25
Kansas	≤3 in child restraint; 4–7 (and <80 or <57″) in child restraint or booster seat	8–13; 4–7 (and >80 or >57″)	$60
Kentucky	≤40″ in child restraint; ≤6 (and between 40″ and 50″) in booster seat	≤6 (and >50″)	$50 child restraint; $30 booster seat
Louisiana	<1 (or <20) in rear-facing child safety seat; 1–3 (or 20–39) in forward-facing child safety seat; 4–5 (or 40–60) in booster seat	6–12 (or >60)	$100
Maine	<40 lbs in child safety seat; 40–80 lbs and <8 yrs in safety system that elevates child so that adult safety belt fits properly; ≤11 (and <100) in rear seat if available	8–17 (or <18 yrs. and >4′9″)	$50 (max. $250 for subsequent offenses)
Maryland	<8 (and <57″ and ≤65 lbs)	8–15 (or ≥57″ or 65 lbs)	$25
Massachusetts	≤7 (and <57″)	8–12 (or ≥57″)	$25
Michigan	≤7 (and <57″); <4 in rear seat if available	8–15 (or ≥57″)	$10 for <4; $25 for 4–8 and under 4′9″
Minnesota	≤7 (and <57″)	≥8 (or >57″)	$50
Mississippi	≤4 in child restraint; 4–6 (and <57″ or <65 lbs) in booster seat	≥7 (or ≥57″ or ≥65 lbs)	$25
Missouri	<4 (or <40) in child safety seat; 4–7 (and 40–80 and <4′9″) in child safety seat or booster seat; ≥4 years (and ≥80 or ≥4′9″) in booster seat or safety belt; if all safety restraints in use, <16 in rear seat	8–16; ≥4 (and >80 or >4′9″)	$50; $10 for >80 lbs or >4′9″
Montana	<6 (and <60)	Not permissible	$100
Nebraska	≤5	6–17	$25 + points
Nevada	<6 (and <60)	Not permissible	$500 (min. $100)
New Hampshire	≤5 (and <55″)	6–17 (or <6 and ≥55″)	$50
New Jersey	<8 (and <80) in rear seat if available	Not permissible	No less than $10 + court fees
New Mexico	<1 in rear-facing infant seat in rear seat if available; 1–4 (or <40) in child safety seat; 5–6 (or <60) in booster seat	7–17	$25

Continued

TABLE 8–2 CHILD RESTRAINTS REQUIRED BY LAW—cont'd

State	Child Restraint Required	Adult Safety Belt Permissible	Maximum Fine for First Offense
New York	≤3 unless >40 lbs and no lap/shoulder belt available; 4–7 unless no lap/shoulder belt available	8–15; or 4–7 (or >40) if no lap/shoulder belt available	$100 + points
North Carolina	≤7 (and <80)	8–15 (or 40–80 lbs in seats without shoulder belts)	$25 + $136 court costs + points
North Dakota	≤6 (and <57″ or <80 lbs)	7–17; ≤6 (and ≥80 and ≥57″); ≤6 (and ≥40) can use lap belt if lap/shoulder belts unavailable	$25 + 1 point
Northern Mariana Islands	<5 (or <70)	>5 (or >70)	$50–$250
Ohio	<4 (or <40) in child safety seat; 4–7 (and <4′9″) in booster seat	8–14	$75
Oklahoma	≤5	6–12; ≥40 lbs can use lap belt if lap/shoulder belt unavailable	$50 *(up to $207.90 with court costs)*
Oregon	≤1 (or ≤20) in rear-facing child safety seat; <40 lbs in a child safety seat; >40 lbs (and ≤4′9″ or less than 8 years old) in safety system that elevates the child so that an adult seat belts fits properly	>4′9″	$142 ($97 plus $45 surcharge)
Pennsylvania	≤7	Not permissible	$100
Puerto Rico	≤4	≥5	$100
Rhode Island	≤7 (and <80 and <57″) in rear seat if available	≤7 (and ≥80 or ≥57″); 8–17	$75
South Carolina	<1 (or <20) in rear-facing infant seat; 1–5 (and 20–39) in forward-facing child safety seat; 1–5 (and 40–80) in booster seat secured by lap/shoulder belt (lap belt alone is not permissible); ≤5 in rear seat if available	1–5 (and ≥80) or ≤5 if child's knees bend over the seat edge when sitting up straight with his or her back firmly against the seat back	$150
South Dakota	<5 (and <40)	5–17 (or ≥40)	$25
Tennessee	<1 (or ≤20) in rear-facing infant seat; 1–3 (and >20) in forward-facing infant seat; 4–8 (and <4′9″) in booster seat; ≤8 (and <4′9″) in rear seat if available; rear seat recommended for 9–12	9–15 (or ≤12 and >4′9″)	$50
Texas	≤7 (and <57″)	Not permissible	$25
Utah	≤7 (and <57″)	8–15 (or ≥57″)	$45
Vermont	<1 (or <20) in rear-facing infant seat in rear seat unless front passenger airbag is deactivated; 2–7 (and >20)	8–17 (and >20)	$25
Virgin Islands	≤5	≥3	$25 to $250
Virginia	≤7; rear-facing devices in rear seat if available; if not, in front seat only if front passenger airbag is deactivated	8–17 (4–8 with physician's exemption)	$50
Washington	<8 (and <4′9″); <13 in rear seat if practical	8–15 (or <8 and ≥4′9″); ≥40 lbs in position where only lap belt available	$124 to driver if passenger <16; $124 to passenger if ≥16
West Virginia	≤7 (and <4′9″)	≤7 (and ≥4′9″)	$20

TABLE 8-2 CHILD RESTRAINTS REQUIRED BY LAW—cont'd

State	Child Restraint Required	Adult Safety Belt Permissible	Maximum Fine for First Offense
Wisconsin	<1 (or <20) in rear-facing infant seat; 1–3 (and 20–40) in forward-facing child safety seat; 4–7 (and 40–80 and <57″) in booster seat; ≤3 in rear seat if available	≤8 (and ≥80 and ≥57″)	$75
Wyoming	≤8 in rear seat if available	Not permissible	$50
Total States	50 + D.C., Guam, Northern Mariana Islands, Puerto Rico, U.S. Virgin Islands		

Unless indicated, # refers to yrs (lbs).
Note: The information presented here is for general information purposes only and is not to be considered legal authority. For clarification on any law, consult the appropriate State Highway Safety Office, http://www.ghsa.org/html/stateinfo/laws/childsafety_laws.html. Adapted from "Child Passenger Safety Laws" by Governors Highway Safety Association, 2011. Copyright 2011 by Governors Highway Safety Association. Reprinted with permission.

PAIN

- Young toddlers do not have the cognitive ability to convey the pain they are feeling.
- The capability to report pain begins approximately at the age of 2.
- Assess for causes of pain such as infection, injury, surgical/procedural, or disease.

CLINICAL PEARL

Use medical play to explain and prepare for medical procedures. A child life specialist (CLS) may assist with this preparation with the nurse. Medical play allows the child to utilize concrete thinking to understand upcoming events. The medical play items prepare the child for how equipment may feel and sound. The preparation will help to eliminate some fear of the unknown. Whenever possible, allow children to keep comfort items (e.g., stuffed animals and blankets) with them during procedures (Figure 8-5).

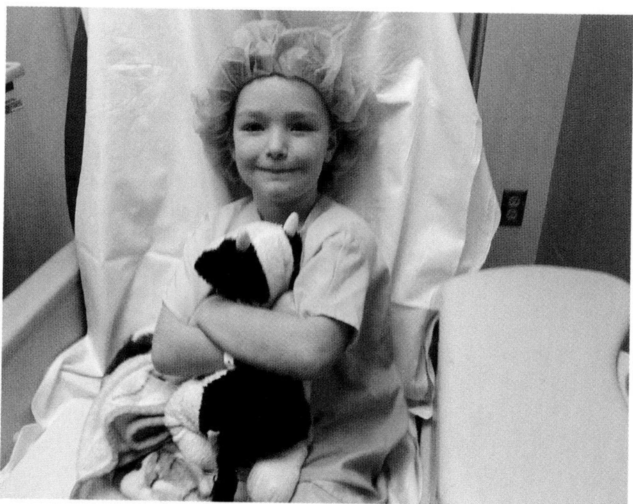

Figure 8–5 Kindergartner prior to surgery.

- Assume pain is present and treat accordingly.

Medication

Provide Appropriate Choices When Giving Medications

Never give children the choice of taking a medication or not. Instead, give them a choice in medication form, such as liquid or chewable, or a choice in what to take the medication with, such as water, juice, or applesauce.

- Assess for elevated heart rate, blood pressure, and respiratory rate. (Reminder: These alone are considered poor indicators of pain.)
- Observe specific behaviors children display in reaction to pain, such as facial expression, movement, and vocalization (**Figure 8-6**).
  - *Furrowed brow and open-mouth-type grimace, or lack of expression*
  - *Restlessness or sleeping and withdrawal (ways to cope with pain)*
  - *Wariness/fear of movement*
  - *Irritability/agitation*
  - *No vocalization to harsh/high-pitched cry*
- Choose appropriate **pain scale**. There are 16 published postoperative pain scales for use with infants and toddlers.
- Evaluate for efficacy of all pain control interventions, including medication, repositioning, and/or consolation measures.
- **Table 8-3** shows some of the differences among pediatric pain scales.

CULTURAL AWARENESS: Pain Scales Are Not Reliable for All Cultures

Some pain scales may not be reliable for children of different cultures due to cultural influence on pain response. In U.S. culture, for example, male children may be told that "big boys don't cry" and therefore may hold back in showing emotions (see Figure 8-6).

Evidence-Based Practice Research

Cohen et al. (2008) reviewed the evidenced-based practice of utilizing pediatric pain scales. Many scales have been validated, but it is most important to identify why the particular scale is being used (Cohen et al., 2008). Some scales have been used in specific environments and for different types of pain (Cohen et al., 2008). The nurse must choose a pain scale that is most appropriate for each individual child.

AGE GROUP CHALLENGES

Potty Training

- Usually begins between the ages of 2 and 3
- Signs of readiness include:
  - *Ability to have dry diaper for a few hours at a time or during a nap*
  - *Regularly timed bowel movements*
  - *Interest in the potty or going to the potty with others*
  - *Physical ability to get to potty and pull up/down pants*
  - *Ability to follow simple directions*
  - *Unhappiness with the feeling of a wet or dirty diaper*
  - *Ability to vocalize when they went and/or if they have to go*
- Signs that the child is not ready include:
  - *Resistance to toilet-training attempts*
  - *Unwillingness to try*
- Rushing a child into potty training will only make the process more lengthy and frustrating.
- Try to avoid potty training during stressful times, such as a move or new baby arrival.
- The teaching process includes the following:
  - *Have the child practice sitting on the potty for a few minutes at a time.*
  - *Practice hand washing; encourage the child to sing a song to wash for the appropriate amount of time.*
  - *Teach proper use of hand sanitizer: must cover hands and dry completely; do not place hands in mouth (can be toxic to children).*
  - *Teach girls to wipe front to back to minimize risk of urinary tract infections.*
  - *Teach boys to urinate in the sitting position first. Once mastered, then move on to standing. May use flushable toilet targets for teaching purposes (do not put toys in the toilet for this purpose).*

FLACC Pain Scale

	Scoring		
Categories	0	1	2
Face	No particular expression or smile; disinterested	Occasional grimace or frown; withdrawn	Frequent to constant frown, clenched jaw, quivering chin
Legs	Normal position or relaxed	Uneasy, restless, tense	Kicking, or legs drawn up
Activity	Lying quietly, normal position, moves easily	Squirming, shifting back and forth, tense	Arched, rigid, or jerking
Cry	No cry (awake or asleep)	Moans or whimpers, occasional complaint	Crying steadily, screams or sobs, frequent complaints
Consolability	Content, relaxed	Reassured by occasional touching, hugging, or talking to; distractible	Difficult to console or comfort

Each of the 5 categories—(F) Face; (L) Legs; (A) Activity; (C) Cry; (C) Consolability—is scored from 0 to 2, which results in a total score between 0 and 10.

From: FLACC Pain Scale, from The FLACC: A behavioral scale for scoring postoperative pain in young children, by S. Merkel et al, 1997, Pediatr Nurse 23(3), pp. 293–297. Copyright 1997 by Jannetti Co., University of Michigan Medical Center. Reprinted with permission.

A

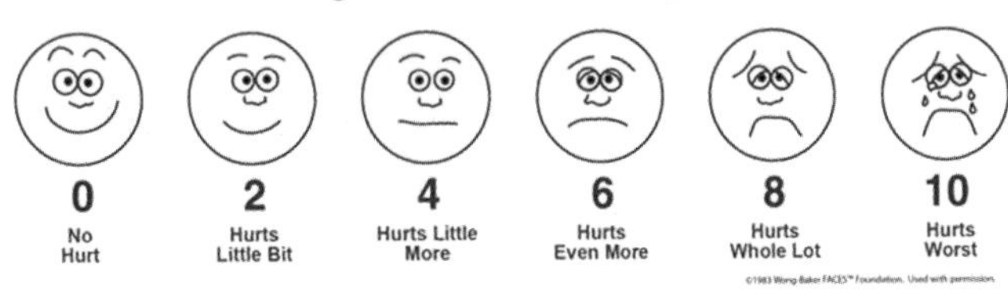

B

Figure 8–6 Pediatric pain scales. (**A**, FLACC Pain Scale, from Merkel, S., et al. [1997]. The FLACC: A behavioral scale for scoring postoperative pain in young children. *Pediatric Nurse, 23*[3], 293–297. Copyright 1997 by Jannetti Co., University of Michigan Medical Center. Reprinted with permission; **B**, Wong-Baker FACES™ Pain Scale, © 1983, Wong-Baker FACES™ Foundation, http://www.WongBakerFACES.org. Used with permission.)

TABLE 8–3 PAIN SCALES TESTED IN TODDLERS AND PRESCHOOLERS

Abbreviated name of pain scale	Name of scale	Appropriate age use	Description
CHEOPS	Children's Hospital of Eastern Ontario Pain Scale	Study done on children ages 1–5; intended for ages 0–4; can be used on children up to 7 years of age	A behavioral scale that gives a number value for cry intensity, facial expression, child verbalization of pain, torso position, touch, and leg movement
CHIPPS	Children and Infants Postoperative Pain Scale	Studied in infants and children ages 0–5; recommended for children ages 0–3	A behavioral scale that assigns a number value for cry intensity, facial expression, trunk position, leg movement, and restlessness
FACES	Wong-Baker FACES Pain Rating Scale	Recommended for children ages 3–7; several studies unable to support reliability for children under 5 years of age	A self-reporting rating scale that assigns a number value to a facial expression to be chosen by a child
FLACC	Faces, Legs, Activity, Cry, Consolability Observational Tool	Studied in children ages 2 months to 7 years; recommended for ages 1–5 or any preverbal child	A behavioral scale that assigns a number value for facial expression, leg movement, activity/restlessness, cry intensity/continuity, and consolability
DEGR	Douleur Enfant Gustave Roussy	Studied on children with cancer ages 2–6	A behavioral scale in which an observer assigns a score of 0 for none to 4 for extreme on 16 different scale items
TPPPS	Toddler-Preschooler Postoperative Pain Scale	Recommended for children ages 1–5	A behavioral scale that assigns a number value for verbal response, facial expression, and body language

- *Encourage*
  - Provide praise and celebrate when the child is done in the potty.
  - Use rewards and incentives—treats, stickers, or new underwear.
  - Don't be severe or punitive when accidents happen.

Separation Anxiety

- Distress caused by a fear of abandonment
- Normal stage of development
- Can begin as early as 8 months of age and end as late as 3 years of age, but peaks between 10 and 18 months (Healthy Children, 2010)
- Lessens over time as child learns that parents will come back
- To reduce separation anxiety, parents/caregivers should:
  - *Distract the child, say goodbye, and leave quickly. The quicker you leave, the quicker the episode will end.*
  - *Practice leaving at home by going to another room and saying you will be back soon.*
  - *Stay calm, be consistent, and give reassurance that you will be back.*

Tantrums and Discipline

- Most common in 1 to 4 year olds
  - *Whining and crying to screaming*
  - *Hitting and kicking to scratching and biting*
  - *Breath holding*
- This is a way for the child to express anger and frustration.
  - *Triggers include:*
    - Hunger
    - Tiredness
    - Being uncomfortable/sick
    - Being overstressed
    - Attention seeking
    - Other problems (mental, physical, or emotional)
- Tantrums usually decrease in number with increase in language skills.
- Caregivers need to stay calm and collected; venting frustration verbally or physically can worsen situation.
  - *Establish and maintain routines.*
  - *Set limits.*
  - *Consequences need to follow poor behavior*
    - Time out or sitting in a chair until calm
    - Taking child to a quiet place

Sibling Rivalry

- **Sibling rivalry** includes jealousy, competition, and fighting among siblings.
  - *To gain attention from parents*
  - *To show dominance over sibling*

- *Some quarreling is normal.*
  - Fighting over toys
  - Calling each other names
  - Telling on each other
- *Toddlers are protective of their toys. Preschoolers are more apt to share.*
- *Don't intervene unless the situation is unsafe.*
  - Encourage them to resolve the problem themselves.
- *If intervention is necessary*
  - Separate the children to their own spaces.
  - Set rules, such as no name calling, no pushing, and no slamming things.
  - Don't choose sides.
  - Assist with proper expression of feelings of anger and frustration.
- *Teach them to be kind to each other.*
  - Apologizing
  - Sharing
  - Comforting each other when hurt

Nutrition

- Transition to milk
  - *Preschoolers 2 years and older should drink 2 glasses of skim or low-fat milk or have 2 other servings of dairy per day (American Dietetic Association [ADA], 2011b).*
  - *Some toddlers may still be breastfeeding. Support the breastfeeding mother by allowing privacy and bonding during feedings.*
  - *Many sources of protein are also common allergens (ADA, 2011a).*
    - Dairy products
    - Seafood
    - Nuts
    - Soy products
  - *Snacks should be healthy enough to provide part of a child's total nutrient intake for the day.*
    - Fruits and vegetables
    - Milk, yogurt, and cheese
    - Whole-grain crackers and cereal
    - Nuts and peanut butter
  - *Toddlers eat approximately 7 times a day, eating more meals than snacks. Preschoolers eat approximately 3 meals a day with quite a few snacks throughout the day.*
  - *Serving larger portions than recommended and/or pressuring a child to eat or clean his or her plate can lead to overeating and increase risk for childhood obesity.*
    - Allow children to self-regulate intake while providing healthy, nutrient-filled choices.
  - *Allow the child to graze throughout the day, as toddlers may not sit for three meals.*

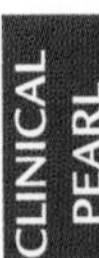

CLINICAL PEARL

According to the American Dietetic Association (2011a), an easy way to calculate an **appropriate serving size** for this age group is 1 tablespoon per year of age.

- *Transition to cups and utensils.*
  - Should be transitioned by age 2
- Encourage self-feeding.
  - To reinforce self-regulation of intake
  - To improve motor function
- Appetite fluctuates in toddlers and preschoolers.
  - Amount of intake can vary with every meal.

Clinical Reasoning

A mother tells you that she is not sure if her child is eating enough each day. She is concerned that the child will not grow properly.

1. What information can assist the nurse to determine if the child is eating enough?
2. What physical assessment data will assist the nurse to determine if the child is eating enough?

- *Difficulty consuming enough iron and zinc*
- *Difficulty fostering healthy eating habits*
  - Finicky eaters
  - Normal to play with food
  - Learning about different textures and tastes
  - May prefer to eat only from a few selected foods
- *Difficulty decreasing amount of intake of juice and sweet drinks*
  - Juice and sweetened drinks should be limited to 4 to 6 ounces per day.
  - The ideal drink choice is plain water.

CRITICAL COMPONENT

Drinking from a bottle throughout the day or at night increases the risk for dental caries (**Figure 8-7**). It may also decrease appetite for solid food and thus increase risk for malnutrition. The American Academy of Pediatrics (n.d.) recommends that a child see the dentist by age 1.

- *Preschoolers may have difficulty sitting at the table due to short attention spans.*
  - They should be encouraged to sit at the table even if not eating to promote good eating habits.
  - Routine is important.

GROWING INDEPENDENCE

Promote Independence with Safety

- Teach toddlers:
  - *Rules and responsibilities*
  - *How to be safe*
  - *How to be a good friend by sharing, being nice, and not hitting others*

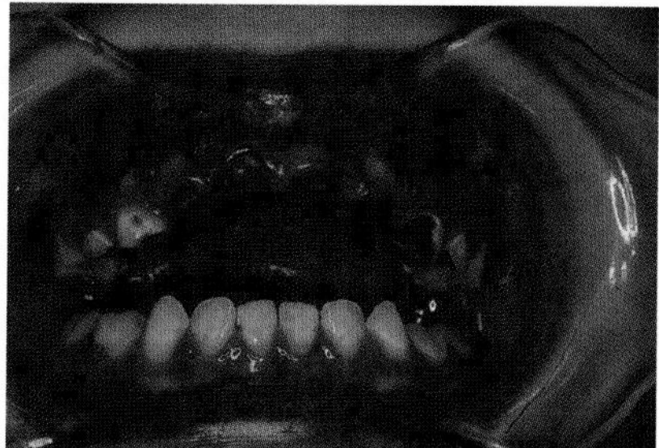

Figure 8–7 Baby-bottle caries.

- *To establish and keep routines so they can begin to do these routine things on their own*
- Give toddlers age-appropriate chores. Allowing them to help teaches responsibility.
- Take time to listen.
  - *Ask them open-ended questions.*
  - *Provide eye contact to show that attention is being given.*
- Encourage children to bathe and dress themselves or assist in these tasks.

CAREGIVER SUPPORT

In Hospital (Acute and Chronic Care)

- Orient caregivers to unit.
- Explain all procedures in a step-by-step manner.
- Go over the plan of care with caregivers daily or as it changes.
- Encourage families to stay informed by asking for test results, updates on patient care, and changes in patient status.
- Encourage the asking of questions and the expression of concerns.
- Instruct caregivers to express when further explanation is needed.
- Urge caregivers to learn about the child's medications.
- Encourage involvement in decision making.
- Reassure caregivers that it is normal to feel scared, helpless, overwhelmed, guilty, sad, worried, confused, frustrated, angry, alone, and tired.
- Remind caregivers to care for themselves. Reassure them that it is fine to go home for a while, whether to relieve stress, take a shower, go to sleep, and/or take care of other responsibilities.

In Home

- Caregivers should have emergency phone numbers available
  - *Nurse advice line*
  - *Number for doctor on call*
  - *Poison control line*
  - *911 availability*

CRITICAL COMPONENT

Assessing for Child Abuse

- Bruised in areas that are not typically bruised during play
- Bruises in different stages of healing
- History of multiple broken bones
- Caregiver speaks up when nurse asks how a bruise occurred
- Caregiver's story does not fit the identified injury
- Multiple hospitalizations and child does not have a chronic health problem

Nurses are required to report suspected abuse by law. The nurse cannot keep a "secret" shared by a child when abuse is suspected.

- Teach caregivers how to care for children at home.
  - *How to care for a fever*
    - Medication
    - Patient cooling techniques
  - *How to prevent dehydration*
  - *Small, frequent sips of fluids*
  - *Electrolyte-replacement beverages*
  - *Broths*
  - *Popsicles*
  - *Diet advancement (as tolerated)*
    - Clear liquids
    - Soft/bland
    - Solids

Signs and Symptoms of Common Childhood Infections

- Fever accompanied by
  - *Moist, productive cough*
  - *Green or blood-tinged nasal discharge*
  - *Pulling at ears*

Simple First Aid

- Wound cleansing
- Use of band-aids
- Topical antibiotics

Signs and Symptoms of Respiratory Distress

- Tachypnea
  - *Breathing rapidly*
  - *Unable to complete sentences*
- Retractions
  - *Ability to see ribs during inhalation*
- Nasal flaring
  - *Nares flare out in an effort to take in air*
- Accessory muscle use
  - *Use of shoulders and abdomen to breathe*
- Tripod positioning
  - *Sitting with head up and out to stent the airway open*
- Stridor, wheezing, and sonorous respirations
  - *Cool mist humidifier*
  - *Warm steam bath*

See Chapter 11 for respiratory information.

When to Call the Doctor

- Follow instructions as provided.
- Call if there has been a negative change from what the doctor has first assessed.

When to Call 911

- Call 911 for all emergencies.
- Child is not breathing properly or adequately.
- Child's face is blue or extremities are blue.
- Call for all perceived emergencies.

PEDIATRIC DISASTER PLANNING

- Equipment standards may vary among first responders (U.S. Department of Health and Human Services, 2010).
- All hospitals are not equipped to provide extensive critical care to pediatric patients.
- More attention has been brought to disaster planning since the New York terrorist attacks on September 11, 2001.
- Weight-based single-dose medications are more difficult to stockpile than adult standard-dose medications.
- Children need to be transported to facilities that can care for their immediate needs.
- Advocating for child safety is the responsibility of all adults.

Review Questions

1. One of the first things to assess in a clinic visit is the chief complaint. When obtaining the chief complaint, the information that the nurse is looking for is:
   A. whether or not immunizations are up to date.
   B. current signs and symptoms or events leading to the visit.
   C. whether or not anyone else in the family is sick.
   D. current medications the child is taking.
2. Separation anxiety is defined as
   A. a normal stage of development.
   B. a toddler's way to express anger and frustration.
   C. specific behaviors small children display in reaction to pain.
   D. distress caused by fear of abandonment.
3. During the early years, it is important to encourage self-feeding and transition to cups and utensils in order to
   A. decrease the risk of dental caries associated with bottle feeding.
   B. reinforce self-regulation of intake.
   C. foster motor skills.
   D. foster independence.
   E. all of the above.
4. Joey and Jason are 3-year-old twins who have come to the clinic today for a well-child check. Their mom reports that they are always fighting over their toys. What do you say to Mom?
   A. They are experiencing separation anxiety from their toys.
   B. Jealousy, competition, and fighting among siblings are characteristic of sibling rivalry, and some quarreling is normal.
   C. Fighting over toys is the leading cause of unintentional-injury-related deaths in 3-year-olds.
   D. All of the above
5. A 5-year-old male is being admitted to the hospital. According to Erikson, in which of the following stages is this child?
   A. Phallic stage
   B. Trust vs. mistrust
   C. Initiative vs. guilt
   D. Preoperational
6. A nurse is making rounds collecting vital signs. Which of the following sets of vital signs is abnormal?
   A. A 5-year-old female: HR 102 beats/min, RR 24 resp/min, BP 90/65
   B. A 2-year-old male: HR 140 beats/min, RR 32 resp/min, BP 86/45
   C. A 5-year-old male: HR 150 beats/min, RR 48 resp/min, BP 70/45
   D. A 3-year-old female: HR 110 beats/min, RR 28 resp/min, BP 76/40
7. What question/questions will appropriately assess if a toddler is ready for potty training?
   A. Is the child unhappy with wearing a wet or dirty diaper?
   B. Is the child eating solid food?
   C. Is the child physically able to get to the potty?
   D. Can the child follow simple directions?
   E. Choices a, c, and d
8. Normal growth and development for a 2-year-old would include which of the following?
   A. Taking turns with friends stacking blocks on top of one another
   B. Writing own name
   C. Beginning to display defiance
   D. Catching a bounced ball and throwing it back overhand
9. Children are anatomically different than adults. What are the differences?
   A. Children have larger tongues and a greater proportion of soft tissue in and around the airway.
   B. Children have less body surface area in relation to total weight.
   C. Children have more elastic and collapsible airways.
   D. All of the above
   E. Choices a and c

10. A 2-year-old female is having a temper tantrum at the day-care center. The best way for the caregiver to handle the situation is to: (select all that apply)
    A. stay calm and collected.
    B. reason with the child and tell her that she is too old to act in this manner.
    C. follow through on appropriate predetermined consequences, such as "time-out."
    D. ignore the child.

References

American Academy of Pediatrics. (n.d.). *Children's oral health.* Retrieved from http://www.aap.org/oralhealth/

American Dietetic Association (ADA). (2011a). *Size-wise nutrition for toddlers.* Retrieved from http://www.eatright.org/Public/content.aspx?id=8055

American Dietetic Association (ADA). (2011b). *When to switch your child from whole milk to low fat.* Retrieved from http://www.eatright.org/Public/content.aspx?id=6442458961&terms=Toddlers+and+whole+milk

Centers for Disease Control and Prevention (CDC). (2009). *Clinical growth charts.* Retrieved from http://www.cdc.gov/growthcharts/clinical_charts.htm

Centers for Disease Control and Prevention (CDC), National Vital Statistics Systems (NVSS), & National Electronic Injury Surveillance System (NEISS). (2006). *CDC childhood injury report.* Retrieved from http://www.cdc.gov/safechild/Child_Injury_Data.html

Christopherson, E. R. (2011). Burns: Hot water safety. In *Pediatric Advisor 2011.1.* Retrieved from http://www.cpnonline.org/CRS/CRS/pa_hotwatr_pep.htm

Cohen, L. L., Lemanek, K., Blount, R. L., Dahlquist, L. M., Lim, C. S., Palermo, T. M., . . . Weiss, K. E. (2008). Evidence-based assessment of pediatric pain. *Journal of Pediatric Psychology, 33,* 939–955. doi:10.1093/jpepsy/jsm103

Healthy Child Care America. (2011). *Crib regulations.* Retrieved from http://www.healthychildcare.org/CribRegulations.html

Healthy Children. (2010). *Soothing your child's separation anxiety.* Retrieved from http://www.healthychildren.org/English/ages-stages/toddler/pages/Soothing-Your-Childs-Separation-Anxiety.aspx

Safe Kids USA. (2009). *Preventing injuries: At home, at play, and on the way.* Retrieved from http://www.safekids.org/our-work/research/fact-sheets/high-risk-fact-safety.html

U.S. Department of Health and Human Services. (2010). *Emergency medical services and pediatric transport.* Retrieved from http://archive.ahrq.gov/prep/nccdreport/nccdrpt4.htm

U.S. Department of Health and Human Services, National Institutes of Health, & National Heart, Lung, and Blood Institute. (2005). *The fourth report on the diagnosis, evaluation, and treatment of high blood pressure in children and adolescents* (NIH Publication No. 05-5268). Retrieved from http://www.cc.nih.gov/ccc/pedweb/pedsstaff/ Pediatric_Blood_Pressure_Management.pdf

9 School-Age Children

Daniel C. Rausch, BSN, RN

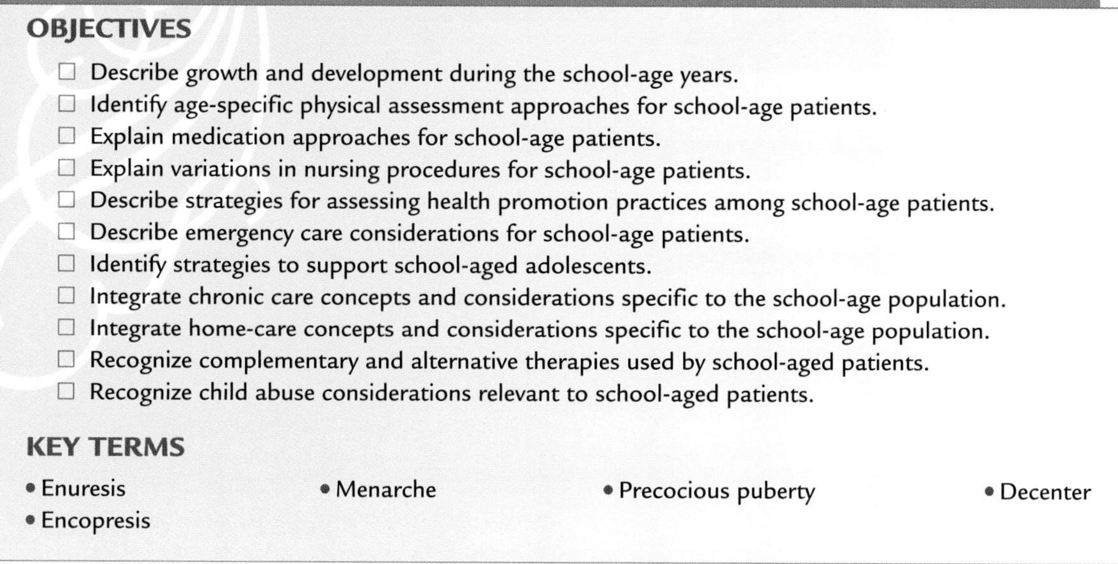

OBJECTIVES

- ☐ Describe growth and development during the school-age years.
- ☐ Identify age-specific physical assessment approaches for school-age patients.
- ☐ Explain medication approaches for school-age patients.
- ☐ Explain variations in nursing procedures for school-age patients.
- ☐ Describe strategies for assessing health promotion practices among school-age patients.
- ☐ Describe emergency care considerations for school-age patients.
- ☐ Identify strategies to support school-aged adolescents.
- ☐ Integrate chronic care concepts and considerations specific to the school-age population.
- ☐ Integrate home-care concepts and considerations specific to the school-age population.
- ☐ Recognize complementary and alternative therapies used by school-aged patients.
- ☐ Recognize child abuse considerations relevant to school-aged patients.

KEY TERMS

- Enuresis
- Encopresis
- Menarche
- Precocious puberty
- Decenter

INTRODUCTION

Children 6 to 12 years old are considered "school age" (**Figure 9-1**). During these years, children are growing at a slower rate than ever before but are still accomplishing important developmental milestones. During this period, a wide variety of changes can be seen in the child in both physical and behavioral aspects. The younger school-age child will be similar to the late-stage preschooler, whereas the older school-age child will be more similar to an adolescent. Each child will move through this stage at a different pace. Careful assessment and adaptability on the part of the nurse are required in caring for patients of this age group.

GROWTH AND DEVELOPMENT

- Physical:
  - *Vital signs (**Table 9-1**)*
    - Pulse oximetry values should be the same as adult values 93%–100%.
    - Pulse oximetry values may be different if there is an underlying cardiac or pulmonary diagnosis.
    - A fever is generally considered to be a temperature greater than 101.4°F or 38.5°C (Asher & Northington, 2008).
  - *Attainment of vital signs should not be difficult with this population. Explain the procedure to the child. Allow the child to choose, as appropriate, which side the blood pressure will be taken on to help the child gain a sense of control.*
  - *Height/weight*
    - The Centers for Disease Control and Prevention (CDC) provides gender- and age-specific grids on which height and weight can be plotted (CDC, 2009; see also CDC Web site at http://www.cdc.gov).
    - Gains 3 kg/year in weight
    - Gains 5 cm/yr in height
    - Girls experience a growth spurt at age 10 to 12.
    - Boys experience a growth spurt at age 12.
    - Weight is obtained using a standing scale unless the child has a condition that does not allow him or her to stand.
    - Similarly, height should be taken standing unless there is a condition that does not allow a standing height. In such cases, a length measurement may be substituted.
  - *Daily fluid requirements*
    - Daily fluid requirements are based on weight (**Table 9-2**).

Don't have time to read this chapter? Want to reinforce your reading? Need to review for a test? Listen to this chapter on DavisPlus at davispl.us/rudd1.

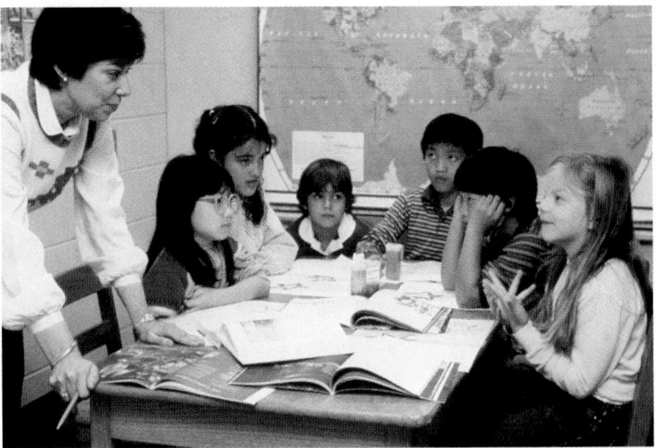

Figure 9–1 School-age children.

- *Normal urine output*
  - Expected urine output is based on patient age and calculated by weight (**Table 9-3**).
- *Pain assessment*
  - A few different pain scales may be used depending on age and developmental level.
  - Any pain assessment must begin by explaining how the pain scales work and assessing the child's ability to properly use the scale.
  - When assessing, specifically teach the levels and ask the child what his or her pain level is, not how he or she feels. Being sick and in the hospital may cause the child to give a higher rating than the actual pain level.
  - A nurse caring for this population should be familiar with the use of a few different pain scales.

CRITICAL COMPONENT

Choice of Pain Scale

Choice of pain scale is dependent upon the nurse's assessment of the child's developmental level.

- FACES may be used for younger school-age children. (See Chapter 8 for information on the FACES scale.)
  - *One downside noted with the FACES scale is that some children will choose the smile face because that is the most desirable. Additionally, if a child is feeling pain, he or she may automatically be drawn to the crying face, number 10.*
  - *Educate the child to point to the face that reflects the level of pain he or she is experiencing.*
- Older school-age children may be able to use a visual analog scale or numeric of 1–10.
- Parents or the child's primary caregiver will be able to assist in the assessment of pain. They will notice minute differences in their children that the nurse may not immediately notice.

TABLE 9–2 Fluid Requirements by Weight

Weight	Fluid Requirement (ml/kg/day)
11–20 kg	1000 ml + 50 ml for each kg above 10 kg
>20 kg	1500 ml + 20 ml for each kg above 20 kg

Adapted from Guid, n.d.

TABLE 9–3 Expected Urine Output

Age	Expected Urine Output
6–7 yrs	1–2 ml/kg/hr
8–12 yrs	0.5–1 ml/kg/hr

Source: Patient.co.uk, 2010.

CULTURAL AWARENESS: Spanish-Language Pain Tools

- There is an increasing number of Spanish-speaking people in the United States, including the pediatric population.
- Spanish-language tools for pediatric pain reporting have not received much research attention.
- The problem with developing these tools is that there are variations in the Spanish language based on country of origin.
  - Colloquialisms vary between countries.
- Another issue is attempting to translate multiple pain scales into universally understood terms (Cleve, Munoz, Bossert, & Savedra, 2001).

TABLE 9–1 VITAL SIGNS TYPICAL FOR AGE

Age	Temperature	Pulse	Respirations	Systolic BP	Diastolic BP
6 yrs	98.6°F	95	20–25	95	55–70
9 yrs	98.1°F	95	17–22	105–110	60–75
12 yrs	97.8°F	85	17–22	118–120	62–76

Adapted from National Institutes of Health, 2008.

- *General survey*
  - General somatic complaints without verified diagnostic clinical data—such as chronic pain, dizziness, sweating, headaches, chest pain, shortness of breath, gastrointestinal (GI) issues/pain such as nausea/vomiting/diarrhea, and back/joint pain—may be an indication of school or home avoidance/problems, anxiety and stress, or depression (Sarafolean, 2000). (See Chapter 14, Mental Health Disorders.)
  - Determine developmental history, family composition, and school performance.
  - Yearly health maintenance visits with a primary care provider are recommended for school-age children (American Academy of Pediatrics [AAP], n.d.).
- *Annual assessments*
  - Height
  - Weight
  - Body mass index
  - Blood pressure
  - Hearing
  - Vision
  - Anemia
- *Immunizations*
  - An immunization schedule, updated each year in January, is available at the Centers for Disease Control Web site (http://www.cdc.gov). (See also Chapter 22, Communicable Diseases.)
- *Skin*
  - Assess for signs of child abuse, such as bruises in various stages of healing, bruises on unusual parts of the body, and cigarette burns.
  - Assess for dryness, rashes, eczema, abrasions, and contusions or scratches.
- *Head*
  - Assess for lice (**Figure 9-2**).
  - Assess hair for dryness and brittleness that can indicate nutritional status.
  - Assess for open lesions/signs of trauma.
- *Eyes*
  - Assess for use of glasses/contacts.
  - Assess visual acuity.
  - Assess for broken blood vessels, jaundice, and dryness.

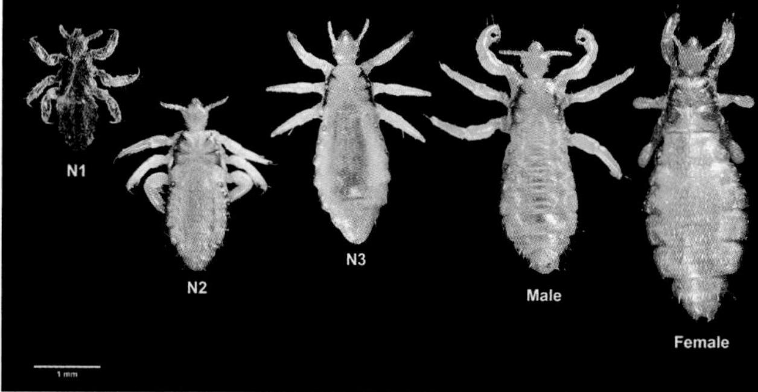

Figure 9–2 Pediculosis (head lice).

- *Ears*
  - Assess for hearing aid use and hearing acuity.
  - Assess for buildup of earwax, which can impair hearing.
  - Assess for an excess buildup of fluid in the canal.
- *Mouth/throat/teeth*
  - During this period, children will start to lose their primary (baby) teeth.
  - New adult teeth will begin to erupt, starting with 6-year molars.
  - Orthodontic treatment may start during this age.
    - *There is a need for increased dental self-care during orthodontic treatment. Be sure that the patient and family are aware of the proper care of braces and removable appliances.*
  - Promote good dental hygiene—children will be starting to care for themselves more independently but may lack motivation to keep it up.
  - Teeth should be brushed after all meals and snacks, and brushing should be assisted/monitored in younger children.
  - Dental checkups should occur every 6 months, with fluoride treatments if fluoride in the water supply is low (AAP, n.d.).
    - *Checkups may occur more often due to increased risk of tooth decay, improper hygiene, or unusual growth patterns.*
  - Assess for loose teeth or removable orthodontic appliances that may need to be removed or observant of during an emergency.
  - Do not assume that the "tooth fairy" visits every home (Dentistry, 2011), as this is influenced by culture.
- *Nose*
  - Assess for a blue or "boggy" appearance of the nasal mucosa, which indicates allergies.
  - Assess for allergic rhinitis.
  - Assess for frequent nosebleeds and mucosal dryness.
  - Assess for airflow, which may be restricted due to acute or chronic sinusitis.
- *Cardiovascular*
  - Assess for any congenital cardiac anomalies by history and auscultation.
    - *With many corrected cardiac defects, the patient may have scars on the chest such as a midline incision or chest tubes.*
  - About 25% to 50% of children have a benign murmur (also called "innocent murmur") that will resolve during this age range (University of Chicago, 2011).
    - *This is often a result of turbulent blood flow at the aorta or pulmonary artery (University of Chicago, 2011). (See also Chapter 12, Cardiovascular Disorders.)*
- *Respiratory*
  - Assess for a history of asthma, which is the number one chronic illness in children. (See Chapter 11, Respiratory Disorders.)
  - Lungs should sound clear. (See Chapter 11, Respiratory Disorders.)
  - Check for signs/symptoms of chronic respiratory issues such as barrel chest and clubbed fingers. (See Chapter 11, Respiratory Disorders.)

- Abnormalities may include crackles, rhonchi, wheezing, retractions, grunting, and nasal flaring.
- Assess skin color to note any oxygenation issues.
  - *These include pallor or cyanosis.*
  - *These could be related to respiratory or cardiac issues.*
- *Gastrointestinal/Genitourinary*
  - Assess for **enuresis**, which is urine incontinence. (See Chapter 16, Renal Disorders.)
  - Assess for **encopresis**, which is the deliberate withholding of stool. (See Chapter 15, Gastrointestinal Disorders.)
  - Evacuation of a small amount of stool may indicate encopresis.
  - Assess for constipation/diarrhea, acute or chronic, and any treatments the patient may be receiving.
- *Reproductive*
  - Girls may experience **menarche**, the start of menses, near the end of this stage. (For information on puberty, see Chapter 10, Adolescents.)
    - *This will be a girl's first period.*
    - *Primary caregivers should be ready to support the child during this time, as it may be emotional and scary.*
    - *Early discussions with the child will help her prepare for this time when it comes.*
    - *Refer to the Tanner Stages to identify what stage of puberty the child is in (Feingold, 1992).*
  - Some children may experience **precocious puberty** (defined as experiencing puberty before age 7 for girls and before age 9 for boys; Kanshiro, 2011).
    - *This may be very difficult for the child. Make sure that appropriate support is given to the child.*
    - *Although a child's primary caregiver may intend to discuss menarche with his or her daughter, precocious puberty may come before this discussion takes place.*
  - Boys
    - *The onset of puberty in boys will be accompanied by:*
      - *An increase in upper body mass*
      - *Increased amount and thickness of hair on the body and genitalia*
      - *Nocturnal emissions, or release of semen during sleep (This is a normal part of puberty and may be seen in the late stage of school age, but more likely in adolescence.)*
- *Neurovascular/musculoskeletal*
  - Increased coordination
  - Increased fine motor skills
  - Increased balance
  - These increases assist in the ability to do more complex tasks, such as riding a bike.
  - Begin scoliosis checks by age 12. (See Chapter 10, Adolescents.)
- *Cognitive*
  - Piaget's cognitive developmental theory (see also Chapter 6, Growth and Development):
    - *Ages 6–9: Preoperational thought, intuitive phase*
    - *Ages 10–11: Concrete operations*
    - *Ages 12–15: Operations*

- Children in this age group will be starting school.
  - *Begin mastering mathematics and reading skills*
  - *Can classify and serialize numbers*
  - *Understand cause and effect*
  - *Have the ability to* ***decenter*** *(see perspectives other than their own)*
- *Psychological*
  - Freud's psychosexual development theory (see also Chapter 6, Growth and Development):
    - *Ages 6–12: Latency stage*
  - Erikson and psychosocial development (see also Chapter 6, Growth and Development):
    - *Ages 6 to 12: Industry versus inferiority*
- *Social*
  - Kohlberg's theory of moral development (see also Chapter 6, Growth and Development):
    - *Pre-conventional level*
      - *Likes to forms clubs with rules and requirements*
      - *Likes to do favorite activities with a best friend*
      - *Usually socializes primarily with children of the same gender*
      - *Follows rules and understands consequences*
      - *Enjoys playing games*
      - *Enjoys having a collection of items, such as video games*

PHYSICAL ASSESSMENT APPROACHES

Lewis (1999) notes the following regarding physical assessment:

- School-age children should be cooperative with the physical assessment.
- Ask the child whether he or she would like the parent or primary caregiver present during the assessment.
  - *Typically, younger school-age children will like to have the primary caregiver present and older school-age children may or may not want the primary caregiver present during the entire assessment.*
- Speak and direct questions directly to the child.
- Give the child rationales for all actions.

> **CLINICAL PEARL**
>
> **Good Touch/Bad Touch**
>
> Use inspection of the genital area as a springboard for discussing good/bad touches.
> Define areas the child should report if anyone touches the child there (breasts, buttocks, and genitalia).

APPROACHES TO MEDICATION ADMINISTRATION

School-age children should be able to assist in the medication administration process.

Medication

Dosing

Medications should have weight-based dosing to provide an appropriate dose.

TYPES OF MEDICATIONS

- Oral medications
  - *Many oral medications can be prepared in a flavored liquid provided by the pharmacy.*
  - *Use caution with flavorings that taste like candy.*
  - *Home medications should be stored in a safe area so that younger school-age children will not get into them.*
  - *Be sure to monitor all administrations of medications to the child.*
  - *Teach the patient's primary caregiver safe medication practices and administration techniques.*

CRITICAL COMPONENT

How Children Take Oral Medications

A small number of children in this age group may start swallowing pills. Be sure to assess how the child prefers to take oral medications, and give the child a choice when possible.

  - *Children of this age will be able to start to assist in and make decisions about medication administration.*
  - *Younger school-age children may choose to take oral liquids from an oral syringe or a medicine cup.*
  - *If appropriate, the nurse may choose a drink or food as a reward.*
  - *If the medication tastes bad, offer a "chaser," numb the tongue beforehand with a popsicle, or have the child pinch his or her nose while ingesting the medication.*
  - *The child's caregiver may administer medications, under nursing supervision, when appropriate.*
- Subcutaneous medications
  - *Use EMLA medicated cream when appropriate.*
  - *EMLA is used to prevent pain associated with needle insertion, intravenous cannulation, and superficial surgery on the skin and genital mucous membranes.*
  - *Assess depth of adipose tissue and muscle mass.*
  - *This will help ensure the nurse uses an appropriate needle size and depth so that the medication is placed subcutaneously and not intramuscularly.*
  - *If the patient has a history of diabetes, the child's caregiver may be experienced at administering subcutaneous injections.*
  - *Older school-age children with diabetes may be starting to administer their own injections. This must occur under parental/caregiver supervision.*
- Intravenous (IV) medications
  - *Use EMLA cream prior to starting IVs.*
  - *A child life specialist will be helpful in explaining procedures in an age-appropriate fashion.*

Medication

Eutectic Mixture of Lidocaine and Prilocaine (EMLA) Cream

EMLA is a medicated cream applied to the skin prior to painful procedures. The mixture contains 2.5% lidocaine and 2.5% prilocaine. It should be in place at least 45 minutes. The longer it is in place, the deeper it will penetrate; 2 hours is best for intramuscular injection. After 4 hours, it begins to lose its effectiveness and should be removed. Another product is known as ELA-Max, which absorbs into the skin more quickly than EMLA.

- Assess for allergic reaction to the medication.
- Apply a large "glob" of the medication to the skin.
- Do not rub it in.
- Apply an occlusive dressing over the medication.
- Do not rub, massage, or disturb the area until ready to perform the procedure.
- Advise the patient's primary caregiver to watch the medicated area so the child does not disturb the cream, pull off the dressing, or consume the cream.
- When dressing is removed, wipe remainder of medication from the skin before cleaning for the procedure (LexiComp Online, 2011).

  - *Medical play can be helpful for this age group.*
  - *Older children may be more compliant if they can make appropriate decisions, such as which side the IV will be put into.*
  - *When inserting an IV, remember that the patient will still need to perform age-appropriate activities such as coloring for younger children and writing, homework, or crafts for older children; if possible, place the IV in the nondominant hand.*

Evidence-Based Practice Research: Use of EMLA Cream

Rogers, T. L. (2004). The use of EMLA cream to decrease venipuncture pain in children. *Journal of Pediatric Nursing, 19*, 33–39. doi: 10.1016/j.pedn.2003.09.005

Research has been conducted since the 1980s regarding the effectiveness of EMLA cream in invasive procedures with children. Invasive procedures include phlebotomy, intramuscular injection, and IV cannulation. One impracticality of EMLA use is the time it takes for effectiveness, which is at least 60 minutes. For a patient getting an injection at an outpatient appointment, this would prolong the time in the office and increase anticipation anxiety. If an injection is known to be needed, EMLA could be applied before arriving at the office. A newer version called ELA-Max can shorten the time to about 30 to 45 minutes, which is still long. EMLA was found to be effective in pain management. However, even with EMLA use, some patients still reported pain during cannulation. EMLA is effective but should not replace other comfort measures, including position, distraction, and an experienced nurse for patients with a "difficult stick" (Rogers, 2004).

VARIATIONS ON NURSING PROCEDURE

- It is important to gain the trust of the child before beginning assessment or procedures.
  - *Explain procedures in an age-appropriate way. Do not lie if a procedure will be uncomfortable or painful; this will lose the child's trust. The child life specialist may be helpful in explaining procedures (see discussion later in this chapter).*
  - *Tell the child and the parents/caregivers what you will be doing before doing it.*
  - *A good approach can be:*
    - **Look**: Assess the child's appearance, muscle tone, and skin.
    - **Talk**: Discuss with the child and the parents/caregivers any recent history or problems. Listen to what the child tells you.
    - **Touch**: Be nonthreatening by using no sudden movements and staying at the level of the child whenever possible.
    - Allow for privacy.
    - Appropriate rewards such as stickers or small toys may be given at the conclusion of the examination.
    - If a procedure needs to be performed, have the instruments ready and inform the child immediately before the procedure. The longer a child is aware that a painful or uncomfortable procedure is coming, the greater the stress that can occur.
    - Do the least invasive parts of the examination first.

HEALTH PROMOTION

- Safety
  - *Bike/scooter/skateboard/sports safety*
    - Educate on use of helmets and pads (**Figure 9-3**).
    - The child can learn how to put on pads and helmets and be able to do this unassisted.
    - Assess for and encourage the use of protective pads and helmets.
  - *Pedestrian safety (**Figure 9-4**)*
    - Walking on sidewalks
    - Looking both ways when crossing streets
    - Walking on the left side of the street, against traffic, for safety
  - *Adult supervision is necessary for many activities.*
    - Children are starting to have independence at this age, and may be able to do many activities with less direct supervision.
    - Children are able to play alone with adults nearby. Children should not be left unsupervised for any extended period of time.
    - By the end of this phase, children will engage in unsupervised activities, such as staying home while their parents/primary caregivers run errands.
    - The child's readiness to be left unsupervised will vary.
    - Additionally, older school-age children may start babysitting.

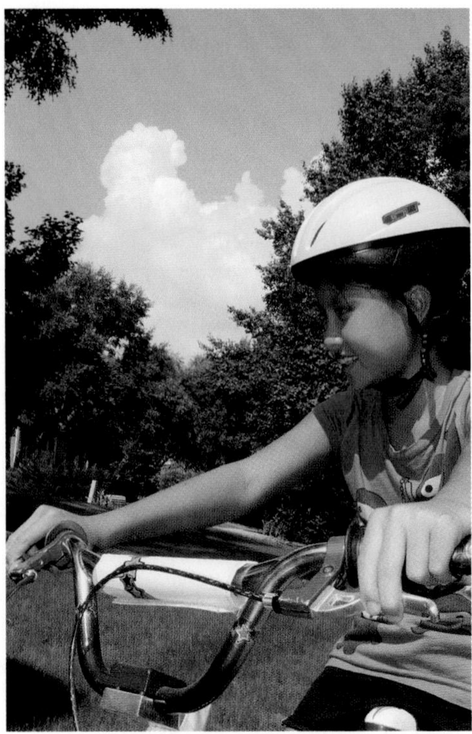

Figure 9-3 Child wearing bike helmet.

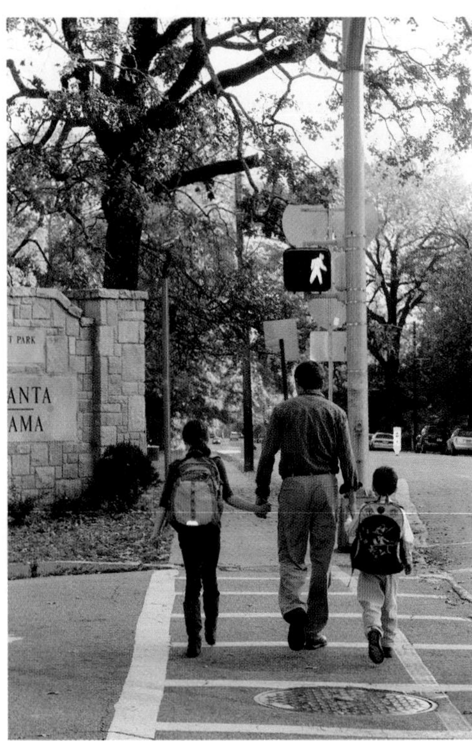

Figure 9-4 Father walking children across the street.

  - *Children will try to be more independent and try more "exciting" and dangerous activities.*
  - *School-age children will be more involved in team activities, such as football, baseball, swimming, and cheerleading.*

Promoting Safety

As children begin to babysit, they should learn about and be comfortable with creating and maintaining a safe environment for the children they supervise and themselves. This includes:

- Knowledge of fire safety
- Care of and observation of children in various stages of growth and development
- Basic first aid and possibly cardiopulmonary resuscitation (CPR)

Many of these skills are taught in babysitting classes offered by hospitals and other organizations, such as the YMCA.

- Nutrition
  - *Decreased caloric requirement compared with previous stages*
  - *Important time to teach children and primary caregivers about proper nutrition*
  - *During the next stage, adolescence, the child's nutritional requirements will increase again.*
- Approximately 18% of school children are obese, defined as >95th percentile by the Centers for Disease Control (CDC), and another 18% are overweight (CDC, 2012a).
  - *A higher body mass index (BMI) in children is linked with increased lipid levels, insulin levels, and blood pressure.*
  - *These can lead to higher risks of atherosclerosis and obesity in adulthood.*
  - *These risks are high for obese children but lower for children who are overweight.*
  - *Overall, overweight children have a greater chance of being overweight as adults.*
  - *The health consequences of obesity in children will have a negative effect on their morbidity and mortality as adults.*
- Exercise
  - *Encourage activity.*
    - Children should have at least 1 hour of activity a day (CDC, 2011).
  - *Encourage normal school-age activities*
    - These can include many outside activities such as ball, jumping rope, bike riding, skating, and playing at a playground.
  - *Encourage participation in school exercise programs.*
    - Most schools will have a physical education program.
  - *As with nutrition, early education and experience with exercise can help to form good habits that can last a lifetime (Pearce, Harrell, & McMurray, 2008).*
- School
  - *Assess for school avoidance/refusal/phobia.*
    - Child displays somatic symptoms such as a "stomachache" without any clinical basis, but only on school days.
    - Child refuses to attend school.
    - An interdisciplinary approach is needed.
    - Teachers, school counselor, parents or primary caregivers, and health-care professionals should be involved.
    - Homeschooling/tutoring may be only option until the issue is resolved.
  - *Bullying*
    - Bullying is significantly more prevalent in the school-age group than in the adolescent group.
    - Studies have found that up to 20% of children report being bullied; other studies have shown as high as 50% (Filippos et al., 2009).
    - Definition: "Bullying is a specific type of aggression in which (1) the behavior is intended to harm or disturb, (2) the behavior occurs repeatedly over time, and (3) there is an imbalance of power, with a person or group perceived as more powerful attacking one perceived as less powerful. This asymmetry of power may be physical or psychological, and the aggressive behavior may be verbal, physical, or psychological. Individuals may be bullies (perpetrators), victims, or bullies/victims" (Filippos et al., 2009 p. 569).
    - Bullying occurs in all countries to a varying degree.
    - Various factors are associated with being a bully, a victim, or both:
      - *Age*
      - *Lower socioeconomic status*
      - *Parents and caregivers having a lower educational level*
      - *Poor health status, increased health needs, and mental health issues*
      - *Physical appearance*
      - *Poor academic achievement or social adjustment*
      - *Sexual orientation*
    - Assess for both physical and psychological signs of bullying.
    - Assist caregivers with finding resources to assist with bullying.
    - Many schools now have programs to deal with bullying and a zero-tolerance anti-bullying policy.
    - For children with special needs, assess the resources available at the school.
- Substance use and sexual activity
  - *Assess for and discourage the use of alcohol, tobacco, and drugs.*
    - Many schools have substance abuse prevention programs, such as DARE.
    - Parents have the strongest influence on teaching children to avoid drugs.
  - *Assess for sexual activity.*
    - Assess for child's understanding and knowledge of sex.
    - Children may be more willing to discuss sexual activity privately, without their parents present.
  - *Sex education may start in many schools during this age range.*
    - Assess caregivers regarding resources for teaching their children about sex.
    - Assess if the caregivers have started to discuss sex with older school-age children.

- Discussing this subject can be difficult for caregivers. Help them to find resources to teach their children and creative ways to open the discussion.
- *"Sexting"*
  - Sexting is a growing issue today.
  - Sexting is the practice of sending nude/explicit videos or pictures on a cell phone or across the Internet or posting to an Internet site. It is considered illegal and children can suffer legal consequences.
    - *Caregivers should ask their children about sexting.*
    - *Caregivers should be aware of any activity that their child participates in on the Internet or on a cell phone.*
    - *Cases that are discovered are being charged as child pornography cases (SafeKids.com, 2009).*

EMERGENCY CARE

- Unintentional injuries and homicides are the two leading causes of death for children 1 to 19 years old (CDC, 2012b).
  - *Child life specialists should be available in the emergency room to help the child through procedures.*
    - The family usually sees the physician as the point person to discuss what is occurring. The physician is often unavailable to talk with the family during the crisis, as he or she is involved in providing and directing care.
    - Social workers and chaplains should be available to the family.
    - Family-centered care remains important during this time.

ACUTE CARE HOSPITALIZATION

- Environment of care
  - *Different facilities will have different types of rooms.*
  - *In any situation, it is beneficial to allow the child and family to have an area for their own items.*
  - *The room should be a safe area for the child.*
  - *All invasive and painful procedures should be performed in a treatment room.*
  - *The child will learn that nothing painful will happen in the safety of his or her own room.*
  - *This will also help prevent child and caregiver fear when clinicians enter the room, as they may worry that any time clinicians enter, they have come to do a procedure.*
  - *Younger school-age children should be taken to the treatment room for any invasive procedure.*
  - *Educate parents/caregivers as to the reason for the use of the treatment room.*
  - *Older school-age children can decide whether or not they want to go to the treatment room or have the procedure, such as IV placement, at the bedside.*
- Role of primary caregivers in care
  - *The nurse should encourage the caregivers to have an active role in the care of the child.*
  - *Caregivers should bring items from home that help the child feel more comfortable and reduce stress.*
  - *Depending on facility policy, children may feel more comfortable wearing their own clothes or pajamas in the hospital.*
  - *Depending on the child's diagnosis, walks with caregivers may be allowed, possibly off the floor.*
  - *Encourage visitation of siblings to promote a normal environment.*
  - *Visiting siblings should be free of illness.*
  - *If siblings are admitted together, try to make sure they get a double room together or in rooms next to each other to make care of the children easier for the primary caregivers.*
    - This will help the children deal with hospitalization as well.
    - Allow siblings to participate in activities with the sick child, if able, so as to help create a more normal environment.
- Role of child life specialist
  - *Child life specialists offer a variety of services.*
    1. Preparation for medical procedures
       - May use medical play to show the school-age child how a procedure is performed.
       - A child's anxiety will be significantly decreased after acting out a planned procedure on a medical doll.
       - Child life specialists may accompany a school-age child to a procedure or test to help provide distraction and coach the child through the procedures.
    2. Celebration of milestones
       - Some children may be in the hospital during major milestones, such as birthdays. Child life specialists may provide an appropriate celebration.
       - Child life specialists will assist with helping children celebrate holidays that they spend in the hospital, such as Christmas.
    3. Therapies
       - Music therapy can provide distraction and a constructive outlet for the stress of hospitalization.
       - Art therapy can also provide distraction and release.
       - Art therapy can help a child create items to decorate the room, creating a more comfortable environment.
       - Therapeutic puppetry
         - *Some hospitals use puppets in therapy because children respond differently to a warm, fuzzy character than they do to adults. For example, Rainbow Babies and Children's Hospital in Cleveland, Ohio, have a puppet mascot named Buddy who can visit children and host shows on the hospital's closed circuit television channel.*
    4. Activity room
       - An activity room may be coordinated by the child life specialist.
       - Children who are not on isolation may go to the activity room to play games, play with toys, or participate in organized activities.
       - Children who are on isolation may have toys brought to their rooms.
       - All toys should be able to be washed with water and disinfectant.
       - No stuffed animals or plush toys can be used with multiple patients.
       - Activities should be overseen by a hospital designate.

5. Medical play for education of illness and procedures
   - The child life specialist can assist with medical play.
   - Dolls can be used to assist in medical play.

- Child's preferences in care
  - *School-age children are starting to express their own preferences and personalities.*
  - *Help school-age children to make appropriate choices.*
  - *Do not offer a child a choice he or she cannot have, such as asking "would you like to take your medicine?" When the child has to take it after answering no, this could cause a loss of trust in the nurse.*
  - *Older school-age children will be seeking more autonomy and may be interested in assisting to perform their care.*
  - *Younger school-age children will be interested in role playing*
  - *All children in this age range will be curious about what is occurring in their care. Be sure to answer any questions honestly and at an appropriate level.*
  - *Younger school-age children will be more concrete thinkers. Avoid using terms that do not accurately describe what will be occurring, such as a "little stick" or "bee sting" for venipuncture.*
- School while in the hospital
  - *If children are well enough, they will need to continue their studies so that they do not fall far behind.*
  - *Some facilities may have a dedicated teacher who will bring the patient to a room for teaching or come to the patient's room to work with the patient.*
  - *The teacher will work with the child's school to get the patient's current assignments.*
  - *Family-centered care (relationship-based care) remains appropriate. (See Chapter 1.)*

CARE WHEN CHRONICALLY ILL

- Normalization of lifestyle
- Limitations
- Reaching milestones
  - *Children with chronic illnesses may reach milestones at a later time than their peers.*
  - *Praise the child for attaining milestones.*
  - *Notify appropriate resources to assist in milestone accomplishments, such as physical or occupational therapy.*
- Role of primary caregivers
  - *Most caregivers will have a very active role in the care of their chronically ill child.*
  - *They will have extensive knowledge of their child's conditions, treatments, and medications.*
  - *Children with chronic conditions may not be able to communicate in the same manner or to the same extent as other children. Caregivers will notice changes in their child that nurses may not notice.*
- Family-centered care
- Caregiver fatigue
  - *Caregivers of children with special needs must devote significantly more time in the care of their child than caregivers of healthy children.*
  - *The time, effort, and expense involved in care can vary greatly.*
  - *These factors can have a significant negative effect on the family and be very stressful for the caregiver.*
  - *It is important that the caregivers have a good support network, such as family.*
  - *It is helpful if the caregivers have assistance and support to be able to "get away" for a while and participate in activities that provide stress relief.*
  - *Some reports show increased marital stress in families of children with special needs (Stanger, & Rimmerman 2001).*

HOME-CARE CONSIDERATIONS

- Children receiving care within the home still need to have some control over their time and activities.
- School work should be kept up to date
- Time for interaction with peers, either in person or over the phone/Internet, should be allotted daily.

CHILD ABUSE CONSIDERATIONS

- Abused children in this age group may fear that they have done something wrong or that they somehow deserve what is happening to them.
- Primary caregivers should make sure that children understand good touch/bad touch.
- Caregivers should listen to children's concerns, ask questions about the adults/peers at school/activities, and monitor for changes in mood or behavior, which may indicate that an abuse episode has taken place.
- Children should also be taught not to go with strangers.
- After-school time should be supervised and structured.
- Children who come home from school to an empty house should be taught to be aware of their surroundings and to lock the door immediately after entering the house. It's also a good idea to have the child call a primary caregiver once safely inside the home (Stirling, 2008).

Clinical Reasoning

Assessing Child Abuse

A patient with cerebral palsy is admitted to your unit. While performing your admission head-to-toe assessment, you note that there are bruises in various states of healing on his forearms and legs. You also notice a few healing burns about 1 cm in diameter on his arms and torso.

1. What concerns do you have?
2. What actions should you perform?

Teacher Notes

The nurse should suspect abuse. Bruises in various stages of healing are a tell-tale sign. Also, the burns are consistent with cigarette burns, which are also often a sign of abuse. In most states it is required by law that the nurse reports any suspicion of abuse to authorities. The patient's physician should be notified and social worker consulted.

Review Questions

1. Which pain scale should a nurse utilize to assess pain in a school-age child?
   A. Visual analog scale
   B. FACES scale
   C. CRIES scale
   D. Both A and B
2. A benign or "innocent" murmur can occur in what percentage of children?
   A. 25%
   B. 1–5%
   C. 95–100%
   D. 75%
3. Which of the following is a correct technique for the application of EMLA cream?
   A. Rub it into the skin until it is no longer visible.
   B. Leave it on the skin for only 5 minutes.
   C. Place a large "glob" on the skin and cover with an occlusive dressing.
   D. Let the child rub it on like lotion.
4. The number one cause of death in school-age children is
   A. cancer.
   B. heart attack.
   C. pneumonia.
   D. arthritis.
   E. unintentional injury.
5. The nurse admits a Spanish-speaking patient. The patient and the parent only understand a few phrases and words in English. The younger sibling (6 years old) speaks fluently to you in English. How should you communicate with this patient?
   A. Have the sibling (the 6-year-old) translate for you.
   B. Utilize the housekeeping worker on your floor, who speaks fluent Spanish.
   C. Use an approved Spanish medical interpreter or approved Spanish medical interpreter hotline.
   D. Get a Spanish dictionary and attempt to communicate more efficiently.
   E. Use only hand signals and body language to explain all care and procedures.
6. Your 12-year-old patient needs to have a new IV started. Which intervention is appropriate?
   A. The patient may choose to use the treatment room or remain in her own room.
   B. The patient may help decide where the IV is located (right arm or left arm).
   C. The patient may have a child life specialist discuss the procedure with her.
   D. The child may listen to music during the procedure.
   E. All of the above
7. What is the best role for parents in the care of their acutely ill school-age child?
   A. Parents should only come during visiting hours.
   B. Parents should be permitted to stay with their child 24 hours a day, providing any care that comforts their child.
   C. Parents should not see their child during the child's stay to prevent crying and distress.
   D. The doctor should decide the visitation schedule.
8. While assessing a special needs patient, you note several bruises in various stages of healing and some small burns on the body. Which of the following is appropriate?
   A. Report your concerns to the social worker and authorities, and maintain a safe environment for the child.
   B. Tell the doctor, but otherwise continue care as usual.
   C. Stay out of it—it is not your business because the bruises did not occur in the hospital.
   D. Question the parents/caregivers until they give you the truth.
9. Expected urine output for a school-age child can vary depending on age, with ______ being considered normal.
   A. 30 ml/hr
   B. 5–10 ml/kg/hr
   C. 30 ml/kg/hr
   D. 0.5–2 ml/kg/hr
10. During a general assessment of a school-age child, which of the following should be observed or noted?
   A. Use of glasses or contacts
   B. Loose teeth and/or orthodontic appliances or braces
   C. Head lice
   D. Waxy buildup in the ears
   E. All of the above

References

American Academy of Pediatrics (AAP). (n.d.). *Bright future guidelines for middle childhood 5 to 10 years.* Retrieved from http://brightfutures.aap.org/pdfs/Guidelines_PDF/17-Middle_Childhood.pdf

Asher, C., & Northington, L. K. (2008). Position statement for measurement of temperature/fever in children. *Journal of Pediatric Nursing: Nursing Care of Children and Families, 23,* 234–236. doi: 10.1016/j.pedn.2008.03.005

Centers for Disease Control and Prevention (CDC (2009). *Clinical growth charts.* Retrieved from http://www.cdc.gov/growthcharts/clinical_charts.htm

Centers for Disease Control and Prevention (CDC). (2011). How much physical activity do children need? Retrieved from http://www.cdc.gov/physicalactivity/everyone/guidelines/children.html

Centers for Disease Control and Prevention (CDC). (2012a). Childhood obesity facts. Retrieved from http://www.cdc.gov/healthyyouth/obesity/facts.htm

Centers for Disease Control and Prevention (CDC). (2012b). Ten leading causes of death and injury. Retrieved from http://www.cdc.gov/injury/wisqars/leadingcauses.html

Cleve, L., Munoz, C., Bossert, E. A., & Savedra, M. C. (2001). Children's and adolescents' pain language in Spanish: Translation of a measure. *Pain Management Nursing, 2,* 110–118. Retrieved from http://www.ncbi.nlm.nih.gov/pubmed/11710087

Dentistry, A. A. (2011). *Regular dental visits.* Retrieved from http://www.aapd.org/ publications/brochures/regdent.asp

Feingold, D. (1992). The Tanner Stages. *Pediatric Endocrinology,* 16–19. Retrieved from http://www.hindawi.com/journals/ijpe/

Filippos, A., Velderman, M. K., Ravens-Sieberer, U., Detmar, S., Erhart, M., Herdman, M., . . . Rajmil, L. (2009). Being bullied: Associated factors in children and adolescents 8 to 18 years old in 11 European countries. *Pediatrics, 123,* 568–578. doi: 10.1542/peds.2008-0323

Guid, F. D. (n.d.). *Pediatric fluid and electrolyte requirements.* Retrieved from https://www.pediatriccareonline.org/

Kanshiro, N. K. (2011). *Precocious puberty.* Retrieved from http://www.ncbi.nlm.nih.gov/ pubmedhealth/PMH0002152/

Lewis, A. (1999). Learning the ABCD's of pediatric assessment. *Nursing, 229,* 32H1. Retrieved from http://journals.lww.com/ajnonline/pages/default.aspx

LexiComp Online. (2011). Retrieved from http://www.lexi.com

National Institutes of Health. (2008). *Pediatric blood pressure charts.* Retrieved from http://www.cc.nih.gov/ccc/pedweb/pedsstaff/bp.html

Patient.co.uk. (2010). *Dehydration in children.* Retrieved from http://www.patient.co.uk/doctor/Managing-Dehydration-in-Children-Paediatric-Fluid-Regimes.htm

Pearce, P. F., Harrell, J. S., & McMurray, R. G. (2008). Middle-school children's understanding of physical activity: "If you're moving, you're doing physical activity." *Journal of Pediatric Nursing: Nursing Care of Children and Families, 23,* 169–182. doi: 10.1016/j.pedn.2007.09.003

Rogers, T. L. (2004). The use of EMLA cream to decrease venipuncture pain in children. *Journal of Pediatric Nursing, 19,* 33–39. doi: 10.1016/j.pedn.2003.09.005

SafeKids.com. (2009). *Sexting tips from ConnectSafely.org.* Retrieved from http://www.safekids.com/sexting-tips/

Sarafolean, M. H. (2000). Depression in school-age children and adolescents: Characteristics, assessments and prevention. *A Pediatric Perspective, 9,* 1–5. Retrieved from http://www.gillettechildrens.org/fileupload/2000-07%20%20Depression%20in%20Children%20%20Vol%2009%20No%2004.pdf

Stanger, V., & Rimmerman, A. (2001). Parental stress, marital satisfaction and responsiveness to children: a comparison between mothers of children with and without inborn impairment. *International Journal of Rehabilitation, 24*(4):317-20.

Stirling, J. (2008). Understanding the behavioral and emotional consequences of child abuse. *American Academy of Pediatrics, 122,* 667–673. doi: 10.1542/peds.2008-1885

University of Chicago. (2011). *Innocent heart murmurs.* Retrieved from http://pediatriccardiology.uchicago.edu/mp/Heart-Murmurs/htmurmurs.htm

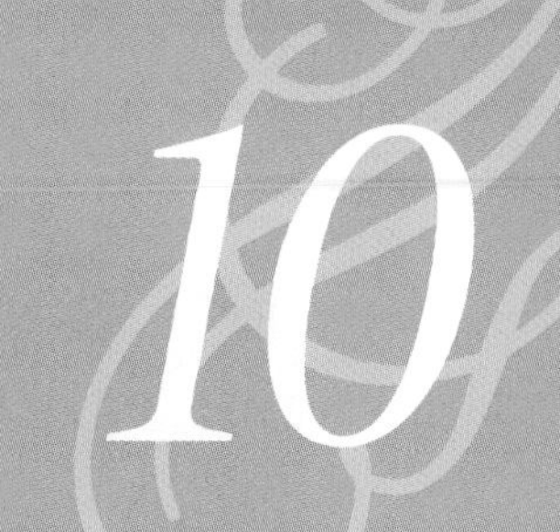

Adolescents

Theresa Puckett, PhD, RN, CPNP, CNE

OBJECTIVES

- ☐ Describe the growth and development that occur during adolescence.
- ☐ Identify age-specific physical assessment approaches for adolescents.
- ☐ Explain medication approaches for adolescent patients.
- ☐ Explain variations in nursing procedures for adolescent patients.
- ☐ Describe strategies for assessing health promotion practices among adolescents.
- ☐ Describe emergency care considerations for adolescent patients.
- ☐ Identify strategies to support hospitalized adolescents.
- ☐ Integrate chronic care concepts and adolescent-specific considerations.
- ☐ Integrate home care concepts and adolescent-specific considerations.
- ☐ Recognize complementary and alternative therapies used by adolescents.
- ☐ Recognize child abuse considerations relevant to adolescents.

KEY TERMS

- bruxism
- malocclusion
- puberty
- gynecomastia
- menstruation
- leukorrhea
- Russell's sign

GROWTH AND DEVELOPMENT

Adolescence is the transition period between childhood and adulthood **(Figure 10-1)**. It is considered to have three stages:

- Early adolescence (ages 11 to 14)
- Middle adolescence (ages 15 to 17)
- Late adolescence (ages 18 to 21)

Although adolescence is often regarded as a period of extreme personal turmoil, most adolescents experience only mild difficulties during this time of life. Developmental warning signs during adolescence include school failure and/or absenteeism and aggressive behavior. The outcomes of this stage of maturity include the development of:

- advanced cognitive abilities,
- autonomy,
- self-identity, and
- social competence (Hornberger, 2006).

Cognitive

- Piaget's cognitive developmental theory (see also Chapter 6, Growth and Development):
  - Ages 10–11: *Concrete operations*
  - Ages 11–15: *Formal operations*
- Develops analytic thinking
- Develops abstract thinking
- Shows concern for politics and social issues
- Begins to have the ability to think long-term and set goals
- Compares self to peers
- Begins to have some awareness of personal limitations
- Begins to have the ability to predict outcomes and consequences
- The prefrontal cortex of the adolescent brain is still developing.
  - *This is the area of the brain associated with critical thinking and decision making.*

Don't have time to read this chapter? Want to reinforce your reading? Need to review for a test? Listen to this chapter on DavisPlus at davispl.us/rudd1.

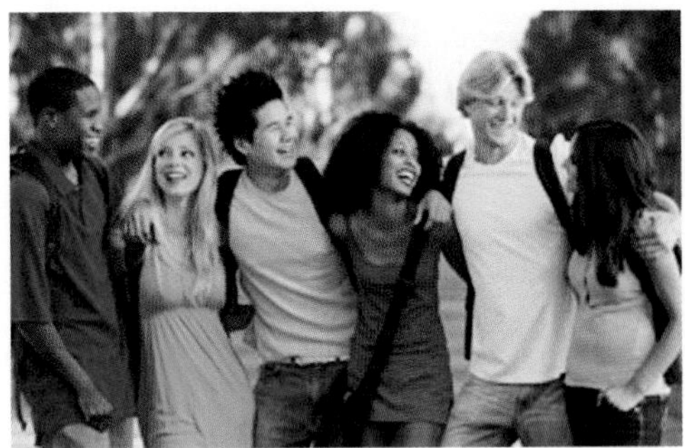

Figure 10–1 Adolescents.

- *The immaturity of this brain area is responsible for the risk-taking behaviors exhibited by adolescents, such as experimenting with substances and engaging in risky sexual activity (Lopez, Schwartz, Guillermo, Campo, & Pantin, 2008).*

Psychological

- Freud's theory of psychosexual development (see also Chapter 6, Growth and Development):
  - Ages 10–12: *Latency stage*
  - Ages 12–18: *Genital stage*
- Erikson's theory of psychosocial development (see also Chapter 6, Growth and Development)
  - Ages 10–12: *Industry versus inferiority*
  - Ages 12–18: *Identity versus role confusion*
  - Age 19: *Intimacy versus isolation*
- Self-conscious
- Compares own body to others
- Interested in sexuality and gender roles
  - *Emergence of sexual feelings and experimentation*
  - *Has a need for privacy*
  - *"Tries on" different styles of dress, communication, and personae*
- Develops personal values
- Wants to be an adult but still needs the support of the family/caregiver
- Self-image is dependent on what others think
- Has mood swings
- Feels as if "on stage" with others around and paying special attention
- Believes that he or she is special and unique
- Has a sense of invincibility
- Is impulsive
- Assumes that others have the same perspective
- Has unrealistic career goals
- Tests limits and rules
- Develops a sense of conscience
- Knows right from wrong
- Can compromise with others when desired

CRITICAL COMPONENT

Adolescence as a Transitional Stage

Adolescence is the transition period between childhood and adulthood.

BIOPSYCHOSOCIAL ASSESSMENT

Adolescence is a period of rapid physical, cognitive, psychological, and social growth. It is the process of becoming an adult. The experience of adolescence is unique for each person. Therefore, growth and development should be assessed individually. Adolescents of the same chronological age may be at different developmental stages. Stressors, such as trauma, loss, illness, and environmental factors can slow or reverse growth and development processes.

General Survey

- Sense of physical awkwardness is normal.
- Determine developmental history, family composition, and school situation.
- Yearly health maintenance visits with a primary care provider are recommended for adolescents between ages 11 and 21 (American Academy of Pediatrics [AAP], n.d.).
- Annual assessments
  - *Height*
  - *Weight*
  - *Body mass index (BMI)*
  - *Blood pressure*
  - *Hearing*
  - *Vision*
- Cholesterol screening should take place once during late adolescence (normal range for ages 11 to 21 is 110 to 175 mg/dl).
- Tuberculosis screening is recommended for at-risk adolescents, including those from countries outside of the United States, those who are HIV positive, and those who are incarcerated or homeless (AAP, n.d.).
- Immunizations
  - *An immunization schedule, updated yearly each January, is available at the Centers for Disease Control (CDC) Web site (hhtp://www.cdc.gov). (See also Chapter 22, Communicable Diseases.)*

Clinical Reasoning

Immunizations for Adolescents

The Society for Adolescent Medicine developed a position statement to address the barriers to successful immunization in adolescents (Middleman, Rosenthal, & Rickert, 2006).

1. What are some barriers to immunization in adolescents?
2. How can the nurse facilitate immunizations in adolescents?

Physical

- Vital signs
  - *Vital sign parameters reach adult values during adolescence.*
    - Heart rate of 85 beats/minute
    - Respiratory rate of 17 to 22 breaths/minute
    - Systolic blood pressure of 118 to 120

- Height/weight
  - *Height and weight can be plotted on gender- and age-specific grids available at the CDC Web site (http://www.cdc.gov).*
  - *Adolescents, particularly girls, are sensitive to height/weight measurements.*
- Daily fluid requirement
  - *Calculation: 1500 ml plus 20 ml for every kilogram above 20 kg*
- Normal urine output
  - *Calculation: 0.5 to 1 ml/kg/hour*
- Pain assessment
  - *Use a numeric scale or a visual analog scale* **(Figure 10-2)**.
- General somatic complaints without verified diagnostic clinical data—such as chronic pain, dizziness, sweating, headaches, chest pain, shortness of breath, gastrointestinal (GI) issues/pain such as nausea/vomiting/diarrhea, and back/joint pain—may be an indication of school or home avoidance/problems, anxiety and stress, or depression. (See Chapter 14, Mental Health Disorders.)

Skin

- The skin becomes thicker and tougher.
- Hormone changes during puberty cause an increase in sweat secretion and oily skin, especially on the face, back, axillae, breasts, and anus.
- Acne may develop. (See Chapter 21, Dermatologic Diseases.)
- Daily washing is important.
- Assess sunscreen use.
- Document birthmarks.
- Check for bruises and burns that could indicate child abuse.
- Check for scratches and eraser burns that could indicate self-harm.
- Document tattoos and piercings.
- Assess and document birthmarks, moles, needle marks, or other skin aberrations.

Promoting Safety

About half (48%) of a sample of 225 adolescents had at least one body piercing (Gold, Schorzman, Murray, Downs, & Tolentino, 2003). Nurses need to educate adolescents and caregivers on the risks associated with body piercing, such as infection, allergic reaction to metal piercings, excessive bleeding, nerve damage, keloids, and dental complications (tongue piercing).

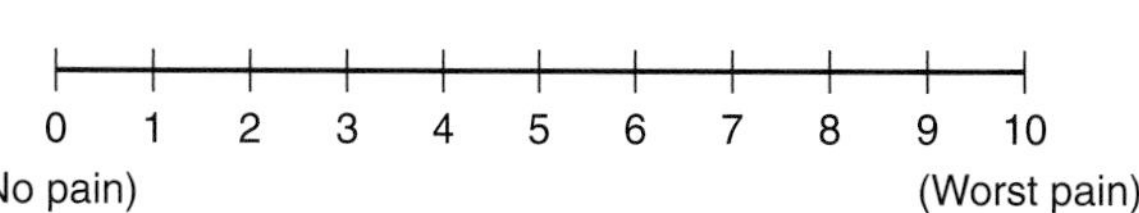

Figure 10–2 Numeric scale.

Head

- Head reaches adult size during adolescence.
- Assess for migraines/stress headaches.
- Hair might be brittle and dry if subjected to frequent color dying.

Eyes

- Visual acuity testing at ages 12, 15, and 18 (AAP, n.d.)
- Assess for glasses and contact lens use, including the use of colored contact lenses for cosmetic purposes.
- Look for signs and symptoms of infection from excessive use of eye makeup.

Ears

- Assess for external ear trauma, piercings/gauges, and signs of infection.
- Assess for evidence of hearing loss, such as not responding to questions or tilting the head to a certain side.
- Assess for use of hearing aids.
- Hearing testing is necessary if positive finding on screening questions (AAP, n.d.).

Mouth, Throat, and Teeth

- Inspect mouth for ulcers that might indicate inhalant or smokeless tobacco use.
- Assess for tongue/lip piercing.
- Dental checkups and tooth cleaning is recommended every 6 months (American Academy of Pediatric Dentistry, 2009).
  - *Red gums may be an indication of periodontal disease.*
  - *Check for dental erosion, tooth loss, and cavities.*
    - Assess for dental grill use, which can cause allergic reactions, gum disease, cavities, and bacterial growth (American Dental Association, 2010).
    - Tooth erosion could indicate that patient has been inducing vomiting.
  - *The third molars (wisdom teeth) erupt between ages 17 and 21.*
  - ***Bruxism**, which is teeth grinding, may be present due to stress.*
  - ***Malocclusion**, which is crowded or misaligned teeth, is common between ages 8 and 16 and may require orthodontic correction.*
- Check the cervical lymph nodes for enlargement and fixation.
- Palpate the thyroid to check for enlargement.

Nose

- Check for nose piercing.
- The nose may appear too large for the face during early adolescence.

Cardiovascular

- The heart grows in strength and size during adolescence.
- Assess for innocent murmurs. (See Chapter 12, Cardiovascular Disorders.)
- Screen for iron-deficiency anemia every 2 to 3 years during adolescence (AAP, n.d.).

Respiratory

- The length and diameter of the lungs increase during adolescence.
- Assess for a history of asthma, which is the number one chronic illness in children. (See Chapter 11, Respiratory Disorders.)
- Lungs should sound clear. (See Chapter 11, Respiratory Disorders.)
- Check for signs/symptoms of chronic respiratory issues, such as barrel chest and clubbed fingers. (See Chapter 11, Respiratory Disorders.)

Gastrointestinal

- Assess nutritional status.
- Assess constipation/diarrhea/vomiting.
- Assess for chronic stomachaches, which could be an indication of stress/anxiety.

Renal

- Assess hydration status.
- Assess for enuresis.
- Assess signs/symptoms of urinary tract infection, particularly among sexually active adolescents.

Reproductive

- Standard assessments include the following:
  - *Breast self-exam monthly*
  - *Clinical breast exam yearly*
  - *PAP test yearly starting at age 21 or within 3 years of becoming sexually active*
  - *Testicular self-exam monthly*
  - *Hernia checks for boys, especially for athletes*
  - *Assess for signs and symptoms of sexually transmitted infections (STIs), such as genital discharge or rash. (See Chapter 18, Reproductive and Genetic Disorders.)*
  - *Assess for signs and symptoms of abuse, such as bruises and skin tears in the genital and anal areas. (See Chapter 14, Mental Health Disorders.)*
- **Puberty** is the process of becoming reproductively mature.
  - *The onset and timing of puberty are highly individual.*
    - Many factors contribute to the variations in puberty onset among individuals.
    - Genetics is the strongest factor associated with the onset and timing of puberty.
  - *The stages of puberty are predictable.*
    - *Girls:* Puberty begins between ages 8 and 13 and is completed in about 4 years **(Figure 10-3)**.
    - *Boys:* Puberty begins between ages 9 and 14 and is completed in about 3.5 years.
  - *During puberty, the secretion of sex hormones increases.*
    - Estrogen
    - Progesterone
    - Androgens
  - *Boys and girls will experience a growth spurt that lasts 24 to 36 months.*
    - Girls will have a growth spurt at ages 10 to 12.
    - Boys will have a growth spurt at ages 12 to 14.
  - *Lean body mass will decrease in girls and increase in boys.*
  - *Adipose body mass will increase in girls and decrease in boys.*
  - *Both sexes will develop coarse hair in the pubic area and under the arms.*
  - *Female breast development begins at ages 8 to 10.*
    - One breast may develop faster than the other.
    - Breast tenderness is common.

CULTURAL AWARENESS: Breast Development

Breast development starts earlier in African American girls than in girls of other cultures (AAP, 2003).

  - ***Gynecomastia** refers to abnormal breast development in boys.*
    - This is a self-limiting condition.
    - It may be related to the increase in sex hormones.
    - It is more common in overweight boys.
  - *Girls begin **menstruation**, the shedding of the uterine lining, approximately 2 years after the onset of breast development.*
    - **Leukorrhea**, a thick white discharge from the vagina, is seen 3 to 6 months before menarche.
    - Periods may be irregular for up to 1 to 2 years after a girl first begins menstruating.
    - Periods will become more regular over time.
    - Girls can become pregnant after the first menstruation.

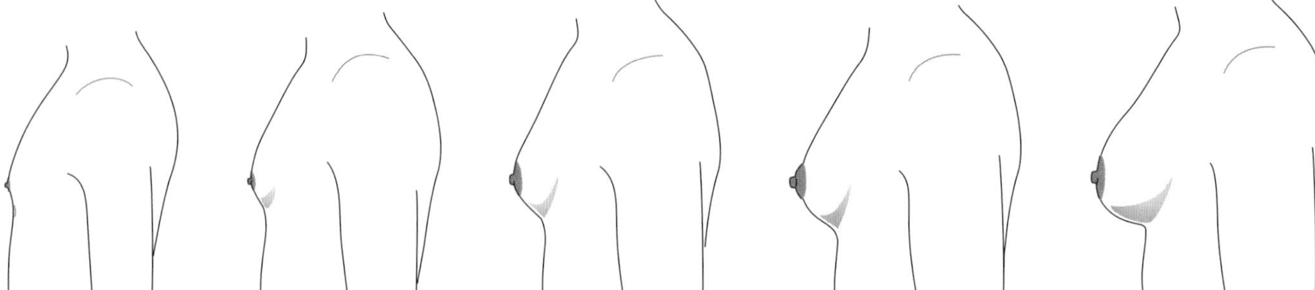

Figure 10-3 Breast development.

- Assess for symptoms of premenstrual syndrome (PMS), such as irritability, anxiety, depression, crying, mood swings, feeling bloated, breast tenderness, and fatigue.
- Assess for precocious puberty (onset prior to age 8) or late-onset puberty (after age 14).
- Assess for the cessation of menstrual periods after an established pattern of regularity, which could indicate a drop in body fat due to excessive exercising, deliberate food restriction/eating disorder, or illness.

■ *Secondary sex characteristics* **(Tables 10-1 and 10-2)**
- Male and female voices deepen.
- Boys develop a more pronounced Adam's apple.
- Amount of pubic hair increases and becomes dark and coarse.
- Hair also grows under arms and on legs.
- The scrotum and the penis enlarge in boys during puberty. (See Chapter 18 for additional reproductive information and Tanner Staging.)

Neurovascular

- The brain is in a period of rapid development.
- Check for equal strength left to right via hand grasps.
- Check deep tendon reflexes **(Figure 10-4)**.

TABLE 10–1 TANNER STAGING (MALE SECONDARY SEX CHARACTERISTICS)

Stage	Pubic Hair	Penis	Testes and Scrotum
1. Preadolescent	No pubic hair except for fine body hair similar to that on abdomen	Same size and proportions as in childhood	Same size and proportions as in childhood
2.	Sparse growth of long, slightly pigmented, downy hair, straight or only slightly curled, chiefly at the base of penis	Slight or no enlargement	Testes larger; scrotum larger, somewhat reddened and altered in texture
3.	Darker, coarser, curlier hair spreading sparsely over pubic symphysis	Larger, especially in length	Further enlarged
4.	Coarse and curly hair, as in adult; area covered greater than in stage 3 but not as great as in adult	Further enlarged in length and breadth, with development of glands	Further enlarged; scrotal skin darkened

Continued

TABLE 10–1 TANNER STAGING (MALE SECONDARY SEX CHARACTERISTICS)—cont'd

Stage	Pubic Hair	Penis	Testes and Scrotum
5. 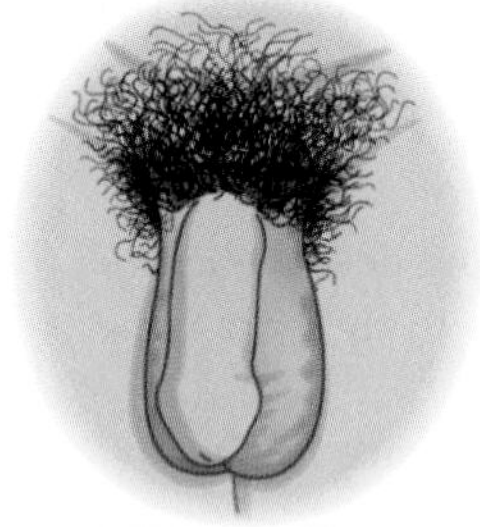	Hair same as adult in quantity and quality, spreading to medial surfaces of thighs but not up over abdomen	Adult in size and shape	Adult in size and shape

From Dillon, P. M. (2007). *Nursing health assessment: A critical thinking, case studies approach* (2nd ed., p. 656). Philadelphia: F.A. Davis.

TABLE 10–2 MATURATION STATES IN FEMALES (SECONDARY SEX CHARACTERISTICS)

Stage 1	
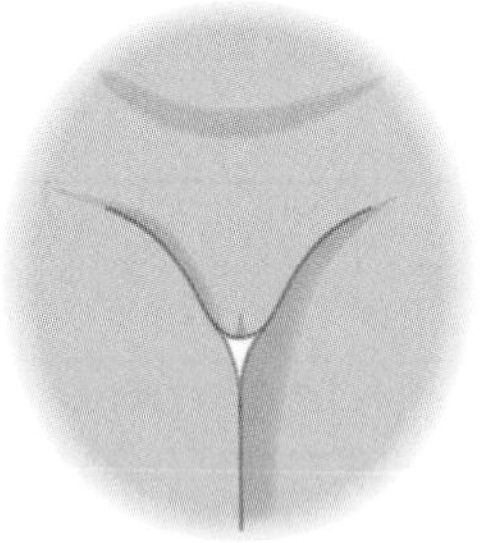	*Preadolescent:* No pubic hair except for fine body hair similar to hair on abdomen
Stage 2	
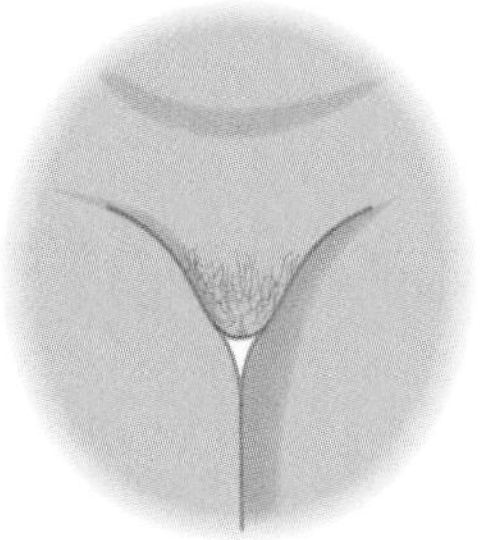	Sparse growth of long, slightly pigmented, downy hair, straight or only slight curled, mostly along labia
Stage 3	
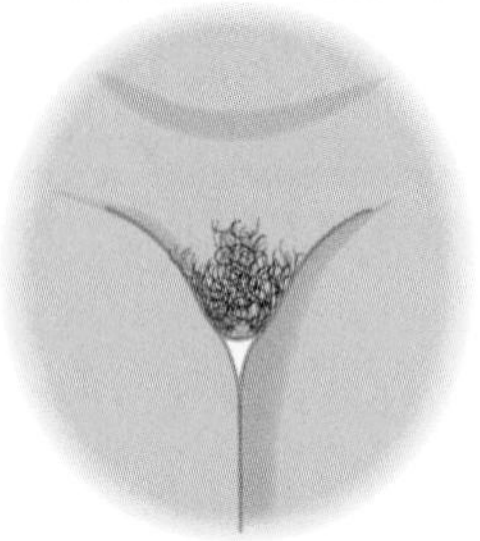	Hair becomes darker, coarser, and curlier and spreads sparsely over pubic symphysis

TABLE 10–2 MATURATION STATES IN FEMALES (SECONDARY SEX CHARACTERISTICS)—cont'd

Stage 4	
	Pubic hair is coarse and curly as in adults; covers more area than in stage 3 but not as much as in adults
Stage 5	
	Quality and quantity are consistent with adult pubic hair distribution and spread over medial surfaces of thighs but not over abdomen

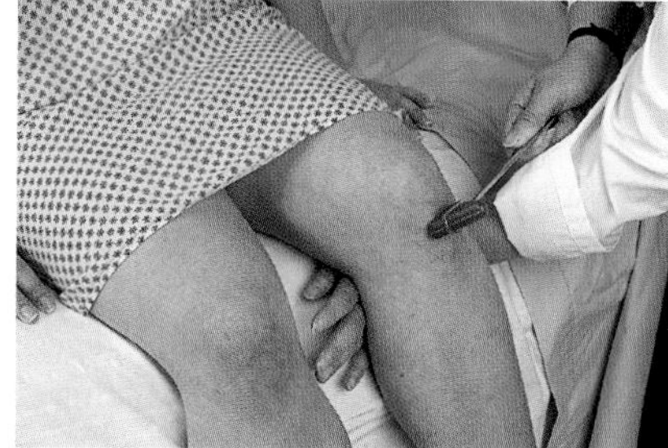

Figure 10–4 Deep tendon reflexes.

Musculoskeletal

- Muscles grow during puberty.
- Feet, hands, arms, and legs grow before the torso, causing adolescents to become prone to clumsiness.
- The shoulders and chest increase in breadth.
- The female pelvis widens during puberty.
- Growth plates at the end of long bones (epiphyses) close by age 20.
- Fractures in the epiphyses before closure jeopardize the long-term growth of long bones.

- Check knuckles for **Russell's sign.**
  - *Abrasions or cuts from sticking fingers down throat to induce vomiting*
- Begin scoliosis checks at ages 10 to 12 **(Figure 10-5).**

Clinical Reasoning

Scoliosis Screening

The U.S. Preventative Task Force (2004) does not recommend scoliosis screening for adolescents. This recommendation contradicts that of Richards and Vitale (2008), which recommends screening for girls starting at ages 10 to 12 and for boys starting at ages 13 to 14 (American Academy of Pediatrics, 2008).

1. What evidence is the Task Force's recommendation based on?
2. What evidence is the Richards and Vitale's recommendation based on?
3. Which recommendation should the nurse follow? Why?

CRITICAL COMPONENT

Body Image

Body image is very important to the adolescent.

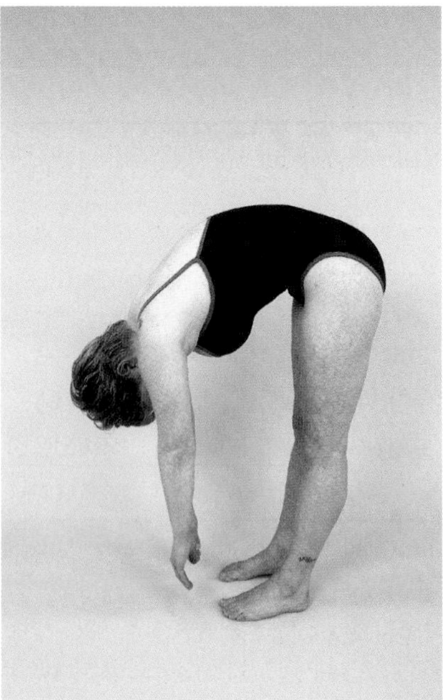

Figure 10–5 How to perform a scoliosis check.

Social

- Kohlberg's theory of moral development (see also Chapter 6, Growth and Development): Conventional level
- Challenges the values, traditions, and beliefs of the family
- Developing own value system
- Wants independence from caregivers
- Conflict between adolescent and caregivers
- Resists adult supervision
- Depends on family in times of crisis
- Has best friend
- Idealizes friendships
- Socializes in cliques of the same sex
- Compares self to others
- Strives for peer acceptance
- Conforms to the norms of the peer group
- Influenced by peer pressure
- Prone to gang membership because of the desire for peer acceptance

CRITICAL COMPONENT

The Influence of Peers

Peers are often more important and influential to adolescents than family members.

- May be employed
- Focused on activities outside of the home

Promoting Safety

Internet safety is important for adolescents. Social networking Web sites have increased adolescents' exposure to unsafe persons. Signs that an adolescent is engaging in risky online behavior include spending a large amount of time online, initiating or receiving calls from individuals unknown to the caregiver, receiving mail/gifts from an unknown person, and quickly changing the monitor screen when the caregiver approaches the computer. More information about Internet safety for adolescents and caregivers is available at the Federal Bureau of Investigation (FBI) Web site (http://www.fbi.gov/publications/pguide/pguidee.htm).

- Explores gender roles
- Seeks out information about sex
- Emergence of sexual feelings
- Explores sexual orientation

CRITICAL COMPONENT

Sexual Identity

When communicating with adolescents, do not assume heterosexuality.

- Starts to develop intimate relationships
- Romances are usually brief but can be very intense.
- May have feelings of being in love
- Has romantic fantasies
- Gay, lesbian, bisexual, transgender, and questioning (GLBTQ) youths are more likely to engage in risky behaviors and to have psychiatric problems than heterosexual youth (Coker, Austin, & Schuster, 2010). See the NAPNAP position statement on health care and GLBTQ youth at http://www.napnap.org/Files/NAPNAPPSHealthRisksandNeedsofLGBTQAdoles_Final2011.pdf.

Spiritual

- Adolescents may start to question or disagree with the religious beliefs of the family.
- Adolescents understand the permanence of death and may ask questions about an afterlife. (See Chapter 4, Cultural, Spiritual, and Environmental Influences on the Child.)

CULTURAL AWARENESS: Religion

For some, adolescence is a time of religious ceremonies that require significant preparation time/activities on the part of the individual, such as the bar or bat mitzvah among Jewish youth and Confirmation for Catholics.

PHYSICAL ASSESSMENT APPROACHES

- Respect privacy.
- Inform the adolescent of your actions and explain the rationales.
- Focus on the positive aspects of the individual.
- Address the adolescent's concerns directly.
- Be cautious about pointing out physical abnormalities.
- Examine the genitals last.
- Use the correct words for anatomy.

> **CLINICAL PEARL**
> **Privacy and Confidentiality**
> Assess the adolescent without the caregiver being present to ensure maximum privacy and confidentiality.

APPROACHES TO MEDICATION ADMINISTRATION

Over 75% of medications are not approved for use in pediatric patients (National Institute of Health, 2010).

- Due to the legalities of testing medications in children through large randomized clinical drug trials, most medications are used "off label" in pediatrics.
- Medications obtain a pediatric label through surveying of prescribers.
- Some medications are labeled for use in adolescents older than age 12, 13, or 17.
- For an updated list of medications that have recently undergone a Food and Drug Administration (FDA) label change to allow for use in pediatric patients, see the FDA Web site (http://www.fda.gov/cder/pediatric).

> **Medication Administration**
> **Aripirazole**
> Aripirazole (Abilify) was relabeled from use in adults only to use in adults and adolescents age 13 to 17 in October 2007 based on survey data from pediatric psychiatrists (Best Pharmaceuticals for Children Act, 2009).

Eyedrops, Nasal Sprays, Ear Drops

- Encourage self-administration.
- Pull the pinna back and up for otic medications.

Oral Medications

- As many as one-third of adolescents cannot swallow whole tablets or capsules (Hansen, Tulinius, & Hansen, 2008).
- Tablets and capsules may need to be crushed.
- An alternative preparation of the medication may be available.
  - *Suspension*
  - *Oral disintegrating tablets*
- Most adolescents master pill swallowing through repeated attempts.
- Learning to swallow pills can lead to a sense of control and ownership over one's own health care.

Medications via Gastrostomy or Nasogastric Tube

- Encourage self-administration.

Rectal Medications

- Encourage self-administration.

Subcutaneous Medications

- Use EMLA cream when available.

IV Medications

- Use EMLA cream when available.

Pharmaceutical Warnings

- Developmental changes affect medication absorption, metabolism, and elimination.
  - *Specifically, the metabolism of medications is affected by puberty.*
  - *Most medications are metabolized faster by a patient in puberty.*
  - *After puberty, medication metabolism decreases to adult levels.*

> **CULTURAL AWARENESS: Biocultural Implications of Medication Metabolization**
> People of Asian descent metabolize some medications slower than average and may need lower and less frequent doses of medication to achieve optimum therapeutic effect (Liao, 2007).

- Adolescents do not always read or understand pharmaceutical warnings found on medicine containers (Goldsworthy, Schwartz, & Mayhorn, 2008).
- Nurses cannot rely on symbols or phrases to warn adolescents of medicine-related risks.
- Adolescents have the best understanding of medication warnings when directly informed verbally by health-care personnel.

VARIATIONS IN NURSING PROCEDURES

- Obtain guardian consent.
- Obtain assent from patient. (See Chapter 2, Standards of Practice and Ethical Considerations.)
- Explain rationales to family and patient.

- Show equipment ahead of time.
- Be honest about the potential for discomfort/pain.
- Maintain patient confidentiality.
- If performing procedures in a setting where multiple adolescents are "lined up" to receive care, such as scoliosis/eye/hearing/lice checks at a school, ensure privacy for each individual and do not announce results in front of others.

HEALTH PROMOTION AND EDUCATION

Health-care encounters provide an opportunity for the nurse to assess and educate adolescents about health promotion.

> CLINICAL PEARL
>
> **"HEADSS"**
>
> Areas of health promotion to assess and educate adolescents about can be summarized with the acronym "HEADSS" (Goldering & Cohen, 1988):
>
> H—Home
> E—Education
> A—Activities
> D—Drugs/Diet
> S—Sexuality
> S—Suicide/Safety

- Assessment of the home
  - *Assess the caregiver–adolescent relationship.*
  - *Assess relationships with siblings.*
  - *Assess support of the extended family.*
  - *Assess where the adolescent lives.*
  - *Ask about substance use in the home.*
  - *Ask about violence in the home.*
  - *Ask about the safety of the neighborhood.*
  - *Ask about community supports and resources.*
- Assessment of education
  - *Assess school performance.*

> **CRITICAL COMPONENT**
>
> **School Performance**
>
> School performance is a strong indication of the adolescent's overall well-being.

  - *Ask about school absenteeism.*
  - *Assess feelings regarding teachers and classmates.*
  - *Assess for bullying.*
  - *Refer to a mental health professional if the adolescent admits to negative thoughts or feelings surrounding school.*
  - *Assess vocational/career aspirations.*
- Assess activities
  - *Mortality*
    - Leading causes of death in adolescence are motor vehicle accidents, homicide, and suicide.
  - *Assess knowledge of injury prevention.*
    - Type and severity of injuries are closely related to developmental stage, psychological needs, and cognitive skills.
    - Practice safe driving, including wearing seat belt, minimizing the number of passengers, not driving when under the influence of alcohol or drugs, and not driving while using a cell phone for texting or talking.
    - Practice gun safety.
    - Practice water safety.
    - Sports injuries: Wear protective gear such as helmet and pads.
  - *Assess for the presence of violence.*
    - Assess for emotional, physical, sexual abuse.
    - Assess for intimate partner violence.
    - Assess for neighborhood safety.
- Assess for drugs/diet
  - *Screen for tobacco use.*
    - Tobacco use includes cigarettes and smokeless "chew."
    - The NAPNAP position paper on the prevention of tobacco use is available at http://download.journals.elsevierhealth.com/pdfs/journals/0891-5245/PIIS0891524504000057.pdf.

> CLINICAL PEARL
>
> **Substance Use**
>
> If an adolescent admits to cigarette smoking, ask about the use of other substances. Nicotine is usually the first drug used by an adolescent and is believed to be a "gateway" to stronger substances such as alcohol and marijuana (Kandel, 2002).

  - *Assess alcohol/substance use:*
    - Illegal substances
    - Prescription drugs
    - Over-the counter-medications
    - Herbal/dietary supplements
    - Propellants/inhalants

> **Evidence-Based Practice Research: Prescription Drug Abuse**
>
> Partnership for a Drug Free America. (2005). *The partnership attitude tracking study.* Retrieved from http://www.drugfree.org/wp-content/uploads/2011/04/PATS-Teens-Full-Report-FINAL.pdf
>
> In a 2005 report from the Partnership for a Drug Free America, 50% of a sample of 7,300 adolescents agreed with the statement that "prescription drugs are safer than illegal street drugs." The report found that 1 in 5 adolescents abuses prescription drugs, with girls being 40% more likely to abuse the drugs than boys (Partnership for a Drug Free America, 2005). What factors contribute to adolescent prescription drug abuse?
>
> 1. Why is there a gender difference in prescription drug abuse among adolescents?
> 2. How can the nurse assess prescription drug abuse in adolescents?

- *Nutrition*
  - Adolescents have an increased caloric need to due rapid growth.
  - For most adolescent boys, 2,800 calories per day is recommended (AAP, 2011).
  - For most adolescent girls, 2,200 calories per day is recommended (AAP, 2011).
  - It is recommended that vitamins and minerals be obtained by eating a well-rounded diet rather than from dietary supplements (AAP, 2011).
  - Encourage healthy dietary habits.
  - Assess for vegan/vegetarian diets and provide education or refer to dietician.
  - Of obese adolescents, 80% will be obese as adults (American Academy of Child and Adolescent Psychiatry, 2008).
  - Obese adolescents are prone to developing hypertension, type II diabetes, dyslipidemia, ankle sprains/ fractures, gastroesophageal reflux, sleep apnea, and fatty liver disease.
- *Safe weight management*
  - Watch for signs of eating disorders such as vomiting, fasting, fad diets, and use/abuse of diet pills and laxatives. (See Chapter 14, Mental Health Disorders.)
  - Assess type and frequency of fast-food consumption.
  - Encourage a low-fat diet, reduced-calorie substitutions, keeping a food log, eating at the table instead of in front of the television, and focusing on the development of a positive self-image.
- *Exercise*
  - Encourage stretching before vigorous exercise to prevent muscle injury.
  - Of 12- to 21-year-olds, 50% get no regular physical activity (President's Council on Physical Activity and Sports, 2011).

- Sexuality
  - *Assess safe sex practices.*
    - Abstinence
    - Birth control options
    - Number of partners
    - Sexually transmitted infections (STIs)
    - Assess condom use.
    - Assess engagement in oral sex and educate about risks such as acquiring sexual herpes virus. Oral sex is often considered "safe" by adolescents.
    - STI testing as appropriate
    - HIV testing as appropriate
  - *For pregnant adolescents (see also Chapter 18, Reproductive and Genetic Disorders):*
    - Assess pregnancy history.
    - Assess feelings about the pregnancy.
    - Encourage patient to tell caregiver about pregnancy.
    - Educate patient about options, such as adoption and terminating the pregnancy.
    - Provide agency information if considering adoption.
    - Educate patient about finding a skilled provider if adolescent is considering abortion.
    - Assist the adolescent in finding an appropriate health-care provider or agency.
    - Encourage early prenatal care.
    - Encourage the attendance of a parenting class if adolescent is planning to assume parenting role.
    - Seek out support resources for pregnant adolescents such as the Women, Infants, and Children (WIC) program, Medicaid, teenage pregnancy classes, groups, and Web sites.
- Suicide/safety
  - *Screen for depression/suicidal ideation/self-harming behavior.*
    - Assess for stressors such as transitioning from high school to college.
    - Teach stress management/relaxation techniques. (See Chapter 14, Mental Health Disorders.)

EMERGENCY CARE

- Common adolescent emergency injuries/issues:
  - *Traumatic injury due to risk-taking behaviors, a sense of immortality, and a lack of connection between cause and effect*
  - *Injuries related to accidental or intentional alcohol/ substance overdose*

> CLINICAL PEARL
>
> **Screening for Substance Use**
>
> In a comparison of three alcohol/substance use screening tools, CRAFFT was found to be the most reliable and valid for use with adolescents (Cook, Chung, Kelly, & Clark, 2005):
>
> 1. Have you ridden in a **C**ar driven by someone (including yourself) who had been drinking or using drugs?
> 2. Do you use alcohol or drugs to **R**elax, feel better about yourself, or fit in?
> 3. Do you use alcohol or drugs when you're by yourself, **A**lone?
> 4. Do you **F**orget things you did while using alcohol or drugs?
> 5. Do your family or **F**riends tell you that you should cut down on your drinking or drug use?
> 6. Have you gotten into **T**rouble while using alcohol or drugs?

  - *Motor vehicle accidents (passenger or driver)*
  - *Sports injuries*
  - *Sexual assault*
  - *Mental health emergencies*
- Primary assessment
  - *ABCs*
  - *Pain*
  - *Skin for evidence of drug use*
  - *Do-not-resuscitate (DNR) status (See Chapter 2, Standards of Practice and Ethical Considerations.)*
  - *Identify patient's guardian.*

- *Identify patient's legal status, such as mature/emancipated minor. (See Chapter 2, Standards of Practice and Ethical Considerations.)*
- *Under the Emergency Medical Treatment and Active Labor Act of 1986, adolescents requiring emergency care may be treated regardless of whether caregiver consent has been obtained. (See Chapter 2, Standards of Practice and Ethical Considerations.)*
- *Contextual information related to the injury/condition*
- *Family/social history*
- *Immunization status*
- *Transportation availability if being discharged from the emergency room*

- Additional considerations
  - *Availability of age- and size-appropriate medical equipment, such as blood pressure cuffs and precalculated emergency drug cards*
  - *Education of nurse in advanced cardiac life support (ACLS) and pediatric advanced life support (PALS) protocols*
  - *Speak with the adolescent privately and ensure confidentiality of the conversation, unless doing so directly threatens the well-being of the adolescent or another person.*
  - *Allow adolescents and caregivers to decide together whether or not to have family members present during procedures such as diagnostic tests or resuscitation.*
  - *Be a patient advocate.*
  - *Provide education of the patient/family.*
  - *Sensitively convey "bad news" to caregivers, who may or may not be present. (See Chapter 5, End-of-Life Care.)*
  - *Facilitate conversations between the adolescent and caregiver(s) regarding sensitive subjects.*
  - *Seek the assistance of a chaplain and/or ethics committee if the adolescent and the caregiver(s) disagree about treatment (O'Malley, Brown, Krug, 2008).*
  - *Child protective services will need to be called in cases of the caregiver refusing life-saving treatment. (See Chapter 2, Standards of Practice and Ethical Considerations.)*
  - *Prepare for the possibility of transferring the patient to a more appropriate facility.*
  - *Ask the adolescent for a secure e-mail address or phone number if providing sensitive follow-up information (O'Malley et al., 2008).*

ACUTE CARE HOSPITALIZATION

- Establish nurse–patient relationship. (See Chapter 3, Family Dynamics/Communicating with Children and Families.)
- Define roles/establish boundaries:
  - *The nurse is not the adolescent's friend, but a professional helper.*
  - *Be consistent and set expectations and consequences for language and behavior.*
  - *Be respectful.*
  - *Be nonjudgmental.*
  - *Develop trust.*
  - *Understand the unique concerns of adolescents.*
  - *Use humor appropriately.*

Clinical Reasoning

Therapeutic Humor

Visit the Web site of the American Association for Applied and Therapeutic Humor (http://www.aath.org), an organization that promotes the use of humor in therapeutic communications with patients.

1. How does this organization define therapeutic humor?
2. How could a nurse use therapeutic humor with adolescent patients?
3. Are there times when the nurse should refrain from using therapeutic humor with adolescent patients? If so, when? Why?

- *Environment of care*
  - The focus of the environment of care should be on providing a sense of control and reducing feelings of anxiety.
  - Be aware that pediatric inpatient units are often geared toward younger children (Tivorsak, Britto, Klostermann, Nebrig, & Slap, 2004).
  - Orientation materials and visitation hours should be different for adolescents than for younger patients.
  - Posters of rock stars, popular actors, and famous athletes are preferred decorations over cartoon characters.
  - Adolescents prefer a more home-like setting rather than a hospital-like setting.
  - Physical space should promote privacy, socialization, and education.
  - Comfortable furniture should be provided, with extra chairs for when family and peers visit.
  - Visible medical equipment in patient rooms is disturbing to adolescents and can increase anxiety; leave only necessary equipment in the patient room or put away in a dresser or closet when not using.
  - Allow for privacy by implementing curtains between bed spaces and locks on the bathroom door.
  - Adolescents gain comfort in being close to the nurse station when acutely ill (Hutton, 2005).
  - Offer a variety of age-appropriate leisure (nonmedical) reading material for distraction, such as teen-orientated magazines.
  - Offer age-appropriate video or computer games and television shows.
  - Offer access to games that release physical energy, such as pool tables, air hockey tables, and table tennis.
  - Provide a separate area for adolescent patients if possible. For example, perhaps the patient lounge

could become "teens only" for an hour every evening.
- A separate teen activity area allows adolescents to feel a sense of control over a space within the hospital unit and decreases the risk of regression to more child-like activities and behaviors.
- Allow adolescents to leave the unit for brief periods if feasible based on condition.
- Offer private telephone access.
- If not on a diet or activity restriction, offer kitchen access so that the adolescent can obtain beverages and snacks independently.
- Adolescents prefer other adolescents as roommates. Avoid wide variation in ages during roommate selection.
- Adolescents prefer one-to-one verbal dissemination of health education/information by a nurse rather than written materials, videos, or Web sites (Hutton, 2005).

- *Nursing interventions*
  - Provide treatments in private.
  - Cluster activities to leave periods of free time for relaxation, homework, or visiting with family and friends.
  - Encourage the adolescent's active participation in meeting health-care needs.
  - Provide appropriate patient education.
  - Show the patient equipment ahead of time.
  - Be honest about pain and side effects.
  - Use pediatric assessment tools when needed.
  - Use size-appropriate blood pressure cuffs.
  - Use age-appropriate pain assessment tools, such as a numeric scale.
  - Use an age-appropriate falls risk tool, such as the Humpty Dumpty Falls Risk Scale (see http://www.mnhospitals.org/inc/data/tools/Safe-from-Falls-Toolkit/s_Hospital_Humpty-Dumpty.pdf).

CARE WHEN CHRONICALLY ILL

- Physical care
  - *Ensure that family and adolescent understand condition/treatments.*
  - *Educate families and adolescents on how to minimize exacerbations of the condition.*
  - *Assure medical control and involvement.*
  - *Assess caregiver burden.*
  - *Promote self-care and functional independence.*
  - *Promote appropriate use of health-care services.*
  - *Coordinate services between health-care providers, school, and home.*
  - *Follow up with families and adolescents after transitioning to adult-focused care.*
  - *Refer families and adolescents to appropriate Internet resources.*
  - *Advocate for chronically ill adolescents.*

Evidence-Based Practice Research: Adolescent Care Preference

Britto, M. T., Slap, G. B., DeVellis, R. F., Hornung, R. W., Atherton, H. D., Knopf, J. M., & DeFriese, G. H. (2007). Specialists' understanding of the health care preferences of chronically ill adolescents. *Journal of Adolescent Health, 40,* 334–341. doi: 10.1016/j.jadohealth.2006.10.020

Fifty-two physicians and 155 chronically ill adolescents completed an 82-item survey about care preferences. The physicians overestimated the adolescents' desire for autonomy and underestimated their desire for a friendly, knowledgeable health-care provider (Britto et al., 2007).

1. What factors account for the discrepancies between what chronically ill adolescents want from a health-care provider and what the physicians think is important to adolescents?
2. How can nurses help close this gap?

- Psychosocial/spiritual care
  - *Use developmental, rather than chronological, age when caring for chronically ill adolescents, as there may be some developmental delays.*
  - *Allow for adolescent completion of tasks as able.* *(See Chapter 4, Cultural, Spiritual, and Environmental Influences.)*

CRITICAL COMPONENT

Sexual Activity Among Chronically Ill Adolescents

Do not assume that chronically ill adolescents are asexual. Assess for sexual activity and safe sex practices.

  - *Promote self-esteem and confidence.*
  - *Foster realistic expectations in parents regarding the adolescent's future personal, academic, and career potential.*
  - *Ensure continued academic success through the use of tutors or other resources.*
  - *Support an adolescent's desire for a vocation/career.*
  - *Assess for grief of losing friends with the same disease. (See Chapter 5, End-of-Life Care.)*
  - *Assess for fear of facing own premature death. (See Chapter 5, End-of-Life Care.)*
  - *Involve in individual and group therapy as appropriate.*
  - *Refer caregivers and adolescents to support groups.*
  - *Refer to chaplain as desired.*

HOME CARE CONSIDERATIONS

There's a growing shift to home care from medical inpatient facilities for adolescents with complex medical conditions. Advances in therapies have decreased the need for hospitalization. In addition, home care decreases financial costs, travel costs, and caregiver burden. Nurses should facilitate the transition from hospital to home. The National Association of Children's Hospitals and Related Institutions Web site offers a tool for families to use when selecting a home care agency (http://www.childrenshospitals.net). Note the following home care considerations:

- Home care increases family and adolescent satisfaction (Kandsberger, 2007).
- Adolescents may have increased opportunities for socializing with peers and participating in school/extracurricular activities as a result of having health-care needs met in the home.
- However, caregivers may feel anxious about having to administer treatments/medications and being responsible for scheduling health-care appointments.
- Some see home as a "safe zone" and do not want it "medicalized" (Kandsberger, 2007).

Clinical Reasoning

Telemedicine

Telemedicine provides an opportunity for delivering home care via telephone/videoconferencing technologies (Young, Barden, McKeever, & Dick, 2006).

1. What are some advantages of using telemedicine for adolescent patients?
2. What are some disadvantages of using telemedicine for adolescent patients?

COMPLEMENTARY AND ALTERNATIVE THERAPIES

Nearly 80% of adolescents have used complementary and alternative (CAM) therapies in their lifetime (Wilson et al., 2006). Herbal and dietary supplements are not regulated by the FDA and have wide variation in content and dose across manufacturers. Although many of these substances are beneficial, interactions with prescription and over-the-counter medications can lead to toxic or sub-therapeutic effects. Family and peer use of CAM influence adolescent use. Internet resources for CAM and adolescents include the National Institutes of Health (NIH) National Center for CAM Web site (http://www.nccam.nih.gov), the NIH Office of Dietary Supplements Web site (http://ods.od.nih.gov), and www.HolisticKids.org.

CLINICAL PEARL

Use of Complementary and Alternative Medicine

Adolescents are often reluctant to discuss their use of CAM. Start out by asking the adolescent about family and peer use of CAM. If the adolescent reports use by a close family member or peer, then he or she is most likely also using CAM.

- Commonly used herbs/dietary supplements among adolescents:
  - *Echinacea, ginseng, ginkgo, garlic, St. John's wort, weight-loss supplements, creatine, vitamins (Kennedy, 2005; Wilson et al., 2006)*
- Commonly used home remedies among adolescents:
  - *Honey, lemon, green tea, chamomile tea (Wilson et al., 2006)*
- Commonly used alternative therapies among adolescents:
  - *Faith healing/prayer, massage therapy, yoga/Tai Chi, air filters/aromatherapy (Wilson et al., 2006)*

Evidence-Based Practice Research: Complementary and Alternative Medicine

Klein, J. D., Wilson, K. M., Sesselberg, T. S., Gray, N. J., Yussman, S., & West, J. (2005).
Adolescents' knowledge of and beliefs about herbs and dietary supplements: A qualitative study. *Journal of Adolescent Health, 37,* 409e–409e7. doi: 10.1016/j.jadohealth.2005.02.003

Focus groups with a total of 81 adolescents found that the participants were familiar with the actual names of herbal and dietary supplements but not with the term "alternative medicine." In addition, the participants related use of herbal/dietary supplements with treating illness rather than with preventative care (Klein et al., 2005).

1. Craft ways to ask adolescents about CAM use.
2. What are some strategies for incorporating CAM into discussions with adolescents about health promotion?

CHILD ABUSE CONSIDERATIONS

- Adolescents may be the victims of physical, emotional, or sexual abuse.
- Adolescents and young adults have higher rates of sexual assault than any other age group (Kaufman, 2008).
- Adolescents are less likely to report abuse than adults because of worry that parents won't let them attend social events anymore, guilt, or lack of memory about the event due to substance use.
- Boys are less likely to report sexual abuse than girls.
- At least one-third of adolescent sexual attacks are perpetrated by a relative or acquaintance (Kaufman, 2008).
- Adolescents with developmental disabilities are more likely to become victims of sexual abuse.
- Alcohol and substance use place an adolescent at greater risk of becoming a victim of sexual assault.
- There is an increasing ability to obtain date-rape drugs, such as flunitrazepam, hydroxybutyrate, and ketamine, over the Internet. As a result, the use of these substances in adolescent acquaintance-rape assaults is on the rise (Kaufman, 2008).

Promoting Safety

Nurses should reinforce safety strategies for avoiding sexual assault, such as going out with a group of friends, staying in public places, and avoiding alcohol/substance use.

- Adolescents are less likely to be physically injured in the attack than adults.

- Nonspecific physical complaints could be an indication of sexual abuse. (See Chapter 14, Mental Health Disorders.)
- Adolescents with a history of sexual abuse are more likely to engage in risky behaviors such as sexual promiscuity and alcohol/substance use.
- Sexually abused adolescents have increased rates of mental health problems, such as depression, anxiety, and post-traumatic stress disorder. (See Chapter 14, Mental Health Disorders.)
- See Chapter 14, Mental Health Disorders, for care of the sexual assault victim.

Review Questions

1. Which of the following is an appropriate response of a nurse to an adolescent's mother questioning why her teen would turn to drugs when he knows it's not permitted in their home?
   A. "All kids try drugs."
   B. "He knows right from wrong."
   C. "The adolescent brain is still developing."
   D. "Adolescents easily give in to peer pressure."
2. When completing an individual biopsychosocial assessment of an adolescent, the nurse would recognize that a delay in growth and development might be caused by
   A. trauma.
   B. unpurified drinking water.
   C. stressors.
   D. all of the above.
3. Which of the following skin conditions might alert a nurse to consider potential child abuse?
   A. Tattoos
   B. Body piercings
   C. Burns
   D. Acne
4. General somatic complaints without confirmed diagnostic data can indicate which of the following in an adolescent patient?
   A. Depression
   B. Insomnia
   C. Hunger
   D. Fatigue
5. The nurse is performing an oral exam. One indication that might cause a nurse to suspect that the adolescent induces intentional vomiting is
   A. bruxism.
   B. protruding wisdom teeth.
   C. gingivitis.
   D. tooth erosion.
6. Chronic stomachaches in adolescents could be a sign or symptom of
   A. anxiety.
   B. the flu.
   C. migraines.
   D. the menstrual cycle.
7. The strongest factor associated with the onset and timing of puberty is
   A. age.
   B. genetics.
   C. onset of sexual activity.
   D. breast development.
8. Which of the following is a similarity in males and females going through puberty?
   A. The secretion of sex hormones decreases.
   B. Lean body mass increases.
   C. Gynecomastia may occur.
   D. Most teens hit puberty at the same age.
   E. Coarse pubic and underarm hair begins to develop.
9. Which of the following would demonstrate that the nurse understands acceptable physical assessment approaches?
   A. The routine pap exam is conducted first.
   B. The adolescent is examined in private.
   C. The nurse explains to the adolescent that all information will be shared with a parent/guardian.
   D. The nurse lists all physical abnormalities for the teen on completion of the exam.
10. A nursing student verbalizes understanding of proper medication administration in adolescents when she tells her instructor which of the following?
    A. "The patient's medicines are only available in capsule form."
    B. "Never crush tablets."
    C. "Alternative medication preparations might be available. I will check with pharmacy."
    D. "Adolescents should be able to swallow any kind of medication."

References

American Academy of Child and Adolescent Psychiatry. (2008). *Obesity in children and teens.* Retrieved from http://www.aacap.org/galleries/FactsForFamilies/79_obesity_in_children_and_teens.pdf

American Academy of Pediatric Dentistry. (2009). *Guideline on periodicity of examination, preventive dental services, anticipatory guidance/counseling, and oral treatment for infants, children, and adolescents.* Retrieved from http://www.aapd.org/media/policies_guidelines/g_periodicity.pdf

American Academy of Pediatrics. (n.d.). *Bright future guidelines for adolescents 11 to 21 years.* Retrieved from http://brightfutures.aap.org/pdfs/Guidelines_PDF/18-Adolescence.pdf

American Academy of Pediatrics. (2003). Timing of puberty in U.S. girls. *AAP Grand Rounds, 9,* 39. Retrieved from http://aapgrandrounds.aappublications.org/content/9/4/39.1.full

American Academy of Pediatrics. (2008). Screening for idiopathic scoliosis in adolescents. Retrieved from www.pediatrics.org/cgi/doi/10.1542/peds.2008-0383. Doi: 10.1542/peds.2002-0383

American Academy of Pediatrics. (2011). Healthy children: A teen's nutritional needs. In D. E. Greydanus (Ed.), *Caring for your teenager: The complete and authoritative guide.* Retrieved from http://www.healthychildren.org/English/ages-stages/teen/nutrition/pages/A-Teenagers-Nutritional-Needs.aspx

American Dental Association. (2010). *Dental grills*. Retrieved from http://www.ada.org/3060.aspx?currentTab=1

Best Pharmaceuticals for Children Act. (2009). *Antipsychotic safety therapeutic working group conference call*. Retrieved from http://bpca.nichd.nih.gov/about/process/upload/Antipsychotic-040109-final-041409.pdf

Britto, M. T., Slap, G. B., DeVellis, R. F., Hornung, R. W., Atherton, H. D., Knopf, J. M., & DeFriese, G. H. (2007). Specialists' understanding of the health care preferences of chronically ill adolescents. *Journal of Adolescent Health, 40,* 334–341. doi: 10.1016/j.jadohealth.2006.10.020

Coker, T. R., Austin, S. B., & Schuster, M. A. (2010). The health and health care of lesbian, gay, and bisexual adolescents. *Annual Reviews of Public Health, 31,* 457–477. doi: 10.1146/annurev.publhealth.012809.103636

Cook, R. L., Chung, T., Kelly, T. M., & Clark, D. B. (2005). Alcohol screening in young persons attending a sexually transmitted disease clinic. *Journal of General Internal Medicine, 20,* 1–6. doi: 10.1111/j.1525-1497.2005.40052.x

Gold, M., Schorzman, C., Murray, P., Downs, J., & Tolentino, G. (2003). Body piercing practices and attitudes among urban adolescents. *Journal of Adolescent Health, 36,* 350–352. Retrieved from http://www.ncbi.nlm.nih.gov/pubmed/15780791

Goldering, J. M., & Cohen, E. (1988). Getting into adolescent heads. *Contemporary Pediatrics, 5,* 75–90.

Goldsworthy, R.C., Schwartz, N.C., Mayhorn, C.B. (2008). Interpretation of pharmaceutical warnings among adolescents. *Journal of Adolescent Health, 42,* 617–625. doi: 10.1016/j.jadohealth.2007.11.141

Hansen, D. L., Tulinius, D., & Hansen, E. H. (2008). Adolescents' struggle with swallowing tablets: Barriers, strategies, and learning. *Pharmacology World Science, 30,* 65–69. doi: 10.1007/s11096-007-9142-y

Hornberger, L. L. (2006). Adolescent psychosocial growth and development. *Journal of Pediatric and Adolescent Gynecology, 19,* 243–246. doi: 10.1016/j.jpag.2006.02.013

Hutton, A. (2005). Consumer perspectives in adolescent ward design. *Issues in Clinical Nursing, 14,* 537–545. doi: 10.1111/j.1365-2702.2004.01106.x

Kandel, D. B. (2002). Stages and pathways of drug involvement: Examining the Gateway Hypothesis. New York: Cambridge University Press. doi: http://dx.doi.org/10.1017/CBO9780511499777

Kandsberger, D. (2007). Factors influencing the successful utilization of home health care in the treatment of children and adolescents with cancer. *Home Health Care Management & Practice, 19,* 450–455. doi: 10.1177/1084822307304827

Kaufman, M. (2008). Care of the adolescent sexual assault victim. *Pediatrics, 122,* 462–470. doi: 10.1542/peds.2008-1581

Kennedy, J. (2005). Herb and supplement use in the US adult population. *Clinical Therapeutics, 27,* 1832–1833. doi:10.1016/j.clinthera.2005.11.004

Klein, J. D., Wilson, K. M., Sesselberg, T. S., Gray, N. J., Yussman, S., & West, J. (2005). Adolescents' knowledge of and beliefs about herbs and dietary supplements: A qualitative study. *Journal of Adolescent Health, 37,* 409e–409e7. doi: 10.1016/j.jadohealth.2005.02.003

Liao, J. K. (2007). Safety and efficacy of statins in Asians. *American Journal of Cardiology, 99,* 410–414. doi:10.1016/j.amjcard.2006.08.051

Lopez, B., Schwartz, S. J., Guillermo, P., Campo, A. E., & Pantin, H. (2008). Adolescent neurological development and its implications for adolescent substance use. *Journal of Primary Prevention, 29,* 5–35. doi: 10.1007/s10935-007-0119-3

Middleman, A., Rosenthal, S., & Rickert, V. (2006). Adolescent immunizations: A position paper of the Society of Adolescent Medicine. *Journal of Adolescent Health, 38,* 321–327. doi: 10.1016/j.jadohealth.2006.01.002

National Institute of Health. (2010). *Pediatric pharmacology research units network*. Retrieved from http://www.nichd.nih.gov/research/supported/ppru1.cfm

O'Malley, P. J., Brown, K., & Krug, S. E. (2008). Patient- and family-centered care of children in the emergency department: Technical report of the American Academy of Pediatrics. *Pediatrics, 122,* e511–e520. doi: 10.1542/peds.2008-1569

Partnership for a Drug Free America. (2005). *The partnership attitude tracking study*. Retrieved from http://www.drugfree.org/wp-content/uploads/2011/04/PATS-Teens-Full-Report-FINAL.pdf

President's Council on Physical Activity and Sports. (2011). *Facts and resources on the health benefits of physical activity*. Retrieved from http://www.fitness.gov/hbpa.htm

Richards, B. S., & Vitale, M. G. (2008). Screening for idiopathic scoliosis in adolescents: An information statement. *The Journal of Bond and Joint Surgery, 90,* 195–198. Retrieved from doi: 10.2106/JBJS.G.01276

Tivorsak, T. L., Britto, M. T., Klostermann, B. K., Nebrig, D. M., & Slap, G. B. (2004). Are pediatric practice settings adolescent friendly? An exploration of attitudes and preferences. *Clinical Pediatrics, 43,* 55–61. doi: 10.1177/000992280404300107

U.S. Preventative Services Task Force. (2004). *Screening for idiopathic scoliosis in adolescents*. Retrieved from http://www.ahrq.gov/clinic/uspstf/uspsaisc.htm

Wilson, K. M., Klein, J. D., Sesselberg, T. S., Yussman, S. M., Markow, D. B., Green, A. E., . . . Gray, N. J. (2006). Use of complementary medicine and dietary supplements. *Journal of Adolescent Health, 38,* 385–394. doi: 10.1016/j.jadohealth.2005.01.010

Young, N. L., Barden, W., McKeever, P., & Dick, P. T. (2006). Taking the call bell home: A qualitative evaluation of tele-homecare for children. *Health and Social Care in the Community, 14,* 231–241. doi: 10.1111/j.1365-2524.2006.00615.x

Common Illnesses or Disorders in Childhood and Home Care

UNIT 4

Respiratory Disorders

11

Jill Morinec, BSN, RN

OBJECTIVES

- ☐ Define key terms.
- ☐ Identify normal assessment findings in the anatomy and physiology of the pediatric respiratory system.
- ☐ Identify differences in the anatomy and physiology of the pediatric and adult patient.
- ☐ Identify the clinical presentation and nursing care of pediatric patients with respiratory disorders.
- ☐ Describe common tests used in diagnosing and treating pediatric respiratory disorders.
- ☐ Identify areas of education for caregivers of children with respiratory disorders.

KEY TERMS

- Ventilation
- Work of breathing
- Flaring
- Retractions
- Hypoxia
- Crackles
- Rhonchi
- Stridor
- Wheezing
- Atelectasis
- Dyspnea
- Hypoxemia

ANATOMY AND PHYSIOLOGY

General

- The upper airway is a passageway that includes the nasopharynx and oropharynx (**Figure 11-1**).
  - *Connected to the ears by eustachian tubes*
    - The nose, pharynx, and larynx, which is covered by the epiglottis, are separated from the lower airway by the trachea.
    - Cilia and mucus in the nostrils warm, clean, and humidify incoming air.
- The lower airway includes the trachea, bronchi, bronchioles, and alveoli.
  - *The left lung has two lobes; the right has three lobes.*
  - *The alveoli are sacs at the ends of terminal bronchioles.*
  - *The alveoli are surrounded by capillaries where oxygen and carbon dioxide diffuse.*
  - *Surfactant is a phospholipid in the alveoli that keeps the alveoli pliable.*
    - Prevents alveoli from collapsing completely at end expiration

Don't have time to read this chapter? Want to reinforce your reading? Need to review for a test? Listen to this chapter on DavisPlus at davispl.us/rudd1.

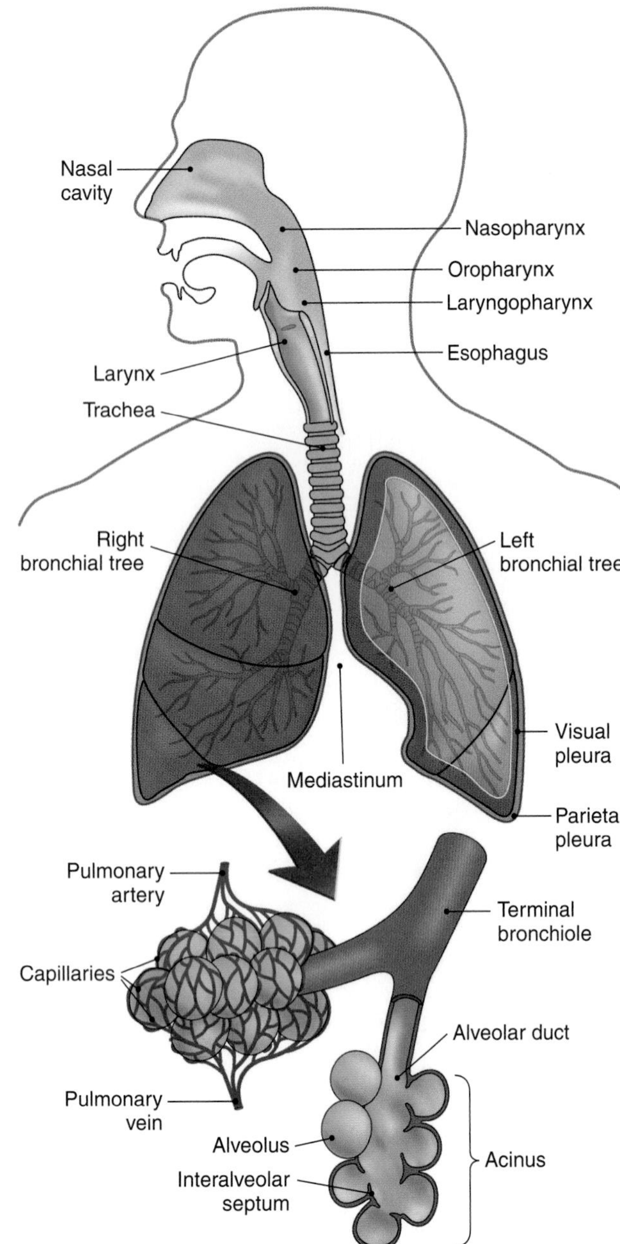

Figure 11–1 Structures of the respiratory tract.

- The lungs are protected by the ribcage, and surrounded by muscles in the thoracic cavity.
  - *The diaphragm muscle separates the lungs from the abdominal cavity.*
  - *The diaphragm contracts, creating a negative pressure, pulling air into the lungs.*
  - *The lungs and chest wall actively expand on inspiration but passively return to resting state with expiration.*
  - *Two pleural membranes*
    - Parietal pleura—lines thoracic cavity, adheres to ribs and superior aspect of diaphragm.
    - Visceral pleura—surrounds each lung; when lungs inflated, lies directly against parietal pleura.
    - Normally separated by only enough fluid to lubricate for painless movement
- Breathing is involuntary; central nervous system controls rate and volume of respiration.
  - *Signals sent by receptors in the lungs and chemoreceptors (pH, $PaCO_2$, PaO_2) in the arterial blood alert the brain*
    - Adjustments made in respirations and heart rate and output to maintain adequate gas exchange
  - *Adequate gas exchange requires equal* ***ventilation*** *and blood distribution.*
  - *Oxygen diffuses across the alveolarcapillary membrane, dissolves in plasma (pressure measured as PaO_2).*
    - Bound to and transported by hemoglobin to the cells for metabolism
  - *Conversely, carbon dioxide, produced by cellular metabolism, dissolves in the plasma ($PaCO_2$) or as bicarbonate.*
    - Travels back to the lungs and across the alveolarcapillary membrane

Developmental Differences in Respiratory System

- A child's upper airway is shorter and more narrow than an adult's.
- A newborn's airway is approximately 4 mm in diameter; an adult's airway is 20 mm.
  - *A 1-mm inflammation circumferentially would decrease a child's airway diameter by 50%, but only by 20% for an adult.*
- Newborns—obligatory nose breathers until 4 weeks of age
- The child's larynx is more flexible than an adult's; it is easily stimulated to spasm.
- The child's intercostal muscles are not fully developed; pronounced abdominal wall movement with respiration is normal until age 6.
- Brief periods of apnea, the absence of respiration, of up to 15 seconds are normal in the newborn period.
- A child's metabolic rate is higher than an adult's, and therefore newborns have a higher oxygen demand; newborns use 4 to 8 liters of oxygen per minute and adults use 3 to 4 liters per minute. A child's respiratory rate is faster, with an irregular pattern.
- Newborns do not have the defense of bronchospasms or constriction to trap foreign irritants, as smooth muscles are not fully developed until about 5 months of age.
- At birth, an infant has about 25 million alveoli, and by age 3, about 200 million.
  - *Alveoli become more complex, and reach about 300 million by adulthood.*
- In children, the bifurcation of the right and left bronchi occurs higher in the airway and the right bronchus enters the lung at a steeper angle in comparison to an adult.
- A child's cartilage surrounding the trachea is more flexible and can compress the airway if the head is not in the proper position.
- The eustachian tubes are shorter and more horizontal in children than in adults.
- A child's lung volume is proportional to chest size; lung growth continues through adolescence.

- A child's tonsils and lymphoid tissues are larger than an adult's.
- The anterior-to-posterior diameter of the chest is equal at birth, decreasing with age.
- Respiratory disorders are classified as upper airway, lower airway, or other respiratory disorders.

ASSESSMENT

General History

- Gestational age
- Past medical history, including onset of current symptoms, pattern of recurrent sore throats, eczema, respiratory problems at birth
- Detailed family history, including chronic respiratory conditions such as asthma
- Exposure to environmental irritants, pets, and smokers living in household
- Feeding and sleeping patterns, growth, and reaching of milestones
- International travel

Physical Examination

- Chest diameter/anterior-posterior diameter

> CLINICAL PEARL
>
> **"Barrel Chest"**
>
> A child's anterior-to-posterior chest diameter is equal until about the age of 2; in older children equality may be a sign of a chronic obstructive lung condition known as "barrel chest" observed in cystic fibrosis or asthma.

- ***Work of breathing***—respiratory effort
  - ***Flaring**, tachypnea, **retractions**, paradoxical breathing (**Figure 11-2**)*
  - *Optimal chest expansion when positioned supine with head of bed elevated to 45-degree angle*
- Position of comfort
  - *Tripod or jaw-thrust, sign of air hunger*
- Symmetrical chest rise
  - *Asymmetrical may indicate tension pneumothorax*
- Color of skin, mucous membranes, nail beds, lips, tip of nose
  - *Acrocyanosis, typical up to 48 hours after birth*

> CLINICAL PEARL
>
> **Assessing Dark-Skinned Infants and Children**
>
> In dark-skinned infants and children, it is best to determine the normal skin color and assess for differences. Erythema will appear as violet or dusky red skin, cyanosis will appear as black skin, and jaundice will appear as darker-than-normal skin. Jaundice is best assessed by looking at the sclera for yellow discoloration.

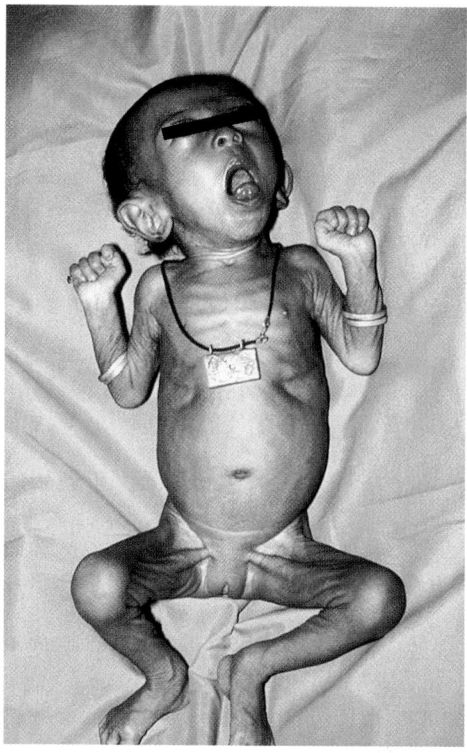

Figure 11-2 Flaring of nostrils during respiratory effort of breathing.

- Simultaneous abdomen and chest rise
- Cough quality, productivity
- Nasal flaring—widening of nares with inspiration
  - *Sign of air hunger*
- Clubbing of finger tips—loss of 160-degree angle of nail bed
  - *May be a sign of chronic **hypoxia**, as seen in cystic fibrosis.*
- Hydration status
  - *Mouth breathing, tachypnea, fever, and anorexia all contribute to dehydration.*

Auscultation

- Anterior and posterior chest, and bilateral mid-axillary for aeration
  - *Respiratory rate—varies based on child's age.*
- Heart rate depends on age; increased with fever, dehydration.
- Adventitious breath sounds
  - ***Crackles** (rales) are fine crackling noises heard on inspiration.*
    - Result as air moves through fluid-filled alveoli, as in pneumonia
    - May not change after coughing
    - The sound can be simulated by rolling hair between your fingers.
  - ***Rhonchi** are low-pitched sounds heard throughout respiration*
    - Air passes through thick secretions throughout respiration.
    - May clear after coughing

- ***Stridor** is a high-pitched sound heard on inspiration. This is often heard when a child has croup.*
- ***Wheezing** is a high-pitched musical sound that can be heard throughout respiration.*
  - Results from air passing through constricted bronchioles or narrowed smaller airways, as in asthma

Percussion

- Lung should resonate when percussed.
  - *Flat or dull sounds in consolidated area*
  - *Tympany with pneumothorax*
  - *Hyperresonance may be heard with the presence of asthma.*

Palpation

- Lymph nodes in head and neck—may be enlarged due to infection.
- Sinuses in older children—assess for tenderness.
- Tactile fremitus—increased with pleural effusion and pneumonia.
  - *Absent in **atelectasis**, pneumothorax, or barrel chest*
- Compare peripheral pulses to central pulses—should be equal.
  - *Severe respiratory distress causes decreased perfusion, results in weaker peripheral pulses.*
- Respiratory distress can progress to respiratory failure; symptoms of each are listed in **Table 11-1.**
- Signs of respiratory failure—muscles of ventilation are fatigued; greater metabolic and oxygen requirements.
- The body can no longer compensate and maintain adequate oxygen and carbon dioxide exchange.
- Respiratory failure can occur if respiratory center is depressed due to overdose of narcotics.
- Emergent interventions imminent

TABLE 11–1 SIGNS OF RESPIRATORY DISTRESS AND RESPIRATORY FAILURE

Signs of Respiratory Failure	Signs of Respiratory Distress
• Tachypnea • Dyspnea • Hyperpnea • Nasal flaring • Use of accessory muscles • Retractions–intercostal in mild distress; suprasternal, subcostal, and supraclavicular seen in moderate distress • Sitting with head of bed elevated • Coughing–intermittent • Adventitious breath sounds • Tachycardia • Dusky nail beds • Hypercapnea • Hypoxia; ability to speak full sentences • Crying–strong	• Mental status change; extreme irritability • Circumoral cyanosis or mottled skin color • Lethargy • Grunting • Head bobbing • Coughing continuously • Retractions–moderate along with the use of accessory muscles • "Quiet" breathing • Sitting forward with arms, knees used for support, tripod • Shallow respirations • See-saw respirations • Hypoxemia–lower than normal oxygen in the blood; is persistent with supplemental oxygen administered • Weak or absent cry • Tachycardia–further elevated heart rate

CLINICAL PEARL

Oxygen flow rate (liters per minute, L/min) of supplemental oxygen does not equal the concentration of oxygen delivered to the child. The oxygen concentration delivered is dependent on the system that is used. See **Table 11-2**.

TABLE 11–2 METHODS OF SUPPLEMENTAL OXYGEN DELIVERY

Oxygen Delivery System	O_2 Concentration Delivered (%)	Flow Rate (L/min)
Nasal cannula	22–40	0.25–4.0
Simple mask	35–50	6–10
Partial rebreather	60–95	>6
Nonrebreather	Approaches 100	10–15
Venturi mask	24–50	Variable
Oxygen hoods	Approaches 100	>10
Oxygen tents	Up to 50	>10

Diagnostic Tests

Arterial Blood Gas

- Evaluates ventilation by measuring pH and partial pressure of oxygen (PaO_2) and carbon dioxide ($PaCO_2$)
- PaO_2 is the amount of oxygen in the lungs available to diffuse into the blood.
  - *Decreased due to hypoventilation, ventilation-perfusion mismatch, or shunting*
- $PaCO_2$ is the amount of carbon dioxide in the blood that can diffuse out of the blood.
  - *Increased due to hypoventilation, marked ventilation-perfusion mismatch*
  - *Decreased due to increased alveolar ventilation*
- pH reveals acid–base balance, which is normally between 7.35 and 7.45 on 1–14 scale.
  - *Acidotic = below 7.4; alkalotic = above 7.4*
  - *Changes due to respiratory or metabolic dysfunction*
  - *Identify respiratory or metabolic compensation mechanisms.*
- Invasive and anxiety provoking for child and parents

Chest X-ray

- Used judiciously due to radiation exposure
  - *Identifies thoracic structures*
  - *Takes different views—AP, lateral, or oblique*
    - Lead protection over gonads

Computed Tomography

- More sensitive; more radiation exposure than chest x-ray (CXR)
- Three-dimensional picture
- Contrast medium used
  - *NPO for 4 to 6 hours*
  - *Child may need sedation.*

Magnetic Resonance Imaging

- Identifies structures and any obstruction of blood flow in blood vessels and tissue.
  - *Powerful magnet; no metal in/on body*
  - *Child may need sedation.*

Bronchoscopy

- Allows direct visualization of trachea, upper parts of bronchi
  - *Used to collect secretion samples, in brush or lesion biopsy, or to remove foreign objects*
    - NPO to prevent aspiration

Pulmonary Function Test

- Measures lung volumes, flow rates, and compliance by measuring expirations
  - *Children 5 years old or older*
  - *Peak flow tests use calculated expiratory flow rates to assess respiratory impairment and effectiveness of therapy.*

Sweat Test

- Uses pilocarpine to stimulate the sweat glands; amount of sodium and chloride produced is measured to identify cystic fibrosis.

Sputum Culture

- Identifies pathogens
  - *Collect in early morning*
  - *Nasal or gastric washings for children too young to produce sputum*
  - *Pulse oximetry—measures the oxygen saturation of blood using infrared light.*

UPPER AIRWAY INFECTIOUS DISORDERS

OTITIS MEDIA (OM)

- Often caused by bacteria
  - *Streptococcus pneumonae, Haemophilus influenzae, and Moraxella catarrhalis*
  - *Can be caused by viruses*
    - Most common causes: respiratory syncytial virus (RSV), rhinoviruses, influenza viruses, and adenoviruses
    - One of most common childhood illnesses
      - *Of all children, 84% will have at least one episode before age 3, with peak incidence between 6 to 12 months of age (Shaikh & Hoberman, 2010).*
  - *Incidence of OM is increased as a result of short, immature upper respiratory tract and the eustachian tubes being connected to the nasopharynx (see* ***Figure 11-3****).*
    - Bottle feeding with the infant supine can cause reflux of formula from the nasopahrynx into the eustachian tube.

Assessment

- Earache, pulling at the ears
- Bulging, red, or opaque eardrum
- Yellow or green or purulent, foul-smelling drainage
- May be accompanied by other nonspecific signs of infection
- High-grade fever
- Anorexia
- Crying
- Sleep disturbances
- Vomiting
- Diarrhea
- Lymph glands enlarged

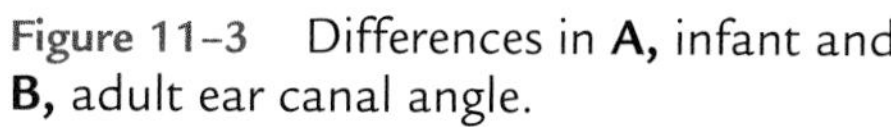

Figure 11-3 Differences in **A,** infant and **B,** adult ear canal angle.

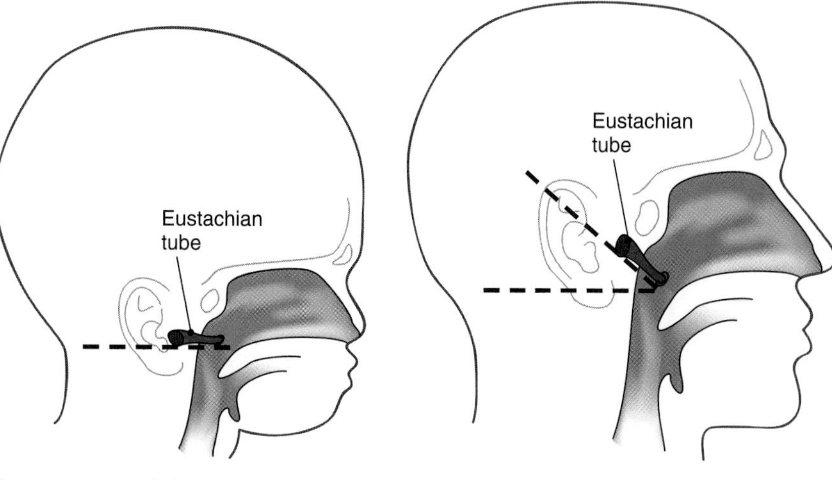

OTITIS MEDIA WITH EFFUSION (OME)

- Eardrum appears retracted, either yellow or gray (**Figure 11-4**)
- No general signs of infection present, but decreased mobility of eardrum
  - *Tinnitus*
  - *Hearing loss*
  - *Mild inability to maintain balance*
- Children who have environmental allergies, are exposed to tobacco smoke, or have eustachian tube dysfunction are more likely to have OM or OME (Torpy, 2010).

Promoting Safety

Antihistamines and decongestants should not be used in treating OME. Studies have shown them to be ineffective in resolution of fluid and to introduce potentially detrimental side effects, including gastrointestinal upset, drowsiness, dizziness, and irritability.

OTITIS EXTERNA (OE), SWIMMER'S EAR

- Outer ear canal infection; pruritis, erythema
  - *Tenderness*
  - *Purulent drainage*

Diagnosis of OM, OME, and OE

- Based on history, signs and symptoms, and pneumatic otoscopy (visualization) that can be confirmed with tympanometry (measured movement of eardrum)

Nursing Interventions

- Management based on accurate and early discernment of OM versus OME
- Antibiotics prescribed conservatively
- Corticosteroids for OE
- Supportive care, analgesics, antipyretics, and adequate hydration

Caregiver Education

- Feed infant in upright position.
- Avoid infant exposure to tobacco smoke.
- Avoid propping a bottle in the infant's mouth.
- Discontinue use of pacifier after 6 months.
- Importance of immunizations—pneumoccoccal vaccine (PCV)
- Only bacterial infections require antibiotics.
  - *Stress the importance of completing antibiotics as prescribed.*
  - *Improvement should be observed within 48 hours.*
  - *Discard any unused antibiotics.*
- Myringotomy—incision in eardrum to relieve pressure, drain fluid.
  - *Tympanostomy—tube placed through eardrum to relieve pressure*
  - *Tubes usually fall out spontaneously within a year.*

SINUSITIS

- Inflammation of the sinuses as a result of viruses, bacteria, or allergens; creates mucus
- Mucus is blocked from draining into nose; acts as pool for pathogens.

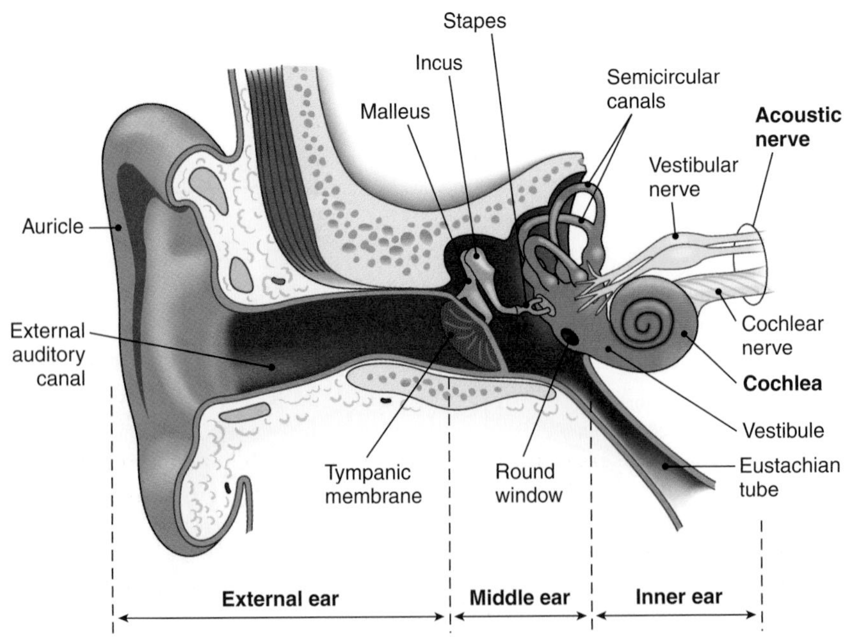

Figure 11-4 Outer and inner ear.

Assessment

- Facial pain
- Headache
- Low-grade fever
- "Cold" symptoms lasting up to 2 weeks
- Thick yellow nasal discharge
- Swelling around eyes
- Fatigue, irritability

Diagnosis

- Clinical presentation

Nursing Interventions

- Antibiotics as prescribed
- Saline nasal drops or decongestants

Caregiver Education

- Teach importance of how to avoid sinusitis during a cold or allergy attack.
- Use oral decongestants or nasal sprays.
- Have child blow nose, one side at a time, blocking the other side.
  - *Developmentally ready around 2 years of age*
- Warm compresses to facial sinus areas
- Cool mist humidifier
- Electrostatic filters on heating and cooling equipment

NASOPHARYNGITIS

- Inflammation of the nasal and pharyngeal mucosa due to bacterial or viral organism
  - *Rhinovirus, enterovirus, adenovirus, metapneumovirus*
  - *Occurs in the early fall and late spring and lasts 7 to 10 days*
  - *Nasal congestion is absent.*
  - *Bacterial infection, often with sore throat and nasal congestion*

Assessment and Diagnosis

- Clinical presentation
- Nasal or throat swabs

Nursing Interventions

- Monitor respiratory status
- Supportive care
- Antibiotics as ordered

INFLUENZA

- Viral infection spread through contact or inhalation of droplets
- The virus is contagious 1–2 days before the onset of symptoms and usually affects the upper respiratory tract.
- Secondary bacterial infections are common with influenza.

> **Promoting Safety**
>
> **Over-the-Counter Medications**
>
> Over-the-counter medications treat only symptoms. Parents/caregivers need to know that medication labeled "pediatric" has been exclusively studied for effectiveness and side effects in children. Parents should read the label to identify "active" ingredients, and follow all "use only as directed" information. Children are more sensitive than adults to medication. Children may have an increase in paradoxical effects. Some drugs, such as aspirin, can cause serious illness or death if given to a child with chickenpox or flu-like symptoms. Cold medicine should not be used in children younger than 4 years of age.

Assessment and Diagnosis

- Abrupt onset
- Fever
- Chills
- Headache
- Flushed cheeks
- Cough
- Malaise
- Cold symptoms
- Possible dry or sore throat, erythematous rash, and diarrhea
- Wheezing may occur if bronchitis is present.

Nursing Interventions

- Symptomatic treatment of viral symptoms
- Adequate hydration
- Antiviral medication, such as amantadine hydrochloride, may reduce symptoms if started within 48 hours of onset of symptoms.
- Annual vaccinations are recommended for high-risk groups.

Caregiver Education

- Supportive care
- Droplet and contact precautions in hospital
- Frequent hand hygiene at home setting; limit visitors
- Encourage fluids for secretion liquification and to prevent dehydration.
- Antiviral medications may cause nausea and may exacerbate asthma.
- Provide rest, quiet, and diversional activities.

TONSILLITIS

- Tonsillitis is inflammation of the palatine tonsils; adenoiditis is inflammation of the pharyngeal tonsils, on the posterior wall of the nasopharynx.
  - *Caused by bacteria or virus*
  - *Incidence of pharyngitis and tonsillitis is highest in children 4 to 7 years of age.*

- *Palatine tonsil size is graded in relation to how much airway obstruction due to protruding tonsils from either side of the oropharynx (**Table 11-3**).*
    - A grade of +1–+2 is normal tonsil size.
    - A grade of+3 is enlarged tonsils seen with infection.
    - A grade of +4 is seen with significant, almost touching or "kissing" tonsils.

Assessment

- Sore throat
- Enlarged tonsils, may be red or covered with exudates
- Difficulty swallowing
- Mouth breathing with halitosis
- Enlarged adenoids may affect speech, and may cause the child to mouth breathe or have snoring or obstructive sleep apnea.
- Peritonsillar abscesses in older children are unilateral, cause severe pain, displace the uvula, and increase risk of dehydration and airway obstruction.

Diagnosis

- History of present illness and physical assessment of pharynx
- Serum analysis reveals leukocytosis
- Throat culture may identify a bacterial cause

Nursing Interventions

- Supportive care
- Antibiotics as ordered
- Tonsillectomy and possible adenoidectomy for chronic inflammation
- After tonsillectomy, place child in side-lying or prone position to drain secretion until he or she is awake.
- Provide gentle oral care only if needed, avoiding surgical site; avoid coughing, using a straw, or blowing nose to avoid bleeding. Encourage popsicles and ice chips while avoiding acidic foods. Dark brown (old) blood-tinged secretions are normal; bright red blood is not.
- Assess for hemorrhage, restlessness, tachycardia, thready pulse, pallor, and repeated swallowing.
- The child may be nauseated from the drainage.
- Attempt to avoid vomiting and minimize crying.

CRITICAL COMPONENT

Post-tonsillectomy Bleeding

A child who is post-tonsillectomy and is continually swallowing is bleeding. Assess for restlessness, frank red blood in the mouth and nose, and increased pulse rate.

TABLE 11–3 TONSIL GRADING SCALE

Grade	Description	Grade	Description
1+ 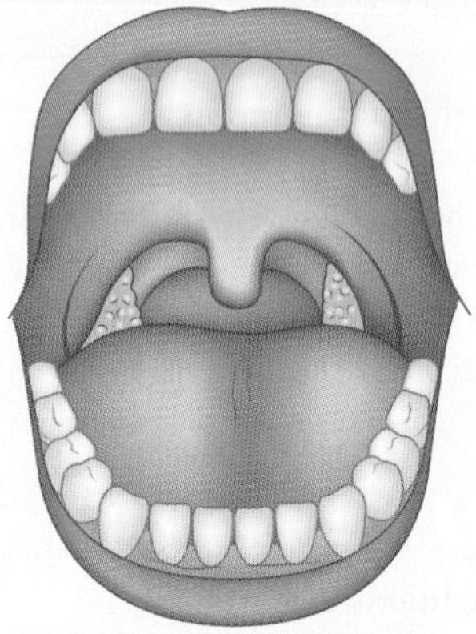 1+	Tonsils extend to arches	3+ 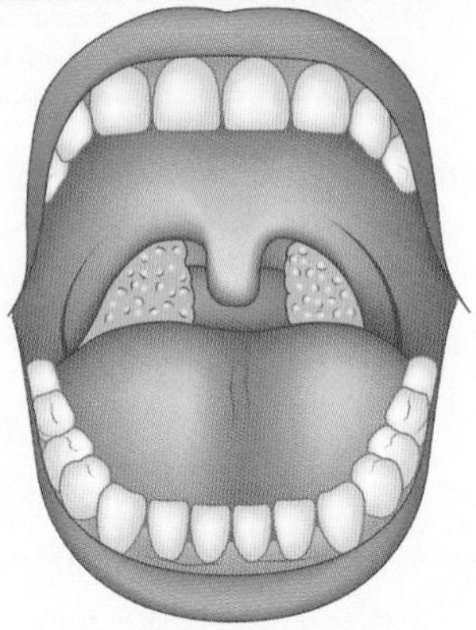 3+	Tonsils approximate the uvula
2+ 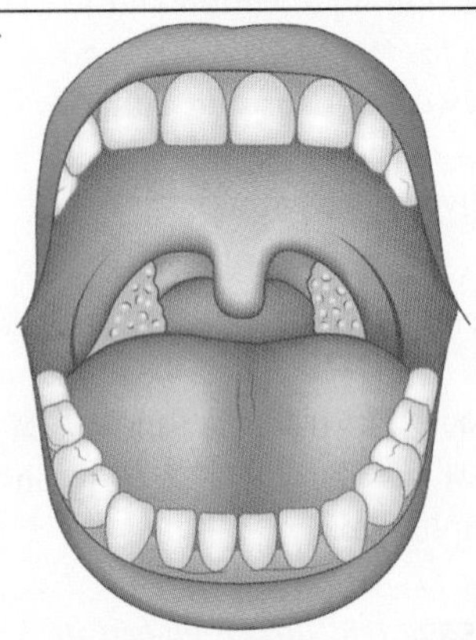 2+	Tonsils extend just beyond arches	4+ 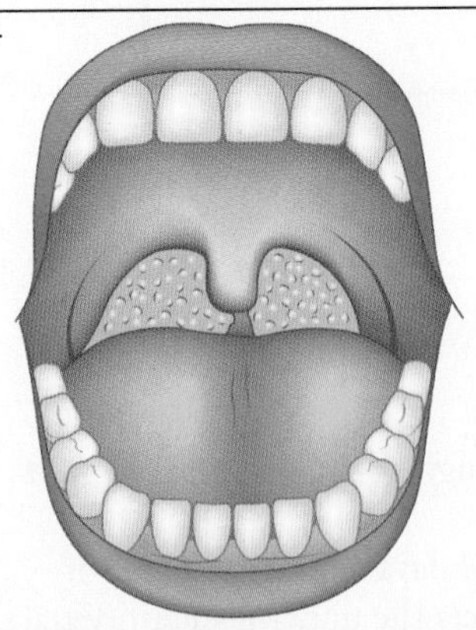 4+	Tonsils meet midline ("kiss")

Source: Dillon, P. M. (2007). *Nursing health assessment: A critical thinking, case studies approach* (2nd ed., p. 305). Philadelphia: F.A. Davis.

- Adequate pain relief is essential to optimize oral intake; encourage child to take pain medicine or get order to change to IV pain medicine.

Caregiver Education

- Instruct parent to report any bleeding immediately—post-operative hemorrhage could occur any time from immediately after the procedure to up to 10 days later.
- Instruct parents that child should avoid acidic, highly seasoned, and hard or sharp foods such as tortilla chips for 2 weeks.
- Instruct parents that child should avoid coughing, clearing throat, gargling, and disturbing tonsils with toothbrush.
- Stress the importance of taking pain medicine before taking fluids or food.

UPPER AIRWAY NONINFECTIOUS DISORDERS

TRACHEOESOPHAGEAL FISTULA (TEF)

- Abnormal communication between the trachea and esophagus (**Figure 11-5**)
- May affect ventilation

Assessment

- Respiratory distress within minutes after birth
- Excessive oral secretions
- Cyanosis
- Coughing spells
- Abdominal distention

Diagnosis

- Prenatal ultrasonography
- Polyhydramnios in utero
- Possible thoracic bubble, and cardiac shift

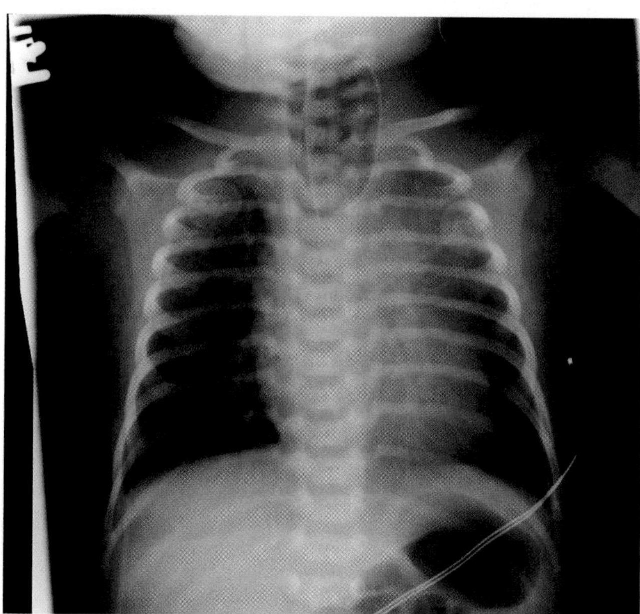

Figure 11-5 X-ray of tracheoesophageal fistula.

Nursing Interventions

- Prepare for surgical repair shortly after birth (hours to days after birth).
- Administer surfactant.
- Assist with extracorporeal membrane oxygenation (ECMO).
- Pre-/postsurgical care
  - *Prevent aspiration—constant oral suction, nasogastric (NG) tube for feeds*
  - *NPO prior to surgery*
  - *Elevate head of bed 30 degrees.*
  - *Oxygen, mechanical ventilation*
  - *Monitor for respiratory distress, arterial blood gases (ABGs).*

Caregiver Education

- Prevent aspiration—feeding, positioning
- Importance of frequent follow-up appointments

LARYNGOMALACIA

- Congenital laryngeal cartilage abnormality
- Redundant laryngeal tissue or curling epiglottis that causes upper airway obstruction

Assessment

- Normal vital signs and oxygen saturation
- Mild tachypnea
- Crowing noise with respirations
- Suprasternal retractions may be present
- Stridor increases when child is supine, crying, or after a feeding.

Diagnosis

- History and laryngoscopy

Nursing Interventions

- Symptoms usually resolve by age 2, without intervention.
- In rare cases, intubation or tracheostomy may be necessary.
- Monitor for acute respiratory distress, stridor, retractions, or **dyspnea**, as well as feeding difficulty.
- Position the neck with slight hyperextension to optimize airflow in flexible airway.
- Provide postsurgical care for the child.

Caregiver Education

- Teach signs and symptoms of baseline versus worsening sounds.
- Teach how to monitor feeding for difficulty sucking and for choking.
- Smaller, more frequent feedings may ensure adequate intake.
- Reassure parents that most children outgrow this disorder by age 2.

SUBGLOTTIC STENOSIS

- Narrowing of airway within the rigid, cricoid cartilage that may be congenital or result from prolonged intubation

Assessment and Diagnosis

- Stridor—inspiratory, expiratory, or both
- Adventitious breath sounds and decreased air movement post-extubation
- Increased work of breathing
- Assess dependency on tracheostomy—the percentage of occlusion that causes increased work of breathing.
- History of recurrent or present croup to identify any additional edema
- Presence of gastroesophageal reflux that may contribute to airway irritation and inflammation

Nursing Interventions

- Close monitoring of respiratory status
- Supplemental oxygen
- Monitoring of intermittent obstructive episodes
- Medications
  - *Oral, IV, or inhaled steroids*
  - *Inhaled epinephrine*
    - Emergency tracheostomy if indicated

Caregiver Education

- Tracheostomy care
- Monitoring breathing; suctioning, especially for mucous plug

CROUP SYNDROMES

ACUTE LARYNGITIS

- Inflammation of the larynx
  - *Can present as sole disorder or be one of multiple respiratory symptoms*
- Laryngitis alone resolves without treatment.
- Loss of voice, or hoarseness
- Rest voice for 24 hours, encourage oral fluids.

ACUTE SPASMODIC LARYNGITIS (SPASMODIC CROUP)

- Viral laryngitis affects children 3 months to 3 years old.
- Pattern of seal-like cough worse at night, absent by day

Assessment

- History of previous attacks lasting 2 to 5 days followed by uneventful recovery
- Night-time barking, seal-like cough
- Afebrile
- Mild respiratory distress
- Stridor scoring to assess difficulty of breathing

Diagnosis

- Clinical signs

Nursing Interventions

- Close monitoring of respiratory status; can progress rapidly
- Cool mist, or going out into cold night air, may relieve spasms.
- Supplemental oxygen if saturation less than 94%.
- Beta-adrenergics (racemic epinephrine)
  - *Aerosolized, rapid-acting, decrease inflammation and mucus, temporary*
  - *Onset 30 minutes; last for 2 hours*
  - *Can lead to tachycardia, hypertension, headache, and anxiety*
  - *Corticosteroids (Dexamethasone) are longer acting, with 36- to 54-hour half-life.*
    - May lead to hypertension and elevated glucose levels

Caregiver Education

- Encourage resting voice.
- Stress the importance of hydration.

EPIGLOTTITIS

- Acute, rapidly progressing inflammation of the larynx and epiglottis
  - *Can be life threatening*
  - *Affects 2- to 8-year-olds*
  - *Usually caused by bacteria, Streptococcus and Staphylococcus*
  - *Can be caused by the virus Haemophilus influenzae type B (Hib) in unimmunized children*

CRITICAL COMPONENT

Possible Bronchospasm and Airway Occlusion

If you suspect a child has epiglottitis, do not inspect the mouth or throat without emergency personnel and intubation supplies on hand because it could stimulate bronchospasm and airway occlusion.

Assessment

- Previously healthy child, suddenly with very ill appearance
- Sudden, high fever
- Severe sore throat
- Four D's—drooling, dysphagia, dysphonia, distressed inspiratory air movement—stridor
- Restlessness, anxiety
- Tachycardia, tachypnea with high fever
- Child may be sitting up and forward, with lower jaw thrust forward, in tripod position.

Diagnosis

- Clinical symptoms
- Lateral neck x-ray—narrowed airway, enlarged epiglottis at base of tongue, appears as inverted thumb ("thumb sign").

- Suspected epiglottitis is a contraindication for visual inspection of mouth and throat.
- If airway secured, perform throat culture; treat for gram positives until cultures return from lab.

Nursing Interventions

- Monitor respiratory status closely; prepare for intubation.
- Encourage child not to cry, to avoid laryngospasms.
- Provide medications as prescribed.
- Hydration—IV fluids
- Emotional support for frightened family
- Supportive treatment—palivizumab prophylaxis (Chavez-Bueno, Asuncion, & Welliver, 2006)

Caregiver Education

- Proper administration of antibiotics
- Encourage oral hydration of child
- Prevention—Hib vaccination

INFECTIONS OF LOWER AIRWAY

BRONCHIOLITIS

- Acute inflammation of bronchioles
  - *Caused by either a virus or bacteria, most often, respiratory syncytial virus (RSV)*
- Viruses enter mucosal cells, rupture cells, create debris and increased mucus production, causing bronchospasms and obstruction.

Assessment

- Mucus may produce wheezing and crackle sounds.
- Apnea
- Nasal congestion
- Fever
- Variant cough
- Inspiratory/expiratory wheeze
- Tachypnea
- Can progress to severe respiratory distress

Diagnosis

- History and clinical signs
- CXR—hyperinflation, patchy atelectasis
- ELISA—identify viral cause
- ABG

Nursing Interventions

- Cardiorespiratory monitoring
- Humidified oxygen or heliox (mixture of oxygen and helium) to increase oxygen diffusion
- Contact precautions—prevent spread of organisms
- Management of mechanical ventilation—positive end expiratory pressure (PEEP)

Evidence-Based Practice Research: Bronchiolitis Caused by Respiratory Syncytial Virus

Durani, Y., Friedman, M. J., & Attia, M. W. (2008). Clinical predictors of respiratory syncytial virus infection in children. *Pediatrics International, 50,* 352–355. doi: 10.1111/j.1442-200X.2008.02589.x.

Because bronchiolitis from Respiratory Syncytial Virus (RSV) has a range of severity, is highly contagious, and is costly to manage prophylactically, Durani, Friedman and Attia (2008) conducted a prospective cohort study to develop a clinical prediction model to identify RSV infections in infants and young children. The study evaluated children 36 months old or younger who came into the emergency department with upper respiratory infection (URI) symptoms and were tested for RSV. Durani and associates (2008) looked at the presence or absence of 13 different clinical symptoms associated with URI and RSV. Analysis of all the data identified that the independent variables of cough, wheezing, and retractions were predictive of RSV infection in infants and young children. The triad of cough, wheeze, and retractions was identified as a predictive model for RSV infection in the winter, with a sensitivity of 80%. This study is important to aid clinicians in early identification of RSV to eliminate unnecessary septic work-ups and avoid the nosocomial spread of RSV (Durani et al., 2008).

1. How could this study help the nurse decide what interventions would be important if a child presented with cough, wheezing, and retractions?
2. Based on the prediction model, what questions would you ask when collecting the patient's health history if the patient presents with wheezing, cough, and retractions?

- Drug therapy—beta-antagonists, steroids, bronchodilators, beta-adrenergics
- Hydration
- Isolation of child to prevent spread
- Pulmonary hygiene—chest physiotherapy, postural drainage, suctioning
- Palivizumab—prophylactic vaccination

Medication

Treatment for Bronchiolitis

Treatment for bronchiolitis is supportive palivizumab, a humanized monoclonal antibody that is used as prophylaxis for RSV. It is given as an intramuscular (IM) injection before the start of the RSV season (usually October to May depending on location) and then every month during RSV season for a total of five injections at the cost of about $1000 for the smallest single dose. Before administering, determine normal partial thromboplastin time (PTT), prothrombin time (PT), and international normalized ratio (INR) and platelet levels. Treatment is recommended for high-risk groups (Buckley, 2010). The Centers for Disease Control and Prevention (CDC) lists the following high-risk groups: infants born at 29 to 35 weeks' gestation who are 3 months or younger at the start of RSV season; infants and children under the age of 2 with congenital heart defects; and infants born at 35 weeks' gestation with chronic lung disease or neuromuscular disorders (CDC, 2009).

Caregiver Education

- Use of bulb syringe
- To avoid spread of RSV, perform hand hygiene, limit contacts.
- Maintain oral hydration and use nasal saline drops to liquefy secretions.
- Monitor temperature, antipyretics.
- Encourage rest.
- Elevate head of bed 30 degrees.
- Assess for respiratory distress, changes in symptoms.

> **CRITICAL COMPONENT**
>
> **Hand Hygiene**
>
> Hand hygiene is crucial. Hands contaminated with respiratory secretions are believed to be the major mode of spread of respiratory infections. Most people wash their hands inadequately. Antibacterial soap and warm water are needed. First wet your hands, and then work up a generous lather for about 30 seconds, or the time it takes to sing "Happy Birthday" twice. Be sure to wash in between fingers and under fingernails. Rinse thoroughly with ends of fingers pointing downward so as not to splash or contaminate anything. Dry hands with paper towels and turn faucet off with paper towel.
>
> Avoid cross-contamination by grouping nursing assignments to include patients with like diagnoses, and by placing susceptible patients in different rooms. Strict attention to maintaining physician-ordered respiratory or contact precautions is vital to prevent cross-contamination.

- Cluster care to allow for rest period.
- Teach when they should notify physician:
  - *Worsening respiratory distress in a high-risk infant less than a year old, increased retractions, increased respiratory rate or adventitious respiratory sounds*
  - *Child appearing more ill, or not eating, drinking, or sleeping*

PNEUMONIA

- Inflammation of lung parenchyma
  - *Caused by viruses, bacteria, mycoplasm, fungus, or aspiration*
- The invading organism travels to lungs via upper respiratory tract or systemically.
- The virus causes cellular destruction and accumulation of debris in bronchioles and alveoli, causing patchy infiltrates.
- Bacteria cause fluid accumulation and cellular debris in bronchioles and alveoli, causing consolidation.
- Impaired gas exchange results from atelectasis and the inflammatory response with both viruses and bacteria.

Assessment

Viral

- Influenza viruses and RSV
- Variant fever, low to high
- Cough, crackles
- Wheezing, more common with RSV
- General malaise, fatigue
- Headaches and stomachaches
- CXR—hyperinflation or consolidation
- Duration—5 to 7 days

Bacterial

- Recent history of upper respiratory infection
- High fever, chills
- Cough
- Abnormal or decreased breath sounds
- Older children may have chest pain, gastrointestinal symptoms.
- Respiratory distress and restlessness
- CXR—consolidation

Diagnosis

- Pulse oximetry—normal or decreased
- Chest x-ray
- White blood cell (WBC) count—slightly elevated in viral (less than 20,000/mm^3) but much higher in bacterial
- Sputum culture—older children
- Nasal washing—younger children and infants

Nursing Interventions

- Provide supportive care for viral pneumonia.
- Monitor oxygenation and hydration.
- Monitor respiratory status.
- Give antibiotics as prescribed for bacterial infections.

Caregiver Education

- Teach safety measures.
  - *Avoidance of aspiration*
    - Elevate head of bed 30 degrees
    - Avoid overfeeding
    - Burp frequently during a bottle feeding
- Teach caregiver the importance of giving antibiotics as ordered; note that antibiotics are not effective for viral pneumonia.
- Inform caregiver that fatigue and cough may linger for a few weeks.
- Pneumococcal vaccine

PERTUSSIS (WHOOPING COUGH)

- Bacterial infection by *Bordetella pertussis;* highly contagious
- Occurs mainly in children under the age of 4
- Occurs most often in spring and summer months
- Decreased incidence with pertussis vaccine
  - *DTaP in infants and children up to age 6*
  - *TDap in children age 7 and older and adults*

Assessment

- Characteristic "whooping" sound after a cough episode, gasping for air

- Three stages
  - *The beginning stage presents as URI, nasal congestion, coughing, rhinorrhea, watery eyes, sneezing; lasts about a week.*
  - *The second stage is marked by intense coughing fits; lasts about a week. Young infants may not exhibit the classic whoop sound but become apneic from partial airway closure.*
  - *The third stage is chronic cough lasting up to 10 weeks or more.*
  - *Known as "100-day cough" (CDC, 2011)*

Diagnosis

- Clinical presentation
- History of incomplete or absent pertussis vaccine
- Polymerase chain reaction (PCR) from nasopharyngeal swab
- Nasopharyngeal culture

Nursing Interventions

- Provide drug therapy as prescribed.
- Monitor respiratory status and give supplemental humidified oxygen.
- Observe droplet precautions.
- Maintain hydration.
- Provide supportive care.

Caregiver Education

- Importance of DTap vaccination
- Preventing the spread of infection
- Inform caregiver that child may have persistent cough for up to 10 weeks after the infection.

TUBERCULOSIS

- Inhaled droplets cause an immune response in the alveoli; result of *Mycobacterium tuberculosis*, an acid-fast bacillus.
- Transmitted in tiny droplets through speaking, coughing, or sneezing
- According to the CDC, 6% of children under age 15 and 11% of young adults ages 15 to 24 were infected with tuberculosis (TB) in 2009 (CDC, 2010).
- Worldwide, over 250,000 children develop TB each year, and 100,000 of these children will die from the infection (World Health Organization, 2011).
- Once in the alveoli, a bacillus triggers an immune response.
- Macrophages form hard tubercles around the bacilli.
- These tubercles can remain dormant or progress to active tuberculosis. TB is not as prevalent in children as in adults.
- Bacilli may spread via the lymphatic or circulatory systems to other sites.
- TB is difficult to diagnose in children, as sputum specimens may be nonconclusive and children may present with vague symptoms as compared to adults.

CULTURAL AWARENESS: Prevalence of Tuberculosis

Tuberculosis is most prevalent in developing countries. The World Health Organization (WHO) noted that the highest incidence of TB was in regions of Southeast Asia and sub-Saharan Africa, with the highest number of TB-related deaths in the sub-Saharan African region (WHO, 2010). The challenges of the HIV epidemic, population growth and migrations, poverty, and sociopolitical instability that affect developing countries affect the treatment of TB. Treatment is long, intensive, and costly, with many potential side effects. Only 20% of people infected with TB complete treatment (WHO, 2006). Lack of adherence to treatment not only precludes a cure, but allows TB to mutate and become drug-resistant. About 460,000 new cases of multi-drug-resistant TB are reported each year (WHO, 2006).

Assessment

- Latent TB—no symptoms, positive skin test, not contagious.
- Active TB
  - *Persistent cough*
  - *Weight loss or inability to gain weight*
  - *Anorexia*
  - *Fatigue*
  - *Low-grade fever*
  - *Night sweats*
  - *Wheezing or decreased breath sounds may be heard in infants.*

Diagnosis

- Challenging, as TB causes a variety of symptoms that change with age
  - *Screening questions for identifying at-risk children*
    - Close contact with person infected with TB?
    - Immigrant from endemic area?
    - Low income or homeless?
    - Immunocompromised?
    - Less than 4 years old?
    - Mantoux test–intradermal purified protein injection; if positive, repeat in 8 weeks.
      - *Positive confirms latent TB*
    - CXR–AP and lateral
      - *Atelectasis*
      - *Enlarged lymph nodes*
      - *Pleural effusion*
      - *Alveolar consolidation*
      - *Presence of tubercles seen in older children*
    - Blood culture
      - *Identifies drug sensitivity*
    - Flexible bronchoscopy
      - *Gastric washings—used for children unable to produce sputum*
      - *May be negative even in active TB*
    - Sputum culture
      - *Serial specimens collected early in the morning*

- *Takes 4 weeks to confirm*
- *Used in children 12 and older who can produce sputum*
- Pleural biopsy—confirms if effusion present
- Lumbar puncture
  - *Confirms TB spread to meninges*

Nursing Interventions

- Provide drug therapy and supportive care.
- Encourage nutrition and rest.
- Monitor respiratory status.
- Observe droplet precautions.
- Maintain hydration.
- Active TB—give antitubercular drugs.
  - *Given in combination for 6 months*
  - *Isoniazid, rifampicin, ethambutol, streptomycin*
    - Latent TB—take same medications, but smaller daily dose for 9 months

Caregiver Education

- Promote nutrition and overall health to avoid infections.
- Prevent exposure and spread of TB.
  - *Take TB medication for at least 2 weeks before exposing noninfected people.*
  - *Family and close contacts should take preventative medication.*
  - *If traveling abroad, get BCG vaccine.*
  - *Wash hands or use sanitizer after exposure to respiratory secretions.*
  - *Infected child should cover mouth and nose with coughs or sneezes.*
- Direct observation of therapy—routine person should ensure child is taking medications as prescribed.
- BCG vaccine—live attenuated strain of Mycobacterium bovis
  - *Not widely used in United States*
  - *Provides incomplete protection*

CRITICAL COMPONENT

Testing for Tuberculosis

If a child is diagnosed with TB, anyone living with the infected child must be tested for TB and treated accordingly.

NONINFECTIOUS DISORDERS OF LOWER AIRWAY

RESPIRATORY DISTRESS SYNDROME

- Seen primarily in premature infants; related to developmental delay in lung maturation
- Alveoli are collapsed at end expiration and cannot respond
- Pulmonary blood is shunted to systemic circulation
- Altered surface tension causes fluid and protein leak from capillaries
  - *Producing hyaline membrane*
  - *Atelectasis*
  - *Hypoperfusion to the lung*
  - *Results in hypoventilation, increased $PaCO_2$, decreased PaO_2, and decreased pH*
  - *Hypercapnia and hypoxia cause arterial vasoconstriction, resulting in further hypoperfusion.*
    - At-risk infants—those with diabetic mothers, second-born twins, delivered by cesarean section, pneumonia infection, perinatal asphyxia
    - Incidence decreases significantly with increased gestational age
      - Direct correlation of severity to prematurity
      - Occurs in infants born at less than 38 weeks' gestation

Assessment

- Within minutes to several hours after birth, exhibit signs of respiratory distress
- Tachypnea
- Retractions, intercostal/subcostal
- Nasal flaring
- Cyanosis
- Grunting
- Fine crackles and diminished breath sounds
- CXR—looks like ground glass; bronchial tree visible and dark (**Figure 11-6**).

Diagnosis

- Respiratory distress starting a few minutes to hours after birth
- CXR—typical appearance
- ABG—**hypoxemia** variable, metabolic acidosis

Nursing Interventions

- Surfactant after birth delivered through endotracheal tube
- Maintain normothermia.

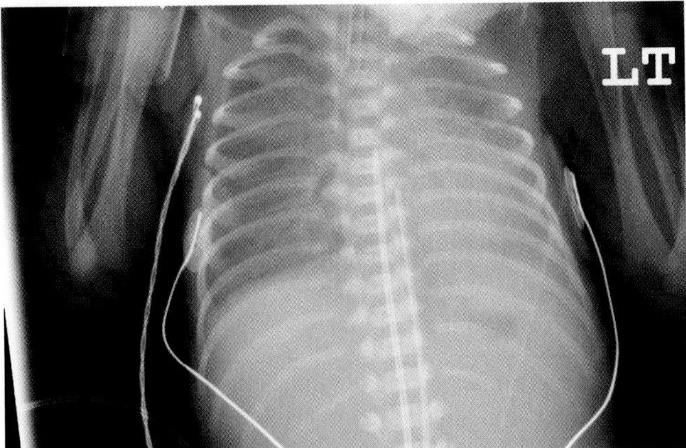

Figure 11-6 X-ray of respiratory distress syndrome.

- Provide supportive care, including nutrition, maintenance of fluid–electrolyte balance, and prevention of infection.
- Provide vigorous respiratory monitoring and support, as well as pulmonary hygiene.
- Support and maintain mechanical ventilation.
  - *Nitric oxide—improves gas exchange and decreases pulmonary inflammation*
  - *High-frequency jet ventilation*
  - *ECMO—artificial heart and lung machine*

Caregiver Education

- Signs and symptoms of respiratory distress
- Oxygen use and safety measures
- Oxygen use usually weaned off by end of first year

CONGENITAL DIAPHRAGMATIC HERNIA

- Life-threatening birth defect that occurs in about 1 in every 2500 to 5000 births (De Buys Rossingh & Dinh-Xuan, 2009)
- Combination of muscle defect between abdomen and thoracic cavity and pulmonary hypoplasia in utero
- Most often seen affecting the left side; lungs that are affected are not fully developed.

Assessment

- Tachypnea, nasal flaring, and retractions
- Circumoral and nail bed cyanosis
- Tachycardia; heart sounds possibly heard on right side of chest
- Irregular chest wall movements
- Decreased breath sounds on affected side
- Bowel sounds heard in the chest
- Visibly sunken abdomen or decreased fullness perceived when palpating abdomen

Diagnosis

- Scaphoid abdomen
- CXR
- Magnetic resonance imaging (MRI)—helpful in determining position of organs

Nursing Interventions

- Immediate respiratory support
- Place child in Semi-Fowler's position on affected side, with the head of the bed elevated.
- Maintain patency of NG tube.
- Monitor IV fluids.
- Monitor and maintain mechanical ventilation, ECMO.
- Provide pre-/post-operative care.
- Monitor for signs of infection and respiratory distress.
- Provide for increased calorie needs and monitor for feeding intolerance.
- Provide support to family in mourning loss of "perfect child."

Caregiver Education

- Positioning of head and thorax higher than abdomen
- Prescribed feeding techniques
- Wound care
- Prevention of infection
- Poor prognosis even after surgical repair
- Refer family to community support groups

CYSTIC FIBROSIS

- Autosomal recessive disorder of exocrine glands marked by increased mucus production and decreased pancreatic enzyme production
- Deletion in chromosome 7 at the cystic fibrosis transmembrane regulator
- Absence of gene decreases chloride-ion and water transport at cellular level
- Affects multiple organ systems
- One of the most common causes childhood death
- The Cystic Fibrosis Foundation (CFF) notes that more than 70% of the population with cystic fibrosis is diagnosed by age 2, and 55% while under the age of 18; the mean survival age is the mid-30s (CFF, 2011).
- Affects the lungs and digestive tract of 30,000 children and adults in the United States, over 70,000 worldwide (CFF, 2011).
- Respiratory system
  - *Excess mucus production in the lungs often leads to secondary bacterial infections; chronic infection leads to tissue damage and, over time, respiratory failure.*
- Digestive system
  - *Thick mucus in pancreatic ducts block enzymes responsible for digestion of nutrients, resulting in loss of ability to absorb fat, proteins, and carbohydrates.*
  - *Decreased or no release of amylase, trypsin, lipase*
  - *Hepatic bile ducts, gallbladder, submaxillary and intestinal glands are obstructed by thick mucus and eosinophilic debris.*
- Metabolic system
  - *Excess sodium chloride production by sweat glands causes hyponatremia.*
- Reproductive system
  - *Ovarian ducts and vas deferens are blocked with mucus, causing sterility.*

Assessment

- History of episodes of recurrent respiratory infections, pneumonia, bronchitis
- Parents report salty taste of child's skin
- Crackles, wheezes, or diminished breath sounds; prolonged expiration
- Digital clubbing—indication of hypoxia, increased rounding and loss of angle at base of nail bed; late sign
- Barrel chest
- Voracious appetite from lost nutrients in undigested food

- Protruding abdomen, "pot belly" with thin extremities
- Stool history—malabsorption; bulky stools or steatorrhea
  - *Pain with movement, presence of blood in stool, constipation, foul odor*
- Girls may have vaginal itching, discharge
- Edema—cardiac or liver failure
- Distended neck veins or heave—cor pulmonale
- Older children may report chronic pain in later stages of disorder
  - *Headaches from hypoxia and hypercarbia; sinusitis*
  - *Musculoskeletal pain from accessory muscle use*

Diagnosis

- Prenatal—DNA testing of amniotic fluid for deletion of delta F508 chromosome; evaluate if decreased
- Sweat chloride test—positive test shows 2 to 5 times normal level of sodium and chloride, must be repeated to confirm.
  - *Sweat chloride concentration of 50 mEq/L is suspicious.*
  - *Positive if increased sodium and chloride over 60 mEq/L on two occasions*
- Pulse oximetry—decreased during exacerbation
- CXR—hyperinflation, atelectasis, infiltrates, bronchial wall thickening
- Pulmonary function test
  - *Decreased forced vital capacity*
  - *Decreased forced expiratory volume*
  - *Increased residual volume*
- Labs
  - *Serum albumin to assess nutritional status*
  - *Metabolic panel to assess hydration status*
  - *Liver enzymes to assess liver function*
- Stool specimen—absence of trypsin
- Fecal fat—72-hour stool collection may show increased fat and decreased albumin levels

Nursing Interventions

- Maintain airway; provide pulmonary hygiene.
- Chest physiotherapy (CP)
  - *Includes postural drainage, chest percussion, vibration, and coughing and deep breathing exercises*
  - *Helps mobilize/eliminate secretions, re-expand lung tissue, and promote efficient respiratory muscle use*
  - *Postural drainage—sequential positioning of patient to allow gravity to work and encourage secretions in the alveolar periphery to move toward the bronchioles and bronchi to be coughed or suctioned out.*
  - *Percussion and vibration*
    - Percussion—using cupped hands to clap on the chest or motorized device; may be done with vibration
    - Vibration—done manually using hands, or a motorized handheld massager; used with percussion or as alternative in patients with chest trauma, severe pain, or who are too frail to tolerate percussion.
  - *Vest—broad wrap that encircles the chest and can go over the shoulders; oscillates (**Figure 11-7A, B**)*
    - Air pressure used to inflate and deflate
    - Often used in asthma and cystic fibrosis patients
    - Alternative use, similar action on lungs as percussion and vibration
  - *Forced exhalation and incentive spirometry*
    - Used in combination to mechanically mobilize/eliminate secretions, re-expand lung tissue, promote efficient respiratory muscle use
    - Used to prevent or manage atelectasis and pneumonia.
  - *CP is contraindicated with chest wall trauma, lung contusion or abscess, pneumothorax, or hemoptysis.*
- Aerosolized medications, bronchodilators, antibiotics, mucolytic agents
  - *Dornase alfa—genetically engineered pulmonary enzyme*
  - *Administered via nebulizer; thins mucus, improves lung function, and decreases risk of infection*
- Low-flow, humidified supplemental oxygen; if too high can depress respirations in chronically hypoxic child
- Monitor respiratory status and for signs and symptoms of infection.
- Antibiotics for infections require higher doses; CF children have higher drug clearance rate.

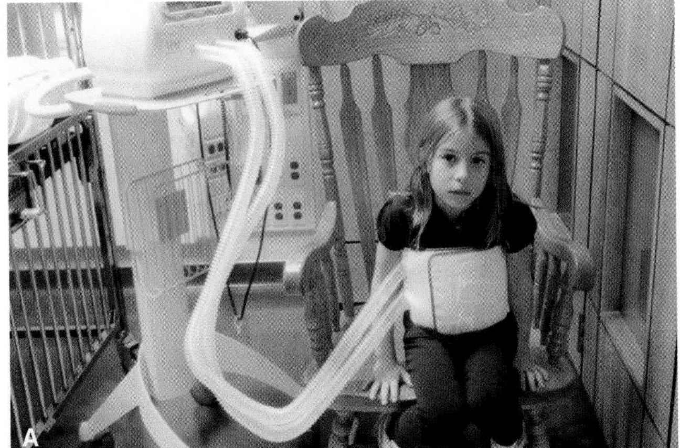

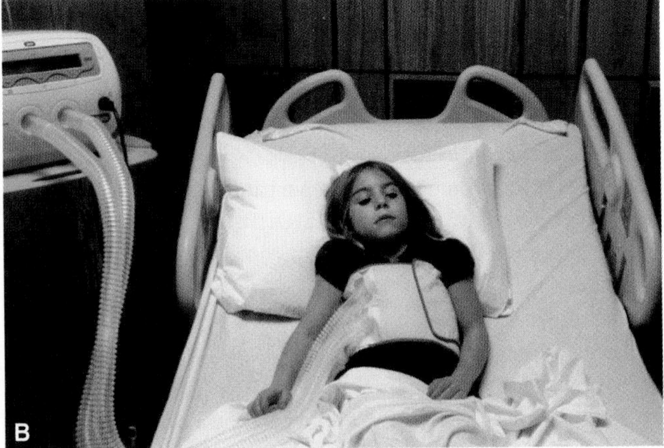

Figure 11-7 **A, B**, Vest for chest physiotherapy.

- Individualized dietary modifications and pancreatic enzyme, multivitamin, and caloric supplements
  - *Prevent gastrointestinal blockages—adequate fluid, adequate fiber, use of stool softeners.*
  - *Fat-soluble vitamin A, D, E, and K supplements*
  - *High-protein diet*
  - *Promote a normal lifestyle for family.*
  - *Postoperative care with single or double lung transplant*

CLINICAL PEARL

Antihistamines

Use of antihistamines is contraindicated in cystic fibrosis because they have a drying effect, making expectoration of mucus more difficult.

Caregiver Education

- Critical importance of chest physiotherapy
  - *Review chest physiotherapy; should be done 3 or 4 times daily.*
  - *CP may induce bronchospasm; precede with intermittent positive-pressure breathing, utilizing aerosol or nebulizer.*
  - *Avoid percussing over the spine or internal organs.*
  - *Chest physiotherapy should be performed with a lightweight shirt or infant blanket covering the chest.*
  - *The child is placed in different positions and cupped-hand percussion is performed on areas of the chest, for at least 2 minutes. It should sound like popping when performed correctly.*
  - *Finish therapy by using base of hand and straightened arm to provide vibration of the lower lobe segment as the child exhales; perform at least 5 times.*
  - *Avoid chest physiotherapy immediately after child has eaten.*
  - *Avoid hospitalization by assisting to clear the respiratory track*
- Teach vest therapy—correct positioning and use.
- Teach postural drainage and sequential repositioning.
  - *Utilizes gravity to promote peripheral pulmonary secretions to move to bronchi and trachea for expectoration*
- Avoid exposure to infections; immediately report increase in cough, change in sputum, or fever.
- Genetic counseling—screening confirms diagnosis and identifies carriers.
- Stress importance of daily physical activity to loosen secretions and encourage optimal lung expansion.
- Teach how to perform nebulizer treatments and use inhalers correctly.
- Review high-calorie foods and high-protein foods.
- Encourage adequate hydration, addressing activity and seasonal changes.
- Suggest daily fat-soluble vitamin supplements.
- Review administration of supplemental pancreatic enzymes before all meals and snacks, and daily vitamins.
- Teach parents and child not to restrict salt in the diet, and that in hot weather a supplement may be needed.
- Provide referrals to emotional and mental health support resources, such religious leaders or psychologists trained in chronic illness.
- Provide information on community resources, the Cystic Fibrosis Foundation, and the American Lung Association, as well as a list of home health-care referrals for visiting nurses and respiratory therapists.
- Annual influenza vaccines are recommended for children with CF and family members.

ASTHMA

- Chronic, obstructive, inflammatory disorder due to hyper-responsiveness of airways, airway edema, airway narrowing, and mucus production
- Genetic, environmental, intrinsic, and extrinsic factors affect asthma, but 20% to 40% of children with asthma have no allergic disease.
- The National Heart, Lung, and Blood Institute (NHLBI) notes that asthma is the most common chronic disease of childhood, affecting 6 million children (NHLBI, 2010).
- Asthma triggers are irritants that stimulate inflammation of the airways.
- Some of these triggers are regularly found in the home (**Figures 11-8 and 11-9**).
  - *Cold air*
  - *Smoke*
  - *Viral infections*
  - *Stress*
  - *Pet dander*
  - *Exercise*
- Bronchospasm caused by constriction of smooth muscle
- Accumulation of secretions
  - *Inflamed and edematous mucous membranes*

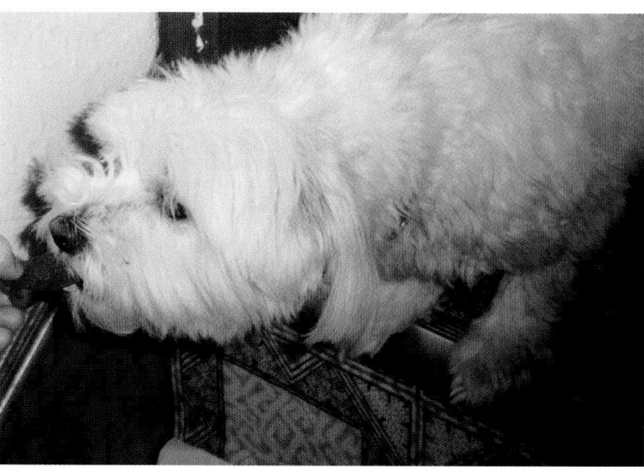

Figure 11–8 Allergen—dog.

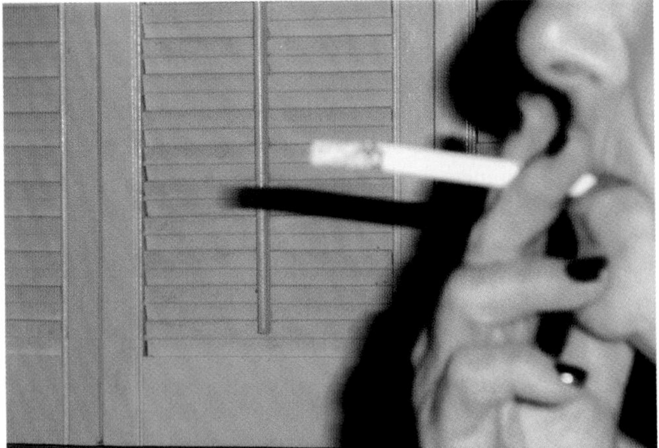

Figure 11-9 Allergen—smoke.

- Immediate or delayed response
  - *Immediate response—sensitized airway mast cells activate immunoglobulin-E, causing release of mediators (histamine, leukotrines, and prostaglandins). Mediators cause bronchoconstriction shortly after exposure, resolving within 1 to 2 hours.*
  - *Delayed response—chemical mediators attract immune system cells (eosinophils, basophils, and neutrophils), which infiltrate and cause release of additional inflammatory materials, damaging smooth muscle cells and causing further edema and mucus obstruction of the small airways.*
  - *Bronchoconstriction can recur and last for several hours.*
  - *Airway hyper-responsiveness can last for weeks or months.*
  - *Blood flows equally to the obstructed alveoli and open alveoli, creating a ventilation–perfusion mismatch and resulting in decreased pO_2 and hypoxia.*

Assessment

- Cough—nonproductive, progressing to frothy; worse at night
- Shortness of breath
- Chest pain, tightness
- Wheezing
- Prolonged expiration
- Food allergies and triggers
  - *High prevalence of asthma in food-allergic children*
  - *Egg and tree nut allergies are most prevalent (Gaffin et al., 2011).*
- History of allergic rhinitis, atopic dermatitis
- Frequent episodes of bronchitis or pneumonia; night coughing
- Mild retractions, accessory muscle use; infants may head bob
- Coarseness or absence of breath sounds is ominous.
- Percussion reveals hyperresonance.
- Barrel chest if chronic asthma
- Exposed to cigarette smoke
  - *Cigarette smoke exacerbates and compounds treatment.*

Evidence-Based Practice Research: Obesity and Asthma

Cottrell, L., Neal, W. A., Ice, C., Perez, M. K., & Piedmonte, G. (2010). Metabolic abnormalities in children with asthma. *American Journal of Respiratory and Critical Care Medicine, 183,* 441–448. doi: 10.1164/rccm.201004-0603OC

Childhood asthma and obesity have reached epidemic proportions worldwide. Researchers have implied a parallel, increased risk and incidence of asthma with increased obesity in children. Obesity has been linked to increased rates of metabolic disorders in children. Obesity has been studied as the precursor to asthma and diabetes, in particular, the mechanical effect of fat on respiratory compliance; the role of nutrients, antioxidants, and saturated fats in both conditions; and the inflammatory airways seen in both conditions. A recent study by Cottrell, Neal, Ice, Perez, and Piedmonte (2010) evaluated a wide range of children, from underweight to morbidly obese. Cottrell et al. (2010) looked at metabolic derangement as the precursor that leads to asthma, diabetes, and obesity. The study showed that all children with asthma, from underweight to obese, had increased tissue insulin resistance and increased triglyceride levels. Comorbidities associated with obesity, hyperlipidemia, and hyperinsulinemia can influence the defense mechanisms of the respiratory tract to be pro-inflammatory. Cottrell and colleagues' study showed that it is conceivable that abnormalities in lipid or glucose metabolism may contribute to the development of asthma (Cotrell et al., 2010).

Clinical Reasoning

You enter the room, where Amy, an 11-year-old girl, neatly dressed with very tight-fitting clothes, is sitting with her mother. The odor of cigarette smoke fills the room. You notice that her abdomen is protruding beneath her shirt and sticking out above her pants. She tells you that she is at the pediatrician's office for a follow-up asthma visit. You greet her and she is smiling while you take her temperature. You ask her to take her shoes off and step on the scale to measure her weight. Suddenly Amy is visibly upset; she starts crying and says "I have been riding my bike and trying to take walks, but nobody ever wants to go with me because I am fat!"

1. How would a nurse set aside any personal feelings concerning smoking and obesity and respond appropriately to Amy?
2. How might this insight help to best support Amy and guide interventions?

Diagnosis

- Crucial to initiate treatment plan and improve quality of life
- Detailed, focused questions on presenting symptoms and precipitation of symptoms
- Family history—parental smoking, asthma, eczema, eosinophilia, any evidence of genetic predisposition to hypersensitivity reactions
- Dermatologic signs—atopic dermatitis
  - *Allergic shiners*
  - *Nasal creases*
  - *Pebbled conjunctiva*

- Tachypnea, with prolonged expiratory phase
  - *Pulse oximetry may be low even with mild symptoms*
  - *CXR—hyperinflation*
  - *ABGs— hypoxemia and hypercarbia*
  - *Pulmonary function tests—spirometry to confirm diagnosis or eliminate others*
    - Used in children at least 5 years old and older
    - Measure forced vital capacity (FVC) and complete exhalation and forced expiratory volume (FEV) over 1 second (FEV1) before and after inhalation of short-acting beta-adrenergic (SABA) agonist.
    - The two numbers are used as a ratio, FEV1/FVC, to determine severity.
    - Risk of exacerbation identified
  - *Peak flow meter—portable, handheld device that measures ability to push air out of the lungs*
    - Not diagnostic
    - Used to monitor therapy
    - Below "personal best"–best level measured when in optimal health
    - Action plan, interventions based on color zones
  - *Allergy testing—identify triggers*
- Spirometry used in children 5 years old and older
- Improvement of symptoms after bronchodilator
- CXR in severe asthma—hyperinflation
- Symptom-based—rhinitis, sinusitis, wheezing
- Eosinophilia—blood and sputum

The NHLBI (2010) put together a program for asthma prevention and education to conduct and review studies about the recognition and treatment of asthma. Initiation of therapy is based on clinical presentation, which is divided into four categories: intermittent, mild persistent, moderate persistent, and severe persistent. A summary of recommendations is provided in **Table 11-4.**

Nursing Interventions

- Assess severity and control of symptoms.
- Use a team approach in the care of the child.
- Provide for elimination or management of triggers.
- Assist in balance between good control of triggers and use of medications.
  - *Rescue medication use should be rare, and daily medications used with resultant minimal side effects.*
- Use a calm approach to child and family, who may be frightened.
- Provide information on spacers/aerochambers, valved holders of metered dose inhalers (MDIs).
  - *Faster delivery time and deposit 50% more medication in airway, rather than in mouth inhaler*
- Assist the parents in educating school personnel—teachers, administrators, and sport coaches. Most childhood sports involve vigorous activity (**Figure 11-10**).

Caregiver Education

- Basic facts about asthma, the role of medications, and patient skills
- Avoiding triggers
- A personal action plan is effective in improving asthma.
  - *A personal, age-appropriate, written plan based on peak flow meter readings, and symptoms, instructing child*

TABLE 11–4 DETERMINING ASTHMA THERAPY BASED ON IMPAIRMENT AND SEVERITY

	Intermittent	Mild Persistent	Moderate Persistent	Severe Persistent
Frequency of symptoms	2×/wk or less, or only with exercise	>2×/wk, but not daily	Daily	Throughout the day
Nighttime awakenings	2×/mo or less	1–2×/mo for 0–4-yr-olds, and 3–4×/mo for older children	0–4-yr-olds, 3–4×/mo; older children >1×/wk	0–4-yr-olds >1×/wk, older children 7×/wk
SABA use	2 days/wk or less	2 days/wk, but no more	Daily	Several times daily
Activity	No limitations	Occasional limitation	Some limitation	Very limited
Lung function	FEV1/FVC greater than 80% in younger children,* normal in older children FEV1 greater than 80%	FEV1/FVC greater than 80% in 5–11-yr-olds, normal in older children FEV1 greater than 80%	FEV1/FVC in 5–11 yr olds is 75–80%, in older children is decreased 5% FEV1 60–80%	FEV1/FVC in 5–11-yr-olds 75%, in older children decreased >5%

Continued

TABLE 11–4 DETERMINING ASTHMA THERAPY BASED ON IMPAIRMENT AND SEVERITY—cont'd

	Intermittent	Mild Persistent	Moderate Persistent	Severe Persistent
Exacerbations	None to one/yr	0–4-yr-olds have ≥2/yr or 4 wheezing episodes/yr lasting 1 day and risk factors present, older children have ≥2 /yr	0–4-yr-olds, if no improvement, consider alternate diagnosis; in older children, >2/yr, risk of exacerbations relative to FEV1, adjust therapy	≥2/yr for all children; for 0–4-yr-olds, if no improvement, consider alternate diagnosis, risk of exacerbations relative to FEV1 Adjust therapy
Medication step	Step 1	Step 2	Step 3	Step 3 for 0–11-yr-olds Step 4 or 5 for older children
Recommended medications	Daily—none, Quick relief—SABA PRN	Daily—low-dose inhaled corticosteroid (ICS) or Cromolyn, Leukotriene receptor antagonist (LTRA) Nedocromil, or Zieuton Quick relief—SABA PRN Consider referral to specialist	Daily—low-dose ICS and long-acting beta2-agonist (LABA) or medium-dose ICS Quick relief—SABA up to TID Consider systemic corticosteroids; recommend referral to specialist	Daily—medium- or high-dose ICS and LABA; consider Omalizumab if child has allergies Quick relief—SABA up to TID Recommend referral

Adapted from the National Asthma Education and Prevention Program. (2007). Expert Panel Report 3: Guidelines for the diagnosis and management of asthma. Summary Report 2007 (NIH publication No. 08-5846). Bethesda, MD: National Heart, Lung, and Blood Institute, National Institutes of Health.

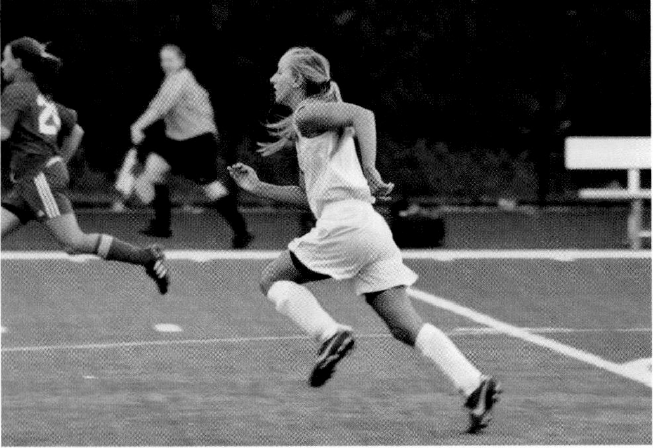

Figure 11–10 Playing soccer, and other vigorous physical activity, is a potential trigger for asthma.

specifically what medications to take and whom to call if asthma symptoms get worse

- Correct use of inhalers and aerochambers
  - *MDI for children 5 years old or older*
  - *Breath-actuated pressurized MDI and dry powder inhalers*
- Importance of using medication as prescribed
  - *Take regular preventive medication, even when free of symptoms (see* ***Table 11-5*** *for a list of asthma medications).*
  - *Avoid overuse of SABA blockers.*

NONINFECTIOUS DISORDERS OF UPPER AIRWAY

FOREIGN BODY ASPIRATION

- Solid or liquid inhaled into respiratory tract most frequently seen in infants 6 months old to 5 years of age

Assessment

- Coughing
- Wheezing
- Stridor
- Gagging
- Possible cyanosis
- Infant or child may be asymptomatic for hours or weeks; eventually irritation, edema, and obstruction will develop, producing symptoms.

TABLE 11–5 ASTHMA MEDICATIONS

Long-Term Control	Quick Relief
Inhaled corticosteroid (ICS)—anti-inflammatory, decreases hyper-responsiveness, inhibits inflammatory cell migration and activation, blocks late reactions to allergens, decreases exacerbations Examples: beclomethasone, budesonide	**Short-acting beta2-agonist (SABA)**—relaxes smooth muscles in the airway; increases water in mucus, promoting clearance; effects seen in 5–10 minutes; drug of choice acute therapy, nebulizer, or MD1 Examples: albuterol, terbutaline, levabuterol
Long-acting beta2-agonist (LABA)—relaxes smooth muscles in airway, duration of action at least 12 hours, used in combination with ICS Examples: salmeteral, famoterol	**Corticosteroid**—decreases airway inflammation, enhances bronchodilation effects of SABA, used in moderate to severe persistent asthma with SABA Example: methylprednisolone (IV or PO)
Leucotrine modifier (LM)—decreases inflammation cascade, alternate choice for mild but persistent asthma, used with ICS for moderate to severe asthma Examples: montelukast, zafirlukast	**Anticholenergic**—inhibits bronchoconstriction, decreases mucus production, used with SABA in acute exacerbation
Mast cell inhibitor—interferes with chloride channels, stabilizes mast cells, alternative for mild but persistent asthma Examples: cromolyn sodium, nedocromil	
Anti-immunoglobulin E antibody (anti-IgE)—used in children 12 years old or older with sensitivity to dust mites, cockroaches, dogs, and cats; used in moderate to severe persistent asthma; anaphylaxis may occur	
Methylzanthine—relaxes smooth muscles in airway, provides continuous airway dilation Examples: PO theophylline, IV aminophylline; monitor serum levels	

Adapted from the National Asthma Education and Prevention Program. (2007). Expert Panel Report 3: Guidelines for the diagnosis and management of asthma. Summary Report 2007 (NIH publication No. 08-5846). Bethesda, MD: National Heart, Lung, and Blood Institute, National Institutes of Health.

- Usually the result of a small toy, grape, peanut, coin, or latex balloon that has become lodged

Diagnosis

- History and clinical signs
- CXR, MRI, or computerized tomography (CT)
- Bronchoscopy—identify and remove object

Nursing Interventions

- After removal of object, observe for laryngeal edema and respiratory distress.
- Antibiotics are only effective in cases of bacterial infection.
- Cool mist and bronchodilators or corticosteroids for 24 to 48 hours

Caregiver Education

- Age-appropriate toys and foods
  - *Cut table food into small pieces.*
  - *Choking interventions—back blows, abdominal thrusts with head lower than chest for infants*
    - Heimlich maneuver for older children

APNEA

- Cessation of breathing for longer than 20 seconds, or any cessation that is accompanied by cyanosis, bradycardia, pallor, and hypotonia
- Apnea of prematurity—most infants born at less than 28 weeks' gestation are affected.
  - *Severity related to prematurity*
  - *Usually resolves by 36 weeks of postconceptual age*
  - *Affected by maternal drug use, thermal instability, infection, conditions of insufficient oxygen delivery, and metabolic and central nervous system disorders*
- Can be early sign of sepsis, respiratory illness, or patent ductus arteriosus
- Obstructive sleep apnea—partial or complete airway obstruction while asleep
  - *Leads to hypoventilation, hypoxia, hypercapnea, and hypertension*
  - *Peak age of 2 to 6 years old*
  - *Obesity and craniofacial abnormalities are contributing factors.*

- Central apnea—condition affecting the brain's respiratory center, the medulla oblongata
  - *Intraventricular hemorrhage, meningitis, seizures, congenital myopathies*
- Different than normal periodic breathing of newborns

Assessment

- Observed cessation of breathing
- Observed infant startling and then awakening from sleep
- Snoring
- Mouth breathing
- Daytime sleepiness
- Hypoventilation, nail bed cyanosis
- Nasal or oral obstruction—enlarged tonsils or tongue
- Obesity

Diagnosis

- Apnea monitor
- Polysomnogram

Evidence-Based Practice Research: Polysomnogram

Aurora, N. A., Zak, R. S., Karippot, A., Lamm, C. I., Morgenthaler, T. I., Auerbach, S. H., . . . Ramar, K. (2011). Practice parameters for the respiratory indications for polysomnography in children. *Sleep, 34,* 379–388. Retrieved from http://www.ncbi.nlm.nih.gov/pubmed/21359087

The American Academy of Sleep Medicine (AASM), as noted in a review of the literature and current diagnostic practice (Aurora et al., 2011), stated that polysomnography should be used to diagnose sleep-related behavior disturbances (SRBDs). Polysomnography (PSG) is an expensive but reliable and clinically significant tool in diagnosing sleep apnea in children when performed and scored in accordance with AASM standards. PSG should be performed when clinical assessment suggests obstructive sleep apnea in children or infants with obesity, chest or facial-cranial anomalies, neuromuscular disorders, and pre- and post-tonsillar-adenoidectomy. PSG is also recommended to titrate positive airway pressure in children undergoing continuous positive airway pressure (CPAP) therapy to manage obstructive sleep apnea. PSG future research should include developing and standardizing clinical use of PSG in children, and PSG use based on respiratory physiologic changes considering age and maturation.

1. Name three things that would improve the outcome of the polysomnogram.

Nursing Interventions

- Cardiorespiratory monitoring with continuous pulse oximetry
- Position head and neck to keep airway patent.
- Supportive care for medical management
  - *Prematurity—administer methylxanthines and doxapram*
  - *CPAP ventilation*
  - *Tonsillectomy*
  - *Weight reduction*
  - *Tracheostomy*
  - *Administer caffeine, theophylline as ordered*

Caregiver Education

- Correct application/use of apnea monitor
- Keep record of episodes in diary or calendar.
- Optimal head and neck positions for airway patency

APPARENT LIFE-THREATENING EVENT (ALTE)

- Episode of apnea accompanied by color change, hypotonia, and choking
- Infants less than 4 months old and a gestational age of 37 weeks or older
- Can occur either while asleep or awake
- Potential causes: gastroesophageal reflux, acute respiratory infection, seizures, feeding aspiration, heart defects, child abuse

Assessment

- Careful history and history of events just prior to event

Diagnosis

- Process of elimination of all other differential diagnoses

Nursing Interventions

- Cardiopulmonary monitoring with continuous pulse oximetry
- Emotional support for family

Caregiver Education

- Infant and child cardiopulmonary resuscitation (CPR)
- Use of apnea monitor
- Optimal feeding position

BRONCHOPULMONARY DYSPLASIA (BPD)

- Chronic respiratory disorder in premature neonates as a result of prolonged oxygen therapy
- Received high-flow oxygen or ventilator assistance on day of birth
  - *Assisted ventilation can injure lungs: a child has less functional surface area with reduced capillary growth to alveoli; ventilation–perfusion mismatch.*
  - *Pulmonary hypertension, increased lung fluid, interstitial fibrosis, and smooth muscle hypertrophy*
- Gestational age of 30 weeks or less
- Immature and decreased number of alveoli
  - *Alveolar sacs develop between the 26th and 28th weeks of gestation.*
- Hyperinflation of immature lungs produces inflammation and scarring in the lungs.
- Contributing factors—infection, patent ductus arteriosus, malnutrition

Assessment

- Increased work of breathing, accessory muscle use
- Tachypnea, increased by 20 to 40 breaths per minute
- Circumoral and nail bed cyanosis
- Retractions—sternal
- Atelectasis
- Prolonged exhalation and use of accessory muscles
- Weight loss or poor weight gain; poor feeding
- Wheezing, coughing
- Hyperextension of the neck
- Nasal flaring
- Right-sided heart failure

> **CRITICAL COMPONENT**
>
> **Malnutrition**
>
> The feeding and activity intolerance of BPD infants make them prone to develop malnutrition, resulting in arrested growth and development. Nursing care should cluster necessary tasks and take a "hands-off" approach.

Diagnosis

- Clinical presentation, if infant requires oxygen 28 days after birth
- CXR—bronchiolar metaplasia, interstitial fibrosis (**Figure 11-11A, B**)

Nursing Interventions

- Promote and monitor respiratory functioning.
- Provide for supplemental oxygen initially; prepare for intubation.
- Assist parents/caregivers in coping with intubated child, who may remain intubated for weeks.
- Provide mechanical ventilation pressures at lowest effective settings
  - *PEEP 6 to7 cm H_2O*
  - *Slightly longer inspiratory time*
  - *Gradual weaning off ventilator*
- Drug therapy as prescribed
  - *Surfactant*
  - *Diuretics to decrease interstitial edema*
  - *Bronchodilators*
  - *Theophylline*
  - *Caffeine to increase lung compliance*
  - *Palivizumab injections to prevent RSV*
  - *Optimize nutritional intake, calories and vitamins*
    - Caloric requirement increased by 150 kcal/kg per day
- Monitor intake and output (I&O) and electrolyte balance.
- Cluster nursing care.
- Encourage parental interaction with infant; provide support and help increase confidence.

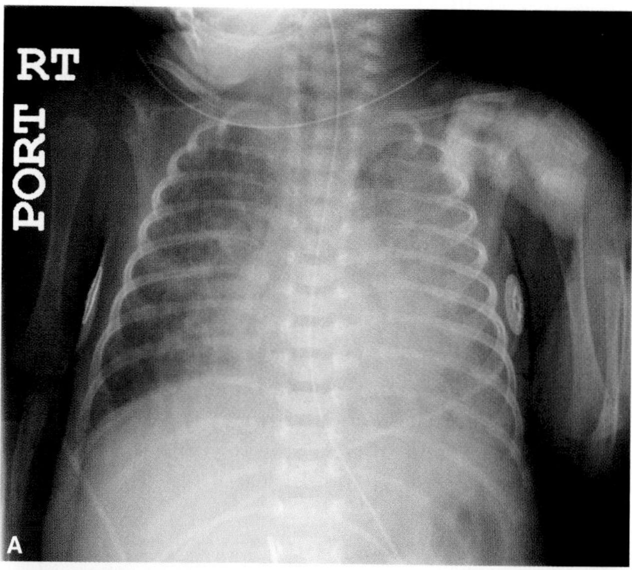

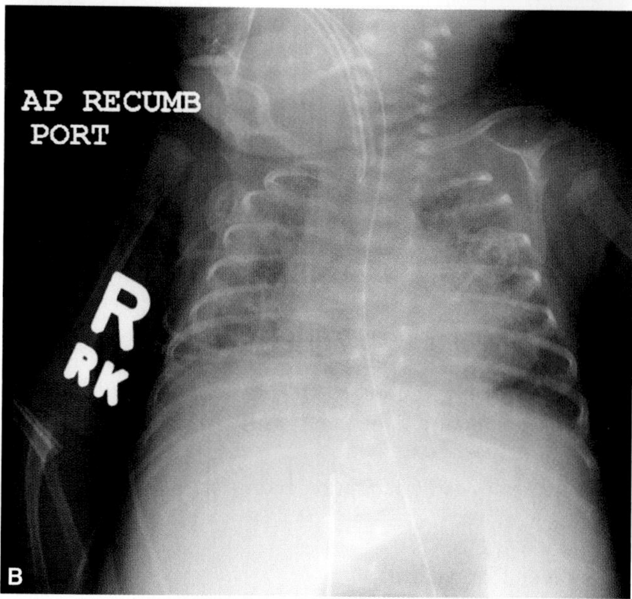

Figure 11-11 **A, B,** X-ray of bronchopulmonary dysplasia.

Caregiver Education

- Oxygen administration
- Stringent hand hygiene
- Ventilator management
- Medication administration
- High-calorie feedings
- Monitoring of I&O

PNEUMOTHORAX

- Extravasation of air from parenchyma into the pleural space as a result of trauma to chest wall or respiratory tract
- Positive pressure in the chest cavity can cause alveoli to rupture.
- Hemothorax—blood in pleural space

- Tension pneumothorax—life-threatening emergency
  - *Air enters the chest with inspiration but cannot exit on expiration.*
  - *Accumulation of air compresses the lung.*
  - *Mediastinal structures are displaced to the contralateral side, impairing venous return to the heart and decreasing cardiac output.*

Assessment

- Decreased or absent breath sounds on affected side
- Decreased chest wall movement and paradoxical breathing
- Sudden or gradual onset of tachypnea
- Retractions, nasal flaring, or grunting depending on amount of air trapped in the pleura
- Decreased oxygen saturation
- Pallor or cyanosis
- Auscultate for tachycardia and breath sounds, absent or diminished on affected side
- Hemothorax—symptoms can be less conspicuous depending on blood loss from cardiac and vascular injuries.

Diagnosis

- CXR
- Clinical presentation

Nursing Interventions

- Oxygen administration
- Cardiopulmonary monitoring with continuous pulse oximetry
- Assist with needle aspiration and/or chest tube placement.

Caregiver Education

- The condition is temporary.
- It is managed in the hospital setting.

SUDDEN INFANT DEATH SYNDROME (SIDS)

- Sudden, unexpected death of an infant under 1 year of age, occurring during sleep. Cause is undetermined even after thorough investigation.
- Can occur any time from 1 week old to 1 year old, with peak incidence from 2 to 4 months of age.
- First symptom is cardiac arrest; infant is found after a nap or nighttime sleep. Autopsy reveals pulmonary edema.

Risk Factors

- Mother under 20 years old
- Low-birth-weight neonate
- Premature birth
- Multiple pregnancy
- Family history of SIDS
- Maternal smoking

Nursing Interventions

- Resuscitation as ordered
- Guide to counseling and community resources; empathy and support
- Prevention of SIDS—position infant/child on back every time for sleeping.
  - *Firm mattress; avoid loose bedding and toys in crib.*

Review Questions

1. Caregivers have just received discharge instructions for their son, who was newly diagnosed with cystic fibrosis. The father confirms understanding of the primary goal of chest physiotherapy (CP) by stating:
   A. "CP allows the lungs to re-expand."
   B. "CP allows for deeper breathing."
   C. "CP prevents hospitalizations."
   D. "CP increases resistance to respiratory infection."
   E. "CP helps mobilize and expectorate secretions."

2. An 11-year-old with cystic fibrosis was admitted with a respiratory tract infection. What would be most accurate to tell the parents?
   A. Decreased ciliary action in the lungs is the cause of infections.
   B. It is okay to hold administration of pancreatic enzymes while the child is ill.
   C. Excessive production of mucus pooling in lungs is a breeding ground for bacteria.
   D. Excessive production of mucus and decreased production of pancreatic enzymes do not cause infection.

3. Which outcome is important to include in the care plan for a child with cystic fibrosis?
   A. Chest physiotherapy performed three times per day
   B. Knowledge: weight-reduction strategies
   C. Adequate gastrointestinal tissue perfusion
   D. Adequate pain control
   E. Age-appropriate weight

4. In assessing a child, you hear wheezing and decreased breath sounds in the bases. The chest x-ray reveals hyperinflation, and Mom tells you that they have two new cats they just rescued. What should be included in nursing interventions?
   A. Nasal pharyngeal suctioning and educating the patient on avoidance of animals
   B. Starting oxygen at 8 L nasal cannula and administering a bronchodilator
   C. Positioning child in left-sided position with head of the bed elevated, and decreasing stimuli
   D. Assessment of level of anxiety of patient and avoiding making the child cry
   E. Getting a complete set of vital signs and preparing the child for possible ABG

5. A 10-year-old presents with shortness of breath, tachypnea, and a nonproductive cough. In talking with the mother, she reveals that the child has asthma and is allergic to walnuts and has had eczema "as long as she can remember." While auscultating the lung fields, what are you most likely to hear?
   A. Crackles on inspiration
   B. Wheezing with prolonged expiratory phase
   C. Stridor on inspiration
   D. Wheezing with staggered expiration

6. You suspect that your patient has asthma. What would be included in assessing for exposure to asthma triggers?
   A. Eczema and dermatitis
   B. Warm moist air with high winds
   C. Exercise, smoke, and pet dander
   D. Stress, obesity, and lack of sleep

7. Which statement is most accurate regarding asthma?
   A. Asthma is a common, chronic disorder of sensitized platelets and chemical mediators stimulating the immune response and mucus obstruction of the small airways.
   B. Asthma is a common disorder of the upper airway that affects the respiratory and cardiac systems that presents with hypoxia, retractions, and high fever.
   C. Cigarette smoke can trigger an exacerbation of asthma, and pulmonary function tests should be done in all children to assess effective weight loss.
   D. Asthma is a chronic inflammatory disorder that is managed with high-dose antibiotics and can last up to 1 week.
   E. Asthma is a recurrent inflammatory disorder triggered by internal and external factors.

8. What information would be important to determine if a wheezing 4-year-old has asthma?
   A. Chest x-ray (CXR), complete blood count (CBC), and blood culture
   B. CXR, CBC, spirometry, and improvement after bronchodilator
   C. CBC, spirometry, and blood cultures
   D. If there are pets, or family members with TB, in the residence where the child lives
   E. CBC, improvement after bronchodilator, and possible triggers

9. A premature infant stops breathing for 15 seconds several times while sleeping. What is the most accurate statement about apnea?
   A. Apnea is cessation of breathing for longer than 20 seconds, associated with cyanosis and bradycardia.
   B. Apnea occurs in half of premature infants born at less than 28 weeks' gestation.
   C. Apnea is normal, only seen in newborns, and lasts longer than 20 seconds per episode.
   D. Apnea is not normal and can be caused by narcotic overdose and atelectasis.

10. What symptoms of a 6-year-old would lead the nurse to suspect the child has apnea?
   A. History of head trauma 4 years ago
   B. Enlarged tonsils, mouth breathing, and reports of waking abruptly
   C. Chronic respiratory infections with delinquent vaccine schedule
   D. Wheezing, age-appropriate weight, daytime sleepiness

References

Aurora, N. A., Zak, R. S., Karippot, A., Lamm, C. I., Morgenthaler, T. I., Auerbach, S. H., . . . Ramar, K. (2011). Practice parameters for the respiratory indications for polysomnograpy in children. *Sleep, 34*, 379–388. Retrieved from http://www.ncbi.nlm.nih.gov/pubmed/21359087

Buckley, B. (2010). American Academy of Pediatrics' RSV prophylaxis guidelines. *Advanced Studies in Pharmacy, 7*, 102–104. Retrieved from http://www.utasip.com/

Centers for Disease Control and Prevention (CDC). (2009). *Respiratory syncytial virus infection (RSV).* Retrieved from http://www.cdc.gov/rsv/clinical/prophylaxis.html

Centers for Disease Control and Prevention (CDC). (2010). *Data and statistics, tuberculosis is one of the world's most deadliest diseases.* Retrieved from http://cdc.gov/tb/ statistics/default.html

Centers for Disease Control and Prevention (CDC). (2011). *Fast facts.* Retrieved from http://www.cdc.gov/pertussis/fast-facts.html

Chavez-Bueno, S., Asuncion, M., & Welliver, R. C. (2006). Respiratory syncytial virus bronchiolitis. *Treatment in Respiratory Medicine, 5*, 483–494. doi: 1176-3450/06/0006-0483

Cottrell, L., Neal, W. A., Ice, C., Perez, M. K., & Piedmonte, G. (2010). Metabolic abnormalities in children with asthma. *American Journal of Respiratory and Critical Care Medicine, 183*, 441–448. doi: 10.1164/rccm.201004-0603OC

Cystic Fibrosis Foundation (CFF). (2011). *About cystic fibrosis.* Retrieved from http://www.cff.org/AboutCF/

De Buys Rossingh, A. S., & Dinh-Xuan, A. T. (2009). Diaphragmatic hernia: Current status and review of literature. *European Journal of Pediatrics, 168*, 393–406. doi: 10.1007/s0043-008-0904-x

Durani, Y., Friedman, M. J., & Attia, M. W. (2008). Clinical predictors of respiratory syncytial virus infection in children. *Pediatrics International, 50*, 352–355. doi: 10.1111/j.1442-200X.2008.02589.x.

Gaffin, J. M., Sheehan, W. J., Morrill, J., Cinar, M., Borras Coughlin, I. M., Sawicki, G. S., . . . Phipantanakul, W. (2011). Tree nut allergy, and asthma in children. *Clinical Pediatrics, 50*, 133–139. doi: 10.2165/00151829-200605060-00011

National Heart, Lung, and Blood Institute (NHLBI), National Asthma Education and Prevention Program. (2010). *Managing asthma long term.* Retrieved from http://www.nhlbi.nih.gov/ guidelines/asthma/asthgdln.pdf

Shaikh, N., & Hoberman, A. (2010). Update: Acute otitis media. *Pediatric Annals, 39*, 28–33. doi: 10.3928/00904481-20091222-03

Torpy, J. M. (2010). Acute otitis media. *Journal of the American Medical Association, 304*, 2194. doi: 10.1001/jama.304.19.2194

World Health Organization (WHO). (2006). *Global tuberculosis control: Surveillance, planning, financing.* Retrieved from http://www.who.int/tb/publications/global_report/en/

World Health Organization (WHO). (2010). *Tuberculosis.* Retrieved from http://www.who.int/mediacentre/factsheets/fs104/en/index.html

World Health Organization (WHO). (2011). Communicable diseases: Tuberculosis factsheets. Retrieved from http://www.searo.who.int/en/Section10/Section 2097/ Section 2106_10681.html

12 Cardiovascular Disorders

Kathryn Rudd, MSN, RN, C-NIC, C-NPT

OBJECTIVES

- ☐ Define key terms.
- ☐ Identify the normal assessment of the anatomy and physiology of the pediatric cardiovascular system.
- ☐ Identify the physical assessment components of pediatric patients with cardiovascular disease.
- ☐ Identify the anatomic features, clinical presentation, stabilization, emergent, and long-term care of the pediatric patient with cardiovascular disease.
- ☐ Identify the nursing interventions necessary to provide the caregiver education needed to care for a child with cardiovascular disease.
- ☐ Describe the common diagnostic tests used in the diagnosing and treatment of cardiovascular diseases in the pediatric population.
- ☐ Develop a nursing care plan for a child with a cardiac condition.

KEY TERMS

- Cardiac output
- Stroke volume
- Congenital heart defect
- Acquired heart defect
- Teratogen
- Thrills
- Wide pulse pressure
- Narrow pulse pressure
- Cyanosis
- Point of maximum impulse
- Hyperactive precordium
- Tachycardia
- Bradycardia
- Murmurs
- Cardiomegaly
- Tetralogy

HEART ANATOMY AND PHYSIOLOGY

- Located in the center of the chest
- About the size of the child's fist
- Heart rate varies with the age of the child from 60 to 160 beats per minute.
- A child's heart pumps as hard as an adult's heart.

Chambers of the Heart

- Four chambers: right and left atria, right and left ventricles (**Figure 12-1A**)
- Right atrium—collects deoxygenated blood from the entire body, except for lungs
- Right ventricle—pumps deoxygenated blood to the lungs via the pulmonary artery
- Left atrium—collects oxygenated blood from the capillary beds of the lungs through the pulmonary veins
- Left ventricle—pumps oxygenated blood through the aorta to the systemic circulation

Heart Valves

- Four valves prevent blood from regurgitating (**Figure 12-1B**).
- Two are atrioventricular (AV) and connect the atria and ventricles.
  - *Tricuspid (three leafs) connects right atria and right ventricle*
  - *Bicuspid (two leafs) connects left atria and left ventricle*
- Aortic and pulmonic valves (semilunar or half-moon shaped—three leaves each)
  - *Pulmonic connects right ventricle and pulmonary artery*
  - *Aortic connects left ventricle and ascending aorta*

Heart Vessels

- Vena cavae—carry blood to the right atrium (**Figure 12-1C**)
  - *Superior vena cava—carries blood from head, arms, and upper body. Lies above the heart.*
  - *Inferior vena cava—carries blood from legs, abdominal cavity, and lower part of the body to the right atrium. Lies below the heart.*

Don't have time to read this chapter? Want to reinforce your reading? Need to review for a test? Listen to this chapter on DavisPlus at davispl.us/rudd1.

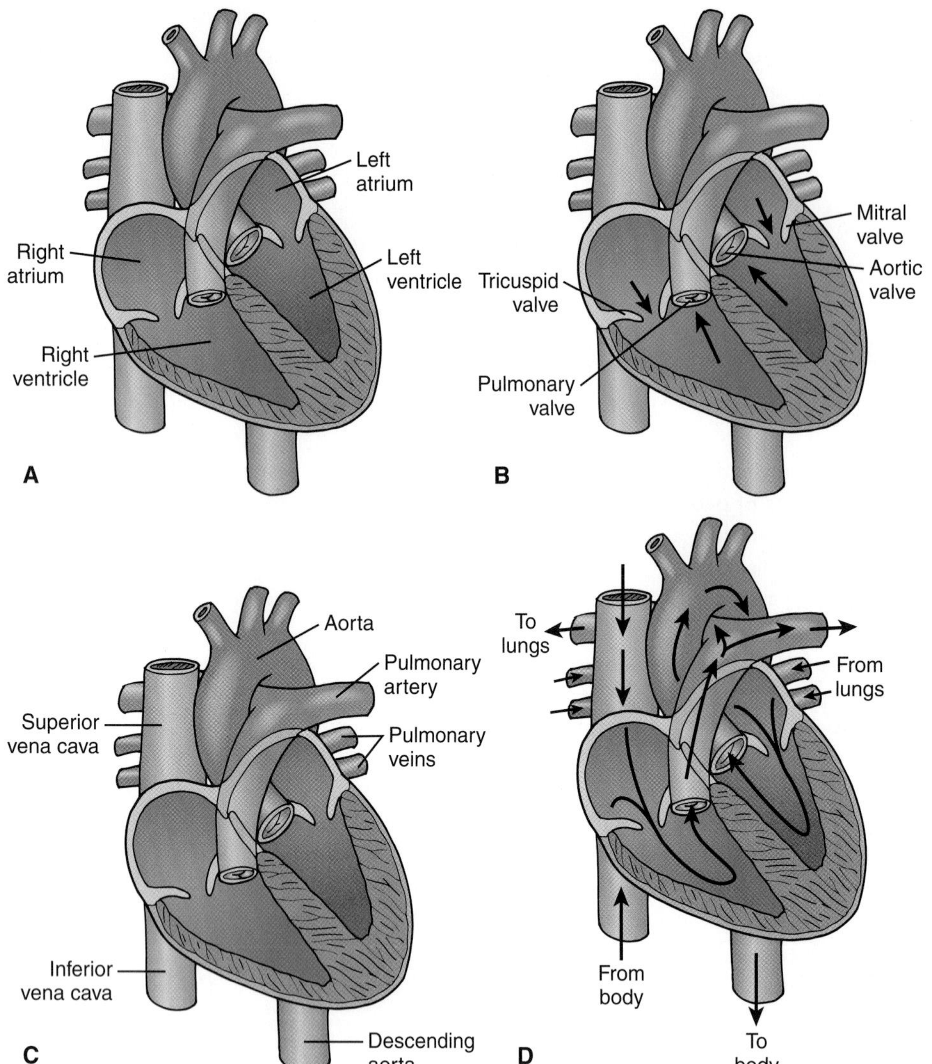

Figure 12–1 Heart structures and blood flow. **A**, Chambers of the heart; **B,** valves of the heart; **C**, vessels of the heart; **D**, normal blood flow.

- Pulmonary artery—carries deoxygenated blood from right ventricle to the lungs to be oxygenated
- Pulmonary vein—carries oxygenated blood from capillary beds of the lungs to the left atrium and the left ventricle
- Aorta—large vessel that carries oxygenated blood from the left ventricle to the rest of the body

Normal Blood Flow

- Blood is pumped out of the heart.
- Blood carries oxygen via hemoglobin to the tissues (**Figure 12-1D**).
- Oxygen is necessary for cell function.
- Tissue perfusion is maintained by sufficient cardiac output.

Cardiac Output

- Amount of blood ejected from the right or left ventricle per minute
- **Cardiac output** = **stroke volume** times heart rate.

Stroke Volume

- Amount of blood pumped out by the left ventricle per minute
- Stroke volume is altered by the size of the heart and the heart rate.
- The Fick calculation is an accurate method to measure cardiac output (**Figure 12-2,** Ward & Hisley, 2009).

$$\text{Pulmonary flow } (Q_p) = \frac{V_{O_2}}{C_{PV} - C_{PA}}$$

$$\text{Systemic flow } (Q_s) = \frac{V_{O_2}}{C_{AO} - C_{MV}}$$

Figure 12–2 Fick calculation.

Pressure Gradients

- Necessary for adequate circulation to lungs and body
- Become disrupted if the cardiac structures fail to develop or close, as well as if they are transposed or become narrowed

Electrical Conduction

- The sinoatrial (SA) node in the right atrium fires at end of diastole to cause depolarization and contraction of the atria (**Figure 12-3**)
  - *Pumps blood into the ventricles*
  - *Responsible for the P wave on the electrocardiogram*
  - *Called the pacemaker of the heart*
- Signal moves down to the AV node located between the atria and ventricles
- P-Q interval on ECG reflects slowed conduction to allow right and left ventricles to fill with blood
- Electrical impulse moves across the fibers called the bundle of His located in the walls of the ventricles
- Fibers divide into right and left bundle branches, Purkinje fibers, in the cell walls of the right and left ventricles. Contraction begins in the walls of the ventricles and is shown in the Q wave of the ECG.
- The left ventricle contracts just before the right ventricle, with the R wave indicating left ventricular contraction and the S wave right ventricular contraction.
- Ventricles relax and wait for the next signal, which is seen as the T wave in the ECG.

Fetal Circulation

- Before birth, 90% of blood bypasses the lungs; the placenta is the organ of respiration (**Figure 12-4**).
- Oxygenated blood is returned via the umbilical vein to the inferior vena cava and to the right atrium.
- Oxygenated blood crosses from the right atrium to the left atrium via the patent foramen ovale (PFO) and is pumped by the left ventricle.
- Deoxygenated blood flows from the superior vena cava to the right atrium and then to the right ventricle, the pulmonary artery, the patent ductus arteriosus (PDA), and the aorta.
- Upon birth and first breath, the patent foramen ovale and patent ductus arteriosus close.

CONGENITAL OR ACQUIRED HEART DEFECTS

- Defects are classified as **congenital heart defects** or **acquired heart defects**.
- Congenital heart defects are genetic in origin, meaning the child is born with the disorder; affect 1 in 170 live births (**Tables 12-1, 12-2**; Nelson & Robin, 2002).
- The defect can be a single lesion or multiple abnormalities.
- Cyanosis occurs when blood flow, either blue or red, to the lungs is insufficient. A large portion of deoxygenated blood is pumped into the systemic circulation when hemoglobin <5 mg/dL (Tsuda, 2009).
- A decrease in oxygen saturation to 85% with normal hemoglobin levels will result in cyanosis (Ward & Hisley, 2009).
  - *Increased pulmonary blood flow—abnormal connection through the septa or the great vessels; increased blood volume on right side of heart with increased pulmonary blood flow and decreased systemic blood flow*
    - Patent ductus arteriosus (PDA)
    - Atrial septal defects (ASDs)
    - Ventricular septal defects (VSDs)
  - *Decreased pulmonary blood flow—pulmonary blood flow is obstructed within the right ventricular outflow. Desaturated blood shunts from right to left across an ASD or VSD into systemic circulation, and the neonate is most likely desaturated and cyanotic.*
    - Tetralogy of Fallot (TOF)
    - Tricuspid atresia (TA)
    - Eisenmenger's syndrome
  - *Obstructive disorders*
    - Coarctation of the aorta (COA)
    - Aortic stenosis (AS)
    - Pulmonary stenosis (PS)
    - Pulmonary atresia (PA)
    - Tetralogy of Fallot with pulmonary atresia
  - *Mixed disorders—blood from systemic and pulmonary circulations is mixed in the heart chambers, desaturation of blood occurs, and cardiac output decreases because of increased volume load on ventricles.*
    - Transposition of the great vessels (TGV)
    - Truncus arteriosus (TA)
    - Total anomalous pulmonary venous return (TAPVR)
    - Hypoplastic left heart (HLH)
    - Ebstein's anomaly
- Acquired heart disease can occur in the normal heart or in the heart with a congenital defect. Acquired heart disease is most often due to:
  - *Infections*
  - *Autoimmune factors*
  - *Genetic factors*
  - ***Teratogens****—any inhaled, ingested, or absorbed agent that has the possibility of altering genetic structure or function*
    - Drugs: alcohol, angiotensin-converting enzyme (ACE) inhibitors, chemotherapeutic agents, smoking, Accutane, Lithium, Coumadin, Dilantin, and others
    - Infections such as cytomegalovirus, rubella, varicella, HIV, toxoplasmosis, herpes, varicella (Rathnau-Minnella, 2008)
    - Maternal factors, such as infant of a diabetic mother (IDM) (Rathnau-Minella, 2008)

CRITICAL COMPONENT

Genetic Factors in Congenital Cardiac Malformations

Genetic factors are the most common causes of congenital cardiac malformations and account for approximately one-fourth of all congenital malformations (Teratogens, 2008).

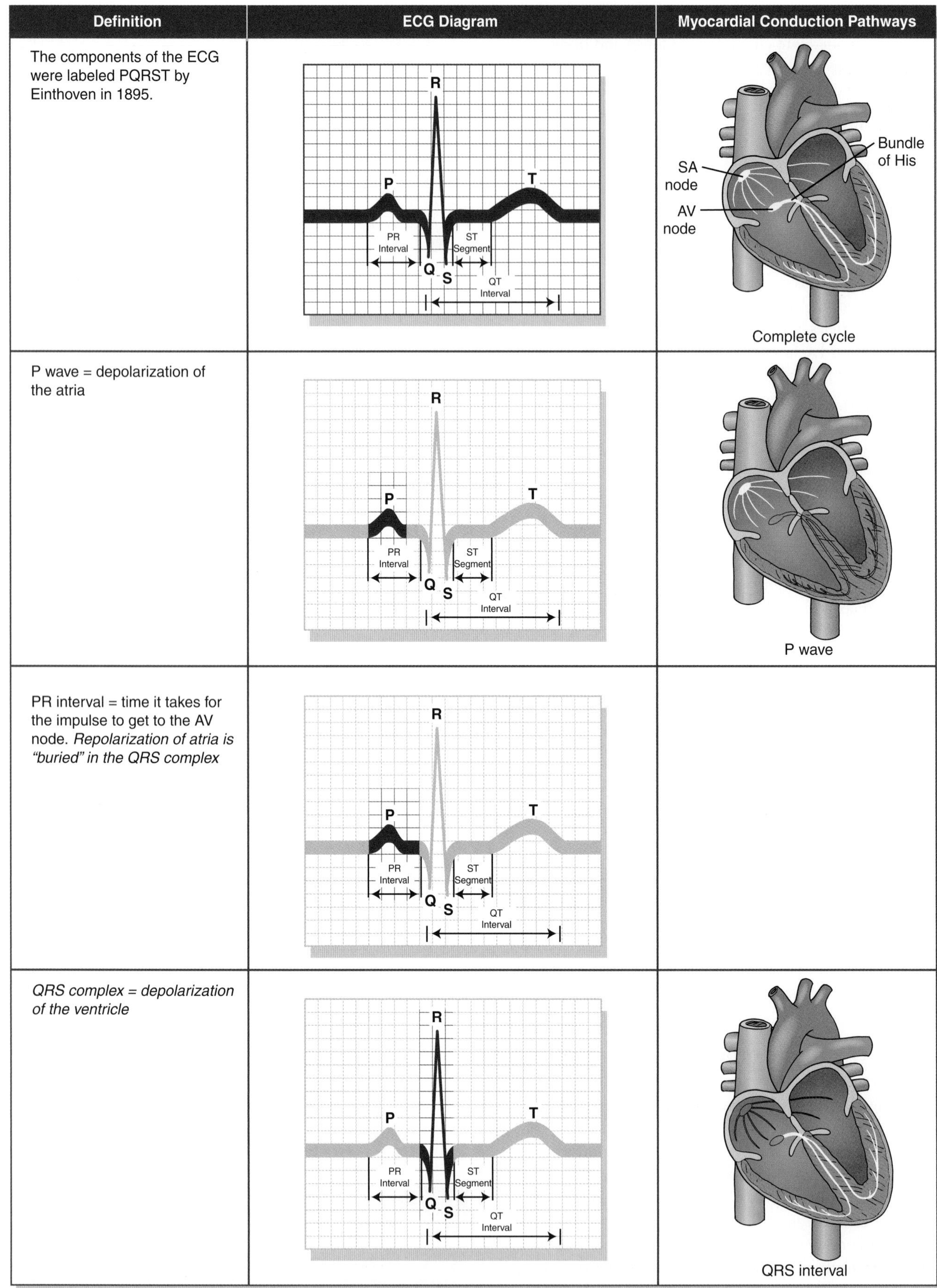

Definition	ECG Diagram	Myocardial Conduction Pathways
The components of the ECG were labeled PQRST by Einthoven in 1895.		Complete cycle
P wave = depolarization of the atria		P wave
PR interval = time it takes for the impulse to get to the AV node. *Repolarization of atria is "buried" in the QRS complex*		
QRS complex = depolarization of the ventricle		QRS interval

Figure 12–3 Conduction of the heart.

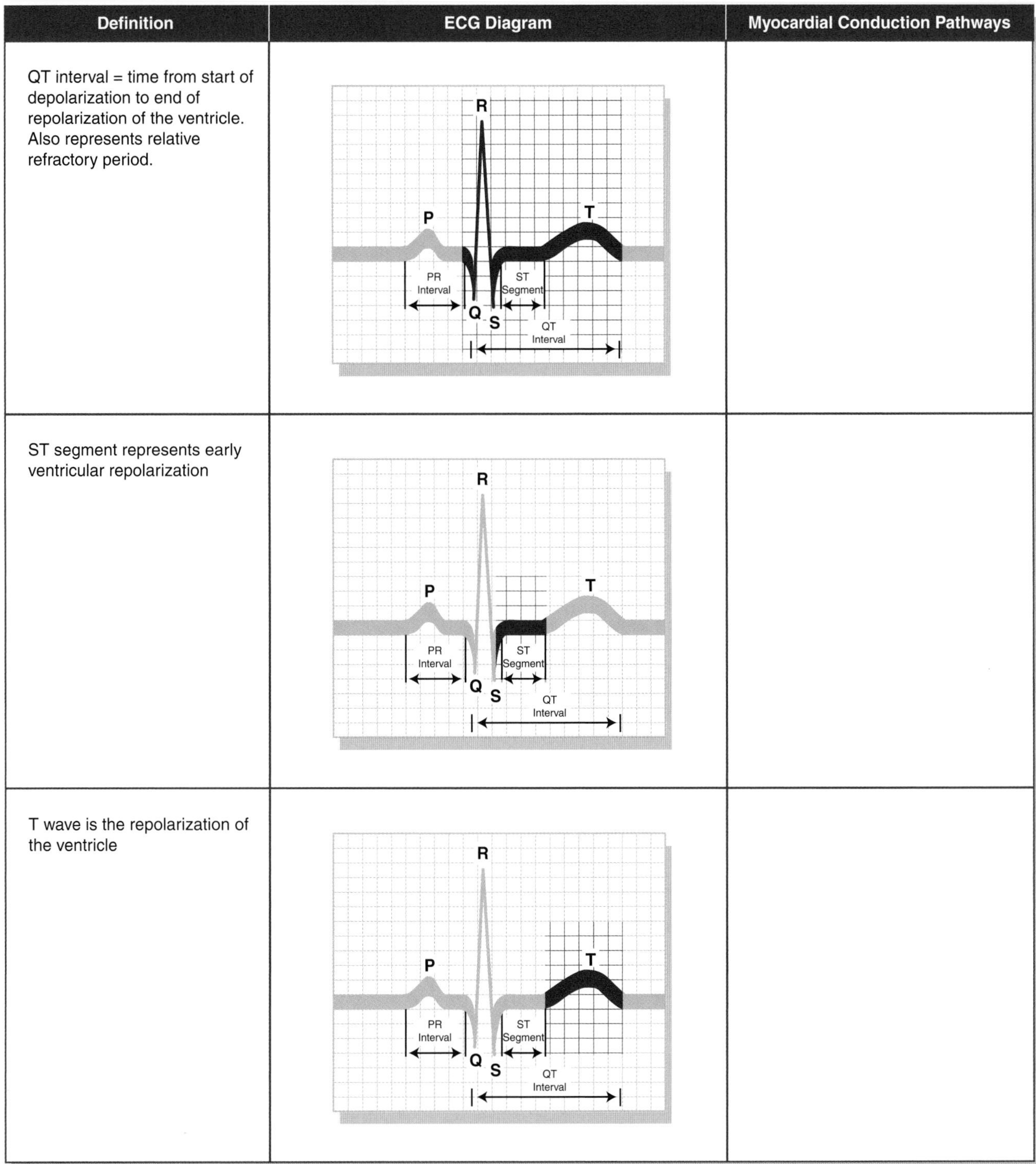

Figure 12-3—cont'd

Assessment

History

General History

- Comprehensive history and physical examination
- Detailed family history, including history of congenital heart disease or genetic disorders
- Prenatal history, including rapid or slow heart rate in utero, diabetes, or lupus
- Detailed history of exposure to infections, exposure to environmental teratogens such as alcohol, cocaine, phenytoin, or lithium
- Gestational age at birth
- Feeding history, weight gain
- Diaphoresis

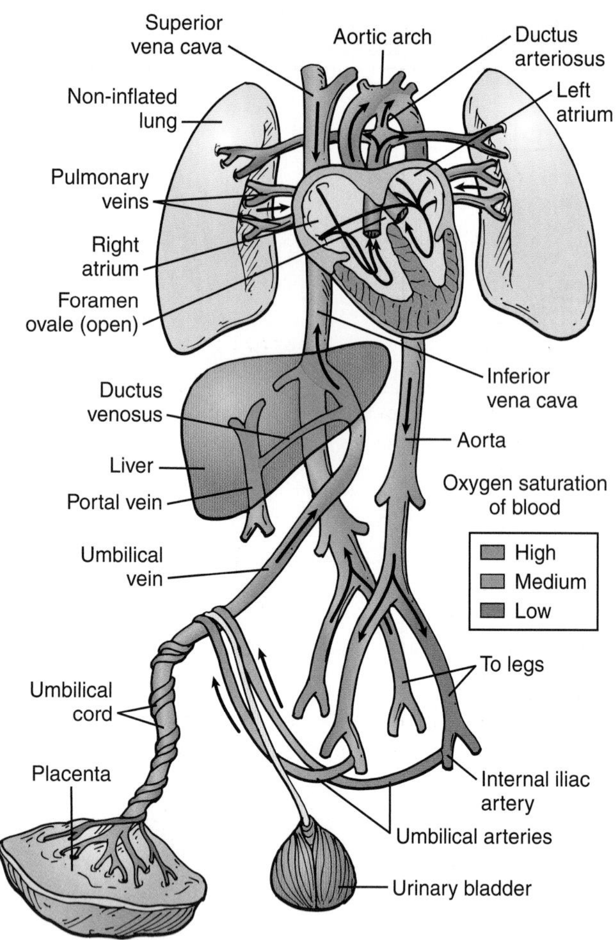

Figure 12–4 Fetal circulation.

- Attainment of developmental milestones
- Respiratory status
- Pain
  - *Chest pain is a rare symptom in the pediatric cardiac patient.*
  - *Myocardial infarction (MI) can occur in disease processes such as Kawasaki disease.*
  - *Chest pain is often due to other conditions, such as costochrondritis, musculoskeletal discomforts, skin conditions, or pleural pain.*

CRITICAL COMPONENT

Family History and Congenital Heart Defects

A family history, especially of siblings, with heart defects indicates a higher risk of congenital heart defects (American Heart Association [AHA], 2007).

Clinical Reasoning

Assessment of Family's Coping Skills

The degree of impact on the family structure is proportionally dependent upon the severity of the heart disease, especially as it relates to financial, social, and emotional burdens (Smith, 2011).

1. What techniques can the nurse utilize to assess the family's ability to cope with the heart disease diagnosis?
2. What are the barriers to obtaining a complete history of the child?

TABLE 12–1 CLASSIFICATION OF CARDIAC DEFECTS

Class	Name	Prevalence (% of all defects)	Types or Forms	Associated Defects
L–R Shunt	Atrial-septal defect	5–10 (50–100)	Secundum or primum or sinus venosus	PAPVR or MVP
	Ventricular septal defect	20–25 (200–250)	Perimembranous, muscular, multiple	PDA, CoA, AV prolapse
	Patent ductus arteriosus	5–10 (50–100)	Large shunt or small	
	AV canal	0.02 (0.20)	Complete or partial; balanced or unbalanced	AV regurgitation; 30% of cases occur with Down syndrome
	Partial anomalous pulmonary venous return	<1 (10)	TAPVR	ASD
Obstructive Lesions	Pulmonary stenosis	5–8 (50–80)	Valvular, subvalvular, supravalvular (PA)	VSD, Noonan syndrome
	Aortic stenosis	0.05 (0.50)	Valvular, subvalvular, supravalvular	Bicuspid aortic valve, Williams syndrome, IHSS
	Coarctation of the aorta	5–10 (50–100)	Preductal, postductal, ascending aorta, descending aorta	Bicuspid AV, aortic hypoplasia, VSD, PDA, abnormal MV

TABLE 12–1 CLASSIFICATION OF CARDIAC DEFECTS—cont'd

Class	Name	Prevalence (% of all defects)	Types or Forms	Associated Defects
	Interrupted aortic arch	0.01 (0.10)	Type of coarctation, types A, B, C	PDA, VSD, bicuspid AV, MV deformity, truncus arteriosus, subaortic stenosis
Cyanotic Defects	Transposition of the great arteries	0.05 (0.50)	D-type, L-type	ASD, VSD, PDA, PS
	Tetralogy of Fallot	0.10 (1.00)	PS or PA or absent PV with PS	May be cyanotic or acyanotic if PS is mild
	Total anomalous pulmonary venous return	0.01 (0.10)	Supracardiac, cardiac draining into right atrium, cardiac draining into the coronary sinus, infracardiac, obstructive	ASD or PFO
	Tricuspid atresia	1–2 (10–20)		ASD, VSD, PDA, CoA, TGA
	Pulmonary atresia	<1 (10)	Variable RV sizes	ASD, PFO, or PDA
	Ebstein's anomaly	<1 (10)	Variable degrees of displacement	WPW, RA hypertrophy, ASD
	Truncus arteriosus	<1 (10)	Types I–IV showing various placements of PA arising from the aorta	Large VSD, right aortic arch, DiGeorge syndrome
	Single ventricle	<1 (10)	DILV or RV	ASD, PS, PA, CoA, VSD, asplenia, polysplenia, TGV
	Double-outlet right ventricle	<1 (10)	Types are by the position of the VSD: subaortic VSD, subpulmonary VSD, remote VSD, subaortic VSD with PS, doubly committed VSD	VSD, PS
	Splenic syndromes	<1 (10)	Asplenia and polysplenia	Various redundant cardiac structures or absence of structures

The numbers in parentheses indicate the number of infants born with defects out of 100,000 live births.
Source: Judith M. Marshall, 2006.

TABLE 12–2 SYNDROMES ASSOCIATED WITH CARDIAC DISEASE

Syndrome/Disease/ Chromosomal Aberrations	Cardiac Defect/Condition	Other Physical Findings
Down syndrome	AV canal, VSD	Down's facies, developmental delay
Noonan syndrome	Pulmonic valve stenosis, LVH	Elfin facies, pectus deformity, joint laxity, undescended testes, spine abnormalities, hypotonia, seizures
Williams syndrome	Supravalvular aortic stenosis, PA stenosis	Williams' facies: small upturned nose, long philtrum (upper lip length), wide mouth, full lips, small chin, and puffiness around the eyes Hypercalcemia, dental abnormalities, renal problems, sensitive hearing, hypotonia, joint laxity, overly friendly personality
DiGeorge or Velo-cardio-facial chromosome	Interrupted aortic arch, truncus arteriosus, VSD, PDA, TOF	Decreased immune response, low-set ears, palate problems, hypoparathyroidism, hypocalcemia

Continued

TABLE 12–2 SYNDROMES ASSOCIATED WITH CARDIAC DISEASE—cont'd

Syndrome/Disease/ Chromosomal Aberrations	Cardiac Defect/Condition	Other Physical Findings
Duchenne's muscular dystrophy	Cardiomyopathy	Generalized weakness and muscle wasting first affecting the muscles of the hips, pelvic area, thighs, and shoulders; calves are often enlarged
Marfan syndrome	Aortic aneurism, aortic and/or mitral regurgitation	Arms disproportionately long, tall and thin with laxity of joints, dislocation of lenses, spinal problems, stretch marks, hernia, pectus abnormalities, restrictive lung disease
Trisomy 18	VSD, PDA, PS	Multiple joint contractures, spina bifida, hearing loss, radial aplasia (underdevelopment or missing radial bone of forearm), cleft lip, birth defects of the eye
Trisomy 13	VSD, PDA, dextrocardia	Omphalocele, holoprosencephaly (an anatomic defect of the brain involving failure of the forebrain to divide properly), kidney defects, skin defects of the scalp
CHARGE	TOF, truncus arteriosus, vascular ring, interrupted aortic arch	*C*oloboma of the eye, *H*eart defects, *A*tresia of the choanae, *R*etardation of *G*rowth and development, and *E*ar abnormalities and deafness
Fetal alcohol syndrome	VSD, PDA, ASD, TOF	Growth deficiencies, skeletal deformities, facial abnormalities, kidney and urinary defects, central nervous system handicaps, organ deformities: genital malformations
VATER (VACTERLS)	VSD and others	*V*ertebral anomalies, vascular anomalies, *A*nal atresia, *C*ardiac anomalies, *T*racheo-esophageal (T-E) fistula, *E*sophageal atresia, *R*enal anomalies, radial dysplasia, *L*imb anomalies, *S*ingle umbilical artery
Turner syndrome	CoA, ASD, AS	Kidney problems, high blood pressure, overweight, hearing difficulties, diabetes, cataracts, thyroid problems, lack of sexual development, "webbed" neck, low hairline at the back of the neck, drooping of the eyelids, dysmorphic, low-set ears, abnormal bone development, multiple moles

Physical Examination

Possible Indicators of Heart Disease in Children

- Failure to thrive (FTT)
- Small for gestational age (SGA)
- Poor weight gain
- Dysmorphic features
- Chest wall deformities, which are a feature of congenital heart disease due to increase in cardiac size, activity, and left-to-right shunting
- Scoliosis
  - *Common in adolescents with congenital heart disease*
- Clubbing and erythema in fingers and toes (**Figure 12-5**)
  - *May result from longstanding cyanosis due to increased formation and enlargement of the capillaries in the periphery to improve circulation*
  - *Excessive growth of soft tissue in fingers and toes*
  - *Result of chronic hypoxia*
  - *Polycythemia results in an increase in red blood cell production to increase oxygen carrying capacity.*

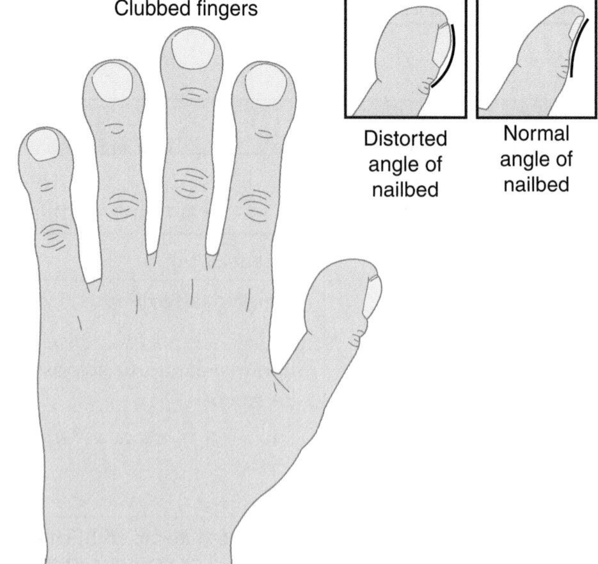

Figure 12–5 Clubbing of the fingers.

- *Polycythemia increases the viscosity of the blood, predisposing to stroke and clot formation (Allen, Driscoll, Shaddy, & Feltes, 2008).*

Respiratory System

- Close evaluation of the respiratory rate and evidence of retractions is important in assessing whether the child has a primary respiratory disorder or cardiac disease.
- Shallow respirations that are rapid with a rate of 50 to 60 breaths per minute in a content infant are abnormal and need to be investigated (Karlsen & Tani, 2003).
- Children with congenital heart disease often have respiratory tract infections, resulting in dyspnea with activity and fatigue (Tsuda, 2009).
- Respiratory symptoms that may indicate pulmonary edema include increased work of breathing, grunting, nasal flaring, and retractions (Tsuda, 2009).

CLINICAL PEARL

Hyperoxia Test

The hyperoxia test, also known as an oxygen challenge test, is used to determine whether the cyanosis being experienced by the neonate is cardiac or respiratory in nature. An arterial blood gas is obtained from the right radial artery when the infant is breathing room air. An arterial blood gas is then obtained following the placement of an infant in 100% oxygen for 10 minutes. The infant with cardiac disease will have a 25 to 40 mm Hg Pao_2 in room air that will not significantly rise in 100% oxygen. This is due to continued mixing of oxygenated and nonoxygenated blood. In an infant with pulmonary disease, the Pao_2 will generally rise to >80 mm Hg unless there is significant pulmonary hypertension present. This is a screening test only, with exceptions that may occur (Acute Care of at-Risk Newborns Neonatal Society [ACoRN], 2009).

Cardiovascular System

See **Table 12-3** for cardiac assessment techniques.

- Level of alertness, activity, and tone
- Chest symmetry and pulsations
- Capillary refill
  - *Pressing a central location (sternum or forehead)*
  - *Normal is less than or equal to 3 seconds*
  - *Prolonged capillary refill indicates poor cardiac output and perfusion (ACoRN, 2009).*
- Pulses
  - *When normal, usually easy to feel in a child*
  - *Infant 160 beats/min, preschool 120 beats/min, adolescent 100 beats/min*
  - *Include radial, carotid, brachial, and femoral pulses*
  - *Should be equal in strength between right and left arms and upper and lower extremities*
  - *Pulses that are bounding in upper extremities and decreased in lower extremities may indicate coarctation of the aorta (COA).*
  - *Pulses that are bounding may suggest systemic hypertension or patent ductus arteriosus.*
  - *Cardiac pulsations are seen in subaortic stenosis.*
  - *Peripheral pulses are indicators of cardiac output, systolic pressure, and diastolic pressure.*
  - *Pulses that are difficult to palpate may indicate poor cardiac output or obstructive outflow lesions (Behrman, Kliegman, & Jenson, 2011).*
  - *Pedal pulses*
  - *Peripheral edema*
  - ***Thrills**—palpation of vibrating sensations due to rapid flow blood from an area of higher pressure to an area of lower pressure; always an abnormal finding (Karlsen & Tani, 2003).*
  - *Temperature of the extremities—cold feet or hands in comparison to torso suggests poor perfusion beyond 8 hours after birth (Tsuda, 2009).*
- Blood pressure
  - *Blood pressure should be assessed by Doppler with the proper size of cuff; use a nonthreatening approach; the child may sit on parent's lap depending upon age.*
  - *Varies with gestational age, weight, or postnatal age*
  - *In newborns, the mean arterial pressure in mm Hg is usually the newborn's completed age in weeks.*
  - *Minimum systolic blood pressure is 70 mm Hg + (2 × age in years).*
  - ***Wide pulse pressures**—diastolic pressures are low and there is a wide gap between diastolic and systolic pressures; indicative of such processes as patent ductus arteriosus.*
  - *Poor cardiac output will result in a low systolic blood pressure with a high diastolic pressure, creating a **narrow pulse pressure**.*
  - *Noninvasive blood pressures are less accurate when the heart rate is greater than 200 beats per minute.*
  - *Four limb extremity blood pressures are indicated if cardiac disease is suspected or murmur is present.*
  - *A preductal right-arm systolic blood pressure greater than 15 mm Hg above the postductal lower limb systolic blood pressure is abnormal (ACoRN, 2009).*
  - *A difference of greater than 10 mm Hg between arms is abnormal (ACoRN, 2009).*
  - *Distended or pulsating neck veins require investigation (Brookes, 2008).*
  - *Hepatomegaly, where the liver is felt more than 3 cm below the right costal margin, indicates increased right arterial pressure and is highly suggestive of congestive heart failure (CHF) (Karlsen & Tani, 2003).*

CLINICAL PEARL

Blood Pressure Cuffs

Undersized blood pressure cuffs will give the nurse a falsely high blood pressure reading, whereas an oversized cuff will give the nurse a falsely low blood pressure reading (Allen et al., 2008).

- Color
  - ***Cyanosis** is the bluish discoloration of the skin, nail beds, tongue, or mucosa.*
  - *Cyanosis is always an abnormal finding.*

TABLE 12–3 CARDIAC ASSESSMENT TECHNIQUES

Assessment Technique	What to Look for	Normal Findings	Abnormal Findings	Rationale
Inspection	Skin color, shape and symmetry of chest, clubbing	Pink, symmetrical chest	Pallor, cyanosis, asymmetry of chest shape and movement, hyperdynamic precordium	Poor cardiac output; deoxygenated circulating blood, ventricular failure or hypertrophy, tachycardia
Palpation	Skin and body temperature, moisture, chest movement, point of maximal impulse (PMI)	Warm, dry, symmetrical movement, PMI at 4th or 5th intercostal space (ICS) at midclavicular line	Cold extremities, dry flaky skin, diaphoresis, thrills or heaves	Poor circulation, heart failure, ventricular hypertrophy
Percussion	Heart shape and size	Normal size and shape for age and weight	Enlarged heart, axis deviation	Heart failure and hypertrophy
Auscultation	Murmurs, other sounds	No murmurs, innocent murmurs; quiet precordium	Murmurs, clicks, rubs, snaps	Structural defects, increased workload of heart and volume overload

Source: Judith M. Marshall, 2006.

- *Central cyanosis is due to problems with the heart or lungs.*
- *Elevated levels of deoxygenated hemoglobin, which is blue in color, are present.*
- *Peripheral cyanosis (acrocyanosis) is often due to interruption in blood flow to the extremity.*
- *Shock can be seen with a prolonged capillary refill time, and pallor is associated with poor perfusion (AAP, 2006).*
- *Pulse oximeter readings of 78% or lower with normal hemoglobin levels will result in outward signs of cyanosis (ACoRN, 2009).*
- *Anemia may not show cyanosis due to decreased levels of hemoglobin; polycythemia may show cyanosis with a smaller amount of deoxygenated hemoglobin.*
- *Quiet pericardium combined with cyanosis is often an indicator of congenital heart disease (Karlsen & Tani, 2003).*
- *Skin that is pale, mottled, or grey in appearance indicates poor perfusion.*

CLINICAL PEARL

Acrocyanosis

Acrocyanosis can occur when there is an interruption of blood flow due to constriction (blood pressure cuff or tourniquet) or vasoconstriction due to temperature changes. Acrocyanosis is very common at birth during the period of transition of the newborn and is seen as bluish discoloration of the hands and feet (Karlsen & Tani, 2003; National Heart, Lung, and Blood Institute http://www.nhlbi.nih.gov/health/health-topics/topics/chd/printall-index.html)

- Urine output is indicative of perfusion to the kidneys.

Auscultation

- Heart sounds heard with diaphragm and bell of the stethoscope (**Figure 12-6**)
  - *S_1 (lub sound) is heard at the 4th or 5th intercostal space at the midclavicular line (MCL)—the closure of mitral (heard at apex of heart) and tricuspid valve (heard at left sternal border [LSB]) (Ward & Hisley, 2009).*
  - *S_2 (dub sound) is heard at the closure of the pulmonic and aortic valves. May be split. Single S_2 is due to absent flow or obstruction in flow to aortic or pulmonic valves (Ward & Hisley, 2009).*
  - *S_3, S_4 gallop—considered normal before the age of 20 (Karlsen & Tani, 2003).*
- **Point of maximum impulse** (PMI)—area of most intense pulsation heard by a stethoscope
  - *In children <7 years of age, located at left MCL and 4th intercostal space*

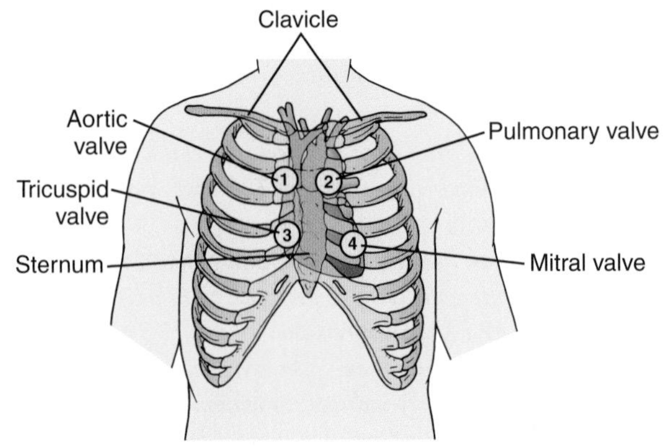

Figure 12–6 Cardiac auscultation landmarks.

- *In children >7 years of age, located along the left sternal border in the 5th intercostal space*
- **Hyperactive precordium** (during auscultation the heart sounds are magnified) or shift in the PMI indicates consideration of dextrocardia or pneumothorax (Karlsen & Tani, 2003).
- Precordial activity
- **Tachycardias**—fast heart rates
- **Bradycardias**—slow heart rates
- Distant or muffled heart sounds
- **Murmurs** are heart sounds that are due to turbulent blood flow. Assess for intensity, location, duration, and quality.
- Diastolic and continuous murmurs are usually pathological (Behrman et al., 2011).
- Innocent murmurs (e.g., systolic, vibratory, musical) are present in many children (**Table 12-4**) due to thin chest walls in the child and hyperactive heart sounds (Karlsen & Tani, 2003).

Diagnostic Tests

Chest X-ray

- Chest x-rays including anterioposterior (AP) and lateral views indicate pulmonary vascularity.
- Cardiac size and shape
- Lung vascular markings
- Position of the stomach (ACoRN, 2009)

Blood Gases

- Metabolic acidosis shows as a decrease in pH and an increase in base excess.
- Base excess is the accumulation of metabolic acids in the blood.
- Monitored by arterial, venous, or capillary blood

Electrocardiogram (ECG or EKG)

- Useful to determine conduction issues
- Needs to be evaluated by a cardiologist

Echocardiogram

- Ultrasound of the heart
- Noninvasive test that indicates structure, size, flow patterns, function, and the blood vessels attached to the heart

Angiography

- Visualizes the structure and function of the ventricles
- Dye is injected via a catheter.

Cardiac Catheterization

- Invasive diagnostic procedure
- Cannulization of a vein, usually in the groin area, to pass a catheter into the heart or major vessels of the heart
- Advanced with the use of x-ray fluoroscopy

TABLE 12–4 MURMURS

Murmurs Grade 1–6 (1 being softest, 6 being loudest)	
Holosystolic	Shunting of blood from an area of higher pressure to an area of lower pressure such as in a ventricular septal defect (VSD), which are harsh murmurs, and atrioventricular regurgitation, which are soft murmurs
Ejection Systolic	As blood flow increases in systole there is turbulence through restricted flow patterns such as in pulmonary stenosis or aortic stenosis
Diastolic	Regurgitation of blood flow from the aorta or pulmonary artery into the ventricles due to pulmonary or aortic insufficiency; always abnormal
Systolic and Diastolic	Result of pressure differences between two structures such as in patent ductus arteriosus
Pansystolic	Heard with congestive heart disease or severe regurgitation of mitral or tricuspid valves
Continuous	Heard with PDAs or AV malformations

Adapted from Karlsen, K. A., & Tani, L.Y. (2003). *S.T.A.B.L.E. cardiac module.* Park City, Utah: S.T.A.B.L.E. Program.

- Interventional catheters—used to open valves or septum in the heart
- Diagnostic catheters—used to measure internal pressures or to visualize circulation
- Electrophysiological catheters—used to evaluate conduction pathways or alter accessory pathways to avoid surgical intervention
- Cardiac catheterization is used to perform myocardial biopsies.
- Temporary measures to be able to delay reparative surgeries
- Provide caregiver education. (Beckman et al., 2005)

Biopsy of the Myocardium

- Frequent in heart transplants
- Monitor for rejection.

Pulmonary Artery Banding

- Palliative measure to decrease pulmonary blood flow
- Prevent pulmonary hypertrophy and pulmonary hypertension
- Utilized as a precursor to cardiac surgery, such as in large ventricular septal defects

Promoting Safety

Cardiac catheterization is used to obtain pressures in the child's heart and vessels, to take x-rays of the heart, to obtain myocardial biopsies, or to perform corrective procedures.

- Nursing care is aimed at alleviating pre-procedure and post-procedure anxiety and complications.
- Preparation and postoperative care will be dependent upon developmental age and parent involvement.
- Child will be given a sedative prior to the procedure to make the child sleepy, and a local anesthetic will be injected in the femoral vein or artery site prior to cannulization of the catheter.
- In catheterization with contrast dye, nursing care should emphasize intake and output.
- Keep extremities straight for 4 to 6 hours with no movement; child should be positioned flat on the back; a sandbag may be used on the extremity.
- A Foley catheter may be used.
- Check pulses above and below catheter site.
- Monitor for bleeding; maintain pressure dressing for 24 hours, then dry occlusive dressing.
- Auscultate for abnormal heart rate or rhythm and compare with pre-operative assessment.
- Monitor for temperature changes or color changes in the arm or leg that is used for the catheterization.
- No tub baths for several days; showers are fine.
- Observe for signs and symptoms of infections such as redness, fever, pain, thrombus formation, dysrhythmias, bleeding, and perfusion. Fever is common following catheterization but should not last longer than 24 hours or go above 100°F.
- Avoid strenuous activity such as lifting, sports, or physical education, although school is appropriate.
- Regular diet
- Return to school within 3 days.
- Follow-up appointments are essential. (LeRoy et al., 2003)

Patient and Caregiver Education

- Physical activity—discuss with the physician, patient, and caregiver if there are any limitations in physical activity.
- Emotional support—child may feel different from peers due to frequent hospitalizations; may result in feelings of isolation, sadness, or just not feeling like a normal child. Behavioral issues may occur due to extreme illness or jealous sibling interactions.
- Provide education to the patient and caregiver about the need for follow-up by a cardiologist for the rest of the child's life. The need to transition to an adult cardiologist should be discussed with teens.
- Endocarditis prevention is necessary for some patients related to dental or medical procedures being performed (see http://www.nhlbi.nih.gov/health/healthtopics/topics/chd/printall-index.htm).

Promoting Safety

To prevent bacterial endocarditis, antibiotics need to be prescribed for all dental and surgical procedures. Patient and caregivers must notify their health-care providers of their valvular history (Bonow et al., 2006).

- Teen girls should be counseled by nurses and physicians related to birth control, as certain congenital heart defects can predispose a teen to higher risks from birth control pills and intrauterine devices.
- Teen girls with certain congenital heart defects may also be at a higher risk of having children with congenital heart defects (see http://www.nhlbi.nih.gov/health/health-topics/topics/chd/printall-index.htm).

CONGENITAL HEART DISEASE WITH INCREASED PULMONARY BLOOD FLOW

PATENT DUCTUS ARTERIOSUS

- See **Figure 12-7**.
- For blood flow, see fetal circulation in Figure 12-4.
- Incidence in term infants is 1/2000 term live births (Dice & Bhatia, 2007).
- In fetal life, pulmonary vascular resistance (PVR) is high due to fluid in the lungs rather than air.
- The organ of respiration in the fetus is the placenta, and the pulmonary artery has a direct connection to the aorta through the ductus arteriosus.
- Following birth, PVR decreases and the ducts close due to the production of bradykinin in the lungs and an increase in neonatal blood oxygen levels (Nelson & Robin, 2002).

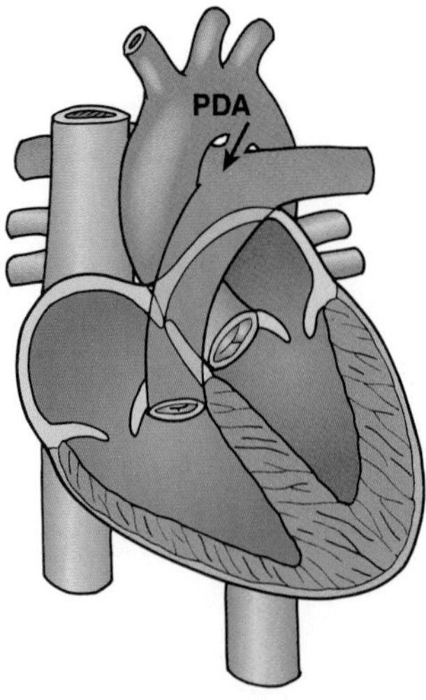

Figure 12–7 Patent ductus arteriosus.

- Left-to-right shunting occurs through the duct that will then connect the pulmonary artery (nonoxygenated) with the aorta (oxygenated).
- The pulmonary artery and the ducts are lined with smooth muscle tissue that normally closes within a few hours to days after birth.
- Most ducts close nearly 100% within 48 hours with full-term infants, and the incidence of them staying open or opening increases as the gestational age of the infant decreases (ACoRN, 2009).
- PDA can take up to a full year to close in some cases.
- Transitioning to extrauterine life results in vasoconstriction of these ducts in response to arterial oxygenation.
- The severity of the disease depends upon the gestational age of the neonate, the size of the ductal opening, and the degree of PVR.

Promoting Safety

Patent ductus arteriosus predisposes the child to the development of bacterial endocarditis due to irritation of the smooth muscle tissue of the pulmonary artery resulting in a more favorable medium for bacterial growth (Walter et al., 2007).

Assessment

- Heart murmur—systolic murmur, mid- to lower-left sternal border, washing machine sound
- Some infants will have no murmur.
- "Wet"-sounding breath sounds
- Tachypnea
- Increased work of breathing, or apnea
- Poor feeding
- Poor weight gain and growth pattern
- Fatigue
- Sweating with feeding
- Excessive fluid weight gain

Diagnostic Tests

- Wide pulse pressures—low diastolic pressures
- Increased vascular markings on the chest x-ray are a late sign due to enlarged heart.
- Poor oxygen saturation
- Bounding pulses
- Enlarged heart
- Prolonged capillary filling time
- Hyperactive precordium
- An echocardiogram will show increased enlargement of left heart chambers (Ward & Hisley, 2009).

Nursing Interventions

- Provide postoperative care following coil embolization or ligation.
- Decrease work of breathing.
- Maintain frequent rest periods.
- Do not cluster care.

Evidence-Based Practice Research: Clustering Care

Holsti, L., Grunau, R. E., Whifield, M. F., Oberlander, T. F., & Lindh, V. (2006). Behavioral responses to pain are heightened after clustered care in preterm infants born between 30 and 32 weeks gestational age. *Clinical Journal of Pain, 22,* 757–764. doi: 10.1097/01.ajp .0000210921.10912.47

Clustering care is effective in promoting the circadian and homeostatic equilibriums of sleep during acute critical care. Recent studies indicate that clustering care over the long term may actually reduce the neonate and infant's periods of growth and adaptability to pain.

- Maintain strict intake and output fluid restrictions.
- Maintain diuretics as ordered.
- Dopamine may be required.
- Maintain digoxin administration as ordered.
- Maintain indomethicin and ibuprofen administration, which is dependent upon weight, renal function, and gestational age.
- Monitor urine output.
- Monitor labs for thrombocytopenia.
- Monitor daily weights.
- Monitor tolerance of feedings.
- Provide preparation of patient for surgical closure.
- Monitor closely following postsurgical closure.
- Monitor wound care.

Medication

Ibuprofen and Indomethicin

Ibuprofen results in complete cessation of ductal flow by facilitating necrosis of the intima of the ductus arteriosus. Indomethicin has been the conventional drug of choice, but some patients have more adverse side effects than with ibuprofen (Calhoun, Murthy, Bryant, Luedtke, & Bhatt-Mehta, 2006).

Patient and Caregiver Education

- Closely monitor oral intake.
- Closely monitor diapers for urine output.
- Monitor for signs and symptoms of irritability, lethargy.
- Keep cardiology appointments.
- Continue diuretics.

ATRIAL SEPTAL DEFECT (ASD)

- Two septal walls fail to form (**Figure 12-8**).
- The septal walls normally close between weeks 4 and 8 of fetal development but may remain open up to 1 year (Ward & Hisley, 2009).
- More blood flows into the right side of the heart from the left atrium, and pulmonary blood flow to the lungs is increased through a hole in the atria.
- May result in pulmonary hypertension.
- Right atrial enlargement can lead to right ventricular hypertrophy.

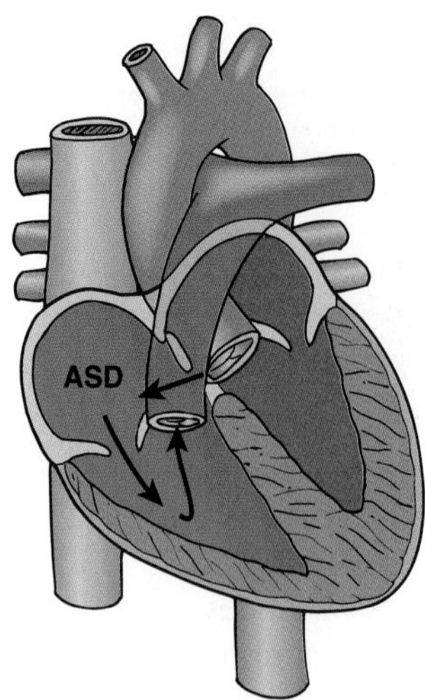

Figure 12-8 Atrial septal defect.

- A left-to-right mixing or shunting of blood may occur at the patent foramen ovale (PFO; a necessary fetal structure) or through the septal defect.
- Increased incidence of stroke in unrepaired atrial septal defects
- Fixed split second heart sound—due to right ventricular overload

Assessment

- Heart murmur
- Known as ejection systolic murmur due to blood being forced through pulmonary valve
- Atrial dysrhythmias
- Higher incidence of emboli
- Recurrent respiratory infections
- Few symptoms in children
- Shortness of breath
- Tires easily with playing
- Poor feeding
- Poor growth if CHF develops due to left-to-right shunting
- Liver enlargement or congestion (Karlsen & Tani, 2003)

Diagnostic Tests

- Echocardiogram shows enlargement of right atrium and right ventricle.
- EKG shows thickening of the heart muscle.
- Chest x-ray shows enlargement of the heart and an increase in blood flow to the lungs.
- Transesophageal ultrasound
- Maintain medications aimed at decreasing the load on the right side of the heart, such as digoxin and diuretics.
- Surgical closure may increase the incidence of pulmonary hypertension resulting in arrhythmias, and surgical patients may experience a higher mortality risk (Karlsen & Tani, 2003).
- Maintain pain medications.
- Closure with cardiac catheterization—transeptal closure across the defect

Nursing Intervention

- Monitor feeding tolerance; offer small frequent feedings with infants and small children.
- Monitor for signs and symptoms of CHF.
- Monitor for increased work of breathing, grunting, retractions, and flaring.
- Monitor growth patterns.

Caregiver Education

- Educate on care of the child following cardiac catheterization, which includes monitoring for bleeding at the catheter insertion site.
- Surgical closures with a patch may result in arrhythmias.
- Monitor for increase in temperature and changes in color or temperature of the catheterized extremity.
- The child may need to be on blood thinners for several months following the procedure.
- Educate on risk for embolization due to dislodgement of the patch.
- The child may need to be on antibiotics for dental work following treatment (Zipes, Libby, Bonow, & Braunwald, 2007).
- Monitor for cyanosis, poor weight gain, respiratory distress, lethargy, and bleeding at insertion site following the procedure.
- Maintain schedule of yearly close follow-ups with cardiologist.

VENTRICULAR SEPTAL DEFECT (VSD)

- Most common congenital heart disease (see **Figure 12-9**)
- Forms at weeks 4 to 8 of fetal development (Ward & Hisley, 2009)
- Right ventricular hypertrophy
- Left-to-right shunting (acyanosis) produces increase in pulmonary blood flow that decreases pulmonary compliance.
- Stiffening of the lungs and ineffective ventilation

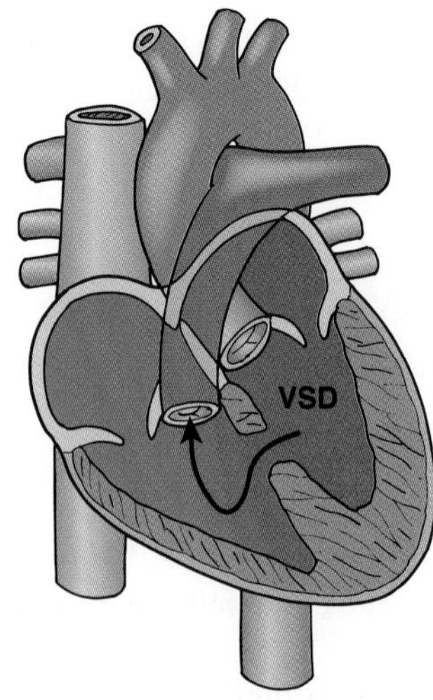

Figure 12-9 Ventricular septal defect.

Assessment

- Often asymptomatic or with a heart murmur
- Shortness of breath
- Feeding difficulties
- Murmur
- Systolic thrill in lower left sternal border
- Failure to thrive
- Recurrent respiratory infections (Ward & Hisley, 2009)

Diagnostic Testing

- Echocardiogram—large left atrium
- Chest x-ray—cardiomegaly of left heart and increased pulmonary vascularity
- Cardiac catheterization

Nursing Intervention

- Same as for atrial septal defect

Caregiver Education

- Similar to atrial septal defect
- Manage postoperative care.

> CLINICAL PEARL
>
> **Ventricular Septal Defects**
>
> In ventricular septal defects, chest x-rays can show the shunting of blood from the left ventricle into the right ventricle. Increased pulmonary blood flow is indicated by an increase in pulmonary vascular markings. The right ventricle of the heart will indicate hypertrophy and **cardiomegaly**, which is an abnormal enlargement of the heart.

CONGENITAL HEART DISEASE WITH DECREASED PULMONARY BLOOD FLOW

TETRALOGY OF FALLOT (TOF)

- Third most common lesion (What are congenital heart defects? n.d.)
- Nonductal cyanotic heart disease (**Figure 12-10**)
- Associated with 22 deletion chromosomes, DiGeorge and Down syndromes
- Occurs more in males than females (Allen et al., 2008)
- Results in a right-to-left type of shunting of blood in the heart, which recirculates venous blood to the body without it having gone to the lungs to be oxygenated.
- **Tetralogy**—"tetra" means *four,* and so this type of cyanotic heart disease has four separate defects within this one syndrome.
  - *Ventricular septal defect (VSD) between right and left ventricles*
  - *Obstructive right ventricular outflow—pulmonary stenosis or obstruction*
  - *Overriding aorta lies directly over VSD and takes blood from both the right and left ventricles; permits oxygenated blood to rest of body*
  - *Secondary thickening of right ventricle (right ventricular hypertrophy) due to restrictive outflow*

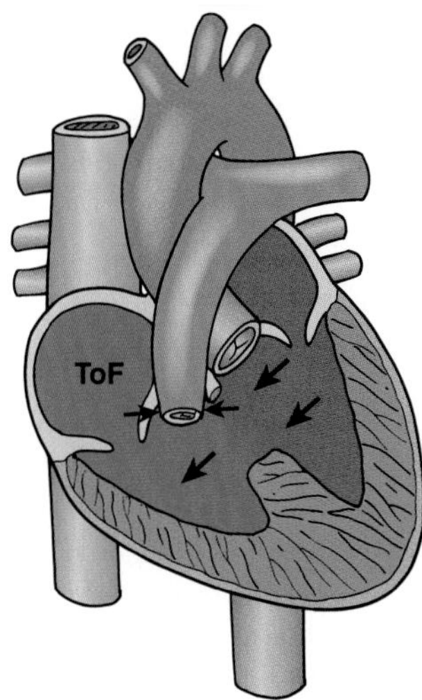

Figure 12-10 Tetralogy of Fallot.

Assessment

- Right-to-left shunting
- "Tet" spells—sudden, marked increase in cyanosis; syncope; can lead to hypoxic brain injury and death
- Pink "tet" spells are due to left-to-right shunting.
- Increased cyanosis with irritability and crying
- Increased irritability due to lack of oxygen
- Clubbing of fingers
- Poor growth is a response to chronic lack of oxygen.

> CLINICAL PEARL
>
> **"Tet" Spells**
>
> Children may squat during a tet spell to improve blood flow from legs back to brain and vital organs, increasing systemic vascular resistance (Bhimji, 2012).

Diagnostic Tests

- Present at birth or within first year of life
- Patent ductus arteriosus (PDA) causes increased blood flow to lungs
- Profound cyanosis is rare.
- Heart murmur may be soft to loud.
- Failure to gain weight
- Fainting
- Dyspnea on exertion
- Polycythemia

- Boot-shaped heart, right ventricular hypertrophy, and small pulmonary artery
- As PDA closes, cyanosis increases.
- Degree of cyanosis dependent on restriction of blood flow to lungs
- Child remains pink with a low degree of mixing; known as "pink tet" (Behrman et al., 2011).

Clinical Reasoning

Hyperoxygenation Test

The hyperoxygenation test is used to monitor the child's oxygenation level in response to being placed on 100% oxygen. Infant will not have respiratory distress and is unresponsive in terms of oxygenation with supplemental oxygen.

1. What is the physiological function of oxygen within the pulmonary vasculature?
2. How does a negative hyperoxygenation status indicate cardiac disease?

Nursing Interventions

- Improve oxygenation through clustering of care.
- Maintain sedative or morphine sulfate to decrease agitation.
- Prevent inconsolable crying.
- Maintain fluid balance.
- Provide oxygen to reduce pulmonary vasoconstriction, but note that this will not improve oxygen saturation or alleviate the cyanosis.
- Maintain vasopressors to increase systemic vascular resistance.
- Maintain prostaglandin E drip to keep PDA open (**Table 12-5**).
- Prepare family for possibility of multiple surgeries, such as modified Blalock-Taussig procedure.

Medication

Prostaglandin E

Prostaglandin E is a potent vasodilator on smooth muscle tissue that keeps open the foramen ovale and the ductus arteriosus. Action is within a few minutes and results in improved pulmonary and systemic blood flow. Nursing interventions include watching for respiratory depression or apnea, flushing, bradycardia, irritability, and diarrhea, and monitoring for bleeding. Dilatation is not specific to the smooth muscle tissue in the heart and occurs systemically. This drug needs to be administered by continuous infusion and requires a separate intravenous site (Deglan, Vallerand, & Sanoski, 2011).

TABLE 12–5 PROSTAGLANDIN E MEDICATION

DRUG	Prostaglandin (Alprostadil)
DOSAGE	Neonatal initial dose: 0.05–0.1 mcg/kg/min IV Maintenance dose: 0.01–0.4 mcg/kg/min IV Infuse IV into large vein or umbilical cord
ACTIONS	Relaxes smooth muscle of the ductus arteriosus, leading to increased pulmonary blood flow with increased blood oxygenation and lower body perfusion; increases Spo_2 and Pao_2
CONTRAINDICATIONS	Respiratory distress syndrome
PRECAUTIONS	Apnea, seizures, fever, hypotension, leukocytosis, fever, and pulmonary overcirculation Infants are usually intubated Prolonged use in hypoplastic left heart syndrome, third spacing: monitor blood oxygenation, arterial pressure

Source: Deglan, J. H., Vallerand, A. H., & Sanoski, C. A. (2011). *Davis's drug guide for nurses* (12th ed.). Philadelphia: F.A. Davis & Co.

Caregiver Education

- Teach the family to calm the infant by holding the infant over the caregiver's shoulders with the child's knees drawn up toward the child's chest.
- Support the caregiver's access to a pediatric cardiologist for the child's lifelong care.

TRICUSPID ATRESIA

- Rare heart condition
- Tricuspid valve is either defective or missing
- Blocks blood flow from right atrium to right ventricle; diminishes blood flow to the lungs
- If there is no VSD, then a PDA must be opened for the child to survive.

Assessment

- Cyanosis
- Shortness of breath
- Delayed growth and poor weight gain
- Murmur due to atrial septal defect that is usually present
- Often associated with pulmonary stenosis
- Clubbing of fingertips in older children

Diagnostic Tests

- Echocardiogram
- Electrocardiogram
- Chest x-ray
- Cardiac catheterization

Nursing Interventions

- Prepare patient for surgery.
- Prepare family for a series of corrective surgeries; Stage II surgery is the Glenn stage, and Stage III surgery is the Fontan procedure (Ward & Hisley, 2009).
- Prepare family for possibility of heart transplant procedure if needed.
- Maintain prostaglandin E1 drip to maintain blood flow to the lungs.

Caregiver Education

- Counsel family that child will need lifelong cardiology care.
- Inform caregivers that further surgeries may need to be performed.
- The child will need to transition to an adult cardiologist.
- Monitor for signs and symptoms of fluid retention, fast heart rate, and chronic diarrhea.
- Monitor for signs of shortness of breath, bluish skin color, or slow growth (Zipes et al., 2007).

EISENMENGER'S SYNDROME

- Occurs with PDA, VSD, or ASD
- Occurs as a result of a hole in the atria (ASD), where high pressures push nonoxygenated blood from right atria into the left atrium due to right ventricular hypertrophy, *or*
- Occurs as a result of a hole in the ventricles (VSD), which results in nonoxygenated blood being pushed into the left ventricle, bypassing the lungs.
- Increased pulmonary vascular resistance exceeds left ventricular pressure.
- Pulmonary hypertension with right-to-left shunting

Assessment

- Shortness of breath
- Fatigue
- Chest pain
- Cyanosis
- Increased red blood cell production

Diagnostic Tests

- Echocardiogram
- Chest x-ray

Nursing Interventions

- Maintain blood pressure control with hypertensive medications.
- Maintain anti-arrhythmics.
- Maintain pulmonary vascular dilation.
- Maintain anticoagulants.
- Prepare patient and family for bypass (ECHMO).

Caregiver Education

- Provide teaching related to treatment issues, such as bypass information.
- Prepare patient/caregiver for possible transfer to another facility for bypass treatment.

CONGENITAL HEART DISEASE WITH OBSTRUCTIVE DISORDERS

COARCTATION OF THE AORTA (COA)

- Narrowing of the aorta between the upper body and the lower extremities, usually distal to left subclavian artery (**Figure 12-11**)
- COA is usually distal to the carotid arteries. Classified as preductal, ductal, and postductal (Ward & Hisley, 2009).
- Increased blood pressure in the upper extremities and head
- Reduction of blood pressure in the lower extremities
- Abnormalities in renin-angiotensin-aldosterone mechanisms
- Aortic valve abnormalities often accompany this disorder.
- Associated with Turner's syndrome
- VSD is common.

Assessment

- Few symptoms
- Systolic ejection murmur

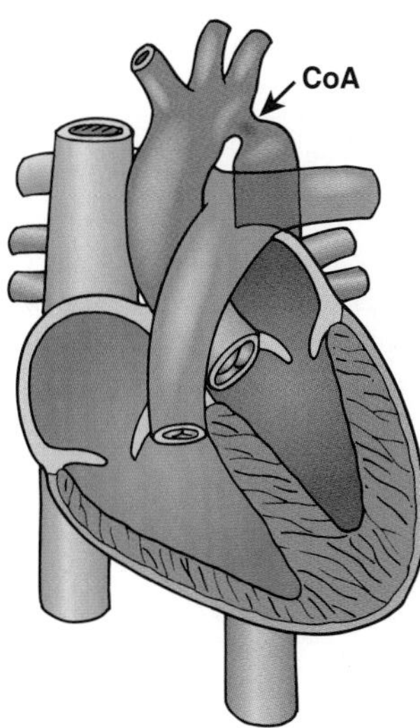

Figure 12-11 Coarctation of the aorta.

- Decreased femoral pulses
- Cardiomegaly and right-sided heart failure secondary to aortic constriction
- In adolescents, may present as hypertension.
- Headache
- Blood pressures are higher in the upper extremities than in the lower—blood pressure in lower extremities is >10 mm Hg less than in the upper extremities (Ward & Hisley, 2009).
- If necessary to check only one extremity, use the right arm with the lower extremity, which is preductal (Ward & Hisley, 2009).
- Hypertension
- Shortness of breath
- Poor feeding, growth, and development
- Signs and symptoms of CHF (Karlsen & Tani, 2003)

Diagnostic Tests

- Chest x-ray or esophagram will show "3 sign" or reverse 3 ("E sign") (Behrman et al., 2011), due to poststenotic dilatation of the aorta.
- Cardiac catheterization
- Rib notching may be present due to collateral vessels eroding the adjacent bones (Ward & Hisley, 2009).
- Balloon dilatation
- Stint placement

Nursing Interventions

- Monitor medications for CHF—Digoxin, Lasix.
- Monitor perfusion.
- Obtain four extremity blood pressures.
- Provide postsurgical care following cardiac catheterization or surgery with graft from a cadaver or resection.

Caregiver Education

- Continue to monitor blood pressure frequently.
- May need to restrict strenuous activity.
- Educate on bacterial endocarditis prevention.

> **CLINICAL PEARL**
>
> **Assessment of Pulses**
>
> Evaluation of pulses for coarctation of the aorta would demonstrate normal or elevated pulses in the upper extremities and decreased pulses in the lower extremities. It is important in this assessment that the right brachial artery be palpated, as the subclavian artery may be involved in giving a false reading on the left brachial artery (AHA, 2008c).

AORTIC STENOSIS

- Obstruction of blood flow from the left ventricle to the aorta, aortic regurgitation (**Figure 12-12**)

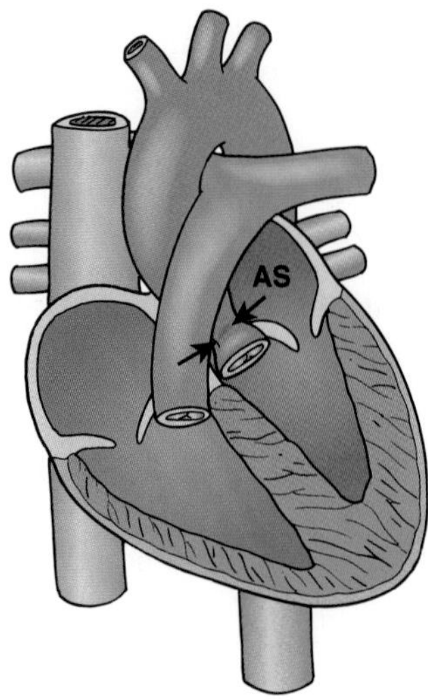

Figure 12–12 Aortic stenosis.

- Causes include valve stenosis or a narrowing of the aorta above the valve from age or congenital disease.
- Stenosis or narrowing increases the workload of the myocardium of the left ventricle, leading to hypertrophy.
- Scarring of the aortic valve occurs from rheumatic fever caused by group A *Streptococcus.*

Assessment

- Chest pain
- Fatigue
- Syncope
- Murmur—systolic ejection
- Shortness of breath
- Narrow pulse pressure with decrease in systolic pressures (Ward & Hisley, 2009)
- Exercise intolerance, which may result in sudden death
- Increased pressure load on left ventricle

Diagnostic Tests

- Electrocardiogram—thickening of the septum and mitral valve abnormalities
- EKG—inverted T waves
- Chest x-ray—cardiomegaly, dilated ascending aorta
- Cardiac catheterization
- Balloon valvuloplasty

Nursing Interventions

- Monitor for signs and symptoms of CHF.
- Prepare for emergency measures for atrial fibrillation.
- Provide caregiver teaching on procedures.
- Provide caregiver home-going teaching.
- Maintain pain management for chest discomfort.
- Maintain prostaglandin E drip to provide patent ductus arteriosus until surgery.

Caregiver Education

- Provide bacterial endocarditis information.

PULMONARY STENOSIS

- Defect in pulmonary artery or pulmonary valve (**Figure 12-13**)

Assessment

- Increased workload of right ventricle
- Congestive heart failure
- Hepatomegaly
- Often associated with other disorders, such as Noonan syndrome or tetralogy of Fallot
- Murmur
- Shortness of breath
- Cyanosis (Karlsen & Tani, 2003)

CLINICAL PEARL

Noonan Syndrome

Noonan syndrome is an autosomal dominant (chance is 1 out of 2) chromosomal defect that mimics Turner syndrome in the webbing of the neck and barrel-shaped chest wall (Rathnau-Minella, 2008).

Diagnostic Tests

- Echocardiogram
- Cardiac catheterization

Nursing Intervention

- Maintain nursing care following catheterization or surgical repair.
- Maintain calm environment to decrease oxygen requirements.
- Monitor blood pressure.

Caregiver Education

- The patient will be hospitalized and balloon angioplasty or valvuloplasty may be needed.
- The patient must return to cardiologist frequently for follow-up.
- Monitor for recurrence of symptoms due to restenosis.

PULMONARY ATRESIA

- Rare congenital defect where pulmonary valve or pulmonary artery does not form properly (**Figure 12-14**; Karlsen & Tani, 2003)
- Pulmonary atresia may also occur with ventricular septal defects and often is associated with patent ductus arteriosus (AHA, 2008b).
- In order to survive, the child must have a patent ductus arteriosus or patent foramen ovale.
- No known causes

Assessment

- Shortness of breath
- Severe cyanosis at birth
- Fatigue
- Tachypnea
- Poor feeding and weight gain

Diagnostic Tests

- Murmur associated with the VSD or PDA
- Electrocardiogram
- Echocardiogram

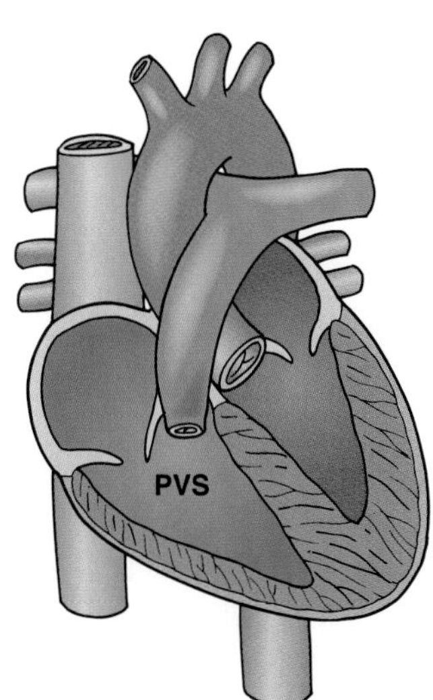

Figure 12–13 Pulmonary stenosis.

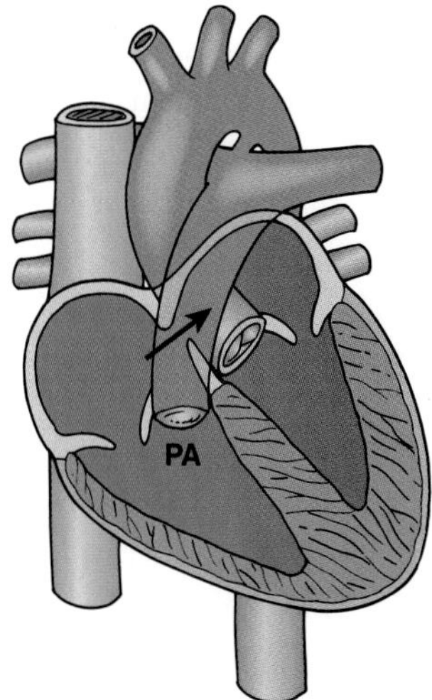

Figure 12–14 Pulmonary atresia.

- Chest x-ray
- Pulse oximeter
- Cardiac catheterization utilized to determine the atresia (Karlsen & Tani, 2003)

Nursing Interventions

- Maintain prostaglandin E drip (PGE1) to keep the ducts open and permit a mixing of the oxygenated and nonoxygenated blood.
- Provide postoperative stabilization if a balloon atrial septostomy is used to keep the foramen ovale open.
- Surgical care may be indicated following surgery (Fontan procedure) in order to repair or replace the valve, or a heart transplant may be necessary (Behrman et al., 2011).

TETRALOGY OF FALLOT WITH PULMONARY ATRESIA

- Occurs with chromosome arm 22q11 deletion (Karlsen & Tani, 2003)
- Associated with VATER syndrome
  - *V—vertebral anomalies*
  - *A—anal anomalies*
  - *T-E—tracheo-esophageal anomalies*
  - *R—renal anomalies (Behrman et al., 2011)*
- May result from maternal diabetes, maternal phenylketonuria, maternal ingestion of retinoic acid
- Symptomatic within a few hours of life
- Severe cyanosis after PDA closes
- In the arteriopulmonary collateral circulation, cyanosis is not as severe (Cavaliere, 2010).

Assessment

- Profound cyanosis
- Peripheral pulses and blood pressure stable until pulmonary blood flow results in bounding pulses
- Normal first heart sound, single second heart sound (Cavaliere, 2010)
- PDA murmur may be heard.
- Delayed growth and development

Diagnostic Tests

- Complete blood count, arterial blood gases
- Echocardiogram, electrocardiogram
- Cardiac catheterization with angiography
- Surgical repair with modified Blalock Taussig procedure and balloon dilatation of the stenotic pulmonary valve (Cavaliere, 2010)

Nursing Interventions

- Monitor for pain, hemorrhage, thrombospasms.
- Maintain oxygenation through monitoring of pulse oximetry (Cavaliere, 2010).
- Maintain hydration through strict intake and output.

Caregiver Education

- Explain importance of follow-up with pediatric cardiologist and the need for future procedures and catheterizations.
- Exercise capacity is limited.
- Maintain caloric intake.
- Monitor for signs and symptoms of heart failure.
- Educate on bacterial endocarditis prophylaxis.

CLINICAL PEARL

Nutrition Supplementation

Children who are in cardiac failure due to pulmonary overcirculation require specific nutritional supplementation in order to maintain sufficient weight gain. Caloric intake may require up to 150 kcal/kg/d (Pasini, Opasich, Pastoris, & Aquilani, 2006).

CONGENITAL HEART DISEASE WITH MIXED DISORDERS

TRANSPOSITION OF THE GREAT VESSELS

- The two great vessels of the aorta and pulmonary artery are reversed (**Figure 12-15**).
- Cyanotic blood flows to the brain, resulting in damage.
- Results in two separate circulatory systems—systemic and pulmonary—that do not mix.
- The aorta receives nonoxygenated blood from the right ventricle that then goes out to the systemic circulation without going to the lungs to become oxygenated.
- The pulmonary artery receives oxygenated blood from the left ventricle that then goes back to the lungs.

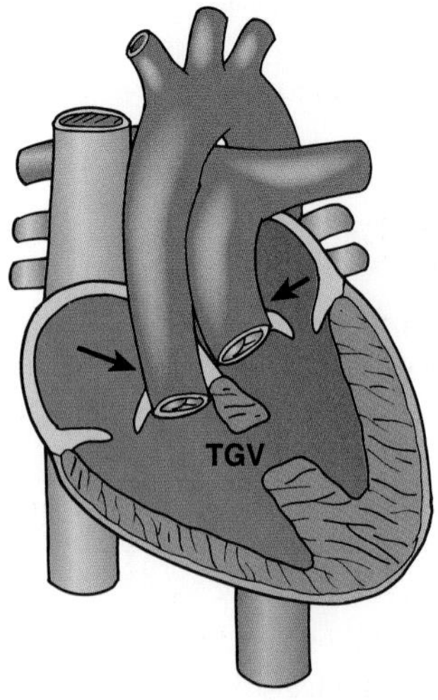

Figure 12-15 Transposition of the great vessels.

Assessment

- Upper extremity with a decreased oxygen saturation versus lower extremity, especially in right arm
- Profound cyanosis, especially with crying
- VSDs allow for mixing of blood.
- PDAs allow for mixing of blood.
- Tachypnea or quiet tachypnea
- Heart murmur
- Signs and symptoms of CHF (Karlsen & Tani, 2003)

Diagnostic Tests

- Negative hyperoxygenation test (ACoRN, 2009)
- Chest x-ray—"egg on a string" visualization, which may be absent in neonate (Ward & Hisley, 2009)
- Cardiac catheterization
- Echocardiogram

Nursing Interventions

- Maintain oxygen saturations in right arm >75% to decrease pulmonary vascular resistance (ACoRN, 2009).
- Maintain medications to treat CHF.
- Maintain fetal circulation through the use of medications.
- Maintain prostaglandin E drip.
- Monitor children placed on captopril/enalopril to relax the coronary arteries.
- Provide postoperative care following corrective Jatene arterial switch procedure.
- Provide postoperative care following Rashkind balloon atrial septastomy. (Karlsen & Tani, 2003)

Caregiver Education

- Patient will be hospitalized and atrial septostomy surgery will be performed to maintain mixing.
- Patient will need to return to cardiologist frequently for follow-up.

TRUNCUS ARTERIOSUS

- Incidence increases in children of women who are exposed to German measles or viral infections (**Figure 12-16**)
- Associated with DiGeorge syndrome or 22q11 (Karlsen & Tani, 2003)
- Associated with infants with Down syndrome, infants of diabetic mothers, and infants of mothers with excessive alcohol consumption during pregnancy (Karlsen & Tani, 2003)
- Complex cardiac anomaly with large VSD and a large single great vessel (truncus) arising over the right and left ventricle (Karlsen & Tani, 2003)
- Truncal valve is stenotic and incompetent.
- Large VSD is present.
- Three types depending upon origination

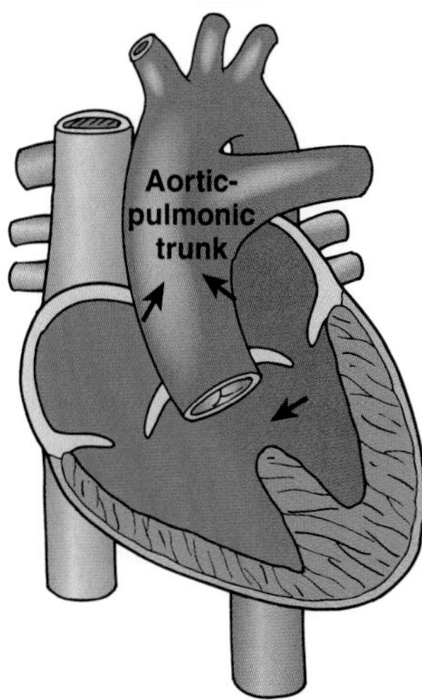

Figure 12-16 Truncus arteriosus.

Assessment

- Mixing of oxygenated and nonoxygenated blood—cyanosis
- Tachypnea
- Diaphoresis
- Increased blood flow leads to increased pulmonary congestion and CHF (Ward & Hisley, 2009).
- Wheezing, grunting, and retractions
- Wide pulse pressures
- Difficulty in feeding
- Loud pansystolic murmur (regurgitating murmur heard throughout systole) and single S_2 (Karlsen & Tani, 2003)

> CLINICAL PEARL
>
> **Pansystolic Murmur**
>
> A pansystolic murmur is turbulence that is heard throughout systole, from the first heart sound to the second heart sound. The sound is due to blood that is heard flowing between the right and left sides of the heart due to the differences in systolic pressures.

Diagnostic Tests

- Chest x-ray indicates enlarged heart with hazy lung fields.
- Echocardiogram shows a single vessel off of the right and left ventricles.
- Cardiac catheterization

Nursing Interventions

- Avoid supplemental oxygen, which decreases pulmonary vascular resistance and leads to excessive pulmonary blood flow (Karlsen & Tani, 2003).
- Monitor child closely with mechanical ventilation.

- Monitor invasive lines; provide inotropes to maximize cardiac function (Ward & Hisley, 2009).
- Maintain nutritional intake.
- Complex surgical repair involving separation of aorta and pulmonary artery with a VSD repair may be necessary.
- Maintain stabilization of vital signs and weaning of oxygen.

Caregiver Education

- Teach signs and symptoms of CHF.
- Educate on importance of follow-up appointments with cardiologist.
- Note that surgery dramatically improves outcomes.
- Monitor for signs and symptoms of tissue changes.

TOTAL ANOMALOUS PULMONARY VENOUS RETURN (TAPVR)

- In this condition all pulmonary veins with oxygen-rich blood follow an abnormal route back to the right atrium instead of the left atrium, making it difficult to distinguish between TAPVR and atrial septal defects (**Figure 12-17**; Karlsen & Tani, 2003).
- Nonobstructive and obstructive
- Three types: interruption occurs beyond left subclavian artery; interruption occurs between left carotid artery and left subclavian artery; or interruption occurs between innominate artery and left carotid artery (Karlsen & Tani, 2003).
- DiGeorge syndrome (Karslen & Tani, 2003)

Assessment

- While PDA is open, patient has few symptoms.
- When PDA closes, profound cyanosis, severe shock, and congestive heart failure result (Ward & Hisley, 2009).

Diagnostic Tests

- "Snowman sign" on chest x-ray (Ward & Hisley, 2009)
- Normal or small heart
- Pulmonary edema on x-ray
- Oxygen saturation levels
- Echocardiogram

Nursing Interventions

- Maintain airway management.
- Maintain strict intake and output; maintain diuretics for CHF.
- Monitor arterial blood gases.
- Provide postsurgical care related to valvular repair.

Caregiver Education

- Educate caregiver on signs and symptoms of restricted blood flow due to continued stenosis (Ward & Hisley, 2009).
- Educate on importance of long-term follow-up with pediatric cardiologist.

HYPOPLASTIC LEFT HEART

- Second most common congenital heart defect (**Figure 12-18**; Karlsen & Tani, 2003)
- Underdeveloped left side of the heart, aorta, aortic valve, left ventricle, and mitral valve leads to pulmonary venous congestion and edema.
- As PDA is open, blood is reaching aorta through this duct.
- Symptoms appear when PDA closes.
- Often associated with absence of corpus callosum (Karlsen & Tani, 2003)

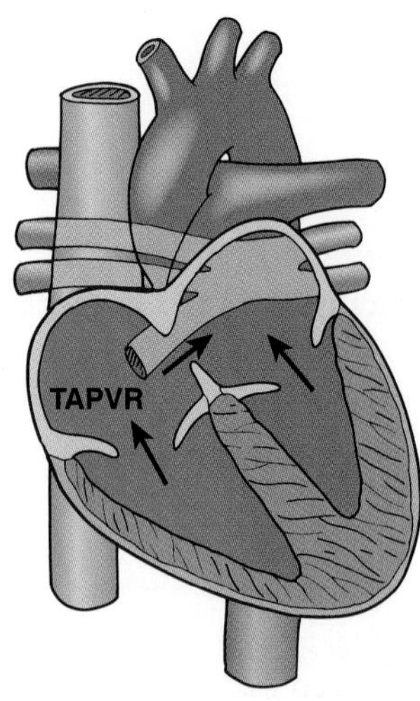

Figure 12–17 Total anomalous pulmonary venous return (TAPVR).

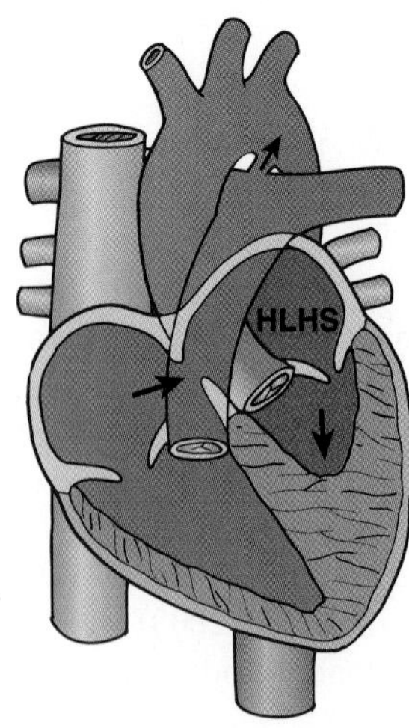

Figure 12–18 Hypoplastic left heart syndrome.

Assessment

- Asymptomatic until ducts close
- Skin ashen in color
- Rapid and difficult breathing
- Difficulty feeding (ACoRN, 2009)
- Usually fatal within the first days or months or life unless treated

Diagnostic Tests

- As PDA closes, baby will become very dusky and ashen.
- Single S_2, gallop (Karlsen & Tani, 2003)
- Echocardiogram
- Chest x-ray

Nursing Interventions

- Maintain prostaglandin E infusion to keep PDA open.
- Provide nursing preparation for surgery—Norwood three-stage procedure to increase ventricular function (Karlsen & Tani, 2003).
- Provide caregiver preparation for severity of condition.
- Anticipate possible transport out of the facility for heart transplant.

Caregiver Education

- Surgical correction or transplantation
- Lifelong follow-up with pediatric cardiologist
- Long-term heart medications
- Bacterial endocarditis protocols (Allen et al., 2008)

EBSTEIN ANOMALY

- Rare defect (**Figure 12-19**)
- Increased incidence with maternal lithium use
- Displacement of the tricuspid valve into right ventricle

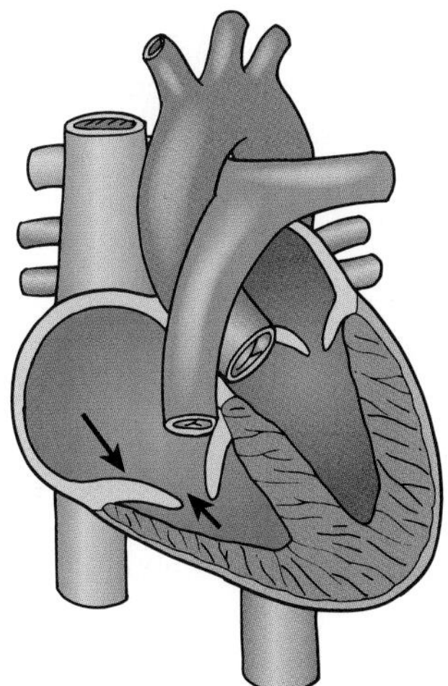

Figure 12-19 Ebstein anomaly.

- Enlarged right atrium and cardiomegaly
- Associated with other congenital heart defects and arrhythmias, such as atrial septal defect, Wolf-Parkinson-White syndrome (cardiac arrhythmia) (Behrman et al., 2011).
- Anomaly is present at birth, but if minor, symptoms may not appear until the child is a teenager or an adult.

Assessment

- Mild to severe cyanosis related to incompetence of tricuspid valve and the blood flow to the lungs
- Often no murmur
- Hepatomegaly
- Splenomegaly
- Feeding problems
- Patient may need immediate surgery.
- A gallop heart murmur may be heard.

Diagnostic Tests

- Chest x-ray will show enlarged, balloon-shaped heart.
- Decreased pulmonary vascular markings
- May predispose child to electrical conduction issues from right atrium to the right ventricle through the bundle of Kent
- Results in increased incidence of Wolf-Parkinson-White (WPW) syndrome and supraventricular tachycardia (SVT) dysrhythmias.
- Cardiac catheterization for conclusive diagnosis (Abdallah, 2008)

Nursing Interventions

- Maintain stabilization of the child's vital signs.
- Maintain prostaglandin E to improve oxygenation through the ducts.
- Maintain the infant on oxygen.
- Maintain inotropes such as Dopamine or Dobutamine to increase blood pressure.
- Prepare patient/caregiver for surgery on an emergent basis—Fontan procedure or transplant

Caregiver Education

- The earlier the symptoms present, the greater the long-term consequences for the child.
- Close monitoring by cardiologist is necessary.
- Depending upon leaky valve, the child may be restricted during sports.

ACQUIRED CONGENITAL HEART DISEASE

CARDIOMYOPATHY

- Chronic progressive disease occurring within the heart muscle itself (primary) or a result of another disease or toxin that affects all organs, including the heart (Behrman et al., 2011)

- Three types: dilated, hypertrophic, restrictive
  - *Dilated or congested—enlarged heart, weak and ineffective pump*
    - Most common form
    - Carnitine deficiency
    - Develop heart failure
    - Blood clots due to slow blood flow
    - Dysrhythmias
  - *Hypertrophic—most common inherited heart defect in the absence of other cardiac disease with left ventricle enlarged; found in infants of diabetic mothers, Noonan's and Pompe's syndromes (Karlsen & Tani, 2003)*
    - Enlarged heart
    - Diastolic dysfunction
    - Exercise intolerance
    - Fainting
    - Leaking valves due to increase septal and ventricle muscle
  - *Restrictive—heart muscle becomes rigid and fails to relax; most rare type*
    - Diastolic dysfunction
    - Fatigue
    - Shortness of breath
- Ventricles primarily affected and become enlarged, thickened, and stiff
- Child is born with normal heart anatomy.
- Heart muscle loses the ability to pump effectively; heart failure and cardiac arrhythmias occur (Behrman et al., 2011).
- Cardiomyopathy is not gender, race, or geographically dependent.
- This is the leading cause of heart transplants in children despite being relatively rare. Causes include:
  - *Chemotherapy*
  - *Viral infections such as Coxsackie-B*
  - *Genetic factors—fatty acid oxidation*
  - *Metabolic disorders (Behrman et al., 2011)*
  - *Persistent rhythm abnormalities*

Assessment

- Congestive heart failure
- Sweating with feedings
- Dizziness
- Weight loss
- Murmur—gallop
- Hepatomegaly with venous congestion
- Fatigue
- Frequent colds, pneumonia
- Dysrhythmias

Diagnostic Tests

- Murmur
- Chest x-ray shows thickening of the cardiac musculature and enlargement.
- Electrocardiogram indicates the degree of enlargement.
- Echocardiogram reveals right- or left-sided enlargement.
- Cardiac catheterization
- Cardiac dysrhythmias

Nursing Interventions

- During acute phase: Maintain intravenous fluids, endotracheal intubation, ventilator, ECMO-artificial heart–lung machine, diuretics, and anticoagulation therapy (Behrman et al., 2011).
- Maintain ACE inhibitors that have positive inotropic properties; they inhibit the chemical angiotensin, which constricts arteries (Behrman et al., 2011).
- Provide valve replacement therapy postoperative.
- Provide heart transplant care if warranted.
- Chronic phase: Anticipate major complications that can include arrhythmias and CHF.
- Anticipate tachycardias (fast heart rates) or bradycardias (slow heart rates).
- Monitor for tachycardias which can develop into fibrillation
- Provide nutritional supplementation with carnitine.
- Monitor children placed on ACE inhibitors, Captopril/enalopril to relax the coronary arteries (Behrman et al., 2011).
- Maintain diuretics except for hypertrophic cardiomyopathy (Zipes et al., 2007).
- Monitor children on Lasix/Aldactone to reduce excess fluid in the lungs.
- Monitor children on Digoxin, which is used to improve cardiac function in those children with a dilated cardiomyopathy by enhancing the pumping effort of the heart (Zipes et al., 2007).
- Digoxin or Verapamil should not be considered for treating sustained tachycardia until ventricular tachycardia has been ruled out (Behrman et al., 2011).
- Monitor children on beta blockers or calcium channel blockers for blood pressure control.
- Monitor for bradycardias when the conduction is interrupted or totally blocked and the child may need to have a pacemaker.
- Monitor for thromboembolus, which may occur due to interrupted blood flow (Zipes et al., 2007).
- An internal cardioverter/defibrillator (ICD) is capable of shocking life-threatening arrhythmias (Zipes et al., 2007).
- Critical patients—those with irreversible heart damage and persistent poor function—may require a heart transplant.

Caregiver Education

- Aimed at the intensive care necessary for a child with a life-threatening condition
- Possible terminal status of the child
- Frequent echocardiograms to monitor size and function of the heart
- Psychological as well as physical preparation
- Activity restrictions to prevent overstimulation of the heart

Evidence-Based Practice Research: Implanting Internal Cardioverter/Defibrillator

ACC/AHA/ESC 2006 guidelines for management of patients with ventricular arrhythmias and the prevention of sudden cardiac death. A report of the American College of Cardiology/American Heart Association Task Force and the European Society of Cardiology Committee for Practice Guidelines (Writing Committee to Develop Guidelines for Management of Patients With Ventricular Arrhythmias and the Prevention of Sudden Cardiac Death). Retrieved from: http://cmbi.bjmu.edu.cn/news/report/2010/cv_gd/77.htm

Implantation of ICDs in pediatric survivors of cardiac arrest is appropriate when a thorough search for a correctable cause is negative and the patient is receiving optimal medical therapy with an expectation of survival for more than a year. Pharmacological and ICDs are appropriate for sustained ventricular dysrhythmias.

http://www.americanheart.org

- Allow the child to discuss feelings, such as concerning the restriction of activity in the previously active child.
- Encourage participation in cardiomyopathy programs (Zipes et al., 2007).
- Active grieving of the parents is expected in this life-threatening situation.

CLINICAL PEARL

Medications for Attention Deficit-Hyperactivity Disorder (ADHD)

The Pediatric Drug Advisory in 2006 issued a Black Box warning to be applied to ADHD medications for children with structural defects, cardiomyopathy, or heart rhythm disorders who are administered these medications and may be at risk for sudden death (AHA, 2008a). Joint statements by the American Academy of Pediatrics and the American Heart Association show that children with heart conditions have a higher incidence of ADHD but that medications used to treat ADHD have not been shown in most cases to cause heart disease or result in sudden cardiac death (American Academy of Pediatrics, 2008).

Medication

Digoxin

- Daily dosing for children with normal renal function
- Ages 2 to 5: 10 to 15 micrograms/kilogram
- Ages 7 to 10: 7 to 10 micrograms/kilogram
- Over age 10: 3 to 5 micrograms/kilogram
- Be aware of the child's baseline parameters, including peripheral pulse, blood pressure, and heart rate.
- Administer 1 hour before or 2 hours after meals; if child vomits dose, do not repeat dose.
- Take apical pulse for a full minute. Hold if pulse is below 60 beats/minute or above 100 beats/minute.
- Note rate, rhythm, and quality. If changes occur, take an electrocardiogram and notify the physician.
- Monitor baseline and periodic ongoing potassium, magnesium, and calcium levels.
- Monitor for signs and symptoms of digoxin toxic effects, including anorexia, nausea, vomiting, diarrhea, and visual disturbances.
- Closely monitor for digoxin toxicity with antibiotic therapy due to changes in intestinal flora.
- Monitor for intake and output in patients with renal disorders (Deglan et al., 2011).

Promoting Safety

Caregiver education for administration of digoxin includes:

- Administer medication at the same time every day and at the correct frequency. Do not double up for a missed dose.
- Notify your physician for >2 pounds per day.
- Notify your physician for advice before administering any over-the-counter medications.
- Do not breastfeed without contacting your physician if you are taking this medication (Deglan et al., 2011).

CONGESTIVE HEART FAILURE (CHF)

- The heart cannot supply enough oxygenated blood to meet the metabolic needs of the body tissues either at rest or work (Ward & Hisley, 2009).
- The heart may fail with high afterloads (COA, AS), valvular regurgitation, or impaired myocardial contractility, as in cardiomyopathy.
- Right-sided heart failure—right ventricle cannot pump blood into the pulmonary artery, resulting in increased pressure in the right atrium and the systemic venous system.
- Left-sided heart failure—blood is backed into the left atrium and the pulmonary veins, resulting in increased lung congestion.
- CHF in pediatric patients with congenital heart disease (CHD) will depend on whether the child has a ductal-dependent lesion, which will most likely present with cyanosis in the newborn period as the ducts begin to close.
- Left-to-right shunting such as in ventricular septal defects may not show CHF until several weeks following birth as a result of chronic pulmonary edema (Everitt & Yetman, 2008).

Assessment

- Edema of the face, hands, and feet, or weight gain
- Cardiac enlargement
- Gallop rhythm
- Tachypnea
- Shortness of breath
- Fatigue
- Poor appetite

- Poor growth
- Sweating with minimal activity

Diagnostic Tests

- History and physical examination
- Chest x-ray indicates an enlarged heart, increase in pulmonary vascularity, and edema.
- Echocardiogram defines anatomy and physiology.
- Electrocardiogram indicates an enlarged atrium.
- Urine and blood tests evaluate blood gas, anemia, and electrolyte balance.

Nursing Interventions

- Maintain oxygenation by elevating the head of the bed.
- Decrease oxygen consumption.
- Monitor intake and output.
- Monitor breath sounds.
- Provide supplemental oxygen.

Caregiver Education

- Surgery may need to be performed for CHD.
- Provide discharge instructions on observation for tachypnea and increased work of breathing.
- Maintain diuretics as ordered (see **Table 12-6** for common diuretics).
- Avoid high-salt-content foods.
- Monitor weight.
- Elevate the head of the bed.
- Provide frequent rest periods.

HYPERLIPIDEMIA

- High potential risk factor for cardiovascular disease
- High concentrations of low-density lipoprotein (LDL) and low concentrations of high-density lipoprotein (HDL)
- May be present early in life

TABLE 12–6 DIURETICS USED TO TREAT CONGESTIVE HEART FAILURE

Action Administer in the Morning	Nursing Interventions	Family/Caregiver Education
SPIRONOLACTONE (ALDACTONE) Potassium-sparing diuretic antagonizes aldosterone receptors of distal convoluted tubule (DCT)	Monitor kidney function with strict intake and output (I&O); watch for alterations in potassium level	Notify physician if child develops diarrhea, vomiting, or signs of dehydration Give missed dose as soon as discovered Do not double up on the doses
HYDROCHLOROTHIAZIDE (DIURIL) Inhibits carbonic anhydrase in the (DCT) Inhibits the cotransport of sodium (Na) and chloride (Cl), thus decreasing sodium chloride (NaCl) reabsorption from the kidneys	Give with meals to prevent gastric upset	Avoid exposure to sunlight Take with food Notify physician if child is dehydrated; vomiting and diarrhea Avoid NSAIDs, as they decrease the effectiveness of this drug Administer medication in the morning
FUROSEMIDE (LASIX) Loop diuretic—acts mainly by inhibiting Na reabsorption in the nephron at the thick ascending limb of Henle's loop	Monitor electrolyte levels, especially potassium; monitor for ototoxicity; may develop renal calculi with prolonged use	May be instructed to feed foods that are high in potassium, such as bananas Give with food—if given once a day, give with breakfast; if twice a day, give at evening meal but not close to bedtime to prevent the need for repeated bathroom trips Report signs of dehydration, allergic responses, shortness of breath
BUMETANIDE-BUMEX Loop diuretic—acts mainly by inhibiting Na reabsorption in the nephron at the thick ascending limb of Henle's loop	Monitor for electrolyte imbalances, especially potassium; may potentiate ototoxic drugs such as aminoglycosides	Report signs of dehydration, vomiting, and diarrhea Avoid exposure to sun May be instructed to feed foods high in potassium, such as bananas

Source: Deglan, J. H., Vallerand, A. H., & Sanoski, C. A. (2011). *Davis's drug guide for nurses* (12th ed.). Philadelphia: F.A. Davis & Co.

- Comorbid with high blood pressure, type I or II diabetes, smoking, overweight, and inactivity
- National Cholesterol Education Program (NCEP) guidelines indicate that if the pediatric patient's LDLs are greater than or equal to 130 mg/dl, the patient has an increased risk of complications resulting from hyperlipidemia (Daniels & Greer, 2008).

CLINICAL PEARL

Screening for Hyperlipidemia

The American Academy of Pediatrics recommends screening children when there is a family history of high cholesterol or premature cardiac disease, combined with at least one major risk factor such as childhood obesity (O'Riordan, 2010).

- Dietary and behavioral changes are necessary for long-term benefits in reduction of cholesterol and prevention of complications.
- The American Heart Association's Step 2 diet recommends 20% fat, of which 7% of this would be saturated fat (AHA, 2008c).
- A limit of 200 mg per day of cholesterol is also recommended.
- Dietary recommendations will only decrease the cholesterol levels by a small percentage.
- Controllable factors need to be addressed throughout life: weight, smoking, hypertension, and inactivity.
- Noncontrollable factors are hereditary factors that significantly impact the incidence of hyperlipidemia.
- Treatment is aimed at controlling manageable factors and the use of statins and niacin for hereditary factors.

Evidence-Based Practice Research: Lipid Screening

Daniels, S. R., & Greer, F. R. (2008). Lipid screening and cardiovascular health in childhood. *Pediatrics, 122,* 198–208. doi: 10.1542/peds.2008-1349

Lipid screening is recommended for:

- All children and adolescents with a positive family history of dyslipidemia
- Overweight children, regardless of family history
- Children who are hypertensive ≥95%
- Patients with diabetes mellitus
- Patients who are 8 or older with an LDL ≥190 mgm/dL (Daniels & Greer, 2008)

HYPERTENSION

- Blood pressure is dependent upon the child's age, gender, and weight.
- Systolic blood pressure in infants is between 70 and 90 mm Hg; adolescents reach adult levels.
- Blood pressure is the force of the blood hitting against the artery walls during contraction of the heart (systole) and during relaxation of the heart (diastole).
- Routine monitoring should begin around age 3.
- Diagnosis of hypertension is not made from one reading.
- Hypertension is diagnosed when blood pressure is >95% for age, weight, height, and sex (Allen et al., 2008).

CLINICAL PEARL

Blood Pressure Percentiles

- Normal blood pressure (BP): less than 90th percentile
- Prehypertension: 90th to 95th percentile with a BP of 120 mm Hg
- Stage I hypertension: 95th to 99th percentile +5 mm Hg
- Stage II hypertension: >99th percentile +5 mm Hg
- "White coat" hypertension is when BP is >95th percentile in the doctor's office but is normal outside the doctor's office (Brookes, 2008).

- Primary hypertension—patient is usually less than 10 years of age; is a disease of exclusion.
- Secondary hypertension—daytime diastolic blood pressure elevations and nighttime blood pressure elevations. May indicate renal or organ involvement.
- Risk factors include genetic causes, obesity, and secondary hypertension issues related to renal perfusion or structural anomalies.
- Syndrome X is the triad of insulin resistance, hypertension, and hyperlipidemia. In recent years this has resulted in a dramatic increase in obesity in young patients.
- Systolic and diastolic BPs are preferred measurements used to diagnose hypertension.
- True BP is measured over a duration.
- Monitor for correct position for BP reading: seated, relaxed, uncrossed arms and legs (Knoerl, 2007).

CULTURAL AWARENESS: Hereditary Risk Factors for Hispanic Americans

Hereditary factors related to heart disease, hypertension, and stroke are the number one killers of Hispanic Americans (AHA, 2008b).

Assessment

- The left side of the heart works harder and may thicken.
- Hypertension can result in stroke and often affects the child's vision due to increased pressure in the blood vessels of the eye.

CULTURAL AWARENESS: Metabolism of Antihypertensive Medications

Racial differences are associated with enzyme polymorphisms in the metabolism of antihypertensives. Nurses should consider the risks for impaired drug metabolism for hypertension based on ethnic or racial affiliation (Kudzma, 2004).

Diagnostic Tests

- Monitored at well-child visits

Clinical Reasoning

Obesity and Hypertension

Obesity is the number one risk factor in the development of hypertension.

1. What is the DASH eating plan?
2. What other risk factors can be modified in the hypertensive child?

Nursing Interventions

- Aim is for reduction of the blood pressure to <95% and resolution of end-organ dysfunction.
- Encourage a routine exercise plan.
- Encourage weight loss if indicated.
- Educate the patient/caregiver on healthy meal choices with lower intake of salt, saturated fat, trans-fatty acids, cholesterol, and carbohydrates, and increased dietary fiber intake.
- Emergency treatment of acute hypertension is the administration of labetalol (0.1 mg/kg) (Deglan et al., 2011).
- Chronic hypertension is usually treated with ACE inhibitors.

CULTURAL AWARENESS: Hot and Cold Theory

Many Hispanics adhere to the hot and cold theory. It is believed that too much exposure to hot or cold results in illness. Hypertension is considered a hot condition (Knoerl, 2007). (See Chapter 4 for further cultural factors.)

RHEUMATIC HEART DISEASE

- Damage to the heart valves
- Systemic inflammatory disease that follows in response to a group A beta-hemolytic streptococcal infection, such as strep throat or scarlet fever, that starts in the throat and if left untreated spreads into bloodstream, usually 20 days after the onset of the illness (Ward & Hisley, 2009).
- If untreated, can lead to bacterial or fungi clumps that can break off and travel to the lungs, brain, kidneys, or other organs.
- Antibodies are produced in response to the organism, and lesions develop in the heart and joints.
- The disease is familial.
- Occurs in lower-socioeconomic situations between the ages of 5 and 15 (Ward & Hisley, 2009)
- Prevalent in the northeastern part of the United States in winter and early spring

Assessment

- Abdominal pain
- Nosebleeds
- Chest pain and heart palpitations
- Waking from sleep with the need to sit or stand up (paroxysmal nocturnal dyspnea)

Diagnostic Tests

- Jones Criteria—first established in 1944 and continually updated. States that there must be two of the major criteria or one of the major and two of the minor criteria present with a streptococcal infection (Special Writing Group of the Committee on Rheumatic Fever, Endocarditis, and Kawasaki Disease of the Council on Cardiovascular Disease in the Young of the American Heart Association, 1992).
  - *Major criteria include symptoms such as polyarthritis, carditis, subcutaneous nodules, nonpruritic ring rash on the trunk or arms, and involuntary nonpurposeful movements known as St. Vitus Dance (Special Writing Group of the Committee on Rheumatic Fever, Endocarditis, and Kawasaki Disease of the Council on Cardiovascular Disease in the Young of the American Heart Association, 1992).*
  - *Minor criteria include a history of rheumatic heart disease, increase in C-reactive protein, low-grade fever less than 99°C, and evidence of heart block (Special Writing Group of the Committee on Rheumatic Fever, Endocarditis, and Kawasaki Disease of the Council on Cardiovascular Disease in the Young of the American Heart Association, 1992).*
- Physical assessment
- Blood tests for the presence of exposure to strep infection
- Electrocardiogram
- Echocardiogram
- Enlarged heart and CHF per chest x-ray

Nursing Interventions

- Maintain administration of inflammatory medications and antibiotics.
- Prepare child for admission to hospital and or surgery.
- Provide detailed education to family regarding prevention, treatment, and reoccurrence of symptoms.

Caregiver Education

- Educate families on the screening of school-age children for sore throats.
- Educate families on the need for completion of antibiotic regimen or prophylaxis as ordered.
- Prepare caregiver for possible hospitalization or heart valve surgery.
- Encourage regular check-ups with cardiologist.
- Encourage immunizations and the annual flu shot.
- Provide education related to prophylaxis antibiotic therapy for dental work.

Evidence-Based Practice Research: Dental Procedures for Children with Heart Disease

American Heart Association. (2007). Prevention of infective endocarditis. Retrieved from http://www.circ.ahajournals.org/cgi/content/full/116/15/1736

If a child requires dental work and has congenital heart disease, a 2007 position statement issued by the American Heart Association recommends prophylactic antibiotics for all dental procedures that involve manipulation of gingival tissue or perforation of the oral mucosa.

SUBACUTE BACTERIAL ENDOCARDITIS

- Can be infective or noninfective
- The endocardium of the heart becomes inflamed with *Viridans streptococcus*, *Streptococcus mutans*, *Streptococcus sanguis*, or *Staphyloccocus*.
- Bacteria or fungi that have entered the body through the mouth, respiratory system, or bloodstream invade and attach themselves to damaged areas of the endocardium.
- Damaged areas of the endocardium allow the bacteria or fungi to easily attach and multiply.
- Healthy hearts do not develop endocarditis, but those patients with damaged heart valves or heart valves are more susceptible (Behrman et al., 2011).
- Entry of organisms can occur with simple cuts, dental work, teeth brushing, respiratory infections, or catheters that are introduced into the body.
- Endocarditis can be life threatening.

Assessment

- Fever
- Fatigue
- Cough
- Heart murmur
- Chills
- Shortness of breath
- Joint pain
- Weight loss
- Flank pain
- Petechiae

Diagnostic Tests

- History and physical examination
- Can mimic other infections
- Blood cultures
- Roth spots—round or oval white spots sometimes seen in the retina in the early stages
- Janeway lesions—flat, painless, red to bluish-red spots on palms and soles of feet (Zipes et al., 2007)
- Osler nodes—painful, red, raised lesions on the palms and soles due to immune complex (Zipes et al., 2007)
- Black lines—splinter-like bits under the nails (Zipes et al., 2007)
- Complete blood count
- Echocardiogram
- Transesophageal echocardiogram—to assess valvular function or vegetation growth

Nursing Interventions

- If untreated, can lead to bacterial or fungi clumps that can break off and travel to the lungs, brain, kidneys, or other organs.
- Monitor for stroke, poor pumping action.
- Maintain intensive antibiotic therapy.
- Monitor for fluid imbalances due to nausea, vomiting, and diarrhea from antibiotics.
- Monitor for CHF symptoms such as shortness of breath, poor weight gain, and edema.
- Monitor for valve failures and cardiac failure.
- Monitor for septic emboli to the lungs.
- Prepare patient for transplanted valves.

Caregiver Education

- High-risk patients with past valve damage, repairs, or defects are at an increased risk and may be treated with prophylactic antibiotics.
- Prepare caregiver for possibility of surgery for valvular replacement.
- Maintain dental health through regular checkups starting as soon as the child's teeth begin to erupt.

KAWASAKI DISEASE

- Also called mucocutaneous lymph node syndrome
- Infantile polyarthritis nodosa results in acute febrile inflammation of the vasculature (Ward & Hisley, 2009).
- Can lead to coronary artery aneurysm
- Leading cause of acquired heart disease in children in the developed world (Behrman et al., 2011)
- Primarily affects children under the age of 5, with peak incidence in children less than 2 years of age (Ward & Hisley, 2009)
- Disease is thought to be due to an infectious organism.
- Mortality in children is based on scarring, stenosis of the main coronary arteries, or myocardial infarction due to coronary thrombosis.
- Not contagious, but is often seen in certain geographic locations and seasonally, with a higher incidence in late winter and early spring
- Often mirrors other infectious diseases such as measles and scarlet fever

Assessment

- Kawasaki disease diagnosis is a diagnosis of exclusion.
- Signs and symptoms that last longer than 5 days include high fever >38.5°C, plus a minimum of four of the clustered symptoms shown in the following Clinical Pearl box.

CLINICAL PEARL

Symptoms of Kawasaki Disease

- Bilateral conjunctivitis
- Painful joints
- Red lips, strawberry tongue, congested oral pharynx
- Enlarged lymph nodes—cervical lymphadenopathy (one lymph node >1.5cm) (Gopinath, Gangadhara, Sadagopan, & Gnanapragasam, 2007)
- Nonspecific groin rash
- Edematous and red hands and feet
- Mimics scarlet fever rash—diffuse polymorphous rash
- Increased white blood cell count
- Extreme irritability
- Cardiac involvement—myocarditis, pericarditis, coronary artery aneurysm, valvular regurgitation, systemic artery aneurysms (Brogan et al., 2002)

Diagnostic Tests

- Diagnosis is through exclusion, as it often mimics other diseases such as scarlet fever, toxic shock syndrome, infectious mononucleosis, and mycoplasma.
- Initial lab results will indicate an increased white blood cell count.
- Lymphocytosis and thrombocytosis
- High fever that is not resolved with antibiotics or antipyretic therapy
- A life-threatening complication of Kawasaki's disease is the development of coronary artery aneurysms.
- A baseline echocardiogram is needed to rule out coronary artery aneurysms.
- Echocardiogram 6 to 8 weeks following the onset of symptoms
- Complications include myocarditis, pericarditis, leaking of the valves, pericardial effusion, and CHF.
- Myocardial infarction occurs in 73% of children within the first year of diagnosis (Brogan et al., 2002).
- Neurologic complications can occur, as well as gastrointestinal complications such as hydrops of the gallbladder (Brogan et al., 2002).

Nursing Interventions

- Maintain anti-inflammatory medications such as high-dose salicylate therapy, which can also be continued for 6 to 8 weeks as an anti-platelet therapy.
- Intravenous gamma globulin is given for the first 10 days after the onset of the symptoms to prevent coronary aneurysms.
- Monitor the child's cardiac status closely for signs and symptoms of CHF.
- Nursing care is aimed at symptom relief (AHA, 2010).

Caregiver Education

- Encourage professional intervention in an infant or child with unresolved fever.
- Kawasaki disease is usually self-limiting.

Promoting Safety

Caregiver education for safety includes:

- Loose clothing
- Cool cloths
- Lip and mouth care
- Clear liquids that are tepid and soft foods to minimize irritation of the oral mucosa
- Parental support for inconsolable child
- Discharge teaching aimed at understanding the progression of the disease
- Prolonged irritability
- Peeling of hands and feet
- Arthritis of weight-bearing joints—stretching and passive range of motion
- Defer live immunizations such as measles, mumps, rubella, chickenpox
- Educate on lifelong possibility of development of cardiac disease.
- Cardiopulmonary resuscitation training (Gopinath et al., 2007)

TOXIC SHOCK SYNDROME

- Rare, life-threatening disease
- Toxins or bacteria induced
- Overstimulation of the immune system
- *Staphylococcus* and *Streptococcus* primary bacteria

Assessment

Symptoms include:

- High fever
- Rash
- Hypotension
- Multisystem organ failure
- Any skin wound, including chickenpox

Diagnostic Tests

- None specific to the disease
- Complete blood count, blood cultures, electrolytes, vital signs
- Chest x-ray

Nursing Interventions

- Maintain intake and output.
- Maintain pain relief.
- Support patient/caregiver.

Caregiver Education

- Call the doctor with high fever, red flat rash, severe nausea and vomiting.
- Take child to hospital if the child is confused or fainting.

> **CLINICAL PEARL**
>
> **Toxic Shock and Tampons**
>
> Always ask the pubescent child if she is menstruating as a screening tool. Toxic shock may develop with the use of tampons that have been left in place for any length of time.

HEART TRANSPLANTATION

- Replacement of diseased heart with a healthy one
- Indicated for children who have serious heart dysfunction, congenital heart disease, cardiomyopathy
- Donated by organ donors or parents of critically ill children
- The United Network for Organ Sharing (UNOS) is responsible for transplant organ distribution in the United States.
- People in most urgent need of a transplant are placed highest on the list and are given first priority when a donor heart becomes available; the list is assessed daily.

Diagnostic Tests

- Blood tests
- Echocardiogram
- Electrocardiogram
- Cardiac catheterization

Nursing Interventions

- Provide preparation of patient for surgery.
- Provide preparation of caregiver for surgery.
- Provide detailed education on medications, signs and symptoms of rejection, and follow-up care.

Caregiver Education

- When organ available, patient will be called to hospital.
- Final blood work will be done to match to organ.
- Child will go to the operating room.
- Transplant will take several hours.
- Long-term medication will be necessary for cardiac management, to reduce risk of organ rejection, and to decrease the load on the heart.
- Educate caregiver on anti-rejection drugs.

> **CLINICAL PEARL**
>
> **Common Signs and Symptoms of Rejection**
>
> - Fever
> - Decreased urine output or fewer wet diapers than usual
> - Elevated heart rate
> - Fast breathing rate
> - Weight gain
> - Fatigue
> - Irritability
> - Poor appetite

CARDIAC DYSRHYTHMIAS -AN EMERGENCY

- Problems with the rate or rhythm of the heartbeat; heart rates that are too fast or too slow affect cardiac output to the brain, heart, and other organs.

Tachycardia

Supraventricular Tachycardia

- Occurs in the atria of the heart
- Heart rate >220 beats/minute
- Random episodes
- Palpitations
- Anxiety
- Lightheadedness
- Treatment
  - *Stimulate vagal response through nasal suctioning.*
  - *Apply crushed ice to the forehead.*
  - *Adenosine (Adenocard)—rapid IV push in a proximal site, repeat within 2 minutes with no response (Deglan et al., 2011)*

Ventricular Tachycardia

- Occurs in the ventricles
- Loss of consciousness
- Sudden death

Torsades de Pointes

- Long QT interval (**Figure 12-20**)
- The QT interval represents repolarization of a cardiac cell.
- Affects approximately 1 in 5000 people (Ward & Hisley, 2009)
- Inherited or induced disorder of the electrical system with prolonged QT intervals

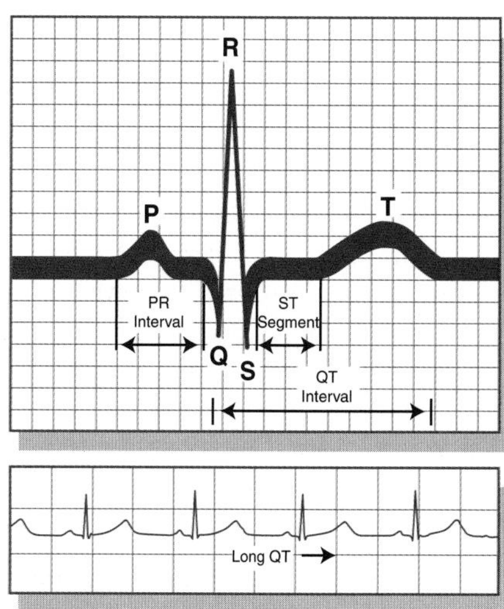

Figure 12-20 Long Q-T interval.

- Sudden, unexpected, life-threatening type of ventricular tachycardia
- Causes include inherited factors, diarrhea, malnutrition, hypomagnesium, hypokalemia, hypocalcemia, and drug induced, such as from anti-arrhythmics or some forms of antibiotic use.
- Rapid fall in blood pressure, fainting, ventricular fibrillation, and death
- Treatment includes removing the causes, such as the drugs; treating the abnormalities, such as with administration of magnesium or potassium; and unsynchronized defibrillation for ventricular fibrillation due to the polymorphic nature.
- Implantation of a defibrillator may be needed.

Bradycardia

- Conduction moves to the SA node down a specific path to reach the ventricles.
- Passes through specialized conducting tissue called the atrioventricular (AV) node
- Sinus bradycardia is when a QRS wave follows a P wave.
- Doesn't transmit = heart block or AV block
- Blocks classified according to the level of impairment: first-degree heart block, second-degree heart block, or third-degree (complete or AV heart block)
- Congenital, injury, or postsurgical
- A pacemaker may be necessary.

Wolf-Parkinson-White (WPW) Syndrome

- Electrical stimulation reaches the ventricles too soon.
- Pre-excitatory syndromes
- Tachycardia
- Syncope
- Chest palpitations
- Death
- Ablation with radio frequency to treat

SHOCK

- Inability of the body to maintain an adequate blood flow and oxygen supply to the tissues needed for metabolism
- Leading cause of childhood morbidity and mortality in the world (Behrman et al., 2011)
- Underlying cause often hard to diagnose
- Three types: hypovolemic, cardiogenic, and septic or distributive (Karlsen, 2006)
  - *Hypovolemic—loss of blood with decrease in hemoglobin; chest x-ray shows normal heart.*
  - *Cardiogenic—damage to the heart muscle resulting in a failure of the pump (ACoRN, 2009).*
  - *Septic or distributive—shifting of fluids from the intravascular space to the extracellular space. It is caused by blood vessel dilatation, often due to sepsis.*
- Shock can affect any end organs in the body.
- This is a medical emergency and is fatal if not treated right away.
- Treatment dependent on identified cause, fluids, blood and blood products, antibiotics, and inotropes to increase blood pressure and delivery of oxygen to the tissues (Karlsen & Tani, 2003).

Assessment

- Confusion or lack of alertness
- Loss of consciousness
- A sudden, rapid heartbeat
- Sweating
- Pale skin
- A weak pulse
- Rapid breathing
- Decreased or no urine output
- Cool hands and feet

Diagnostic Tests

- Monitoring of blood pressure
- Chest x-ray
- Echocardiogram
- Arterial blood gases

Nursing Interventions

- Provide emergency interventions.
- Maintain medications, intravenous access, and fluids to increase volume and blood pressure.
- Maintain oxygen supplementation.

Caregiver Education

- Provide education to call 911 for signs and symptoms of shock.
- Provide education related to intake and output of the child.

Review Questions

1. The Jones Criteria are used to diagnose which of the following?
   A. Septic shock
   B. Rheumatoid arthritis
   C. Systemic lupus erythematosus
   D. Bipolar disorders
2. The nurse responds to the child's monitor alarm, which sounded this morning. When the nurse views the ECG, it shows a heart rate of 240 beats/minute. The nurse verifies that this rate is correct. This ECG indicates
   A. bradycardia.
   B. tachycardia.
   C. supraventricular tachycardia.
   D. second-degree heart block.

3. Transposition of the great vessels involves which of the following structures?
   A. Pulmonary veins and pulmonary artery
   B. Aorta and pulmonary veins
   C. Inferior vena cava and superior vena cava
   D. Aorta and pulmonary artery

4. Primary or essential hypertension is suggested when the blood pressure is
   A. <90th percentile.
   B. <50th percentile.
   C. between 95th percentile and 5 mm Hg above 99th percentile.
   D. >99th percentile plus 5 mm Hg.

5. The caregiver caring for a child following a cardiac catheterization should monitor
   A. heart rate and rhythm.
   B. color of hands and feet.
   C. excessive salivation.
   D. respiratory depression.

6. The caregiver of a child with tetralogy of Fallot (TOF) notes that her child consistently squats, and asks why. The nurse should provide the following information to answer this caregiver's question:
   A. "Your child is squatting because he wants you to carry him."
   B. "Your child is squatting because TOF results in leg pain."
   C. "It increases the circulation to the child's lungs."
   D. "The knee–chest position results in increased inferior vena cava pressure."

7. The most common congenital heart defect is
   A. coarctation of the aorta.
   B. ventricular septal defect.
   C. tetralogy of Fallot.
   D. truncus arteriosus.

8. Too small of a blood pressure cuff will result in
   A. a falsely low BP reading.
   B. a correct BP reading—the cuff size has no effect on the blood pressure.
   C. an increased systolic BP.
   D. a falsely high BP reading.

9. In assessing a heart murmur in an infant with a patent ductus arteriosus (PDA), the nurse is most likely to note a
   A. "washing machine" murmur.
   B. harsh clicking sound.
   C. soft, squeaking murmur.
   D. gallop murmur.

10. A cardiac assessment performed by the nurse includes which of the following?
   A. Heart rate, respiratory rate, color, blood pressure, pulse oximetry, and pulses
   B. Heart rate, color, blood pressure, pulse oximetry, and pulses
   C. Heart rate, respiratory rate, color, and pulses
   D. Heart rate, respiratory rate, color, and liver edges

References

Abdallah, H. (2008). *The Children's Heart Institute.* Retrieved from http://www.childrensheartinstitute.org/medicate/medshome.htm

Acute Care of at-Risk Newborns Neonatal Society (ACoRN). (2009, September). *2010 update.* Vancouver, British Columbia: Author.

ACC/AHA/ESC 2006 guidelines for management of patients with ventricular arrhythmias and the prevention of sudden cardiac death. A report of the American College of Cardiology/American Heart Association Task Force and the European Society of Cardiology Committee for Practice Guidelines (Writing Committee to Develop Guidelines for Management of Patients With Ventricular Arrhythmias and the Prevention of Sudden Cardiac Death). Retrieved from: http://cmbi.bjmu.edu.cn/news/report/2010/cv_gd/77.htm

Allen, H. D., Driscoll, D. J., Shaddy, R. E., & Feltes, T. E. (Eds.). (2008). *Moss and Adams' heart disease in infants, children, and adolescents* (7th ed., Vol. 2). Philadelphia: Lippincott Williams & Wilkins.

American Academy of Pediatrics. (AAP). (2006). 2005 American Heart Association (AHA) Guidelines for Cardiopulmonary Resuscitation (CPR) and Emergency Cardiovascular Care (ECC) of Pediatric and Neonatal Patients: Pediatric Advanced Life Support. Retrieved from: http://pediatrics.aappublications.org/content/117/5/e1005.extract. doi: 10.1542/peds.2006-0346

American Academy of Pediatrics (AAP). (2008). American Academy of Pediatrics/American Heart Association Clarification of Statement on Cardiovascular Evaluation and Monitoring of Children and Adolescents with Heart Disease Receiving Medications for ADHD. Retrieved from http://www2.aap.org/pressroom/aap-ahastatement.htm

American Heart Association (AHA). (2007). *Prevention of infective endocarditis.* Retrieved from http://www.circ.ahajournals.org/cgi/content/full/116/15/1736

American Heart Association (AHA). (2007). *Genetic Basis for Congenital Heart Defects: Current Knowledge.* A Scientific Statement from the American Heart Association Congenital Cardiac Defects Committee, Council on Cardiovascular Disease in the Young: Endorsed by the American Academy of Pediatrics. Retrieved from http://circ.ahajournals.org/content/115/23/3015.full doi: 10.1161/_CIRCULATIONAHA.106.183056

American Heart Association (AHA). (2008a). *Cardiovascular monitoring of children and adolescents with heart disease receiving medications for attention deficit/hyperactivitydisorder.* Retrieved from http://circ.ahajournals.org/cgi/content/full/117/18/2407

American Heart Association (AHA). (2008b). *Heart facts 2006: Latino/Hispanic Americans.* Retrieved from http://americanheart.org

American Heart Association (AHA). (2008c). *Recommendations for blood pressure management.* Retrieved from http://www.hyper.ahajournals.org/cgi/content.full/45/1/142

American Heart Association (AHA). (2010). *Kawasaki disease.* Retrieved from http://www.americanheart.org

Beckman, R. H., Hellenbrand, W. E., Lloyd, T. R., Lock, J. E., Mullins, C. E., Rome, J. J., & Teitel, D. F. (2005). Task force 3: Training guidelines for pediatric cardiac catheterization and interventional cardiology. *Journal of the American College of Cardiology, 4,* 7–17. doi: 10.1016/j.jacc.2005.07.017

Behrman, R. E., Kliegman, R. M., & Jenson, H. B. (2011). *Nelson textbook of pediatrics* (19th ed.). Philadelphia: W.B. Saunders.

Bhimji, S. (2012). Tetralogy of Fallot. Retrieved from http://emedicine.medscape.com/article/2035949-overview

Bonow, R. O., Carabello, B. A., Chatterjee, K., de Leon, A. C. Jr., Faxon, D. P., Freed, M. D., . . . Shanewise, J. S. (2006). ACC/AHA 2006 guidelines for the management of patients with valvular heart disease: A report of the American College of Cardiology/American Heart Association Task Force on Practice Guidelines. *Circulation, 114*, e84–e231. doi: 10.1161/CIRCULATIONAHA.106.176857

Brogan, P. A., Bose, A., Burgner, D., Shingadia, D., Tulloh, R., & Michie, C. (2002). Kawasaki disease: An evidence based approach to diagnosis, treatment and proposals for future research. *Archives of Disease in Childhood, 86*, 286–290. doi: 10.1136/adc.86.4.286

Brookes, L. (2008, February 19). New U.S. national hypertension guidelines (JNC 8) scheduled for 2009. American Society of Hypertension, 19th Annual Scientific Meeting. Retrieved November 7, 2011, from http://www.sld.cu/galerias/pdf/servicios/hta/new_us_national_hypertension_guidelines.pdf.

Calhoun, D. A., Murthy, N., Bryant, B. G., Luedtke, S. A., & Bhatt-Mehta, V. (2006). Recent advances in neonatal pharmacotherapy: Pharmacologic management of patent ductus arteriosus. *The Annals of Pharmacotherapy,40*, 710–719. Retrieved from http://www.medscape.com /viewarticle/530060_3

Cavaliere, T. A. (2010). *Resource guide for neonatal cardiac care.* Glenview, IL: National Association of Neonatal Nurses.

Daniels, S. R., & Greer, F. R. (2008). Lipid screening and cardiovascular health in childhood. *Pediatrics, 122,* 198–208. doi: 10.1542/peds.2008-1349

Deglan, J. H., Vallerand, A. H., & Sanoski, C. A. (2011). *Davis's drug guide for nurses* (12th ed.). Philadelphia: F.A. Davis & Co.

Dice, J. E., & Bhatia, J. (2007). Patent ductus arteriosus: An overview. *Journal of Pediatric Pharmacology Therapy, 12(3),* 138-146. Doi:10.5863/1551-6776-12.3.138

Everitt, M. D., & Yetman, A. T. (2008). Congestive heart failure in the pediatric patient with congenital heart disease. *Pediatric Health, 2,* 33–45. doi: 10.2217/17455111.2.1.33

Gopinath, K., Gangadhara, R., Sadagopan, S., & Gnanapragasam, J. (2007). Kawasaki disease: An incomplete presentation. *The Internet Journal of Pediatrics and Neonatology, 7.* Retrieved from http://www.ispub.com/ostia/index.php?xmlFilePath=journals/ijpn/vol7n1/kawasaki.xml

Holsti, L, Grunau, R. E., Whifield, M. F., Oberlander, T. F., & Lindh, V. (2006). Behavioral responses to pain are heightened after clustered care in preterm infants born between 30 and 32 weeks gestational age. *Clinical Journal of Pain, 22,* 757–764. doi: 10.1097/01.ajp .0000210921.10912.47

Karlsen, K. A. (2006). *The S.T.A.B.L.E. program* (5th ed.). Park City, UT: S.T.A.B.L.E. Program.

Karlsen, K. A., & Tani, L.Y. (2003). *S.T.A.B.L.E. cardiac module.* Park City, UT: S.T.A.B.L.E. Program.

Knoerl, A. M. (2007). Cultural considerations and the Hispanic cardiac client. *Home Healthcare Nurse, 25*, 82–86. Retrieved from http://www.nursingcenter.com/library/journalarticle.asp?article_id=694540

Kudzma, E. C. (2004). Culture competence: Cardiovascular medications. *Progressive Cardiovascular Nursing, 16*, 152–161. Retrieved from http://www.medscape.com/viewarticle/415058_3

LeRoy, S., Elixson, E. M., O'Brien, P., Tong, E., Turpin, S., & Uzark, K. (2003). Recommendations for preparing children and adolescents for invasive cardiac procedures: A statement from the American Heart Association Pediatric Nursing Subcommittee of the Council on Cardiovascular Nursing in collaboration with the Council on Cardiovascular Diseases of the Young. *American Heart Association, 108*, 2550–2564. doi: 10.1161/_01.CIR.0000100561.76609.64

Nelson, D., & Robin, N. (2002). Advances in the genetics of pediatric heart disease. *Contemporary Pediatrics, 19*, 85–100. Retrieved from http://www.modernmedicine.com/modernmedicine/article/articleDetail.jsp?id=126571

O'Riordan, M. (2010*). One in five kids with abnormal lipids.* Retrieved from http://www.medscape.com/viewarticle/716402

Pasini, E., Opasich, C., Pastoris, O., & Aquilani, R. (2006). Inadequate nutritional intake for daily life activity of clinically stable patients with chronic heart failure. *The American Journal of Cardiology, 93*, 41–43. Retrieved from http://www.ncbi.nlm.nih.gov/pubmed/15094105

Rathnau-Minnella, C. H. (2008). *The ABCs of genetics. Self-study course* (2nd ed.). Glenview, IL: National Association of Neonatal Nurses.

Smith, M. (2011). Congenital heart disease and its effects on children and their families. *Pediatric Nursing, 23*, 30–35. Retrieved from http://www.deepdyve.com/lp/royal-college-of-nursing-rcn/congenital-heart-disease-and-its-effects-on-children-and-their-WCUaW0UqM0

Special Writing Group of the Committee on Rheumatic Fever, Endocarditis, and Kawasaki Disease of the Council on Cardiovascular Disease in the Young of the American Heart Association. (1992). Guidelines for the diagnosis of acute rheumatic fever: Jones Criteria, 1992 update. *Journal of the American Medical Association, 268*, 2069–2073.

Teratogens. (2008). Retrieved from http://www.gbmc.org/genetics/harveygenetics/prenataldx/PatientInformation/teratogens.cfm

Tsuda, T. (2009). *Diagnosis and management of low cardiac output in infants.* Lecture presented for NIC University. Retrieved from http://www.nicuniversity.org/lectureDetail.asp?courseid=NICU0008

Walter, W., Taubert, K. A., Gewitz, M., Lockhart, P. B., Baddour, L. M., Levison, M., . . . Durack, D. T. (2007). AHA guideline. Prevention of infective endocarditis. *Circulation, 116*, 1736–1754. doi: 10.1161/CIRCULATIONAHA.106.183095

Ward, S. L., & Hisley, S. M. (2009). *Maternal-child nurse care: Optimizing outcomes for mothers, children, & families.* Philadelphia: F.A. Davis Co.

What are congenital heart defects? (n.d.). Retrieved from http://www.nhlbi.nih.gov/health/health-topics/topics/chd/print-all-index.html

Zipes, D. P., Libby, P., Bonow, R. O., & Braunwald, E. (Eds.). (2007). *Braunwald's heart disease: A textbook of cardiovascular medicine* (8th ed.). St. Louis, MO: Saunders.

13

Neurologic and Sensory Disorders

Tina Goodpasture, MSN,RN, FNP

OBJECTIVES

- ☐ Define key terms.
- ☐ Identify the normal assessment of the pediatric nervous system.
- ☐ Describe normal growth and development of the brain and spinal cord.
- ☐ Identify disorders that can result in intellectual and developmental delays in children.
- ☐ Identify common neurological congenital abnormalities of the nervous system.
- ☐ Recognize seizure disorders and treatment for seizure types.
- ☐ Recognize disorders resulting in temporary loss of consciousness.
- ☐ Identify headache disorders in children.
- ☐ Identify neurocutaneous disorders in children.
- ☐ Identify common movement disorders in children.
- ☐ Identify common causes of pediatric stroke.
- ☐ Identify neuromuscular disorders in children.
- ☐ Identify types of neuropathy that occur in children.
- ☐ Identify types of infections that affect the neurological system.
- ☐ Identify common behavioral concerns in children.

KEY TERMS

- Neuron
- Myelin
- Peripheral nervous system
- Central nervous system
- Gray matter
- White matter
- Development
- Seizure
- Neurocutaneous
- Dysmorphic
- Neural tube
- Syncope
- Neuromuscular
- Tone
- Neuropathy

ANATOMY AND PHYSIOLOGY

- The **neuron** is the central component of the nervous system.
- **Myelin** is a protective covering that provides insulation for electrical impulses from nerve cells.
- The nervous system has two parts: the **peripheral nervous system** and the **central nervous system**.

Peripheral Nervous System

- The peripheral nervous system has two parts: the somatic or voluntary nervous system and the autonomic or involuntary nervous system.
- The somatic system has two kinds of nerves: afferent and efferent nerves.
  - *Afferent nerve fibers carry information from receptors in the body to the brain.*
  - *Efferent nerve fibers carry information from the brain to the body.*

Autonomic Nervous System

- The autonomic nervous system is responsible for involuntary nerve actions that control body function such as heart rate, breathing, digestion, perspiring, urination, salivation, and sexual arousal.

Don't have time to read this chapter? Want to reinforce your reading? Need to review for a test? Listen to this chapter on DavisPlus at davispl.us/rudd1.

- The two divisions of the autonomic nervous system are the sympathetic and parasympathetic nervous systems.
  - *The sympathetic system is responsible for action, such as the "fight-or-flight" response.*
  - *The parasympathetic system is responsible for rest and recuperation of the body systems.*

Central Nervous System

- The central nervous system is composed of the brain and the spinal cord.
- The brain is divided into three main sections: cerebrum, cerebellum, and brainstem.

Brain

- The cerebrum is the largest section and is responsible for complex functions such as actions and thoughts **(Figure 13-1)**.
- The cerebrum is divided into two hemispheres and four lobes.
- The hemispheres are separated by the longitudinal fissure and communicate with each other via the corpus callosum.
- The four lobes are named for the bones that cover them.
- Below the **gray matter** is a layer of **white matter**, which is composed of bundles of myelinated nerve cells that carry nerve impulses to neurons.
- The surface of the brain is a layer of gray matter called the cerebral cortex.
  - *There are three types of functional areas in the cerebral cortex: motor areas that control voluntary movement, sensory areas that control conscious awareness of sensation, and association areas that integrate information.*
  - *Conscious behavior involves the entire cortex. There is no functional area that acts independently.*
- Each brain hemisphere is divided into four lobes: the frontal lobe, the parietal lobe, the temporal lobe, and the occipital lobe.
  - *The frontal lobe is responsible for managing emotions, judgment, impulse control, social behavior, and some motor functions.*
  - *The parietal lobe is responsible for perception and interpretation of touch, pressure, temperature, and pain, as well as some muscular movements.*
  - *The temporal lobe is responsible for perception and recognition of auditory information, memory, and speech.*
  - *The occipital lobe is responsible for processing visual information.*
- Hemispheres act in a contralateral fashion, which means that they control the opposite side of the body.
- The cerebellum is a small structure that lies under the larger cerebrum and serves to coordinate motor activity and equilibrium.
- The brainstem is the lower portion of the brain.
  - *It connects with the spinal cord and houses the connections between the motor and sensory portions of the brain and the rest of the body.*
  - *It houses 10 of the 12 pairs of cranial nerves.*
  - *It controls automatic behaviors necessary for the body to survive.*
  - *It contributes to the regulation of the heart rate and respirations, as well as the body's ability to manage consciousness and sleep patterns.*

Cranial Nerves

- There are 12 pairs of cranial nerves **(Table 13-1)**.
- All but two pairs emerge from the brainstem.

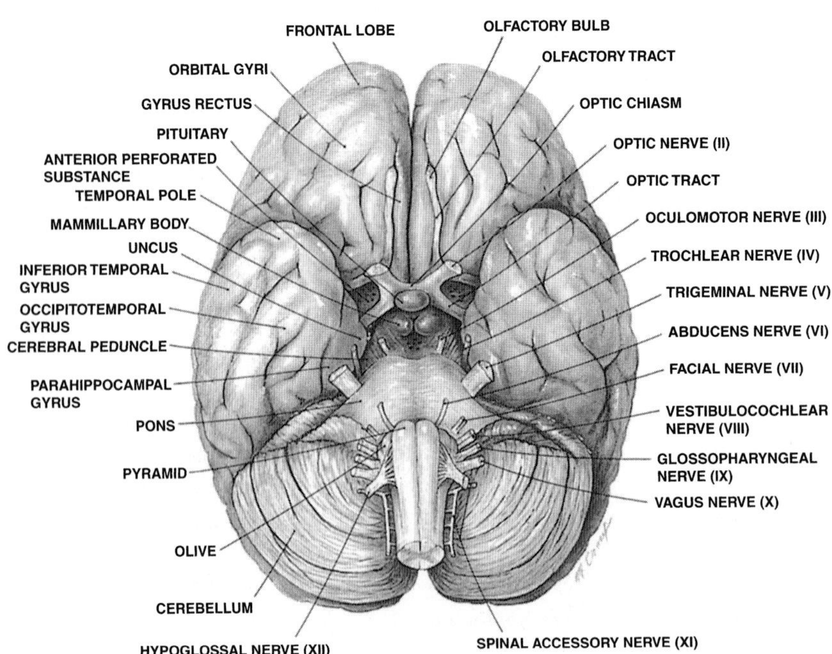

Figure 13–1 Ventral surface of the human brain.

TABLE 13–1 CRANIAL NERVES

Cranial Nerve	Function
Olfactory (I)	Sensory—smell
Optic (II)	Sensory—vision and visual reflexes
Oculomotor (III)	Motor—extraocular eye movement, eyelids, papillary constriction, accommodation of lens
Trochlear (IV)	Motor—extraocular eye movement
Trigeminal (V)	Sensory—facial sensation, corneal reflex, chewing Motor—biting and jaw movements
Abducens (VI)	Motor—extraocular eye movement
Facial (VII)	Sensory—facial sensation, taste Motor—facial expression, salivation, lacrimation
Vestibulocochlear (VIII)	Sensory—equilibrium and hearing
Glossopharyngeal (IX)	Sensory—sensation of middle ear; pharynx, palate, and posterior tongue; taste from posterior tongue Motor—swallowing, salivation
Vagus (X)	Sensory—pharynx, larynx, thorax, abdomen Motor—swallowing and speech, heart rate, gag reflex Autonomic—parasympathetic response to thorax and abdomen
Spinal accessory (XI)	Motor—head rotation, shoulder muscles
Hypoglossal (XII)	Motor—tongue

- Some cranial nerves are involved in the function of special sensory functions (such as vision and hearing), whereas others control motor movements in the face and neck.

Ventricles and Meninges

- The ventricles are cavities in the brain that produce cerebrospinal fluid.
- Cerebrospinal fluid serves to provide nourishment and cushioning to the brain and the spinal cord.
- The meninges are the system of membranes that makes up the covering of the central nervous system and are composed of three layers: dura mater, arachnoid, and pia mater.
  - *The dura mater—means "tough mother"; a thick, strong membrane that surrounds the venous system that takes blood from the brain to the heart.*
  - *The arachnoid—has a thin and spidery appearance; is a loose-fitting sac that serves to help cushion and protect the central nervous system.*
  - *The pia mater—means "soft mother"; a thin membrane that completely covers all the surfaces of the brain and spinal cord, holding blood vessels and capillaries.*

Spinal Cord

- The spinal cord is protected by the bones of the vertebrae and is divided into five sections: cervical, thoracic, lumbar, sacral, and coccygeal **(Figure 13-2)**.
  - *Cervical—nerves in the neck that supply movement and feeling to top of the head, base of the skull, neck muscles, shoulders, elbows, arms, wrists, hands, fingers, esophagus, heart, coronary arteries, lungs, chest, breast, and diaphragm.*
  - *Thoracic—nerves in the upper back that supply the blood to the head, brain, eyes, ears, nose, sinuses, mouth, esophagus, heart, lungs, breast, gallbladder, liver, diaphragm, stomach, pancreas, spleen, kidneys, small intestines, uterus, appendix, buttocks, and colon.*
  - *Lumbar—nerves in the lower back that control and provide regulation for the uterus, large intestines, buttocks, groin, reproductive organs, colon, upper legs, knees, and sciatic nerve.*
  - *Sacral—nerves that control and regulate the buttocks, reproductive organs, bladder, prostate, sciatic nerve, lower legs, ankles, feet, and rectum.*
  - *Coccygeal—nerves that control and regulate the rectum.*
- The spinal cord is covered by meninges and has five layers
  - *Dura mater*
  - *Subdural space*
  - *Arachnoid space*
  - *Subarachnoid space*
  - *Pia mater*
- The spinal cord has gray matter in the center of the cord, and white matter in the outer aspect.
  - *The spinal cord gray matter functions to provide communication between the peripheral and central nervous systems.*
  - *Spinal cord gray matter is not covered by a myelin sheath.*
  - *The spinal cord white matter functions to hold columns or tracts that carry information to and from the brain.*

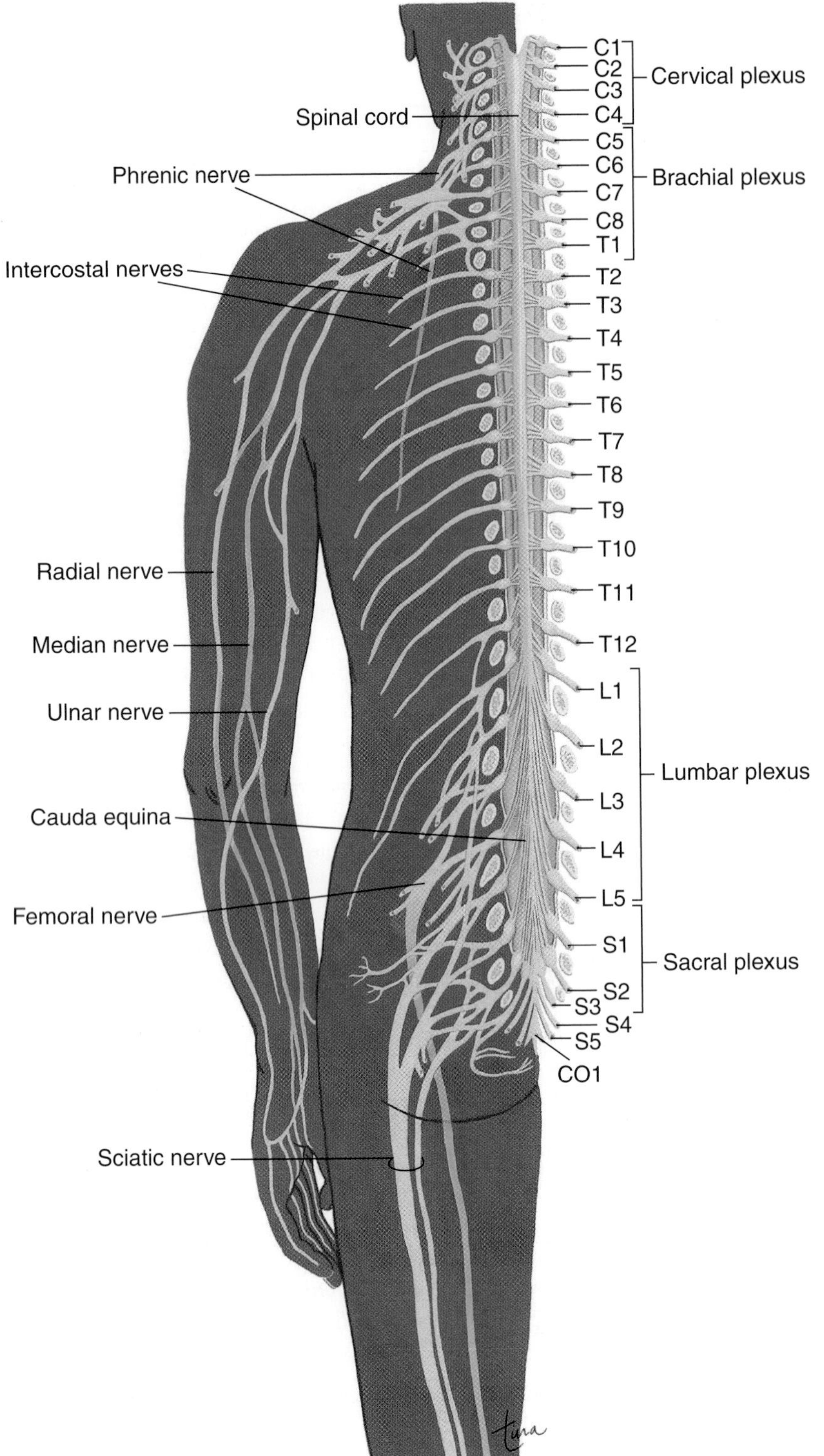

Figure 13–2 The spinal cord and vertebral bodies.

- The ascending tracts carry sensory information toward the brain.
- The descending tracts carry motor information from the brain to the body.

Reflexes

- Reflexes are involuntary movements that occur in response to a stimulus.
- Reflexes occur at the brainstem or spinal-cord level.
- Deep tendon reflexes occur at the level of the spinal cord **(Table 13-2)**.
  - *Provide information about the communication between the central nervous system and the peripheral nervous system.*
  - *A decreased reflex response usually indicates a problem with the peripheral nervous system.*
  - *A brisk or exaggerated reflex response indicates a problem with the central nervous system.*

TABLE 13-2 DEEP TENDON REFLEXES

Reflex	Source Spinal Nerves
Biceps reflex	C5,C6
Brachioradialis reflex	C5, C6, C7
Extensor digitorum reflex	C6, C7
Triceps reflex	C6, C7, C8
Patellar reflex or knee-jerk reflex	L2, L3, L4
Achilles reflex or ankle jerk reflex	S1, S2
Babinski reflex or plantar reflex	L5, S1, S2

- *The deep tendon reflexes are sometimes called stretch reflexes.*
- *The deep tendon reflexes are controlled by the spinal nerves.*

- Primitive reflexes are controlled by the brainstem **(Table 13-3)**.
  - *Primitive reflexes are also called survival reflexes or newborn reflexes.*
  - *They are automatic, stereotyped movements in infants.*
  - *Primitive reflexes are present at birth in full-term newborns and most disappear in the first months of life.*
  - *In premature infants, some primitive reflexes are not present or are suppressed by treatment necessary for them to survive.*

TABLE 13-3 PRIMITIVE REFLEXES

Reflex	Onset	Action	Expected Age of Disappearance
Asymmetrical tonic neck reflex or "fencing" reflex	Birth	When the infant is lying in a supine position and the head is turned to the side, the infant responds by extending the arm and leg outward on the side to which the head is turned; the arm and leg on the opposite side remain flexed	At 6 months when the child is awake Abnormal if the infant holds the posture for more than a few seconds or if it is present after 6 months of age Indicates a lesion in the hemisphere of the brain opposite the direction to which the face is turned
Palmar grasp reflex	Birth	A finger or small object placed in the infant's hand elicits an involuntary flexion or grasp; the grasp tightens when the finger or object is moved away	Weakens by 3 months Should be completely absent by 6 months of age Abnormal if the grasp is asymmetric or if it persists past 6 months
Placing reflex	Birth	When the infant is held upright and the foot is allowed to touch a firm surface, the hip and foot will flex as the infant withdraws the foot	Disappears by 5 months of age Abnormal if asymmetric or persists past 5 months of age
Moro reflex or startle reflex	Birth	Occurs with sudden movement, noise, or change of light The back arches, the arms flex and move away from the body, and then return to the body; often accompanied by crying	Typically disappears by age 6 months Abnormal if absent Abnormal if asymmetric and may indicate birth trauma to the nerves of the arm
Blinking	Birth	A light puff of air will result in the infant closing the eyes	Should be a permanent reflex
Babinksi sign	Birth	When the sole of the foot is stroked, the toes fan out	Should disappear between 9 and 12 months of age
Rooting reflex	Birth	When the cheeks or side of the mouth is touched, the infant turns the head and begins sucking	Disappears by 3 to 4 months of age
Stepping	Birth	Infant held above surface and feet lowered to touch surface moves feet as if to walk	Disappears after 3 to 4 months
Swimming reflex	Birth	When placed face down in water, makes coordinated swimming movements	Disappears by 6 months
Sucking reflex	Birth	When an object touches the mouth, the infant should suck automatically	Disappears after 3 to 4 months
Parachute reflex	By 10 months of age	When the infant is held in the prone position and the body is moved abruptly, headfirst in a downward direction, the infant extends both arms and legs symmetrically	Should persist Abnormal if this fails to develop of or if it is asymmetric

Continued

TABLE 13–3 PRIMITIVE REFLEXES—cont'd

Reflex	Onset	Action	Expected Age of Disappearance
Traction	By 5 months of age	When the infant is pulled by the hands to a sitting position from a supine position, the infant should resist by pulling against the examiner and raise the head	Should persist Abnormal if there is head lag
Trunk righting	By 8 months of age	While sitting, the infant is gently but firmly pushed to one side, past midline; the infant should flex the trunk toward the force of the push and extend the arm and hand away from the force	Should persist Abnormal if this fails to develop of or if it is asymmetric
Head righting	By 4 months of age	When the infant is gently swayed from side to side in a vertical position, the head should remain vertical despite the body's change in position	Should persist Abnormal if this fails to develop of or if it is asymmetric

Source: Behrman et al., 2007; Volpe, 2001.

- *Some primitive reflexes remain throughout life, such as blinking.*
- *Absent primitive reflexes indicate interruptions in sensory and motor processes in the brain and spinal cord.*
- *If primitive reflexes persist past the age at which they should disappear, it indicates that the child will have problems with normal* ***development****, as the frontal lobe of the brain has not inhibited these reflexes and the cerebral cortex has not assumed the role of directing more complex, voluntary functions.*
- *In brain-injured patients, the primitive reflexes may resurface if the frontal lobe is no longer suppressing them. This is called the frontal release sign.*

NEUROLOGICAL DEVELOPMENT

- Begins during the embryonic period
- Development continues on a fairly predictable schedule through adolescence. This predictable pace of development is known as *developmental milestones.*
- The majority of changes occur in infancy and early childhood, until the child is about 6 years of age. Development occurs at a slower pace through adolescence.

Disruptions in Neurological Development

- Disruptions in the neurological development of infants and children can have various etiologies:
  - *Genetic*
  - *Metabolic*
  - *Infectious*
  - *Trauma*
  - *Degenerative disorders*
  - *Anatomic brain malformations*
- Associated conditions
  - ***Seizures***
  - *Sensory impairments*
  - *Problems with physical growth*
  - *Psychiatric and behavioral disorders*

Intellectual and Developmental Delay

- *Developmental delay* is largely a descriptive term, not a specific diagnosis.
- A developmental delay is any situation in which the child is not meeting age-appropriate milestones as expected in one or more areas of development:
  - Fine motor skills, *which are small muscle movements, usually movements of the fingers that require hand and eye coordination*
  - Gross motor skills, *which are large muscle movements associated with movement of the entire body*
  - Language *(both receptive and expressive language)*
  - Social skills, *which are appropriate social interactions, such as bonding and then separating from parents, and age-appropriate play with others*
  - Adaptive skills, *which are skills needed for independence, such as feeding, dressing, bathing, and toileting*
- Types of developmental delays
  - *An individual milestone*
  - *Mixed milestones*
  - *Global developmental delay: all milestones are delayed.*
- The presentation of developmental delay is age-dependent.
- The most common parental concern is delayed development of expressive language.

ASSESSMENT

General History

- Detailed medical and social history of the child
- History of the mother's pregnancy, labor, and delivery
- Child's birth history
  - *Gestational age*
  - *Birth weight*
  - *APGAR scores*
- General health of the child
  - *Accidents*

- *Illnesses*
- *Surgical history*
- *Ages when milestones were achieved*
- *History of regression of milestones*

■ Concerns regarding behavior
- *Interaction with others*
- *Aggression*
- *Repetitive behaviors*
- *Attention*
- *Activity level*

■ Social history
- *Parenting variations*
  - Loss of parent through abandonment, incarceration, death
  - Alterations in parenting through separations and divorce
  - Foster parenting
  - Professional parenting, such as group homes
  - Adoptive parents
  - Elderly parents (grandparents)
  - Adolescent parents

■ Socioeconomic issues
- *Homelessness*
- *Poverty*
- *Availability of medical services (rural health)*
- *Race and ethnicity*
- *Cultural differences*
- *Literacy of parents*

Physical Examination

■ Head circumference abnormalities
- Microcephaly—*the head circumference is more than two standard deviations below average for the child's age, sex, race, and period of gestation.*
- Macrocephaly—*the head circumference is more than two standard deviations above average for the child's age, sex, race, and period of gestation.*

CULTURAL AWARENESS: Differences in Head Circumference

Head circumference may have differences in some populations. For instance, infants from China, Vietnam, Thailand, and Southeast Asia have a smaller head circumference and growth rate. Select the appropriate chart for the child you are screening and observe for the presence or absence of growth in the percentile for the child's age and sex (Centers for Disease Control and Prevention [CDC], 2011).

■ Muscle tone abnormalities
- *Increased muscle tone: hypertonia*
- *Decreased muscle tone: hypotonia*

■ Muscle atrophy or wasting

■ Large or clustered skin lesions, called **neurocutaneous** lesions

■ **Dysmorphic** features, such as low-lying ears, flattened nose, abnormal eyelid creases

■ Abnormalities in the cranial nerves, such as decreased vision or hearing, or inability to use the tongue

CLINICAL PEARL

Assessment of Motor Skills

Watch children at play before attempting to examine or interact with them. Information about their fine motor, gross motor, and adaptive skills can be observed when children are at play. In addition, offer age-appropriate toys as part of the assessment to see if the child manipulates the toy appropriately.

■ Documentation of the presence of physical findings of known genetic disorders, such as facial or hand features of a child with Down syndrome

■ Achievement of developmental milestones in infants and children is best screened by using a standardized developmental screening tool **(Table 13-4)**.

■ This helps to improve early detection of children at risk for developmental delay and to determine the direct intervention required.

Diagnosis

■ Chromosome testing

■ Metabolic screening

■ Thyroid function screening

TABLE 13-4 DEVELOPMENTAL SCREENING TOOLS

Name of Developmental Screening Tool	Ages
Ages and States Questionnaire (ASQ)	Infants to 5 years
Denver Developmental Screening Test-II (DDST-II)	1 month to 6 years
Early Screening Inventory-Revised (ESI-R)	3 months to 6 years
Bayley Infant Neurodevelopmental Screen (BINS)	3–24 months
Brigance Screens	21–90 months
Batelle Developmental Inventory	Birth to 8 years
Child Development Inventories or Child Development Review	3–72 months
Child Development Review—Parent Questionnaire (CDR-PQ)	18 months to 5 years
Infant Development Inventory (IDI)	0–18 months
Parent Evaluations of Developmental Status (PEDS)	Birth to 8 years
The Bzoch-League Receptive-Expressive Language Test (REEL-2)	Infants to 3 years

Source: Centers for Disease Control and Prevention (CDC), 2011; National Early Childhood Technical Assistance Center, 2008.

- Magnetic resonance imaging (MRI)
  - *An MRI of the brain should be performed in the following situations:*
    - Dysmorphic features
    - Sudden loss or regression of skills
    - Traumatic injury
    - Multiple developmental days without obvious cause (Shevell et al., 2003)

Promoting Safety

- The child will be given age-appropriate sedation for the MRI, as no movement is permitted in order to obtain clear images.
- Nursing care is aimed at alleviating anxiety and complications.
- Vital signs must be monitored and compared to pre-sedation values.
- Level of alertness and safety must be monitored as the child awakens from sedation.
- Intake and output must be monitored. The child should be able to drink adequate liquids and demonstrate sufficient urinary output before discharge.
- Parents must be taught what to expect after sedation. Often children cry and react paradoxically to sedatives.

Treatment

- Multidisciplinary approach
  - *Physical therapy*
  - *Occupational therapy*
  - *Speech therapy*
  - *Educational services*
  - *Audiology*
  - *Psychology*
  - *Social work*
- Treatment of any associated condition, such as thyroid disorders and failure to thrive, will also be indicated.
- The family of a child with developmental delay requires additional support due to stressors:
  - *Time*
  - *Emotion and grief*
  - *Finances*

CRITICAL COMPONENT

Early Diagnosis of Developmental and Behavioral Disabilities

In the United States, 17% of children have a developmental or behavioral disability. Unfortunately, less than 50% of these children are identified before school age. By this time, considerable delays have already occurred, and thus treatment begins much later in life than is optimal for the best outcome (CDC, 2011).

CONGENITAL ABNORMALITIES OF THE NERVOUS SYSTEM (NEURAL TUBE DEFECTS)

- Congenital abnormalities of the nervous system are called **neural tube** defects **(Figure 13-3).**
- Neural tube defects are defects that occur in the brain and spinal cord during the fetal period.
- They are thought to be due to folic acid deficiency in pregnant women. It is recommended that all women of child-bearing age take folic acid supplements prior to and during pregnancy.
- Normally, the closure of the neural tube occurs around the 28th day after fertilization.

CLINICAL PEARL

Folic Acid Supplements

Because neural tube closure occurs before most women know they are pregnant, it is important to teach adolescent girls to begin taking folic acid supplements of at least 0.4 mg per day before pregnancy occurs (Ellenbrogen & Roberts, 2009).

- The two most common defects are spina bifida, in which the spinal column doesn't close completely, and

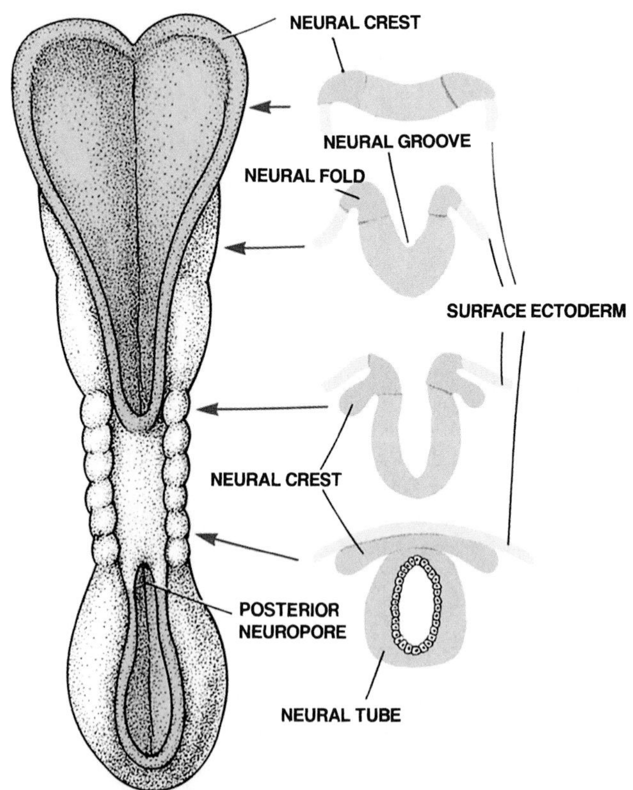

Figure 13-3 The neural tube.

anencephaly, in which most of the brain does not develop (Ellenbrogen & Roberts, 2009).

SPINA BIFIDA

- Children with spina bifida can have paralysis of the legs.
- Problems with control of the bowel and bladder are also common.
- Types of spina bifida
  - Spina bifida cystica—*a section of the spinal cord and the nerves that come from the cord is exposed and visible on the outside of the body.*
    - Also called myelomeningocele
    - Causes partial or complete paralysis below the spinal opening (Ellenbrogen & Roberts, 2009)
  - Meningocele—*the membrane that surrounds the spinal cord is enlarged, creating a mass.*
    - The spinal cord is covered by skin.
    - May not be visible on exam, but seen by ultrasound or MRI
    - Can be removed surgically
    - Does not always cause disability (Behrman, Kliegman, Jenson, & Stanton, 2007)
  - Spina bifida occulta—*a section of the spinal vertebrae is malformed but the spinal cord and nerves are normal.*
    - The defect is not visible.
    - It is usually found accidentally.
    - A version of spina bifida occulta is tethered cord syndrome, in which there are tissue attachments that limit the movement of the spinal cord within the spinal column (National Institute of Neurological Disorders and Stroke [NINDS], 2011e).

CRITICAL COMPONENT

Protection of Open Spinal Cord Defects

When a child is born with an open spinal cord defect, the nurse must exercise caution to keep the defect covered and protected until surgical correction can occur (Behrman et al., 2007).

ANENCEPHALY

- Anencephaly is a condition in which most of the brain does not develop
- Those affected are usually stillborn or die shortly after birth (Volpe, 2001).

OTHER TYPES OF NEURAL TUBE DEFECTS

- *Chiari malformation*—structural defects in the cerebellum, which is the part of the brain that controls balance (NINDS, 2011c).
  - *The bony space at the lower portion of the skull is smaller than normal.*
  - *The cerebellum and brainstem are pushed downward.*
  - *The pressure on the cerebellum can block the flow of spinal fluid.*
  - *Symptoms may include:*
    - Dizziness
    - Muscle weakness
    - Numbness
    - Vision problems
    - Headaches
    - Problems with balance and coordination
  - *Types of Chiari malformation*
    - Type 1
      - *Usually no symptoms*
      - *Frequently diagnosed by accident during an evaluation for another condition*
    - Type 2
      - *Also known as Arnold-Chiari malformation*
      - *Larger, downward herniation of the cerebellum*
      - *May be accompanied by a myelomeningocele*
    - Type 3
      - *Associated with occipital encephalocele, in which a portion of the brain protrudes through an opening on the back of the head (Volpe, 2001)*
- *Encephalocele*—a portion of the brain protrudes through an opening in the skull.
  - *Common locations*
    - A groove in the middle of the skull
    - Between the forehead and nose
    - On the back side of the skull
  - *The severity can vary, depending on the size and location.*

Assessment

- General physical examination
- Documentation of dysmorphic features or obvious malformations
- Assess presence or absence of developmental milestones

Diagnosis

- In addition to physical examination, an MRI of the brain or spinal cord is necessary for diagnosis and determining the extent of the malformation.

Treatment

- Nursing interventions are aimed at supportive care.
- A multidisciplinary approach is needed.
  - *Physical therapy*
  - *Occupational therapy*
  - *Speech therapy*
  - *Educational services*
- Parents need support, as parenting children with neural tube defects cause stress.
  - *Time*
  - *Emotions*
  - *Grief*
  - *Finances*

CONGENITAL MALFORMATIONS

- Congenital malformations usually occur during fetal development.
- Causes
  - *Genetic influences*
  - *Exposure to medications known or suspected to cause birth defects, also known as teratogens*
  - *Infections*
  - *Radiation*
  - *Maternal drug and alcohol use during pregnancy*
  - *Unknown*
- Congenital malformations can occur in the brain or in the bony structures of the skull and face.
  - Agenesis of the corpus callosum—*the structure or bridge that connects the two hemispheres of the brain is partially or completely missing (Volpe, 2001).*
    - The most common brain malformation
    - Children with agenesis of the corpus callosum can have normal intelligence with only some mild differences in learning or may display severe mental retardation, hydrocephalus, and seizures.
    - This defect can occur by itself or in conjunction with other defects of the brain. It can also occur with other defects, such as malformations of the face.
  - Dandy Walker malformation—*malformation of the cerebellum and the fluid-filled spaces around it (Feinichel, 2001; Volpe, 2001).*
    - There is enlargement of the fourth ventricle and increased intracranial pressure.
    - Agenesis of the corpus callosum is frequently associated with Dandy Walker malformations.
    - There are often malformations of the heart, face, limbs, fingers, and toes as well.
  - Lissencephaly—*means "smooth brain."*
    - Absence of the folds, grooves, and fissures in the brain
    - Severely neurologically impaired
  - Microcephaly—*the circumference of the head is more than two standard deviations below normal.*
    - The brain has not developed properly or has stopped growing.
    - May be present at birth or may develop when the child grows but the head does not.
    - Associated with Down syndrome, chromosomal abnormalities, metabolic processes, maternal substance abuse, and maternal cytomegalovirus, rubella, or chicken pox exposure
    - Often display cognitive, motor, and speech delays
    - Can have dysmorphic facial features, growth retardation or dwarfism, hyperactivity, and seizures
  - Schizencephaly—*the presence of abnormal slits or clefts in the hemispheres of the brain (Volpe, 2001).*
    - Clefts in both hemispheres will usually result in developmental delays and problems with purposeful movement, including paralysis.
    - Clefts in one hemisphere will usually result in paralysis on one side of the body, but the child may have normal intelligence.
    - May be associated with microcephaly, hydrocephalus, poor muscle tone, and seizures
  - Craniosynostosis—*premature closure of sutures on infant's head that results in abnormal head shape (see Chapter 7 for further details).*
    - Often associated with facial deformities
    - Surgical correction is performed in infancy.

Assessment

- General physical examination
- Documentation of dysmorphic features or obvious malformations
- Assess presence or absence of developmental milestones.

Diagnosis

- In addition to physical examination, an MRI of the brain is necessary for diagnosis.
- X-rays and computed tomography (CT) scan of the skull and facial bones are used in craniosynostosis to determine the location of premature closure of the sutures and to plan for surgical correction.

Treatment

- The treatment and prognosis of these disorders depend on the particular type of disorder.
- Some children may require surgery, such as shunts or surgeries to repair craniofacial problems.
- Others may require supportive care, such as medications to treat seizures or physical and speech therapy, to help them achieve developmental milestones.
- Parents need support, as parenting children with neural tube defects can cause stress.
  - *Time*
  - *Emotions*
  - *Grief*
  - *Finances*

HYDROCEPHALUS

- Hydrocephalus occurs when cerebrospinal fluid (CSF) collects in an abnormal pattern in the brain **(Figure 13-4)**.
- This can cause an enlargement in the ventricles, called ventriculomegaly, which in turn may cause harmful pressure on the other fragile tissues of the brain.
- There are four ventricles in the brain, connected by narrow channels that allow the CSF to drain and be reabsorbed into the bloodstream. If there is an increase in the normal amount of CSF, the result is hydrocephalus.

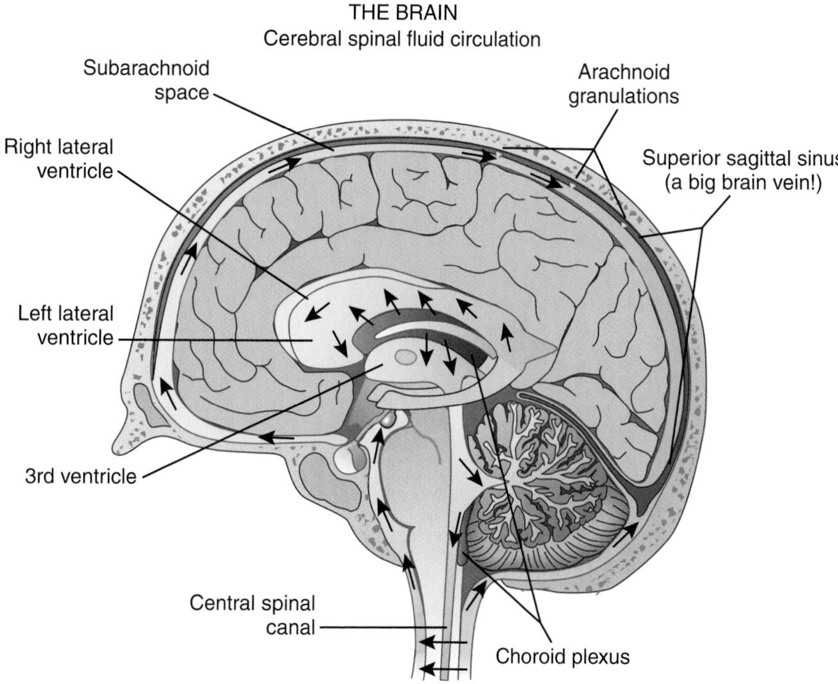

Figure 13-4 The circulation of spinal fluid.

Types of Hydrocephalus

- *Congenital*–when the blockage occurs prior to birth.
- *Acquired*—occurs at the time of birth or at some point afterward.
  - *Two types*
    - *Communicating hydrocephalus*–the flow between the ventricles is not impaired and the cerebrospinal flow is blocked after it leaves the ventricles.
    - *Noncommunicating hydrocephalus*–the cerebrospinal fluid flow is blocked at some point along the narrow channels that drain the ventricles. This can also be called obstructive hydrocephalus (Espay, 2009).
  - *There are two forms of acquired hydrocephalus that primarily affect older adolescents or adults:*
    - *Hydrocephalus ex-vacuo*–occurs after injury to brain tissue, such as after stroke or trauma. It can cause the brain tissue to shrink.
    - *Normal pressure hydrocephalus*–most common in the elderly and has symptoms of significant problems with walking, memory, and bladder control.

Symptoms of Hydrocephalus

- Vary according to the age of onset
- Depend on how rapidly and how severely the CSF accumulation occurs
- Infants can tolerate increased CSF and ventricular enlargement better than adults because the bones of the skull have not fully closed, thus allowing the body to better accommodate the building pressure.
- Symptoms in infants include:
  - *Rapid increase in head circumference or an unusually large head size*
  - *Vomiting*
  - *Lethargy*
  - *Irritability*
  - *Seizures*
  - *A downward deviation of the eyes called "sunsetting"* ***(Figure 13-5)***
- Children and adolescents have different symptoms, which may include:
  - *Headache*
  - *Vomiting*
  - *Papilledema (swelling of the optic disc)*
  - *Blurred or double vision*
  - *Sunsetting eyes*
  - *Lethargy*
  - *Problems with balance*

Clinical Reasoning

Changes in the Fontanels

Open sutures and fontanels in infants help to compensate for increases in intracranial pressure. Nurses should gently palpate the fontanel and be alert to changes, such as a sunken fontanel or a tense and bulging fontanel (Behrman et al., 2007).

1. When a nurse assesses a posterior fontanel in a 7-month-old infant, what are normal findings?
2. It is normal for a fontanel to be firm and bulging if the infant has what condition?
3. A mother brings her 2-week-old infant to the emergency department. She tells you that the baby has been nursing poorly, has had several loose stools, and has been sleeping more than usual. The nurse would suspect that the infant may be dehydrated based on the mother's description and what presentation of the fontanels?

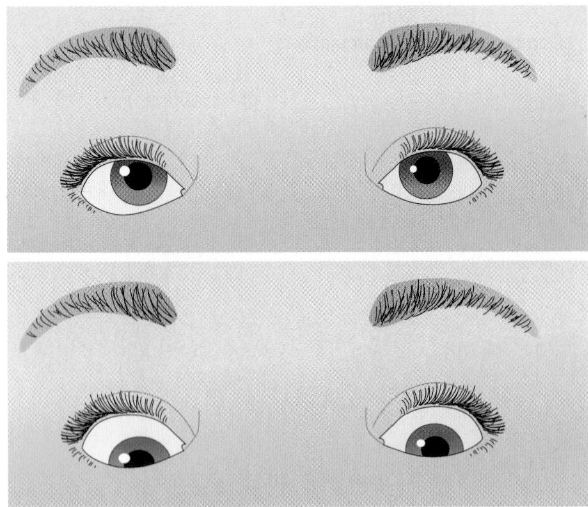

Figure 13–5 "Sunsetting" eyes in hydrocephalus.

- *Slowed developmental progress or changes in memory*
- *Irritability*
- *New onset of urinary incontinence*

CLINICAL PEARL

Shunt Catheters and Hydrocephalus

If a child has an implanted ventriculoperitoneal shunt but develops symptoms of hydrocephalus, a CT scan of the brain with x-rays of the chest and abdomen must be performed to assess the patency and function of the shunt catheters.

Assessment

- General physical examination
- Documentation of dysmorphic features
- Assess presence or absence of developmental milestones.
- Serial head circumference measurements are required to monitor head growth. Rapid or linear head growth is an indicator of developing hydrocephalus.

CLINICAL PEARL

Measuring Head Circumference

Head circumference should always be measured at the fullest part of the head, above the eyebrows and ears, and around the back of the head (Behrman et al., 2007).

Diagnosis

- In addition to physical examination, MRI of the brain is necessary for diagnosis.

Treatment

- Hydrocephalus is usually treated surgically, with a shunting system. This shunt diverts the flow of CSF from the brain to another part of the body, where it can be drained and absorbed by the bloodstream.
- The success of treatment for hydrocephalus varies and is dependent upon the severity of the malformation.

CRITICAL COMPONENT

Symptoms of Shunt Infection or Malfunction

The nurse caring for a patient who has had a ventriculoperitoneal (VP) shunt implant should be alert to signs and symptoms of shunt infection or malfunction. Signs of these problems can include rapid onset of vomiting, severe headaches, irritability, lethargy, fever, redness at the surgical wound sites, or leaking cerebrospinal fluid at the head along the shunt valve area (Behrman et al., 2007; Espay, 2009).

SLEEP DISORDERS

- Sleep disorders in children are common and affect not only the child's rest but behavior and learning ability as well.
- Sleep disorders in children are also disruptive to parents and other siblings.
- Most children stop these behaviors as they mature, but while they occur they are disruptive to both the child and the family.
- Types of sleep disorders in children are:
  - *Problems with going to sleep (insomnia); can be transient or chronic*
  - *Problems with staying asleep (sleep arousals during the night or awakening very early in the morning)*
  - *Sleeping at inappropriate times*
    - *Hypersomnia*—excessive sleepiness.
    - *Narcolepsy*—excessive sleepiness along with daytime sleep attacks.
  - *Obstructive sleep disorder*
    - *Sleep apnea*
  - *Limb movements in sleep*
    - *Periodic limb movement disorder*—unusual limb jerking that limits restfulness.
    - *Restless leg syndrome*—leg discomfort such as pain or crawling sensations that limit sleep.
  - Parasomnias—*abnormal behaviors associated with sleep*
  - Night terrors—*awakening in the first one-third of the night, usually between midnight and 2 a.m., screaming in fear, disoriented upon awakening; parents unable to comfort the child (Parker, Zuckerman, & Augustyn, 2005).*
    - May be triggered by fever, emotional stress, or sleep deprivation
    - The child does not recall the event the following day.
    - Common in boys aged 5 to 7 years but can occur in all children aged 3 to 7 years.
    - Can also occur in older children and adolescents with emotional stress and with alcohol intake.

- *Sleepwalking*
  - Can include other physical activity during sleep, even complex activity such as dressing or undressing
  - Occurs in non-REM (REM = rapid eye movement) sleep
  - Occurs early in the night
  - Tends to run in families
  - Most common at ages 4 to 8 years
  - The child looks awake and eyes are open.
  - May have nonsensical speech
  - Is usually brief, lasting just a few minutes, but can last up to 30 minutes
  - If awakened, the child will be confused and disoriented.
  - May go back to sleep in an unusual place
- *REM sleep behavior disorder*
  - Acting out dreams violently
  - Tends to occur near morning
- *Nightmares*
  - Occur in the early morning
  - The child remembers details of the dream.
  - The child is not confused upon awakening (Parker et al., 2005).

Assessment

- A general physical assessment should be performed to evaluate for conditions that would cause disruptions in sleep, such as abrupt changes in blood sugar, gastroesophageal reflux disease (GERD), and seizures.
- A careful history of the child's habits should be obtained.
  - *Prior sleep habits*
  - *Daytime napping*
  - *Stressors such as the death of a loved one, bullying at school, anxiety*
  - *Caffeine intake*
  - *Medications that cause sleep disturbance*
  - *Weight gain and obesity*

> CLINICAL PEARL
>
> **Screening for Sleep Disorders**
>
> All children should be screened for sleep disorders, and children who are obese should have specific screening for sleep apnea. Parents may report heavy snoring or choking sounds during sleep, as well as daytime fatigue, irritability, or learning problems in school.

Diagnosis

- A diagnosis can be made from a thorough history in most cases.
- A polysomnogram or sleep study may be necessary to evaluate the problem.

> CLINICAL PEARL
>
> **Ruling Out Other Causes of Sleep Disorders**
>
> A preverbal infant or nonverbal older child should be assessed to rule out discomfort causing sleep disturbance, such as GERD or ear infection.

Treatment

- Treatment is aimed at the cause of the problem.
- Sleep hygiene or habits to promote sleep should be instituted.
- Hypnotic sleep aids should not be used in children.
- Safety measures should be instituted for sleepwalking behaviors, such as blocking stairways and clearing walkways to prevent falls.
- There is no treatment for sleepwalking, but children can be injured during sleepwalking behaviors. For this reason, the safety measures just mentioned should be instituted.

SEIZURE DISORDERS

- Seizures occur because of sudden abnormal electrical activity in the brain.
- A single seizure is a symptom of abnormal electrical activity in the brain.
- Recurrent seizures, and particularly recurrent seizures accompanied by electroencephalogram (EEG) findings of persistent abnormal brain activity, are diagnostic of epilepsy.
- The various types of seizures are classified according to the origination of the seizure in the brain and the affect upon the child.
- **Table 13-5** describes the types of seizures.

PARTIAL SEIZURES

- Partial seizures, also called focal seizures, occur in just one part of the brain.
- These seizures begin in one location in the brain and spread to other regions.
- The symptoms of focal seizures vary according to the location of origin of the seizure and the area to which the seizure spreads.
  - *Mild twitching movements of one part of the body or clonic (jerking) movements of an extremity without loss of consciousness*
  - *Unusual smells, tastes, or tingling sensations*
  - *Memory changes and emotional distress, such as feelings of fear, an also occur.*
- These seizures are usually brief and do not involve total loss of awareness.
- Sometimes a partial seizure can spread widely to various parts of the brain, and the partial seizure becomes secondarily generalized, meaning that tonic-clonic (alternating periods of rigidity and jerking) movements and loss of consciousness occurs after the focal seizure behavior spreads.

TEMPORAL LOBE EPILEPSY

- Temporal lobe epilepsy is the most common partial seizure or localization-related epilepsy (Feinichel, 2001; Goldstein, 2004).

TABLE 13–5 SEIZURE TYPES

GENERALIZED SEIZURES	SYMPTOMS
CAUSED BY ELECTRICAL IMPULSES MOVING THROUGH THE ENTIRE BRAIN	
Generalized tonic-clonic, also known as "grand mal"	Rhythmic jerking of the extremities with muscle rigidity and loss of consciousness
Absence	Brief loss of consciousness
Myoclonic	Brief, isolated jerking movements
Clonic	Repetitive, rhythmic jerking movements
Tonic	Muscle rigidity
Atonic	Loss of muscle tone
PARTIAL SEIZURES	**SYMPTOMS**
CAUSED BY ABNORMAL ELECTRICAL IMPULSES MOVING THROUGH A SMALL PART OF THE BRAIN	
Focal	Motor symptoms—jerking, muscle rigidity, spasms, head turning Sensory symptoms—unusual sensations affecting vision, hearing, smell, taste, or touch Psychological—alterations in memory of emotions All occur without loss of consciousness
Complex partial	Automatisms such as lip smacking, chewing, sucking, repetitive and involuntary movements, walking, restlessness Consciousness is altered but the person remains awake
Partial secondary generalization	Partial seizure symptoms that evolve into loss of consciousness and convulsive movements

- Temporal lobe seizures are often resistant to treatment with medication.
- Temporal lobe epilepsy is associated with a specific lesion in the temporal lobe called hippocampal sclerosis.
- The hippocampal sclerosis can sometimes be surgically removed, which can stop or diminish seizure activity.
- The abnormality in the temporal lobe can be a congenital brain malformation.
- It can also result from early childhood head trauma that resulted in a loss of consciousness, complex or prolonged febrile seizures, infections such as encephalitis or meningitis, or temporal lobe tumors.
- Onset is usually age 10 to 20
- The EEG shows anterior temporal spikes or sharp waves that occur when both awake and asleep.
- These seizures can be resistant to treatment with medication.

JUVENILE MYOCLONIC EPILEPSY

- Juvenile myoclonic epilepsy is an epilepsy syndrome in which myoclonic seizures or rapid brief jerks of the arms and legs occur, most frequently in the early morning, soon after awakening (Feinichel, 2001).
- Some children have staring behavior or absence seizures with the myoclonic seizures.
- Some go on to have a tonic-clonic seizure after the myoclonic seizures.
- One of the most common epilepsy syndromes in children
- Surfaces between late childhood and early adulthood, usually around puberty
- More common in children who experience absence seizures
- More common in children with family members who have generalized seizures
- These seizures can be photosensitive, or triggered by flickering light, such as strobe lights, television, video games, sunlight shining through trees, or sunlight reflecting off snow or water.
- The EEG shows a specific pattern of spikes and waves. Flashing lights are often shown to children undergoing an EEG to test for this pattern.

BENIGN ROLANDIC EPILEPSY

- Benign Rolandic epilepsy is an epilepsy syndrome in children between the ages of 3 and 13, with the average age being 6 to 8 years.

CLINICAL PEARL

Postictal Paralysis

A phenomenon known as *Todd's paresis* or *postictal paralysis* can be seen after a seizure. This is a weakness on one side of the body that is temporary and can last from a half hour to 36 hours. The paralysis can be partial, affecting only one limb, or it can be complete, affecting the entire side of the body. It is not known why this temporary paralysis occurs. The paralysis tends to occur more frequently after generalized seizures and febrile convulsions. It is important for the nurse to be alert to this phenomenon. The child's affected limbs should be protected from injury until the paralysis has resolved, and the parents will need to be reassured that the condition is temporary.

- More common in boys than girls
- More common in children with close relatives with epilepsy
- The child exhibits twitching, numbness, or tingling in the face and tongue.
  - *The seizure interferes with speech.*
  - *Drooling may occur as well.*
  - *The seizure lasts less than 2 minutes.*
  - *The child remains fully conscious.*
- Tonic-clonic seizures may occur, usually during sleep.
- The EEG shows a pattern of spikes, called centrotemporal spikes.
- This epilepsy syndrome is also known as benign childhood epilepsy with centrotemporal spikes (BCECTS).

GENERALIZED SEIZURES

- Generalized seizures used to be called "grand mal" seizures and are characterized by abnormal activity that occurs on both sides of the brain in a disorganized fashion.
- The patient usually experiences tonic (rigid) as well as clonic (bilateral rhythmic jerking of the extremities) movements, with total loss of awareness.

ABSENCE SEIZURES

- A common type of a generalized seizure that produces loss of awareness but does not cause tonic-clonic movements is an absence seizure.
- These used to be called "petit mal" seizures.
- Absence seizures in childhood are known as childhood absence epilepsy.
- These occur in children, and appear as if the child is staring into space.
- Other signs of absence seizures:
  - *Subtle lip movements or lip smacking*
  - *Fluttering eyelids*
  - *Chewing motions*
  - *Small movements of hands or fingers*
- The seizures last only a few seconds, and may occur hundreds of times per day.
- There is no known cause for absence seizures, but they can be provoked by hyperventilation.
- Absence seizures can be dangerous because the lapse in awareness can result in injury.
- The child may have problems with learning because he or she misses information in school when the seizures occur.
- Seizures are frequently not recognized by teachers or parents, and the child may even be punished for "daydreaming."
- Absence seizures can be controlled with anti-epileptic medication.
- Most children outgrow these seizures by their teen years, but 50% of children with absence seizures will then develop juvenile myoclonic epilepsy.
- Complications of absence seizures:
  - *Progression of the seizure disorder to a more generalized seizure disorder*
  - *Absence status epilepticus, in which the child has a prolonged absence seizure that lasts several minutes instead of a few seconds*

Evidence-Based Research Practice: Medications for Treating Childhood Absence Epilepsy

Buchhalter, J. (2011). Treatment of childhood absence epilepsy. *Epilepsy Currents, 11,* 12–15. Retrieved from http://www.ncbi.nlm.nih.gov/pmc/articles/PMC3063575/

In a clinical trial investigating the use of ethosuximide, valproic acid, and lamotrogine in the treatment of childhood absence epilepsy, ethosuximide and valproic acid were found to be more effective than lamotrogine. Ethosuximide showed fewer adverse side effects.

FEBRILE SEIZURES

- Febrile seizures are convulsions triggered by a rise in body temperature.
- These seizures are common in children of ages 3 months to 5 years.
- Twice as common in boys as in girls
- Do not cause brain injury
- Usually last less than 5 minutes
- Do not occur frequently
- Do not increase the risk of epilepsy

MYOCLONIC SEIZURES

- Myoclonic seizures are sudden, brief jerks of muscle groups.
- Loss of consciousness may be very brief and may not be noticed by parents or caregivers.
- Myoclonic seizures may occur in clusters, either several in a row or several in a day.

LENNOX-GASTAUT EPILEPSY

- Lennox-Gastaut epilepsy is a type of epilepsy characterized by multiple different types of seizures.
  - *Tonic seizures and atonic seizures are common.*
  - *The seizures are often intractable, or difficult to control.*
  - *The EEG shows a characteristic pattern of background slowing along with spike and wave bursts.*
  - *Most children with Lennox-Gastaut epilepsy exhibit some degree of mental retardation.*
  - *The cause is not usually identified.*
  - *The syndrome persists from childhood through adulthood, with some subtle changes in the types of seizure.*

INFANTILE SPASMS

- Infantile spasms are a type of myoclonic epilepsy.
- Occurs in infants from 3 to 12 months of age.
- Consists of sudden flexor or extensor movements of the neck, trunk, and extremities.
- The EEG shows a characteristic pattern called hypsarrhythmia.
- Usually occurs upon awakening or going to sleep
- Seizures can occur 100 or more times per day.
- The cause is not always known.
- The standard of care is to start treatment within 4 weeks of onset of seizures.
- West syndrome is a syndrome that encompasses infantile spasms, the EEG pattern of hypsarrthymia, and mental retardation.

ATONIC SEIZURES

- Atonic seizures involve a sudden loss of muscle tone and loss of consciousness.
- The head alone may drop or the child may lose all tone and fall.
- Also called "drop attacks."
- The seizure may be brief, lasting just a few seconds, or may be longer, lasting several minutes.
- The child is usually drowsy after a long atonic seizure.

STATUS EPILEPTICUS

- Status epilepticus is a condition in which the brain is in a state of constant seizure.
- Generally described as a seizure that lasts 30 minutes or more
- Can also be described as recurrent seizures without regaining consciousness between seizures for greater than 30 minutes (or less than 30 minutes if treatment has been given to stop the seizures)
- Some evidence suggests that seizures that last 5 minutes have the potential to be unable to stop on their own and may progress to status epilepticus (Ochoa & Riche, 2008).
- Always considered a medical emergency (Bader & Littlejohns, 2004)
- More common in very young children and in the elderly

> **CLINICAL PEARL**
>
> **Assessing Movements**
>
> For young infants, to determine whether movements are normal-for-age tremulous movements or seizure activity, check for subtle signs of seizures such as lip smacking, tongue thrusting, or rapid eye movements. The nurse can also gently grasp the extremity—tremulous movements will stop, seizure activity will not.

Assessment

- General physical examination
- Note the presence of any dysmorphic features.
- Document presence or absence of developmental milestones.

Diagnosis

- The diagnosis of a seizure disorder is first made on the history of the event—what happened prior to, during, and after the seizure.
- An EEG should be performed with the child awake and asleep.
- An MRI of the brain should be performed if the EEG is abnormal, showing an irritable focus in the brain.

> **CLINICAL PEARL**
>
> **Performing an EEG**
>
> A good time to do an EEG on a young child is at a naptime. The procedure is frightening to children, and this way they will sleep through the procedure. The EEG will also indicate if there is a relationship between sleep and the seizure activity.

Treatment

- Treatment is aimed at the frequency and type of seizures.
- Anti-epileptic medications may be used to reduce the seizure frequency and severity.
- For febrile seizures, it is important to identify the source of the infection causing the fever and adequately treat the fever in susceptible children.
- If a seizure lasts longer than 5 minutes and includes loss of awareness, parents can be taught to administer rectal diazepam gel (Diastat) at home to attempt to stop the seizure.
- If the seizure does not respond to the administration of rectal diazepam gel and continues longer than

5 minutes, the parents should be taught to call 911 to summon help.
- Lengthy seizures may require intravenous medications to stop the seizure.
- Lengthy seizures may also require respiratory support and administration of supplemental oxygen.

Nursing Interventions

- The child should be turned to his or her left side when experiencing a seizure.
- Clothing that is tight around the neck should be loosened when the child is experiencing a seizure.
- The child should be protected from injury by the movements of the seizure.
- The child should be comforted and allowed to rest after the seizure has ended.
- The child should not be restrained during the seizure.
- Nothing should be placed in the mouth of a person having a seizure.
- Children may be incontinent of urine or stool during the seizure.
- Some children may vomit during or after the seizure.
- Brief periods of confusion may occur after the seizure.
- Many children complain of headache after a seizure.
- Prolonged seizures that last greater than 5 minutes may require emergency care, such as respiratory support and intravenous medication to abort the seizure.
- If the child has epilepsy or recurrent seizures, antiepileptic medication may be administered. These medications are selected based on the seizure type and frequency **(Table 13-6)**.

Promoting Safety

Nurses should help parents plan for safety in the event of seizures occurring in the future, such as always wearing helmets and protective gear when playing sports. The nurse should promote water safety by instructing parents to allow children to bathe with supervision (with unlocked doors and within earshot of parents), and teens should not be allowed to shower or bathe unless another responsible person is in the home. Swimming should never occur without direct supervision. Instruct parents to provide a bed of lower height for the child with seizures if possible—sleeping on an upper-level bunk bed should be avoided.

TABLE 13–6 ANTIEPILEPTIC MEDICATIONS

Drug	Indication	Brand Name	Dosage	Side Effects	Monitoring
Acetazolamide	Menstrual-related seizures	Diamox	5 mg/kg/day, titrating up to 20 mg/kg/day (tablets)	Anorexia, weight loss, sleepiness, tingling in the hands and feet, increased urination, headache	Blood urea nitrogen (BUN), creatinine, complete blood count (CBC) at baseline and at least every 6 months thereafter
ACTH, corticotropin	Infantile spasms	Acthar gel	5–40 U/day IM for 1–6 weeks, 40–160 U/day IM for 3–12 months if indicated (injectable)	Increased appetite, weight gain, irritability, edema, hypertension, risk of infections	Monitor food intake and weight Monitor glucose and electrolytes weekly during therapy
Carbemazepine	Partial and tonic-clonic seizures	Carbatrol, Epitol, Tegretol	10–20 mg/kg/day, titrating up to 35 mg/kg/day (tablets, chewable tablets, long-acting tablets, liquid suspension)	Sleepiness, rash, ataxia, headaches, nausea and vomiting, aplastic anemia, agranulocytosis, changes in liver function, hyponatremia, syndrome of inappropriate antidiuretic hormone (SIADH), water intoxication	Monitor CBC, liver enzymes, BUN, creatinine, urinalysis, and lipid panel. Monitor for depression, suicidality, behavior changes May make absence and myoclonic seizures worse

Continued

TABLE 13–6 ANTIEPILEPTIC MEDICATIONS—cont'd

Drug	Indication	Brand Name	Dosage	Side Effects	Monitoring
Clobazam	Tonic-clonic, complex partial, and myoclonic seizures	Frisium	0.5 mg–1.0 mg/kg/day, titrating up to no more than 40 mg/day (tablets)	Ataxia, sleepiness, diplopia, dysarthria, may affect liver function	*Not available in the U.S. CBC and liver enzymes at baseline and annually thereafter
Clonazepam	Tonic-clonic, partial, absence, and myoclonic seizures; Lennox-Gastaut syndrome; infantile spasms	Klonopin	25 mcg/kg, titrating up to 1–2 mcg/kg/day (tablets, oral dispersible tablets)	Sleepiness and sedation common Irritability, aggression, and restlessness can occur	Tolerance can develop—monitor administration carefully
Diazepam	Status epilepticus	Diastat	0.2 mg/kg (gel, rectal delivery system)	Sedation, ataxia, blurred vision	Used for emergency treatment of prolonged seizures
Divalproex (Valproic Acid, Valproate)	Absence, tonic-clonic, partial, and myoclonic seizures	Depakote, Depacon Depakene	10–15 mg/kg/day, titrating up to 30–60 mg/kg/day (tablets, liquid suspension, capsules, injectable)	Weight gain, hair changes/loss, changes in liver function, rash, elevated ammonia level, tremor, anemia, low platelets	CBC and liver function tests at baseline and monthly thereafter Ammonia levels if lethargy occurs Monitor weight Birth defects if taken in pregnancy
Ethosuximide	Absence seizures	Zarontin	7.5 mg/kg, titrating up to 45 mg/kg/day Maximum of 1.5 gm/day per day if necessary (capsules, liquid suspension)	Nausea, vomiting, headache, drowsiness, rash, anemia	CBC at baseline and at least every 6 months thereafter
Felbamate	Partial seizures and tonic-clonic seizures in Lennox-Gastaut syndrome	Felbatol	15 mg/kg/day, titrating up to 45 mg/kg/day. Maximum 3,600 mg/day (tablets, liquid suspension)	Aplastic anemia, liver failure, anorexia, weight loss, nausea and vomiting, headache, dizziness, insomnia	CBC and liver enzymes at baseline and monthly thereafter
Fosphenytoin sodium	Status epilepticus seizures or intravenous substitution for oral phenytoin in some cases	Cerebryx	Load with 15–20 mg PE/kg then administer 3 mg PE/kg/min up to 150 mg PE/min IV for status epilepticus Can be given 4–6 mg PE/kg/day IM or IV in divided doses for short-term therapy (injectable only, measured in Phenytoin Equivalents—PE)	Nystagmus, dizziness, headache, sleepiness, ataxia, itching, tingling sensations, cardiac arrest, hypotension, central nervous system depression	BP, ECG, respirations continuously during and every 20 min after loading CBC, liver enzymes, folate if prolonged treatment Also monitor for depression, suicidality, behavior changes
Gabapentin	Partial seizures	Neurontin	10–15 mg/kg/day, titrate to 50 mg/kg/day (tablets and capsules)	Sleepiness, dizziness, ataxia, fatigue, rash, behavior changes, peripheral edema	Creatinine at baseline Monitor for depression, suicidality, behavior changes

TABLE 13–6 ANTIEPILEPTIC MEDICATIONS—cont'd

Drug	Indication	Brand Name	Dosage	Side Effects	Monitoring
Lamotrogine	Partial seizures, tonic-clonic seizures in Lennox-Gastaut, primary generalized tonic-clonic seizures	Lamictal	0.15 mg/kg/day, titrate up to 3 mg/kg/day in divided doses (tablets, chewable tablets, oral dispersible tablets)	Rash, dizziness, sleepiness, headache, diplopia, blurry vision, nausea and vomiting May worsen myoclonus	*Rash usually occurs within the first 6 weeks of treatment Need to titrate dose slowly More common if taken along with Depakote
Levetiracetam	Partial seizures, juvenile myoclonic epilepsy, primary generalized tonic-clonic seizures	Keppra	20 mg/kg/day, titrate up to 60 mg/kg/day (maximum 3000 mg/day) (liquid suspension, tablets)	Dizziness, tiredness, weakness, increased infections, anger, irritability, anorexia, agitation, diplopia, ataxia, rash, depression, thoughts of suicide	Creatinine at baseline Monitor for depression, behavior changes, suicidality
Lorazepam	Status epilepticus	Ativan	0.05–0.1 mg/kg IV, may repeat 0.05 mg/kg x1 after 10–15 minutes if seizures continue (injectable, tablets)	Sleepiness, irritability, hyperactivity, cognitive slowing, blurred vision, confusion, respiratory depression, blood dyscrasias	Respirations (when given IV for status epilepticus), CBC, liver enzymes for prolonged treatment
Oxcarbazepine	Partial seizures	Trileptal	16–20 mg/kg/day to start, titrate up to maximum of 60 mg/kg/day (tablets and liquid suspension)	Dizziness, sleepiness, fatigue, tremor, diplopia, headache, nausea, vomiting, abdominal pain, ataxia, visual changes, hyponatremia, rash, confusion, cognitive slowing	Creatinine at baseline, sodium levels periodically Monitor for depression, behavior changes, suicidality
Phenobarbital	Primary generalized tonic-clonic seizures, status epilepticus	Phenobarbital	3–5 mg/kg/day for infants 5–8 mg/kg/day for young children For status epilepticus, 10–20 mg/kg IV, then 5–10 mg/kg IV q 15–30 min Maximum 40 mg/kg IV (injectable)	Sleepiness, cognitive and behavior changes, rash, liver function changes, anemia	CBC and liver function at baseline and at least every 6 months thereafter
Phenytoin	Tonic-clonic seizures, complex partial seizures, status epilepticus	Dilantin, Phenytek	Dosage based on age, start with 5 mg/kg/day and titrate accordingly (capsules, chewable tablets, injectable)	Rash, ataxia, diplopia, slurred speech, confusion, gingival complications, coarsening of facial features, changes in liver function, anemia	CBC, liver enzymes, folate at baseline and at least every 6 months thereafter.

Continued

TABLE 13–6 ANTIEPILEPTIC MEDICATIONS—cont'd

Drug	Indication	Brand Name	Dosage	Side Effects	Monitoring
Pregabalin	Partial seizures	Lyrica	Not applicable for children May use in older adolescents 50 mg to start, titrate up to 600 mg/day (capsules)	Dizziness, sleepiness, ataxia, peripheral edema, weight gain, blurred vision, diplopia, rash, confusion, dry mouth, tremor, thrombocytopenia, rhabdomylosis, suicidality	Creatinine at baseline. Monitor for depression, suicidality, behavior changes
Primidone	Seizure disorder	Mysoline	15–20 mg/kg/day, may increase up to 250 mg three times per day (tablets)	Ataxia, vertigo, nausea, vomiting, fatigue, irritability, emotional labiality, diplopia, rash, drowsiness, osteopenia, thrombocytopenia, megaloblastic anemia, lupus erythematosus, suicidality	Creatinine at baseline, CBC, metabolic panel, drug levels, folate every 6 months Monitor for suicidality
Rufinamide	Lennox-Gastaut syndrome	Banzel	10 mg/kg/day, titrating up to 45 mg/kg/day (tablets)	Sleepiness, ataxia, tremor, diplopia, nystagmus, nausea and vomiting	Suicidal thoughts, shortened QT interval—do ECG at baseline and with dose changes
Tiagabine	Partial seizures	Gabatril	Start at 4 mg per day titrating up to 2–56 mg/day For use in children greater than 12 years old (tablets)	Dizziness, abdominal pain, nausea, vomiting, diarrhea, rash, irritability, tremor, depression, confusion, weight gain, cognitive slowing, status epilepticus, central nervous system depression, incapacitating weakness, suicidality	Monitor for depression, behavior changes, suicidality, weight gain
Topiramate	Partial seizures, primary generalized tonic-clonic and tonic-clonic seizures in Lennox-Gastaut syndrome	Topamax	1–3 mg/kg/day to start, titrating up to 5–9 mg/kg/day Maximum 400 mg/day (tablets)	Anorexia, weight loss, tingling in hands and feet, cognitive slowing, kidney stones, acute glaucoma, heat stroke	BUN, creatinine, sodium bicarbonate at baseline and every 6 months thereafter Monitor weight and adequate hydration Monitor for depression, behavior changes, suicidality
Lacosamide	Partial seizures	Vimpat	Not applicable for children May start with 50 mg BID, titrating up to 400 mg/day in older adolescents (tablets)	Dizziness, headache, diplopia, nausea, vomiting, fatigue, sleepiness, tremor, nystagmus, diarrhea, depression, cognitive slowing,	Creatinine and EKG at baseline, then periodically thereafter Monitor for depression, behavior changes, suicidality

TABLE 13–6 ANTIEPILEPTIC MEDICATIONS—cont'd

Drug	Indication	Brand Name	Dosage	Side Effects	Monitoring
				itching, PR prolongation, atrial fibrillation, atrial flutter, syncope, suicidality	
Zonisamide	Partial seizures	Zonegran	Not applicable for children May use in adolescents >16 years old Start with 100 mg/day, titrating up to maximum of 600 mg/day (capsules)	Sleepiness, dizziness, fatigue, anorexia, nausea, headache, irritability, agitation, cognitive slowing, depression, diplopia, ataxia, tingling, rash, weight loss, dry mouth, kidney stones, pancreatitis, rash, constipation, depression, suicidality	Sodium bicarbonate, BUN, creatinine at baseline and every 6 months thereafter CBC at least annually Monitor for depression, behavior changes, suicidality

Source: Deglan, Vallerand, & Sanoski, 2011.

CLINICAL PEARL

Seizure Action Plan

Nurses can help parents to feel more in control by helping them to develop a seizure action plan (**Figure 13-6**). This is a medical plan of treatment and recovery that can be utilized by parents, caregivers, and teachers (Epilepsy Foundation, 2008).

SYNCOPE

- **Syncope**, or fainting, is a common condition that affects children and adolescents in which a brief loss of consciousness and posture occurs, caused by a temporary decrease in blood flow to the brain.
- There are many causes of fainting. If blood does not circulate properly or if the autonomic nervous system does not work properly, changes in blood pressure and heart rate can cause fainting.
- The child regains consciousness and becomes alert quickly, but may have a few moments of confusion after a syncopal event.
- Types of syncope
  - Vasovagal syncope—*the most common type of syncope; blood pressure drops quickly, reducing the blood flow to the brain. Standing results in a flow of blood in the lower extremities, and the autonomic nervous system needs to act in conjunction with the heart to normalize blood pressure. Also known as neurocardiogenic syncope.*
  - *Postural tachycardia syndrome (POTS)*
    - Characterized by a rapid heartbeat and then fainting when the person stands up from a seated position. Because of the complex nature of this condition, it is managed by both neurology and cardiology.
  - Orthostatic hypotension *or* orthostatic intolerance—*occurs when the body has slowed responses to changes in position or in response to exercise, heat intolerance, or stress.*
  - Cardiac syncope—*loss of consciousness due to a heart condition that interferes with blood flow to the brain.*
    - Abnormal heart rhythms
    - Obstructed blood flow in the heart or cardiac blood vessels
    - Heart valve disease
    - Aortic stenosis
    - Heart failure
  - *Psychogenic syncope—a person faints in response to anxiety or panic.*
  - Metabolic syncope—*a person faints in response to metabolic conditions such as hypoglycemia or hyperventilation (Hamancioglu, 2006; Schwartz et al., 2005).*

Assessment

- General physical examination
- Detailed history of the event

Diagnosis

- Diagnosis can sometimes be made based on the history of the event.
- An EEG and electrocardiogram (EKG) should be performed to evaluate for other conditions.
- Blood tests to evaluate for metabolic problems such as diabetes should be performed.
- In about 30% of cases, the cause cannot be determined.

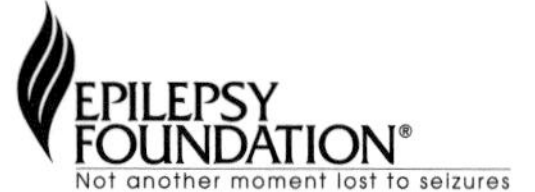

Seizure Action Plan

Effective Date

This student is being treated for a seizure disorder. The information below should assist you if a seizure occurs during school hours.

Student's Name | Date of Birth

Parent/Guardian | Phone | Cell

Other Emergency Contact | Phone | Cell

Treating Physician | Phone

Significant Medical History

Seizure Information

Seizure Type	Length	Frequency	Description

Seizure triggers or warning signs: Student's response after a seizure:

Basic First Aid: Care & Comfort

Please describe basic first aid procedures:

Does student need to leave the classroom after a seizure? ❐ Yes ❐ No

If YES, describe process for returning student to classroom:

Basic Seizure First Aid

- Stay calm & track time
- Keep child safe
- Do not restrain
- Do not put anything in mouth
- Stay with child until fully conscious
- Record seizure in log

For tonic-clonic seizure:

- Protect head
- Keep airway open/watch breathing
- Turn child on side

Emergency Response

A "seizure emergency" for this student is defined as:

Seizure Emergency Protocol
(Check all that apply and clarify below)

❐ Contact school nurse at ______________

❐ Call 911 for transport to ______________

❐ Notify parent or emergency contact

❐ Administer emergency medications as indicated below

❐ Notify doctor

❐ Other ______________

A seizure is generally considered an emergency when:

- Convulsive (tonic-clonic) seizure lasts longer than 5 minutes
- Student has repeated seizures without regaining consciousness
- Student is injured or has diabetes
- Student has a first-time seizure
- Student has breathing difficulties
- Student has a seizure in water

Treatment Protocol During School Hours (include daily and emergency medications)

Emerg. Med. ✓	Medication	Dosage & Time of Day Given	Common Side Effects & Special Instructions

Does student have a **Vagus Nerve Stimulator?** ❐ Yes ❐ No If YES, describe magnet use:

Special Considerations and Precautions (regarding school activities, sports, trips, etc.)

Describe any special considerations or precautions:

Physician Signature ______________ **Date** ______________

Parent/Guardian Signature ______________ **Date** ______________

DPC772

Figure 13-6 Seizure action plan. *(With permission from the Epilepsy Foundation, Washington, D.C.)*

Treatment

- Treatment is aimed at supportive care.
- Prevention of future syncope events is also important.

HEADACHES AND MIGRAINES

- Headaches are a common pediatric complaint.
- About 75% of children will experience a headache before 15 years of age.
- About 10% occur before the age of 10 years (Lopez & Rothrock, 2008).
- Headaches in children are usually benign, but they are frightening to the child and to his or parents.
- They account for missed participation in school, sports, and social activities, as well as parents missing days from work to care for the child.

Types of Headaches

- Primary headaches
  - *The headaches occur spontaneously, and not because of any other health problem or trauma.*
  - *Includes migraine and tension headaches (Silberstein, Saper, & Freitag, 2008; Young & Silberstein, 2004)*
- Secondary headaches occur as a result of some other condition:
  - *Infection*
  - *Head injuries such as concussions*
  - *Chronic sinus disease*
  - *Problems with blood vessels in the head (such as aneurysms)*
  - *Tumors*
  - *Other medical conditions, such as diabetes (Silberstein et al., 2008; Young & Silberstein, 2004)*

> **CLINICAL PEARL**
>
> **History of Headaches**
>
> It is important to gather a complete history of the headaches, because the headache presentation is often the best clue to the source of the headaches. Information such as time when the headaches occur, whether headaches awaken the child from sleep, whether sudden vomiting without nausea occurs, whether the child has had a recent injury, and whether the headache is accompanied by a fever or stiff neck are all sources of vital information when assessing a child's history of headaches.

Tension Headaches

- Feelings of tightness or pressure around the head
- A steady pain as opposed to a pounding or throbbing pain
- Mild or moderate pain
- Do not usually prevent children from participating in their usual activities
- Are not usually associated with any other symptom, such as nausea or vomiting
- Some children report increased sensitivity to noise.
- Typically last 30 minutes to a few hours, but can also be chronic and occur every day
- Usually lessen during school holidays

Migraine Headaches

- Severe and have disabling symptoms of severe throbbing or pounding unilateral pain
- Worsen with exertion
- Sensitivity to light and sound is common.
- Nausea, vomiting, and stomach pain can occur.
- Some children have an "aura" or warning that the headache is going to occur.
  - *Flashing lights*
  - *Colored spots in their vision*
  - *Blurry vision*
  - *Dizziness*
  - *Vague feeling of malaise*
  - *May last from a few hours to several days*
  - *May be an inherited family condition*
  - *Sleep may be needed for the headache to be fully relieved.*
  - *Sometimes patterns can be noted, such as occurrence after prolonged exertion in athletes or with menstrual cycles (Silberstein et al., 2008; Young & Silberstein, 2004).*
- Abdominal migraines are migraine variants that occur in children.
  - *Unknown cause*
  - *More common in girls*
  - *Symptoms*
    - Acute, severe midline abdominal pain
    - Nausea
    - Vomiting
    - Pallor
    - Anorexia
  - *Duration*
    - From 1 hour to up to 3 days
    - Treatment is aimed at supportive care and identification of migraine triggers.
- Cyclic vomiting is a migraine variant characterized by recurrent attacks of violent or prolonged vomiting.
  - *No headache is associated with cyclic vomiting.*
  - *May last for hours*
  - *Treatment is aimed at supportive care and identification of migraine triggers.*
  - *Amitriptyline, a tricyclic antidepressant, is helpful in preventing cyclic migraines in some children (Feinichel, 2001; Lopez & Rothrock, 2008).*

Assessment

- A general physical assessment should be performed.
- A detailed history of the headache should be obtained.

Diagnosis

- Diagnosis is often made based on the history of the event.

- Headache diaries are helpful in assessing the frequency and severity of the headaches.
- Headache diaries may also help identify potential headache triggers.
- An MRI or CT scan of the brain is not indicated unless there is an abnormal finding on the examination of the child.
- A serum lactate level can exclude a mitochondrial disorder in children with cyclic vomiting, as the level is elevated in mitochondrial disorders and normal in cyclic vomiting.

Treatment

- Treatment is aimed at supportive care and at prevention of the headaches.
- Avoid headache triggers when possible.
  - *Common headache triggers in children:*
    - Skipping meals, with the most common being breakfast
    - Inadequate fluid intake
    - Sleep deprivation
    - Stress
  - *Parents and children are encouraged to keep a diary of the headaches in order to better classify the headaches and identify potential triggers.*
- Some children have a significant headache disorder and need prescription medications aimed at prevention of migraines. These include:
  - *Beta blockers such as Propranolol*
  - *Seizure medications such as Depakote and Topamax*
  - *Antidepressants such as Amitriptyline, Pamelor, Effexor*
- Some children need prescriptions to abort severe migraines. These include:
  - *Triptan medications such as Imitrex, Zomig, and Maxalt*
  - *Anti-emetics such as Phenergan and Zofran*
  - *Analgesic medications such as Tylenol and Advil*
- Some children will need to stop activities and sleep for the headache to completely resolve.

> **CLINICAL PEARL**
>
> **Headache Diary**
>
> A diary of the child's headaches is valuable for identifying triggers, helping to determine the headache type, and helping the child to feel in control of the condition.

NEUROCUTANEOUS DISORDERS

- Neurocutaneous syndromes are disorders in nerve cells that lead to abnormal growth of tumors in various parts of the body.
- They are caused by the abnormal development of cells in the embryonic stage.
- The disorders are characterized by distinctive neurocutaneous lesions.
- Some of these conditions can be diagnosed at birth but may not cause problems until later in life.
- Common neurocutaneous disorders that are seen in infants and childhood include:
  - Neurofibromatosis—*tumors grow on nerve cells (NINDS, 2011a).*
  - Sturge-Weber syndrome—*angiomas develop on the thin membrane that later surrounds the brain and spinal cord and the skin of the face, usually in the ophthalmic and maxillary divisions of the trigeminal nerve (Berhman et al., 2007).*
  - Tuberous sclerosis—*tumors grow in the brain, kidneys, heart, lungs, eyes, and on the skin (Berhman et al., 2007).*
  - Ataxia-telangiectasia—*degeneration in the portion of the brain that controls motor movements and speech (Berhman et al., 2007).*
- Symptoms vary from mild to severe, and can cause not only external skin lesions but also internal tumors, seizures, and learning problems.

NEUROFIBROMATOSIS

- Neurofibromatosis is one of the most common neurocutaneous syndromes.
- It can cause tumors to grow on nerve cells, called neurofibromas.
- These tumors cause skin changes, bone deformities, and eye problems.
- Seizures can also occur because of lesions that may occur in the brain.
- Neurofibromatosis is usually inherited, but up to half of cases occur because of spontaneous changes or mutations within a person's genes.
- The child of a parent with neurofibromatosis has a 50% chance of inheriting the disorder.
- The two different forms of this disorder are
  - *Neurofibromatosis type 1 (NF1)*
  - *Neurofibromatosis type 2 (NF2)*
- Neurofibromatosis type 1, or NF1, accounts for approximately 90% of all cases and is also known as von Recklinghausen disease.
- Children with NF1 often inherit the disease from a parent.
- The classic sign of NF1 is skin pigment findings known as "café-au-lait" spots (Zitelli & Davis, 2007).
  - *These light brown or coffee-colored patches may be present at birth and can look like freckles at first.*
  - *Axillary freckling in a young child is high suspicious for NF1 (Zitelli & Davis, 2007; NINDS, 2011b).*
  - *The lesions increase in size and number during the first few years of life.*
  - *A child diagnosed with NF1 will usually have at least six café-au-lait spots that are larger than ½ inch in diameter.*
  - *The lesions are flat, do not cause pain, and do not progress to tumors.*

- Lisch nodules may also be found in patients with NF1 (Zitelli & Davis, 2007).
  - *The nodules are tiny, benign tumors found on the iris of the eye.*
  - *In some cases, tumors can develop along the optic nerves and affect vision.*

Assessment

- General physical examination
- Thorough skin examination
- Measurement and documentation of skin lesions

> **CLINICAL PEARL**
>
> **Measuring Lesions**
>
> A small clear ruler is helpful for measuring the size of lesions such as café-au-lait spots without obscuring the lesion being measured.

Diagnosis

- Diagnosis is based on clinical findings.
- A baseline MRI of the brain should be performed and then repeated as the child grows to monitor for tumors.
- An MRI of the brain and optic nerve should be performed in children with Lisch nodules.
- An EEG should be performed if seizures occur.
- A blood test can be performed to evaluate for a defect in the NF1 gene.

Treatment

- Treatment focuses on managing the symptoms.
- Sometimes the neurofibromas are surgically removed if they are causing pain or causing problems with a vital organ.
- Seizures can usually be controlled with medication.
- A child may need specialized educational plans if learning is a problem.
- Psychological therapy may be needed for children and adolescents with self-esteem problems due to the visible tumors (see Chapter 18, Reproductive and Genetic Disorders, for further details).

ATAXIA TELANGIECTASIA

- Ataxia telangiectasia is a progressive degenerative disease that ultimately involves most body systems (Behrman et al., 2007).
- It is a recessive genetic disease, which means that both parents carry the gene but they do not have the disorder.
- Ataxia telangiectasia is typically diagnosed when the child is approximately 2 years old.
- Cerebellar degeneration occurs, causing ataxia and slurred speech.
- This condition progresses until the child is unable to sit or stand unsupported.
- Most children require a wheelchair for mobility.
- Telangiectasias are tiny red veins that appear in the corners of the eyes or on the exposed ears and cheeks when the child is in sunlight.
- The appearance of the veins is a significant symptom in the diagnosis of this disease.
- Disruptions in the immune system are extremely common in children with ataxia telangiectasia.
- Recurrent respiratory infections and pneumonia are common.
- Some cancers are more common in this population, particularly leukemia.

Assessment

- General physical examination
- Thorough skin examination
- Evaluation of presence or absence of developmental milestones

Diagnosis

- Diagnosis is based on clinical findings.
- A baseline MRI of the brain should be performed.
- A blood test can be performed to evaluate for a genetic marker.

Treatment

- The treatment focuses on managing the symptoms.
- Screening for other health problems should be performed.
- A multidisciplinary approach is needed due to the complex nature of this disorder.

MOVEMENT DISORDERS IN CHILDREN

- There are two main types of movement disorders in children.
  - *Excessive movement, or hyperkinetic movement*
  - *Diminished movement, or bradykinetic movement*
- The most common in children is hyperkinetic movement.
  - *Abnormal, repetitive, and involuntary movements, such as:*
    - *Tics*—sudden, repetitive, involuntary movements.
    - *Tremors*— involuntary trembling movements.
    - *Dystonia*—muscle contractions cause twisting movements of the muscle groups, resulting in abnormal postures.
    - *Chorea*—muscle contractions result in quick, rhythmic movements that resemble dancing movements.
- Bradykinetic movements are less common in children and are more commonly seen in adults, such as the very slow and rigid movements of a person with Parkinson's disease.

- Ataxia and spasticity are movements but they are not classified as a movement disorder but rather a motor dysfunction.
- Movement disorders are thought to be caused by disorder in the communication from the brain to the muscles that results in unintentional movements. Children with tics do not intend to blink their eyes rapidly or clear their throats excessively, but the communication that occurs from the brain causes them to do so.
- The most common movement disorder in children is tics.
  - *Motor tics are most frequently seen.*
    - Motor tics are sudden, brief involuntary movements.
      - *Eye blinking*
      - *Grimacing*
      - *Neck jerks*
      - *Movements of the shoulder*
      - *Nose twitches*
      - *Grinding of the teeth*
      - *Tensing of the muscles of the chest or abdomen*
  - *Vocal tics may also occur and are sounds such as:*
    - Sniffing
    - Clearing of the throat
    - Grunting
    - Squeaking
    - Humming sounds
    - Clicking the teeth together
    - Sucking sounds
- A child may have complex motor tics with more than one body part involved.
- Complex vocal tics may be repetition of words or syllables, spoken syllables or words, shouts, or obscenities.
- Complex motor and vocal tics are often mistakenly thought to be voluntary by the public and can be disturbing to the family of the child (American Academy of Child and Adolescent Psychiatry, 2004).
- Parents often assume that their child has Tourette's syndrome, a more complex tic disorder, when in actuality the child has a condition known as transient tic of childhood.
- The distinction between these two conditions is noted by the length of time the tic has been present and the type of tic seen.
  - *Transient tic of childhood is typically a disorder of motor or vocal tics that may last for several months but not greater than 1 year.*
  - *Tourette's syndrome is a disorder of complex motor and vocal tics that have been present for more than 1 year and began before the child's 18th birthday (Kenney, Kuo, & Jimenez-Shahed, 2008).*
- It is possible for motor tics to become chronic in some children, whereas chronic vocal tics are rare.
- If the child has only one type of tic for more than 1 year, it is termed a *chronic tic disorder*, not Tourette's syndrome (which requires for both motor and vocal tics to be present).
- Tics usually appear before the age of 10, with the most common age at diagnosis being 6 to 7 years.
- The most common motor tic is eye blinking.
- The most common vocal tic is sniffing or clearing of the throat.
  - *It is often misdiagnosed as allergy manifestations.*
- Tics may worsen at around age 12, and usually disappear completely by age 18.
- Tics will worsen with anxiety in most children.
- Tics can sometimes occur as a secondary symptom as a result of
  - *Infections*
  - *Medication effects*
  - *Developmental*
  - *Genetic disorders*
  - *Neurocutaneous disorders*
  - *Degenerative disorders*
  - *Stroke*
  - *Head trauma*
- Most children learn to manage the tic on their own, with supportive parents and teachers who do not focus on the behavior.
- By their mid-teens, most have developed social relationships with people who show acceptance of the tic as part of the person.
- The behavior tends to diminish until it is absent by the time the child is 18 years old.

Assessment

- General physical examination
- In evaluating a movement disorder, ask:
  - *If the frequency of movement in question is abnormal*
  - *If the character of the movement is abnormal*
  - *If anything in the environment is causing the disorder (such as a foreign body in the eyes of a child, thus causing the tic-like movement of the eyes)*
  - *If the movement can be voluntarily suppressed*

Diagnosis

- Diagnosis is based on clinical findings and history of the tics.

Treatment

- Treatment focuses on supportive care.
- Most children learn to manage the tic on their own, with supportive parents and teachers who do not focus on the behavior.
- By their mid-teens, most have developed social relationships with people who show acceptance of the tic as part of the person.
- Medications to suppress the tic can be considered if the tic is emotionally distressing to the child or if the tic causes pain or discomfort.
- Screening for other health problems should be performed.

PEDIATRIC STROKE

- Stroke or cerebrovascular accidents are more common in adults but can occur in children.
- They can occur:
  - *In utero*
  - *During or shortly after birth*
  - *As a result of trauma or illness*
- Neonatal hemorrhages are unfortunately common in premature infants due to the fragile nature of their neurovascular networks (**Figure 13-7**).
- Malformations of brain structures or blood vessels are often the cause of strokes in young children.
- Infections or illnesses, such as meningitis, encephalitis, and sickle cell disease states, are other causes of strokes.
- The effects can be mild, with only some mild weakness in an extremity, or devastating, with profound and severe neurologic impairment (American Heart Association [AHA], 2009; Bader & Littlejohns, 2004).

Assessment

- A thorough examination and vigilance on the part of the nurse are necessary to assess for subtle changes in motor or sensory function.

Diagnosis

- Diagnosis is made on the basis of areas of bleeding in the brain, as verified by CT or MRI imaging of the brain.
- For premature infants and neonates, hemorrhages in the brain can be seen on cranial ultrasound.

Treatment

- Treatment is aimed at the cause of the stroke, as well as at the symptoms and residual effects.
  - *Intensive physical, occupational, and speech therapies are required.*
  - *The family needs support, as caring for children with these conditions is emotionally, physically and financially exhausting.*
- Screening for the development of hydrocephalus in indicated, as this is a common complication of pediatric stroke.

INFECTIONS OF THE NERVOUS SYSTEM

- Infections of the nervous system have four main causes.
  - *Bacterial*
  - *Viral*
  - *Fungal*
  - *Parasitic infections*
- The most common infection is meningitis (**Figure 13-8**).
  - *Meningitis is an infection of the meninges, which are the coverings of the brain and spinal cord (NINDS, 2011d).*
  - *Can be a precursor to encephalitis, which is an acute inflammation of the brain.*
  - *Brain abscess can occur.*
  - *This can be a life-threatening infection.*
  - *Meningitis is treated as a medical emergency.*
  - *Symptoms include:*
    - Severe headache
    - Stiff neck
    - Sudden high fever

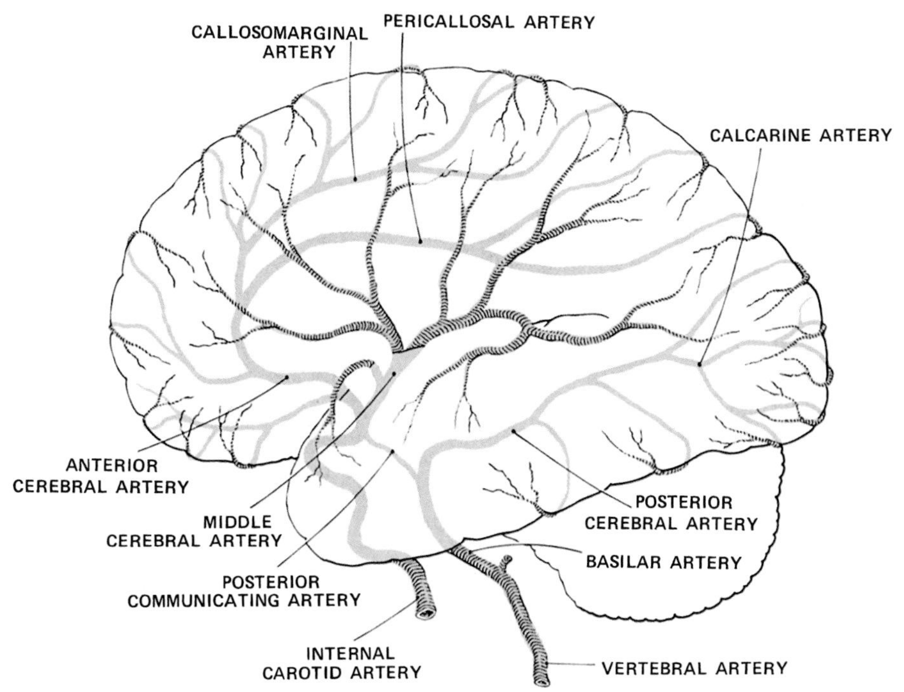

Figure 13-7 The arteries in the brain.

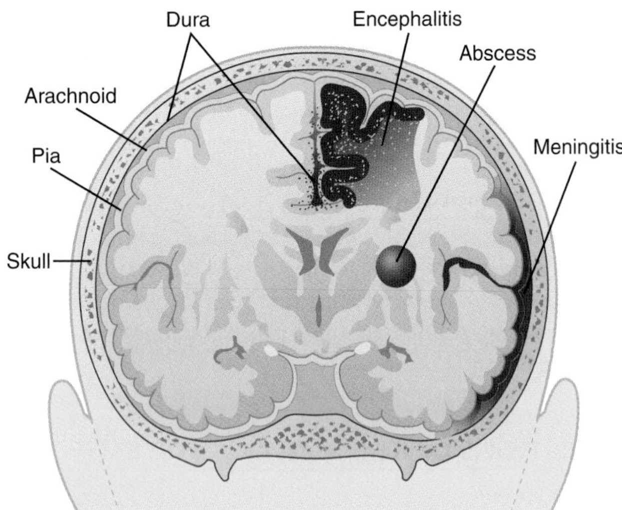

Figure 13–8 Major sites of infection in the brain. *(From Davis, L. E., King, M., & Shultz, J. L. [2005].* Fundamentals of neurologic disease. *New York: Demos Medical Publishing, Inc.)*

- Bulging fontanel in infants
- Altered mental status

- *Infants and young children may have more subtle symptoms of irritability and sleepiness.*
- *If a rash is present, it can indicate the existence of a specific bacterial infection.*

Assessment

- Thorough physical examination
- Thorough history of the child's illness
- Physical signs of neck rigidity
  - *Kernig's sign*
    - With the child lying on his or her back, flex the hip and knee 90 degrees. If the Kernig's sign is positive, pain will prevent the child from extending the knee (Behrman et al., 2007; Schwartz et al., 2005).
  - *Brudzinski's sign*
    - Flexion of the neck causes involuntary flexion of the knee and hip (Behrman et al., 2007; Schwartz et al., 2005).

Diagnosis

- Diagnosis is made based on symptoms and lab data.
- Complete blood count shows elevation in white blood cell count.
- Lumbar puncture or spinal tap is performed to obtain spinal fluid for testing.
- Cerebrospinal fluid is tested for the presence of protein and white blood cells, and cultured to identify a causative agent.
  - *An elevated protein count and low glucose level in spinal fluid indicates bacterial meningitis.*
  - *The protein count is normal to low and the glucose level is normal to high in viral meningitis (Bader & Littlejohns, 2004).*

CRITICAL COMPONENT

Lumbar Puncture

The nurse will need to help the child to be properly positioned for a lumbar puncture. Because of the degree of flexion needed for access to the lumbar spine, the nurse should be alert to respiratory compromise in the infant or child (Bader & Littlejohns, 2004).

Treatment

- Treatment is aimed at rapid recognition of the cause of the infection.
- Administration of broad spectrum antibiotics
- Supportive care of the child
- Rapid deterioration is possible in patients with meningitis.
- The nurse must be vigilant to recognize even the most subtle symptoms.
- As the causative agent is identified, the treatment is revised to be more specific to that organism.
- Meningitis of any type can leave children with deficits.
  - *Hearing loss*
  - *Learning problems*
  - *Seizures*
  - *Mental retardation*
- Bacterial meningitis is fatal if untreated.
- Even when treated, bacterial meningitis may have grave effects, depending on the age of the child and the causative organism.
- About 30% of newborn infants die from bacterial meningitis, even with treatment (Volpe, 2001).
- Viral meningitis is rarely fatal and usually resolves without anti-viral medications.
- Fungal meningitis can be fatal without treatment, and unfortunately the treatment is not without its own risk to the child.
- Protozoan or parasitic infections can be treated with some specific medications, such as anti-malarial drugs, as well as some antibiotics.
- Prevention of nervous system infections is possible in some cases.
- A vaccine is available for some types of bacterial meningitis.
- In the case of infants being born to mothers known to be infected with specific organisms, prophylactic antibiotics are considered to be the standard of care.
- Prevention of infection by protozoan organisms should be implemented when possible. For close contacts of patients with some types of bacterial meningitis, appropriate antibiotic therapy should be administered.

CLINICAL PEARL

Fever and Lethargy as Symptoms of Meningitis

Meningitis should always be suspected in acutely ill infants and children with fever and lethargy until proven otherwise (Schwartz et al., 2005).

NEUROMUSCULAR DISORDERS

- **Neuromuscular** disorders are the cause of muscular weakness and abnormal **tone** in infancy and childhood.
- These disorders are diagnosed based on which area of the neuromuscular system is affected.
- The most common neuromuscular disorders are:
  - *Cerebral palsy*
  - *Muscular dystrophy*
  - *Myasthenia gravis*
  - *Spinal muscle atrophy, which is a degenerative disorder of the anterior horn cell of the spinal cord*

CEREBRAL PALSY

- *Cerebral palsy* is the name given to a group of conditions that affect motor development in children.
- It can be quite mild, with abnormal tone and weakness in one extremity.
- It can be severe, affecting all extremities, growth and development, and the intellectual capabilities of the child.

MUSCULAR DYSTROPHY

- Muscular dystrophy is a disorder that results in muscular weakness and a decrease in muscle tone over time (Davis, King, & Shultz, 2005; El-Bohy & Wong, 2005).
- There are several types of muscular dystrophy.
  - *Becker's muscular dystrophy*
    - Inherited disorder that causes progressive weakness in the pelvis and legs over time
    - Symptoms are usually noted around age 12.
    - Disability tends to occur at a fairly slow rate.
    - Cardiomyopathy, or weakness in the heart muscles, can occur.
  - *Duchenne's muscular dystrophy*
    - More rapidly progressing
    - Usually diagnosed before the age of 6 years
    - More common in males
    - A leading cause of rapid disability in young children
    - Cardiomyopathy, or weakness in the heart muscles, can occur.
    - A finding is Gowers' sign, which is seen when children who are in a squatting position have to use their hands and arms to "walk up" their own bodies, pushing as they go, in order to stand. This is due to weakness in the proximal muscles (the hips and thighs) of the lower limbs (Davis et al., 2005).
  - *Fasiculohumeral muscular dystrophy*
    - Less disabling than other neuromuscular disorders
    - Diagnosed due to weakness in the shoulder and facial muscles
    - Weakness can occur in the limbs but this is less common and tends to occur only later in life as the condition worsens.
    - It is also a genetic disorder.

MYASTHENIA GRAVIS

- Myasthenia gravis is an autoimmune disorder
- Antibodies block acetylcholine receptors at the neuromuscular junction or the site where the neuron causes muscles to react (Davis et al., 2005).
- It affects voluntary muscles in the eyes, mouth, throat, and extremities.
- Three types of myasthenia gravis:
  - *Congenital*
    - The rarest form is congenital; in this disorder, genes must be transmitted from each parent in order for the child to have the disorder. Symptoms begin in infancy and do not go into remission.
  - *Transient neonatal*
    - This form occurs when a women with myasthenia gravis gives birth.
    - The baby has symptoms of the disease as a result of myasthenia antibodies crossing the placenta to the fetus.
    - This occurs in about 10% to 15% of babies born to mothers with myasthenia gravis and disappears without recurrence in the first few weeks of life (Volpe, 2001).
  - *Juvenile*
    - Juvenile myasthenia gravis is most common in female adolescents, particularly Caucasians.
    - This life-long condition is usually diagnosed in the mid-teens and goes in and out of remission.
    - About 10% of all cases of myasthenia gravis begin as juvenile myasthenia.

Assessment

- The symptoms of myasthenia gravis are predominantly weakness and fatigue.
- Persons with this disorder are unable to keep their eyelids raised and develop a condition called ptosis, or drooping eyelids.
- Mouth and throat muscles are weakened, and thus affected individuals cannot smile responsively, nor can they use a straw for drinking liquids.
- Swallowing becomes difficult in untreated cases.

CLINICAL PEARL

Symptoms of Myasthenia Gravis

Parents often report that the child looks tired or sad. These are cues to screen for myasthenia gravis, as the child may be developing ptosis of the eyelids or the inability to smile.

Diagnosis

- A blood test is performed to evaluate serum acetylcholine receptor antibodies.
- Electromyography (EMG) may be performed to confirm muscle activity.
- A Tensilon test may be performed, in which a medication called edrophonium chloride is injected intravenously to see if myasthenia gravis symptoms temporarily resolve.

CLINICAL PEARL

Medications and Myasthenia Gravis

Some medications can exacerbate weakness in a child with myasthenia gravis. These drugs include aminoglycosides, procainamide, quinidine, curare, succinylcholine, some channel blockers, and beta blockers. The nurse should have a thorough awareness of medications that are being administered to the child (Myasthenia Foundation of America, 2008).

Treatment

- Treatment is aimed at supportive care.
- Cholinesterase inhibitors may be used, which act to prevent the acetylcholine receptor from being blocked or broken down, thus allowing it to act as a neurotransmitter.
- Immunosuppressants can also be used in some cases if the patient is unresponsive to or intolerant of cholinesterase inhibitors.
- Sometimes a surgical procedure is required to remove the thymus gland, which works to provide T cells, which are necessary for autoimmunity. The thymus loses most of its function after adolescence, so this procedure is usually done in adulthood.

CRITICAL COMPONENT

Respiratory Function

Nurses must be alert to respiratory function changes in children with myasthenia gravis. Thorough assessment of breath sounds, respiratory rate, and oxygenation is critical (Bader & Littlejohns, 2004).

SPINAL MUSCLE ATROPHY

- Spinal muscle atrophy is a degenerative disorder of the anterior horn cells of the spinal cord (Behrman et al., 2007; Feinichel, 2001).
- Results in weakness and wasting of voluntary muscles
- Spinal muscle atrophy is the most common recessive genetic disorder that is lethal in children (Menkes, 1995).
- In milder forms of the disease, it is the second most common neuromuscular disorder in childhood.
- Recent research has indicated that there may be a genetic component due to an abnormality on chromosome 5.
- A characteristic initial finding is often proximal lower extremity weakness.
- Three types of spinal muscle atrophy (SMA):
  - *SMA Type 1 is also known as Werdnig-Hoffman disease.*
    - Most severe form
    - Begins in utero or early infancy
    - Infants have few spontaneous movements.
    - They are unable to lift their heads.
    - They have trouble sucking and swallowing.
    - They exhibit a loss of deep tendon reflexes.
    - Fasciculations, or constant, wormlike movements of the tongue, are noted.
    - Fasciculations can sometimes also be seen in the deltoid, biceps, and quadriceps muscles.
    - The respiratory muscles are weak, and death occurs by age 3 years due to respiratory compromise.
    - Infants who display symptoms at birth usually have a shorter life span and die before they are 12 months old.
  - *SMA Type 2 is noted later in infancy.*
    - Usually noted between the ages of 6 and 24 months
    - Deep tendon reflexes are absent.
    - Muscle fasciculations may or may not be present.
    - Life span for those with SMA Type 2 is 20–30 years.
  - *SMA Type 3 is a juvenile form of the disease.*
    - Also known as Kugelberg-Welander disease
    - Onset of the disease is between ages 3 and 17 years.
    - Early symptoms are nonspecific and include delayed motor milestones.
    - Atrophy of proximal muscles may be present.
    - SMA Type 3 is a milder form of the disease and children live into adulthood.

Assessment

- Thorough physical examination
- Thorough history of the child's illness

Diagnosis

- Diagnosis is derived from symptoms.
- Blood can be tested for genetic markers.
- EMG is performed to document muscle responses.
- A muscle biopsy is performed if blood tests are negative and the EMG is suggestive of spinal muscle atrophy.

Treatment

- Treatment is aimed at supportive care.
- The family of a child with spinal muscle atrophy requires additional support due to stress.
  - *Time*
  - *Emotions*
  - *Grief*
  - *Finances*

NEUROPATHY SYNDROMES

- **Neuropathy** is a condition in which peripheral nerves are damaged (**Figure 13-9**).
  - *Neuropathy can be an inherited disorder.*
  - *Or may be the result of*
    - A metabolic or endocrine disorder such as diabetes

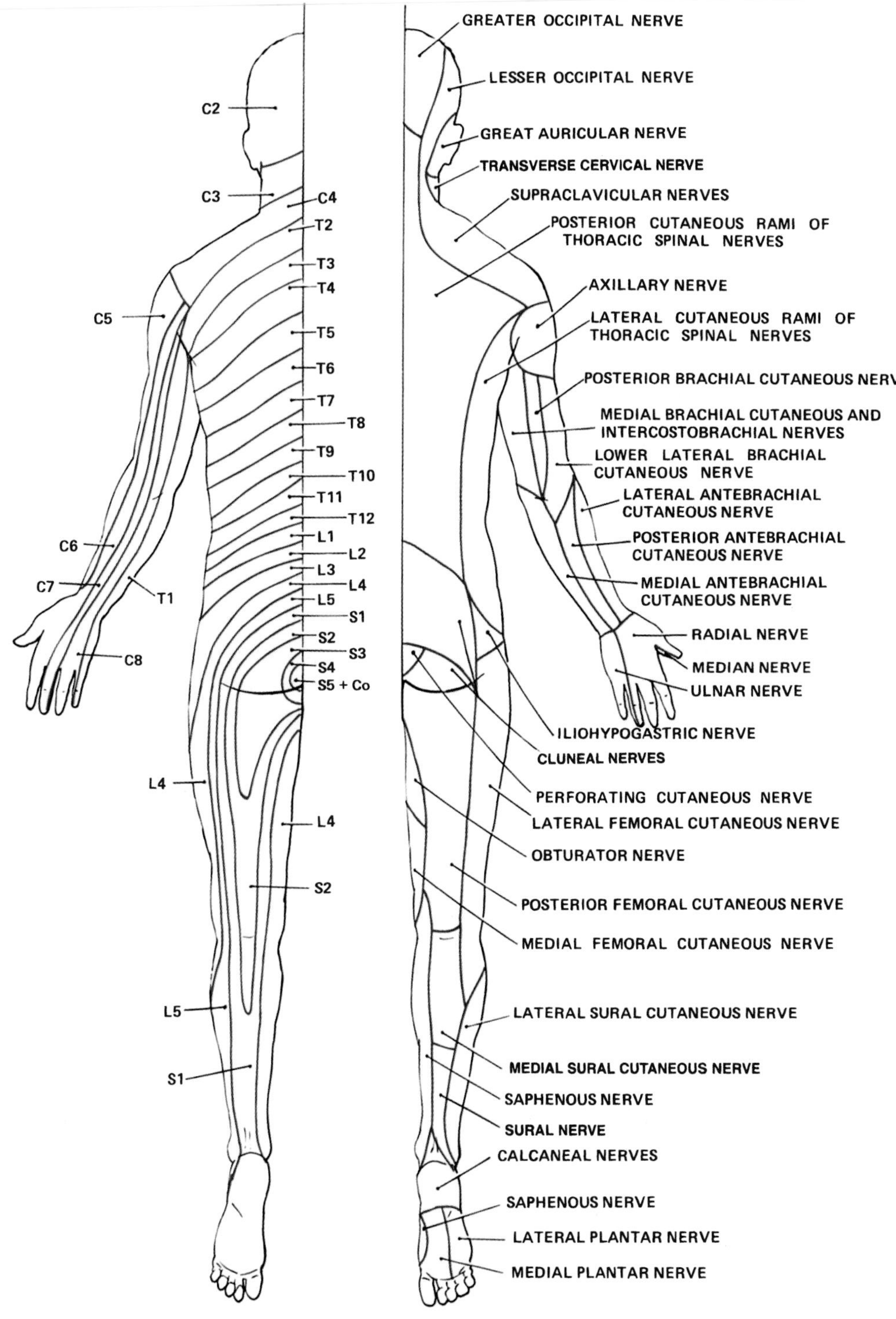

Figure 13-9 Pattern of innervations of the body by dorsal roots and peripheral nerves. *(From Gilman, S., & Newman, S. W. [2003].* Manter and Gatz's essentials of clinical neuroanatomy and neurophysiology *[10th ed.]. Philadelphia: F.A. Davis.)*

- Toxins such as chemotherapy
- Inflammation
- Vitamin deficiencies
- Trauma

- *Sometimes the cause cannot be determined, and is thus termed "idiopathic."*

- Symptoms
  - *Decreased sensation*
  - *Pain*
  - *Tingling*
  - *Problems with balance*
  - *Weakness in the extremities*
  - *Weakness can also occur in any other location in which autonomic nerves exist in the body.*
    - This leads to conditions such as abnormalities in the heart rate and respiratory rate, inability to perspire, problems with food absorption, constipation, and bladder dysfunction.

GUILLIAN–BARRÉ SYNDROME

- Guillian–Barré syndrome is an acute, inflammatory, demyelinating polyneuropathy that affects the peripheral nervous system (Davis et al., 2005; Schwartz et al., 2005).
- *Demyelinating* means that the protective myelin covering on nerve cells is being broken down, thus interrupting the smooth flow of impulses.
- The hallmark of Guillian–Barré is ascending paralysis, in which weakness occurs distally in the lower limbs and spreads to the upper extremities and torso.
- A complete loss of deep tendon reflexes occurs in patients affected by Guillian–Barré syndrome.
- This condition can be severe and affect the child's ability to breathe.
- Death may occur if the pulmonary system is severely compromised.
- Most patients recover fully but the course of the disease is slow, showing improvement after 4 weeks and often taking up to a year to achieve full recovery.
- About 20% of those affected have lingering affects after 1 year if the disease course was severe or treatment was delayed.

Assessment

- Thorough physical examination
- Thorough history of the child's illness
- Deep tendon reflexes may indicate a loss of reflexes along with the ascending paralysis.

Diagnosis

- Diagnosis is made based on symptoms and diagnostic test results.
- EMG is done to test the electrical activity in the muscles.
- Nerve conduction velocity (NCV) testing is done to measure the speed of electrical signals traveling through a nerve.
- Lumbar puncture is done to assess protein and white blood cell count. In Guillian–Barré, the protein count is elevated and the white blood cell count is normal.

Treatment

- Treatment is aimed at supportive care.
- *Plasmapheresis*—a procedure in which plasma is removed from blood cells and then the blood cells are returned to the patient. This is thought to remove autoantibodies from the blood and thus reduce the severity and duration of the syndrome.
- *Intravenous gamma globulins*—gamma globulins are substances that the body uses to help naturally fight the syndrome; they are given intravenously on a schedule until the patient shows normalization.
- Most patients recover fully, but the course of the disease is slow, showing improvement after 4 weeks and often taking up to a year to achieve full recovery.
- About 20% of those affected have lingering affects after 1 year if the disease course was severe or treatment was delayed.

Review Questions

1. Common characteristics seen in children with autism include
   A. clinging to parents.
   B. impaired language skills.
   C. stereotypic behaviors such as hand flapping or rocking movements.
   D. both b and c.
2. Common characteristics seen in children with ADHD include
   A. inattention.
   B. impulsive behavior.
   C. dyslexia.
   D. both a and b.
3. A nurse caring for a 13-year-old boy notices that he has involuntary muscle jerks and makes vocal grunting sounds that are more noticeable when he is nervous. The nurses realizes that he likely has
   A. seizures.
   B. Tourette's syndrome.
   C. multiple sclerosis.
   D. a behavioral disorder.
4. When caring for a 4-year-old girl, the nurse notes that her anterior fontanel is open and soft. This finding is
   A. normal for her age.
   B. abnormal for her age.
   C. normal in children of some ethnicities.
   D. none of the above.
5. You are the nurse in a busy emergency department. A father brings in his 1-year-old daughter and tells you that she has a fever of 104 rectally, is somewhat sleepy, and has a stiff neck. Which of the following should be your response?
   A. Ask him to take her to her pediatrician, as the emergency department is crowded and busy.
   B. Ask him to complete paperwork and have a seat until called, as the child has pink cheeks and is holding onto a toy.
   C. Tell him to take her home and give her a baby aspirin.
   D. Assume that she may have meningitis and immediately take her to a private exam room to begin assessment and treatment.

6. A 16-year-old girl loses consciousness, falls to the floor, and begins jerking her arms and legs. As the school nurse, you know that she is having a seizure and it is important to do everything as follows, *except*:
   A. gently roll her to the side.
   B. time the length of the seizure.
   C. put a padded spoon in her mouth to keep her from biting her tongue.
   D. monitor her airway.

7. In an infant, brain growth can be screened by performing what task?
   A. Measuring head circumference
   B. Plotting the height and weight on a growth chart
   C. Age-appropriate play with the baby
   D. None of the above

8. You are the triage RN in a family practice office. A mother brings in her 10-year-old daughter and tells you that she has had a headache, vomiting, and intolerance to light for the past hour. Information you would want to gather about this child would include
   A. previous history of head injuries.
   B. previous history of headaches.
   C. recent history of febrile illness.
   D. all of the above.

9. Which cranial nerve innervates the structures necessary for hearing?
   A. CN 5
   B. CN 11
   C. CN 8
   D. CN 3

10. You are the RN starting your shift on a pediatric unit. You are taking care of a 7-month-old infant who has been alert and behaving in an age-appropriate manner on the previous shift. When you perform your first assessment, his parents tell you that in the last hour, he has become sleepier and did not cry when the lab technician drew blood a few minutes ago. Your response is to
    A. encourage the parents to keep the room quiet to allow him to sleep.
    B. document it and plan to recheck him in an hour.
    C. tell his parents to make him wake up because it is not time for him to go to bed.
    D. realize that lethargy in an infant is always an ominous neurological sign and immediately assess him.

References

American Academy of Child and Adolescent Psychiatry. (2004). *Tic disorders*. Retrieved from http://www.aacap.org/cs/root/facts_for_families/tic_disorders

American Heart Association (AHA). (2009). *Pediatric stroke*. Retrieved from http://www.strokeassociation.org/presenter.jhtml?identifier=3030392

Bader, M. K., & Littlejohns, L. R. (2004). *AANN core curriculum for neuroscience nursing* (4th ed.). St. Louis, MO: W. B. Saunders.

Behrman, R. E., Kliegman, R. M., Jenson, H. B., & Stanton, B. F. (2007). *Nelson textbook of pediatrics* (18th ed.). St. Louis, MO: W. B. Saunders.

Buchhalter, J. (2011). Treatment of childhood absence epilepsy. *Epilepsy Currents, 11*, 12–15. Retrieved from http://www.ncbi.nlm.nih.gov/pmc/articles/PMC3063575/

Centers for Disease Control and Prevention (CDC). (2011). *Child development—developmental screening*. Retrieved from http://www.cdc.gov/ncbddd/child/devtool.htm

Davis, L. E., King, M., & Shultz, J. L. (2005). *Fundamentals of neurologic disease*. New York: Demos Medical Publishing, Inc.

Deglan, J. H., Vallerand, A. H., & Sanoski, C. A. (2011). *Davis's drug guide for nurses* (12th ed.). Philadelphia: F.A. Davis.

El-Bohy, A. A., & Wong, B. L. (2005). The diagnosis of muscular dystrophy. *Pediatric Annals, 34*, 525–530. Retrieved from http://www.ncbi.nlm.nih.gov/pubmed/16092626

Ellenbrogen, R. G., & Roberts, T. S. (2009). *Neural tube defects in the neonatal period*. Retrieved from http://emedicine.medscape.com/article/979902-overview

Epilepsy Foundation. (2008). *Seizure action plan*. Retrieved from http://www.epilepsyfoundation.org/programs/schoolnurse/upload/seizure-action-plan.pdf

Espay, A. J. (2009). *Hydrocephalus*. Retrieved from http://emedicine.medscape.com/article/1135286-overview

Feinichel, G. M. (2001). *Clinical pediatric neurology*. St. Louis, MO: W. B. Saunders.

Gilman, S., & Newman, S. W. (2003). *Manter and Gatz's essentials of clinical neuroanatomy and neurophysiology* (10th ed.). Philadelphia: F.A. Davis.

Goldstein, J. L. (2004). Evaluating new onset of seizures in children. *Pediatric Annals, 33*, 368–374. Retrieved from http://www.ncbi.nlm.nih.gov/pubmed/19449511

Hamancioglu, K. (2006). Is syncope cardiovascular in origin? *Practical Neurology, 5*, 42–49. Retrieved from http://pn.bmj.com/

Kenney, C., Kuo, S., & Jimenez-Shahed, J. (2008). *Tourette's syndrome*. Retrieved from http://www.aafp.org/afp/2008/0301/p651.html

Lopez, J. I., & Rothrock, J. F. (2008). *Headache, pediatric perspective*. Retrieved from http://emedicine.medscape.com/article/1179166-overview

Menkes, J. H. (1995). *Textbook of child neurology* (5th ed.). Philadelphia: Williams & Wilkins.

Myasthenia Foundation of America. (2008). *Myasthenia gravis: A manual for the health care provider*. Retrieved from http://www.myasthenia.org/LinkClick.aspx?fileticket=b8Af4U6u9Ak%3d&tabid=82

National Early Childhood Technical Assistance Center. (2008). *Developmental screening and assessment instruments with an emphasis on social and emotional development for young children ages birth through five*. Retrieved from http://www.nectac.org/~pdfs/pubs/screening.pdf

National Institute of Neurologic Disorders and Stroke (NINDS). (2011a). *NINDS neurofibromatosis information page*. Retrieved from http://www.ninds.nih.gov/disorders/neurofibromatosis/neurofibromatosis.htm

National Institute of Neurologic Disorders and Stroke (NINDS). (2011b). *Neurofibromatosis fact sheet*. Retrieved from http://www.ninds.nih.gov/disorders/neurofibromatosis/detail_neurofibromatosis.htm

National Institute of Neurologic Disorders and Stroke (NINDS). (2011c). *Chiari malformation fact sheet*. Retrieved from http://www.ninds.nih.gov/disorders/chiari/chiari.htm

National Institute of Neurologic Disorders and Stroke (NINDS). (2011d). *Meningitis and encephalitis fact sheet*. Retrieved from http://www.ninds.nih.gov/disorders/encephalitis_meningitis/detail_encephalitis_meningitis.htm

National Institute of Neurologic Disorders and Stroke (NINDS). (2011e). *Tethered cord fact sheet*. Retrieved from http://www.ninds.nih.gov/disorders/tethered_cord/tethered_cord.htm

Ochoa, J. G., & Riche, W. (2008). *Epileptic drugs: An overview*. Retrieved from http://emedicine.medscape.com/article/1187334-overview

Parker, S., Zuckerman, B., & Augustyn, M. (2005). *Developmental and behavioral pediatrics, a handbook for primary care* (2nd ed.). Philadelphia: Lippincott Williams & Wilkins.

Schwartz, M. W., Bell, L. M., Bingham, P. M., Chung, E. K., Friedman, D. F., Mulberg, A. E., & Tanel, R. E. (2005). *The 5-minute pediatric consult* (4th ed.). Philadelphia: Lippincott Williams & Wilkins.

Shevell, M., Ashwal, S., Donley, D., Gingold, M., Hirtz, D., Majnemer, A., . . . Sheth, R. (2003). Practice parameter: Evaluation of the child with global developmental delay. Report of the Quality Standards Subcommittee of the American Academy of Neurology and the Practice Committee of the Child Neurology Society. *Neurology, 60*, 367–380. doi: 10.1212/01.WNL.0000031431.81555.16

Silberstein, S., Saper, J. R., & Freitag, F. G. (2008). *Diagnostic and therapeutic challenges in acute migraine*. Retrieved from http://cme.medscape.com/viewprogram/1708_pnt

Volpe, J. (2001). *Neurology of the newborn* (4th ed.). St. Louis, MO: W. B. Saunders.

Young, W. B., & Silberstein, S. D. (2004). *Migraine and other headaches*. New York: Demos Medical Publishing.

Zitelli, B. J., & Davis, H. W. (2007). *Atlas of pediatric physical diagnosis* (5th ed.). Philadelphia: Elsevier.

14 Mental Health Disorders

Andrea Warner Stidham, PhD, RN
Theresa L. Puckett, PhD, RN, CPNP, CNE

OBJECTIVES

- ☐ Discuss three current trends in pediatric psychiatry.
- ☐ Describe multiaxial diagnosis.
- ☐ Describe learning disabilities in children, as well as recommended treatments.
- ☐ Discuss reactive attachment disorder in children, as well as recommended treatments.
- ☐ Explain two mood disorders diagnosed in children, as well as recommended treatments.
- ☐ Explain five anxiety disorders diagnosed in children, as well as recommended treatments.
- ☐ Identify three disruptive disorders diagnosed in children, as well as recommended treatments.
- ☐ Discuss one impulse-control disorder diagnosed in children, as well as recommended treatments.
- ☐ Discuss schizophrenia in children, as well as recommended treatments.
- ☐ Identify four pervasive developmental disorders diagnosed in children, as well as recommended treatments.
- ☐ Identify three eating disorders diagnosed in children, as well as recommended treatments.
- ☐ Describe three current treatment modalities in pediatric substance abuse treatment.
- ☐ Describe dual diagnosis in children.
- ☐ Discuss child abuse assessment, diagnosis, and recommended treatments.

KEY TERMS

- Autism
- Hallucination
- Multiaxial assessment
- Psychoeducation
- Anhedonia
- Bullycide
- Cognitive behavioral therapy (CBT)
- Interpersonal psychotherapy (IPT)
- Alexithymia
- Suicidality
- Anxiolytic
- Perseveration
- Tangential
- Obsession
- Compulsion
- Delusion

INTRODUCTION

Childhood and adolescence are periods of great transition and reorganization. Wide variation exists regarding what is normal developmental behavior. However, children can and do develop mental health disorders. Some disorders start in childhood and last a lifetime. Others resolve during childhood. As with any chronic illness, caregivers of children with mental illness need support and may grieve the loss of who they thought their child was and would become.

- About 20% of the child population is estimated to have a mental disorder resulting in mild functional impairment (U.S. Department of Health and Human Services, 1999).

CULTURAL AWARENESS: Incidence of Mental Illness

Incidence of mental illness is higher in subcultures of the population, such as incarcerated juveniles and lesbian, gay, bisexual, transgender, questioning, and intersex children.

- Between 5% and 9% of the child population have a mental disorder resulting in extreme functional impairment (U.S. Department of Health and Human Services, 1999).
- Of pediatric hospital admissions, 7% are for mental health reasons, with depression being the primary diagnosis (AHRQ, 2011).

Don't have time to read this chapter? Want to reinforce your reading? Need to review for a test? Listen to this chapter on DavisPlus at davispl.us/rudd1.

- Approximately 80% of adolescents will experience at least one depressive episode (U.S. Department of Health and Human Services, 1999).
- In the United States, six children per day kill themselves.
- Anna Freud, Sigmund Freud's youngest child, is considered the founder of pediatric psychiatry.

WHAT IS MENTAL ILLNESS?

- A distorted view of self
- Often unable to maintain personal relationships
- Loss of the ability to respond to the environment in ways that are in accord with oneself or society's expectations
- Characterized by thought or behavior patterns that impair functioning and cause the individual distress
- Loss of a person's ability to respond to the environment in manners that align with individual, family, or societal expectations
- Impaired judgment
- Lack of insight regarding own abilities and consequences of actions

> CLINICAL PEARL
>
> **Mental Illness and Developmental Age**
>
> Developmental age needs to be considered when assessing behavior and thought patterns.

Results of Mental Illness

- Cognitive distortions leading to lowered self-esteem
- Inability to form and/or maintain meaningful personal relationships
- Physical disability, morbidity, and/or death

Risk Factors for Mental Illness

Mental health disorders can occur across all social classes and families; however, there are risk factors for developing mental disorders in childhood. These include:

- Physical problems
- Intellectual disabilities (such as mental retardation)
- Low birth weight
- Family history of mental illness or addictive disorders
- Multigenerational poverty
- Caregiver separation, abuse, or neglect

ETIOLOGY OF MENTAL ILLNESS IN CHILDREN

Genetic Influences

- Multiple genes, interacting with environmental factors, seem to confer risk of mental illness. Up to this point, no single gene has been pinpointed as causing mental illness.
- Major psychiatric disorders, such as depression, anxiety disorders, schizophrenia, and bipolar disorder, are found among family generations. Research indicates that **autism**, learning and language disorders, attention deficit-hyperactivity disorder (ADHD), and enuresis (bedwetting) seem to be genetically transmitted.
- Having a parent or sibling with a mental illness indicates increased risk for developing mental illnesses among other closely related family members.

Psychological Influences

- Stressful life events (e.g., caregiver illness, relocating, death of family member)
- Personality/temperament (e.g., how the child's temperament elicits reactions from parents or caregivers, accurate processing of social clues, sense of self-efficacy, ability to problem solve)
- Gender (some psychiatric disorders affect males and females disproportionally, for example, depression for girls and ADHD for boys)
- Age (children respond differently to events according to developmental maturity)

Social/Environmental Influences

- Parents (warm or supportive versus disregarding or neglectful)
- School adjustment (positive experiences versus negative experiences)
- Socioeconomic status (poverty and/or homelessness serve as barriers to normal developmental maturity and are risk factors for developing psychiatric disorders)
- Culture (view of diagnosis and treatment of mental illness can serve as barrier or protective factor in the development of mental illness)
- Religion (view of diagnosis and treatment of mental illness can serve as barrier or protective factor in the development of mental illness)
- Interpersonal relationships (positive, supportive relationships can serve as a protective factor in the development of mental illness)

Neurochemical Influences

- Norepinephrine deficiencies can cause:
  - *Impaired attention*
  - *Problems concentrating*
  - *Problems with memory*
  - *Slow information processing*
  - *Depressed mood*
  - *Psychomotor retardation*
  - *Fatigue*
- Serotonin deficiencies can cause:
  - *Anxiety*
  - *Panic*
  - *Phobia*
  - *Obsessions*

- *Compulsions*
- *Food cravings*
- *Bulimia*

- Dopamine deficiencies can cause:
  - *Decreased ability to experience pleasure*
  - *Increased irritability and aggression*
  - *Decreased cognitive functioning*
  - *Decreased motivation*

EMOTIONAL INTELLIGENCE

Emotional intelligence (EQ) stems from the prefrontal cortex and allows an individual to identify, analyze, understand, and regulate behavior. Children who have been abused or neglected or have a psychological disorder often lack EQ skills.

Clinical Reasoning

Importance of Emotional Intelligence

EQ allows individuals to appropriately interpret and respond to social cues from others.

1. Which is more important to the long-term success of a child, IQ or EQ?

TRENDS IN PEDIATRIC PSYCHIATRY

- Medication wash—taking a child off of all medications and seeing how he or she does "naturally"; usually done in an inpatient setting
- More pediatric bipolar disorder being diagnosed in children, even in those previously diagnosed with ADHD
- Few providers specializing in pediatric psychiatry means that children sometimes do not get care
- More children admitted to inpatient psychiatric facilities due to worry over parents' financial concerns
- More children dealing with anger issues
- Younger and younger suicidal/self-harming children being seen in practice
- More clinical drug trials on pediatric participants
- Children are not as resilient as previously thought.

Clinical Reasoning

Adolescent Brain Development

New research shows that the adolescent brain is still in development until the early 20s, and that it matures from back to front. In addition, at around age 11 or 12 many brain connections are lost and the brain rewires itself to have more adult patterns of thinking (Winters, 2008).

1. What is the relationship between frontal lobe development and risk taking?
2. What are the nursing implications of this new research on adolescent brain development?

ASSESSMENT

Mental health assessment must occur within family, social, and cultural contexts and be considered within the context of the child's development. Assessment includes evaluation of the child's biologic, social, and psychological factors. Mental health assessment generally takes place in the schools and primary care offices. Families are essential partners in the provision of child mental health services.

CLINICAL PEARL

Puberty and Mental Health Illness

When taking a mental health history, the parents will often report that the child's symptoms started or got worse around the time of puberty.

Mental Status Examination

- The health-care provider will assess the child specifically for skills related to language as well as cognitive, emotional, and social functioning. A mental status examination is conducted and includes the following:
  - *Appearance, motor activity, self-concept, and behavior*
  - *Social interaction, general intelligence, memory, and orientation*
  - *Attention span and comprehension, speech, and language*
  - *Mood/feelings and insight and judgment*
  - *Thought processes and content*
  - *Auditory* ***hallucinations*** *(hearing voices that no one else hears)*
  - *Visual hallucinations (seeing things that no one else sees)*
  - *Delusional thoughts (such as thinking oneself to be a king)*
  - *Self-harm by banging head, cutting self, or by other means*
  - *Substance use/abuse*
  - *Sudden change in behavior*
  - *Sudden change in school performance*
- The health-care provider will ask several questions of both the child and caregiver to determine:
  - *What caused the patient/family to seek help at this time*
  - *Psychiatric history (formal mental health services, family history of mental illness)*
  - *Current and past health status (symptoms child is experiencing and length of time they have been present)*
  - *Medications*
  - *Neurologic history (handedness, dizziness, seizures, hyperactivity)*
  - *Responses to mental health problems (what helps or aggravates symptoms)*
  - *Developmental history (pregnancy, delivery, Apgar scores, developmental milestones)*
  - *Attachment, temperament, behavior problems*
  - *Self-concept (identity, self-esteem)*
  - *Risk assessment (suicidal, homicidal ideation, substance use/abuse)*

- *Risk of suicide, including: past history or suicidal thoughts/attempts, thoughts of/and or presence of a plan, lethality of the plan, and access to the means described in the plan*
- *Risk of assaulting others and/or past history of assaulting others*
- *History of aggression toward animals*
- *History of arson*
- *History of running away*
- *Family relationships (parents, deaths/losses, conflicts, siblings)*
- *Relationships with peers and others in social settings (drug and alcohol use/abuse, dating, friends, participation in school-related activities)*
- *School performance (adjustment, attendance, relationships with teachers)*
- *Temper tantrums*

CLINICAL PEARL

Assessing Risk for Suicide

When assessing suicidality, ask about a plan and whether the patient has means to carry out the plan. If the child does have access to a stash of pills or a weapon, it is the nurse's responsibility to work with the family and appropriate authorities to eliminate access.

- The three mental health conditions most common in children are:
  - *Learning disabilities*
  - *ADHD*
  - *Behavioral conditions (For additional information please see www.cdc.gov/nchs/hdi.htm)*
- Common childhood problems include:
  - *Death and grief*
  - *Parental separation and divorce*
  - *Sibling relationships*
  - *Physical illness*
  - *Adolescent risk-taking behaviors*
  - *Separation anxiety*
  - *Temper tantrums*
  - *School phobia*
  - *Bullying*
  - *Growth and development issues*

CRITICAL COMPONENT

The Effect of Certain Behaviors on Quality of Life

Behaviors that interfere with quality of life at home and school need to be evaluated by a professional.

- Nursing interventions to help a child through a common childhood problem are:
  - *Provide support*
  - *Encourage expression of feelings*
  - *Provide information*
  - *Answer questions honestly*
  - *Assess for anger-related problems and suicidality*
  - *Refer for individual and family therapy as needed*
- Before the child is diagnosed with a mental health disorder, a physical assessment, including lab work, should be completed to rule out the following conditions that could produce symptoms similar to those of mental health problems:
  - *Organic disorders*
  - *Sensory disorders*
  - *Medication-induced symptoms (e.g., weight loss, drug-induced psychosis)*
  - *Thyroid abnormalities*
  - *Mental retardation*
  - *Brain tumors*
  - *Lead poisoning*

Multiaxial Assessment

Mental health assessment occurs on many levels and in different settings to assess individual functioning. The *Diagnostic and Statistical Manual of Mental Disorders* (DSM) is a guide of all diagnosable mental illnesses (American Psychological Association [APA], 2000). This manual is updated periodically. The current version is DSM-IV-TR (fourth edition text revision). The DSM-V is in development and due for forthcoming publication. The DSM-IV-TR offers guidelines for **multiaxial assessment**, or assessment of various areas of individual functioning. Multiaxial assessment includes five *axes* that identify important areas of symptom presentation:

- Axis I: Clinical Disorders (AKA: the clinical disorder)
- Axis II: Personality Disorders, Mental Retardation, and Learning Disabilities
- Axis III: General Medical Conditions
- Axis IV: Psychosocial and Environmental Problems
- Axis V: Children's Global Assessment Scale (C-GAS) Score

The Children's Global Assessment Scale (C-GAS) score helps clinicians quantify how well an individual is functioning in his or her everyday life on a 0–100 scale. The higher the score on the C-GAS, the higher functioning the individual is in managing daily life. Scores below 60 are concerning and indicate a low level of functioning. Clinicians often list current and potential C-GAS scores on Axis V.

Limitations of the DSM with Children

- Has 75% interrater reliability (Grisso, 2004)
- Of children currently diagnosed with a mental health disorder, 75% to 80% will not meet the criteria for the disorder a year from now (Grisso, 2004).
- Gender, age, race, and developmental level also effect how mental disorders are manifested and can be measured, but this is not addressed in the DSM (McNeish & Newman, 2002).
- High comorbidity rates in children reflect a "general psychopathology" consistent with immature development and the consequent lack of ability to differentiate disorders into discrete categories (Grisso, 2004).

SETTINGS OF CARE IN PEDIATRIC PSYCHIATRY

- School counselor
- Home therapist
- Outpatient psychiatrist/psychologist
- Group home
- Residential treatment

> **CLINICAL PEARL**
>
> **Residential Treatment**
>
> Residential treatment is expensive and often not covered under private insurance. Sometimes caregivers have to give up custody rights over the child in order for the county or state to fund residential treatment.

- Partial hospitalization program (PHP)
- Intensive outpatient program (IOP)
- Inpatient psychiatric unit

INPATIENT PSYCHIATRIC THERAPY

Inpatient psychiatric therapy is considered when the patient is at immediate risk of harming self or others. Admissions are either voluntary (guardian agrees to the admission) or involuntary (child is "pink-slipped" by a physician or police). Laws surrounding inpatient psychiatric treatment vary by state. Other uses for inpatient treatment include:

- It is better than the juvenile detention center. Sometimes incarcerated juveniles state that they are suicidal in order to leave the detention center for a while.
- As a dumping ground. Frustrated guardians may see the hospital as an out. Children come to the hospital with every worldly possession in tow.
- Lots of personalized attention. Children who crave attention tend to enjoy being hospitalized on the inpatient psychiatric unit.
- Respite care. Tired guardians who need a break may seek hospitalization for the child.

Risks of Inpatient Psychiatric Admission

- Learning new (negative) behaviors from peers
- Hearing about subjects that the child has not been exposed to previously, such as drugs and sex
- Physical/psychological violence from peers

Therapeutic Milieu

- The environment of care is called the milieu in psychiatric care.
- The milieu itself is a treatment modality (Peplau, 1989).
- All aspects of the milieu should contribute to care and recovery.
- Structured components of the milieu are group therapy, community meetings, and **psychoeducation** classes
- Unstructured components of the milieu include interactions between patients, staff, visitors.

Health-Care Providers in the Therapeutic Milieu

- Professionals who work in the therapeutic milieu include:
  - *Psychiatric nurse*
  - *Psychiatric advanced practice nurse (adult, family, child CNS or NP)*
  - *Psychiatric social worker*
  - *Psychologist*
  - *Psychiatrist*
  - *Medical doctor*
  - *Occupational therapist*
  - *Certified addiction counselor*
  - *Milieu therapist*
  - *Mental health worker/technician*
  - *Activity therapist*

Rules of the Milieu

- Refer to patients by first name only.
- Patients should not have shoelaces, belts, piercings, or anything else that could be used to hurt themselves or others.
- Pin numbers or a code word may be used to ensure patient confidentiality. Do not give information to someone who does not have the pin number/code word.
- No outside food is allowed in the milieu.
- Check all belongings/items that come in to ensure patient and staff safety.
- Check every patient at least every 15 minutes to ensure safety.
- Watch for own personal safety. Do not wear necklaces/scarves that can be used to choke you.
- Be mindful of all items taken onto the milieu. Pencils, staples, and silverware can be used by patients to hurt self or others.
- Do not hand out personal information, such as your phone number or e-mail address.

Admission Process

- Direct patient to change into a hospital gown.
- Check all belongings.
- Retain contraband items.
- Skin check: Document all rashes, cuts, and scars that a patient has upon admission.
- Psychological and risk assessment: Address the child and parent.
- History and physical
- Labs (complete blood count with differencial CBC w/diff, comprehensive metabolic panel [CMP], thyroid stimulating hormone [TSH], urine or blood toxicity, urinalysis, and pregnancy test if applicable)

Types of Restrictions with Interventions for Inpatient Psychiatric Patients

Suicide Precautions

- Frequently reassess for suicidal thoughts.
- Have child wear a cloth or paper gown.
- Monitor patient one on one.
- Room near nurse's station
- Finger foods only

Assault Precautions

- Frequently assess for signs of escalation.
- No roommate
- Do not allow patient off the unit.

Elopement Precautions

- Monitor exits and doors.
- Monitor patient whereabouts frequently.
- Have child wear hospital gown and slippers.

Boundary Precautions

- Watch child for inappropriate verbal or physical interactions with others.
- No roommate

Restrict to Unit

- Child is not allowed to leave the unit due to psychological or medical condition.

Typical Day

- Shower/clean room/breakfast
- Goal group
- Psychoeducational groups
- Art group
- Physical activity
- Visiting/phone calls
- Reflections

Discharge Process

- Distribute satisfaction surveys.
- Ensure that patient can contract for safety.
- Arrange follow-up appointments
- Make sure that patient/family has needed prescriptions.

PEDIATRIC THERAPEUTIC APPROACHES

Key Influences

- Key factors that influence therapeutic approaches with children:
  - *Children need to be prepared for the future.*
  - *Children need to develop self-awareness.*
  - *Children use more nonverbal communication than verbal communication.*

Goals of Therapy

- Improve communication skills.
- Build self-esteem.
- Stimulate development.
- Build an emotional repertoire.
- Improve emotional vocabulary.
- Encourage assimilation of traumatic events.
- Enable detachment from an emotional experience.

General Approaches to Therapy with Children

- Keep it fun.
- Let the child be in control.

Types of Therapy Used with Children

- Play therapy
- Art therapy
- Music therapy
- Pet therapy
- Cognitive-behavioral therapy
- Dialectical behavior therapy
- Hypnosis

Tools Used in Therapy with Children

- Board games
- Group games
- Recreational equipment/approaches
- Arts and crafts
- Animals
- Worksheets
- Behavior charts
- Timers to teach patience/impulse control
- Videos
- Video games
- Relaxing music/sounds
- Weighted vests/body socks
- Visual supports

SCHOOL FOR CHILDREN WITH MENTAL ILLNESS

- Teachers and other school staff need to be trained in how to recognize and address children with mental health disorders.
- Caregivers often feel frustrated by a lack of services and tired from being the child's advocate within the system.
- Nurses should support caregivers and help them to be the best advocates for their children.
- Children with mental health disorders have certain rights under the Americans with Disabilities Act (ADA), such as nondiscrimination for selection into a school or program. Only children who are a direct threat to others may be excluded from school or certain programs within the school.

- A Section 504 plan may be implemented to identify the accommodations needed by the child in order to be able to fully participate in a program/activity in school.
- The Individuals with Disabilities Education Act (IDEA) ensures that children with mental illness have access to early intervention and special education services as needed.
- Children with mental illness may need an individualized educational plan (IEP) at school in order to be successful. An IEP describes goals for the child and identifies the services needed in order to attain the goals (**Figure 14-1**). Periodic meetings between parents, teachers, the school counselor/psychologist, special education teacher, and others at the school ensure that services are modified as needed so that educational goals can be reached.

PSYCHIATRIC AND BEHAVIORAL DISORDERS

LEARNING DISABILITIES

Learning disabilities (LDs) are neurologically based and may be caused by a number of factors, including:

- Interuterine conditions such as maternal cigarette, alcohol, or drug use
- Genetics
- Environmental factors
- Diagnosis of ADHD or autism

CRITICAL COMPONENT

Learning Disabilities and Intelligence

Persons with a diagnosed learning disability are often of average or above average intelligence.

Nursing Interventions

- Be patient.
- Assess learning needs.
- Assess how child learns best.
- Design learning interventions accordingly.

Caregiver Education

- Teaching for caregivers of a child with a suspected or diagnosed learning disability:
  - *Be patient with the child.*
  - *Be an advocate for the child.*
  - *Request testing through the school.*
  - *Seek help as soon as a disability is suspected.*
  - *Pursue an IEP as needed.*

BEHAVIOR PROBLEMS

Children with or without a mental illness may exhibit undesirable behaviors.

What Is "Behaviorally Challenged"?

- Failing to initiate behaviors requested by an adult in a reasonable time frame
- Failure to complete the directive
- Failure to follow previously learned rules of conduct in a situation
- Yelling
- Complaining
- Defiance
- Tantrums
- Throwing objects
- Insults
- Swearing
- Steals
- Lies
- Argues
- Annoys
- Teases
- Ignores adults
- Fails to complete chores
- Engages in physical fights
- Fails to complete schoolwork
- Refuses to go to school
- Ignores self-care
- Talks back
- Disrupts others

Causes of Behavior Problems

- Inconsistent discipline
- Inconsistent monitoring of the child's behavior
- Harsh discipline methods
- Dysfunctional/inconsistent child/family member interactions
- Mental health diagnosis

Outcomes of Behavior Problems

- Family conflict
- School problems
- Issues with peers
- Frustrated caregivers
- Frustrated child
- Caregivers feel hopeless, helpless
- Fewer family activities
- Fewer interactions between the caregivers and child
- Caregiver and child feel isolated

Help for Caregivers

Caregivers should get help when

- Behavior is developmentally inappropriate.
- Behavior is causing impairment at home, school, or with peer relationships.
- Behavior is causing a significant amount to emotional distress to self/parents.

National Center for Learning Disabilities, Inc.
The power to hope, to learn, and to succeed

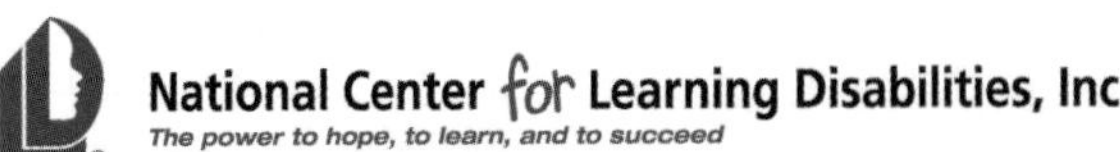

IEP Checklist for Parents

Use this list to determine if your child's IEP contains all of the components required by IDEA. Remember to provide your input to the school in advance of your child's IEP meeting.

			Notes:
❑ Yes	❑ No	Is the information in your child's present level of performance (PLOP) clearly stated and supported with objective information and assessment or evaluation data, such as information from standardized testing, curriculum based measurements or performance on district or state-wide assessments?	
❑ Yes	❑ No	Does the present level of performance (PLOP) section of the IEP contain information about the academic, developmental and functional needs of your child?	
❑ Yes	❑ No	Are your concerns and expectations for your child included in the present level of performance (PLOP) section of the IEP?	
❑ Yes	❑ No	Are your child's annual goals clearly stated and can they be measured?	
❑ Yes	❑ No	Knowing the effects of your child's disability, do the annual goals directly relate to your child's needs as stated in the present level of performance (PLOP)?	
❑ Yes	❑ No	Is the specific way(s) to master the annual goals clearly stated?	
❑ Yes	❑ No	Is the method(s) to monitor and evaluate your child's progress toward the annual goals clearly stated?	
❑ Yes	❑ No	Does the IEP indicate the amount of time your child will spend in general education?	
❑ Yes	❑ No	Are the special education services and related services recommended for your child supported by scientific research that supports their effectiveness? If not, what evidence has the school provided to indicate that the services and instructional methods proposed for your child have been found to be effective for children with similar learning difficulties and of similar age?	
❑ Yes	❑ No	Does the IEP state who will be responsible for implementing the services listed?	
❑ Yes	❑ No	Are the appropriate related services addressed on the IEP?	
❑ Yes	❑ No	Do you know how the IEP content will be communicated and shared with the staff responsible for their implementation?	
❑ Yes	❑ No	Are all of the appropriate accommodations listed?	
❑ Yes	❑ No	Does the IEP indicate how your child will participate in state and district testing?	
❑ Yes	❑ No	Have any potential consequences of your child's assessment participation been explained to you? Have you discussed whether your child may or may not be allowed to move on to the next grade or graduate with a regular diploma?	

Figure 14–1 An individualized education plan (IEP) describes goals for the child and identifies the services needed in order to attain the goals. *(© 2011 The National Center for Learning Disabilities, Inc. All rights reserved. For more information, visit LD.org).*

Types of Help Available

- School counselor
- Individual/family counseling
- Inpatient treatment
- Parent coaching

Nursing Interventions

Nursing interventions for the child who is behaviorally challenged include:

- Monitor behavior consistently.
- Praise the good.
- Be consistent (social predictability is key).
- Focus on giving positive attention.
- Defiance and aggressiveness produce the consistency the child craves and therefore these behaviors increase.
- Use immediate and consistent punishments for noncompliance.
- Recognize and terminate escalating behaviors.
- Confront negative interactions.
- Provide incentives for compliance.
- Do not regress to name-calling/threats.
- Utilize joint problem-solving and negotiation techniques.
- Communicate in positive terms.
- Identify and reframe your expectations, especially if the child has a mental health diagnosis.

STRESS AND CHILDREN

Stress is a normal part of life. Children need to experience some stress in order to practice coping skills and gain confidence in handling future stressors.

Factors That Predispose Children to Stress

- Cognitive immaturity
- Lack of judgment/insight
- Home setting
- School setting
- Peers
- Events
- Family changes
- Emphasis on achievement
- Pace of life
- Media influences
- Lack of basic needs being met
- Anticipated events such as changing schools and starting menstruation

Manifestations of Stress

Physical

- Headaches
- Stomachaches
- Cardiovascular disorders
- Gastrointestinal upset
- Enuresis (bedwetting)
- Encopresis (incontinence of stool)
- Decreased immune functioning

Behavioral

- Acting inward, such as self-harming, isolating, abusing substances, or overeating
- Acting outward, such as engaging in verbal/physical altercations with peers or adults

Psychosocial

- Anxiety
- Depression
- Irritability
- Anger

Nursing Interventions

Nursing strategies for stress management in children and adolescents include encouraging the following:

- Exercise
- Journaling/drawing
- Deep breathing
- Meditation
- Hypnosis
- Prayer
- Talking with an adult or peer

> **CLINICAL PEARL**
>
> **Capabilities Versus Expectations**
>
> Focus on the child's capabilities, not on your expectations.

Caregiver Education

When to get help:

- Child is an immediate threat to self or others
- Talk of suicide
- Suicidal gestures
- Symptoms interfere with relationships
- Symptoms interfere with school/home/work

Crisis Intervention

A crisis is a time-limited critical incident such as the death of a parent or the loss of a home due to fire. Crisis is personal; what is considered a crisis to one person may not be a crisis to another. The four main concepts of crisis intervention are:

- Safety—of the patient and of the health-care professionals involved with the case.
- Catharsis—patients in crisis have an overwhelming need to express feelings.
- Empathy-based listening—for example, "help me to understand how you're feeling."

- Entropy—do not add any more chaos into the situation. As the child escalates, the nurse should become even more calm by talking softer and controlling body language.

Use of Restraints with Children

Evidence-Based Practice Research: Restraint Use with Children

Azeem, M., Aujla, A., Rammerth, M., Binsfeld, G., & Jones, R. (2011). Effectiveness of six core strategies based on trauma informed care in reducing seclusions and restraints at a child and adolescent psychiatric hospital. *Journal of Child & Adolescent Psychiatric Nursing, 24*, 11–15. doi: 10.1111/j.1744-6171.2010.00262.x

Restraints are used as an intervention when the child is hurting him- or herself or others and should always be a last resort. Policies surrounding the use of restraints vary by institution and state. Pediatric deaths have been associated with the use of restraints.

1. What alternatives can be used instead of restraints?

Application of Restraints

When applying restraints:

- Obtain a physician's order.
- Check for contraindications to restraint, such as a physical health issue or history of prior abuse.
- Do not restrain face down.
- Do not restrain with arms over head.
- Make sure that two fingers can be placed in between the restraint and the limb. Recheck circulation of the extremities every 15 minutes.
- Take vital signs every 15 minutes. Pay careful attention to respiratory status.
- Offer fluids/toilet every 15 minutes.
- Provide range of motion every 15 minutes.
- Assign a staff member to provide one-to-one observation of the patient.
- Discontinue as soon as the child is in control or has fallen asleep.
- Debrief with the child and staff after the episode.

Use of Seclusion with Children

Seclusion should be used as a last resort when the child is at risk or is actually harming others (Azeem et al., 2011). If the child is harming him- or herself, do not seclude the patient. If the child starts to punch or kick the wall or head-bang, seclusion must be discontinued immediately.

- When implementing seclusion:
  - *Obtain a physician's order.*
  - *Check for contraindications to restraint, such as a physical health issue or history of prior abuse.*
  - *Take vital signs every 15 minutes.*
  - *Offer fluids/toilet every 15 minutes.*
  - *Provide range of motion every 15 minutes.*
  - *Assign a staff member to provide one-to-one observation of the patient.*
  - *Discontinue as soon as the child is in control or has fallen asleep.*
  - *Debrief with the child and staff after the episode.*

Promoting Safety

Nurses can avoid the use of seclusion and restraints by using preventive measures, including awareness of the child's trauma history, forming and using plans to keep patients safe, using comfort rooms, maintaining communication with caregivers and families, and using deescalation approaches (Azeem et al., 2011).

PERSONALITY DISORDERS

- Personality influences everything that the person thinks, feels, and does—like a lens through which one views life.
- Personality is developed by age 2 years. Therefore, early childhood experiences influence whether the child will have a personality disorder as an adult.
- Personality disorders (PDs) are often not diagnosed in childhood. However, pediatric nurses should be aware of them, as children may show features of a personality disorder.
- The personality issues most often detected in childhood are MacDonald's triad and borderline personality disorder.

Theories of Personality Disorders

- Psychodynamic/developmental—someone with a personality disorder is stuck in a developmental age of about 7 years old.
- Cognitive/behavioral—behaviors are learned. Patients with a PD have learned maladaptive behaviors. These behaviors can be improved through self-awareness and behavior modification techniques.
- Biological/neurochemical—PDs are the result of atypical brain chemistry and can be treated with psychopharmacology, diet, and exercise.

MacDonald Triad—the Precursor to Antisocial Personality Disorder

Young children who display bedwetting, cruelty to animals, and pyromania (MacDonald's triad) will likely have antisocial personality disorder as an adult.

CLINICAL PEARL

Risk Factors for MacDonald's Triad

When assessing enuresis, also ask about behavior toward animals and fire-setting.

Borderline Personality Disorder

Adolescents can exhibit traits consistent with borderline PD. These traits can include:

- Feeling as though bordering between sanity and psychosis
- Staff splitting (attempting to manipulating staff to think that other staff members are not providing the best care)
- Self-mutilating behaviors/suicidal gestures and attempts
- Affective instability—shifts in moods
- Identity disturbance
- Role absorption—narrow definition of self
- Painful incoherence—internal disharmony
- Inconsistency in thoughts, feelings, and actions
- Unstable interpersonal relationships
- Fear of abandonment
- Unstable, insecure attachments
- Overidealized/intense relationships
- Cognitive dysfunctions such as dissociation, disturbed thinking patterns, impaired problem solving, and impulsivity

Nursing Interventions

Nursing management of a patient with borderline PD includes:

- Monitor for suicidal ideation, gestures, and attempts.
- Monitor for deliberate self-harm.
- Establish a routine.
- Be consistent.
- Do not be manipulated.
- Offer support.
- Encourage individual and group therapy.
- Administer antidepressants and other medications as ordered.

IMPAIRED EXECUTIVE FUNCTIONING

- Executive functioning is higher-order thinking that is necessary for:
  - *Planning*
  - *Organizing*
  - *Sequencing*
  - *Using memory and information*
  - *Self-regulation of emotions and behavior*
- The components of executive functioning include:
  - *Working memory and recall*
  - *Activation, arousal, and effort*
  - *Controlling emotions*
  - *Internalizing language*
  - *Complex problem solving*

Symptoms of Impaired Executive Functioning

A child with impaired executive functioning skills may exhibit

- Forgetfulness
- Distorted sense of past events
- Altered sense of time
- Altered sense of self-awareness
- Altered sense of future

Impairments in executive functioning may exist with or without another clinical disorder. Many children with ADHD have issues with executive functioning.

Nursing Interventions

Nursing interventions for a child with impaired executive functioning include:

- Be concrete.
- Use visual aids.
- Reduce workload.
- Give extended time on tests.
- Increase support/supervision.

ATTACHMENT DISORDERS

- The quality of the parent–child relationship is the cornerstone of future interpersonal relationships.
- Attachment is biologically driven and is manifested by the need to touch and be close to a parental figure (Harlow, Harlow, & Suomi, 1971).
- Both mothers and fathers play a role in childhood attachment.
- Disrupted attachments occur when the infant is unable to respond appropriately to a caregiver, when a caregiver does not respond appropriately to an infant, or a combination of the two.
- Infants need thousands of successful cycles of expressing a need and then having the need met in order to achieve attachment.
- Disrupted attachments can result in feeding disorders, failure to thrive, anxiety disorders, or reactive attachment disorder.
- Reactive attachment disorder is characterized by the failure of a child younger than the age of 5 to initiate or respond appropriately to caregivers and/or social situations. As a result, caregivers then disregard the child's physical and/or emotional needs.
- A child may have diffuse attachments (inhibited type) or indiscriminate sociability (disinhibited type).
- Children at risk for attachment disorders include those who are abused, neglected, or adopted.

Primal Wound Theory of Attachment Disorders

- A child separated from his or her mother at birth loses mother and a sense of self, as these are the same from the child's perspective (Verrier, 1993).
- The child will suffer from a sense of losing oneself.
- This is very hard to overcome, even years later.

Treatment

Treatment and management of reactive attachment disorder of infancy or early childhood (Newman & McDaniel, 2005) includes:

- Rebirthing
- Rage reduction

- Avoid power struggles.
- Don't reward manipulative behaviors.
- Work toward emotional regulation.

MOOD DISORDERS

A mood disorder is an expression of depression in children.

- Infants
  - *Sad expression or lack of expression*
  - *Look away when spoken to*
  - *Lack of interest in play*
  - *Problems sleeping or eating*
  - *Separation from primary caregiver, such as during prolonged hospitalizations where parent visits infrequently or foster care experience*
  - *Increased risk with babies of depressed mother*
- Toddlers/Preschoolers
  - *Irritable*
  - *Act out*
  - *Suddenly begin getting in trouble at preschool or day care*
  - *Do not experience pleasure*
  - *Low self-esteem*
  - *Guilt*
- School-age/Adolescents
  - *Act outward*
  - *Act inward*
  - *Hopeless about the future*
  - *Angry*
  - *Defiant*
  - *Depressed adolescents are likely to use behaviors such as poor school performance, cutting, and suicidal gestures as attempts to communicate depression (Grisso, 2004).*

DEPRESSION

- Children are less likely than adults to experience psychosis with depression.
- Depressed children are more likely than adults to manifest symptoms of anxiety and somatic symptoms.
- Mood may be irritable, rather than sad (acting out instead of acting in)
- Suicide is a real risk, which peaks during mid-adolescence.
- Mortality from suicide increases steadily throughout the teenage years.
- Patient may be diagnosed with major depression, dysthymic disorder, or depressive episode NOS (not otherwise specified).
- Patients age 10–21 should be assessed for depression at every well-child visit (American Academy of Child and Adolescent Psychiatry [AACAP], 2007).

Risk Factors for Developing Depression

- Prior episode of depression
- Family history of depressive disorder
- Lack of social support
- Stressful life event
- Current substance use/abuse
- Medical comorbidity

CLINICAL PEARL

Assessing Depression Using SAD FACES

Assess for depression with the following tool:

S—Sleep disturbances
A—**Anhedonia** (inability to experience pleasure)
D—Despair
F—Fatigue
A—Appetite changes
C—Concentration
E—Emotional sensitivity
S—Suicidal ideation

Suicidality in Children

Risk Factors for Suicide

Children experiencing depression are at risk for suicide. Even young children can have thoughts of suicide. Motivations behind suicidal thoughts/gestures/attempts include:

- A desire to die
- A desire to hurt others (i.e., to upset or "get back at" caregiver)
- A desire to escape a painful home or school situation, such as being bullied or abused
- A desire to punish oneself due to feeling guilty about something

Deterrents to Suicide

- Having family support
- Believing that suicide is wrong from a religious standpoint
- Having hope for future

Bullycide

- **Bullycide** is suicide due to becoming depressed and hopeless because of being bullied by peers

Indications for Medications

- Child not responding to psychotherapy
- Severe symptoms that interfere with daily living
- History of recurrent depressive episodes
- Psychotic

Evidence-Based Practice Research: Treating Depression in Children

David-Ferndon, C., & Kaslow, N. J. (2008). Evidence-based psychosocial treatments for child and adolescent depression. *Journal of Clinical Child & Adolescent Psychology, 37*, 62–104. Retrieved from http://www.ncbi.nlm.nih.gov/ pubmed/18444054

Cognitive behavioral therapy (CBT) currently has the most research evidence for the treatment of depression in children, and CBT and **interpersonal psychotherapy (IPT)** are preferred therapies for adolescent depression. Treatments can be administered in a variety of different formats, including individual and group therapy (David-Ferndon & Kaslow, 2008).

CLINICAL PEARL

Treating Symptoms with Medication

Two rules of medicating children for psychiatric symptoms:

1. Skills before pills—try therapy first.
2. Start low, go slow—use low doses and titrate up slowly as needed.

Psychotropic Medication and Children

- The effects of most psychotropic medications are not well studied in children.
- Most psychiatric drugs are used off-label or for age groups not recommended by the Food and Drug Administration (FDA).
- Suicidal risks may increase in the initial days of treatment when first started on an antidepressant medication.
- In most cases, children need smaller doses of medication spaced throughout the day.

Antidepressants

- Take 2–4 weeks to work
- Goal of treatment: to restore normal levels of neurotransmitters
- Act on serotonin, dopamine, or norepinephrine
- Of patients, 70% respond to treatment (defined as a 50% decrease in symptoms) (AACAP, 2007).
- Many have severe sexual side effects.
- These drugs do not cure depression; they reduce symptoms.
- They improve motivation and psychomotor retardation before they improve mood.
- Antidepressants are divided into the following classifications:
  - *Tricyclic antidepressants (TCAs)*
  - *Monoamine oxidase inhibitors (MAOIs)*
  - *Norepinephrine and dopamine reuptake inhibitors (NDRIs)*
  - *Serotonin and norepinephrine reuptake inhibitors (SNRIs)*
  - *Selective serotonin reuptake inhibitors (SSRIs)*
  - *Atypical antidepressants*

Selective Serotonin Reuptake Inhibitors (SSRIs)

SSRIs are the first-line agents used to treat depression in children. They have less risk of side effects compared to other classifications of antidepressants. These drugs work by blocking the reuptake of serotonin in the synaptic gap. Examples of SSRIs used in children include Prozac, Zoloft, and Lexapro. Side effects of SSRIs include gastrointestinal (GI) distress, sedation, anticholinergic effects such as dry mouth and constipation, sexual dysfunction, and orthostatic hypotension.

- Serotonin syndrome
  - *Serotonin syndrome is an iatrogenic toxidrome that is the result of taking too many agents that block the reuptake of serotonin. These agents could be prescribed medications, over-the-counter medications, and herbal supplements such as St. John's Wort.*
  - *Serotonin syndrome is usually mild, but can cause death.*
  - *Symptoms include thermal dysregulation, confusion, agitation, fever, shivering, diaphoresis, tremor, and diarrhea.*
  - *Treatment includes discontinuing one or more of the offending drugs and providing supportive care.*
- Serotonin discontinuation syndrome
  - *Serotonin discontinuation syndrome can occur when the patient suddenly stops taking an SSRI.*
  - *Symptoms include dizziness, feeling confused, flu-like symptoms, tremor, insomnia, agitation, anxiety, lability, and crying spells*

Predictors of Medication Noncompliance

- Poor insight into symptoms/disease
- Negative attitude toward medications by child and/or family members
- Substance use/abuse by the child or caregiver
- Acute illness of the child or caregiver
- Inadequate discharge plan/lack of follow-up care
- Poor therapeutic relationship with the child and/or caregiver

Nursing Interventions

Nursing interventions for the child taking antidepressant medications include:

- Provide patient and family medication education.
- Monitor for compliance with medication regimen.
- Monitor blood pressure.
- Assess for suicidality.

Other Treatments for Depression in Children

Besides psychopharmacology, children experiencing depression may attend individual or group therapy and may even receive electroconvulsive therapy (ECT).

- ECT is the last-resort treatment for a pediatric psychiatric patient and will usually be used only for adolescents. It is the delivery of electrical current through the brain.
- A grand mal seizure is induced, which enhances dopamine sensitivity in the brain and reduces the reuptake of serotonin. Patients usually undergo a series of treatments, such as three times per week for 6 weeks.
- Nursing considerations for the patient undergoing ECT include:
  - *Informed consent from caregiver*
  - *Assent from child*
  - *Restriction of food/fluids for 6 to 8 hours prior to treatment to prevent aspiration*
  - *Completion of a preoperative checklist*
  - *Administration of a muscle relaxant*
  - *Assess vital signs during procedure.*
  - *Assess patient for confusion and short-term memory loss after procedure.*
  - *Place patient on falls precautions after procedure until patient physically and psychologically returns to baseline.*

Deliberate Self-Harm

Children who are depressed may exhibit self-harming behaviors such as head-banging or cutting. This usually occurs as the result of a high level of psychiatric pain, especially when the patient feels like he or she is unable or unwilling to communicate feelings (**alexithymia** = "I have no words for my feelings").

Nursing Interventions

Nursing interventions for the child who self-harms include:

- Assess patient frequently for signs of psychiatric pain.
- Assess skin frequently for signs of self-harm.
- Encourage expression of feelings.
- Maintain a safe environment free of objects that can be used for self-harm.

BIPOLAR DISORDER

Types of Bipolar Disorder

- Bipolar Type 1—alternating between major depression and mania
- Bipolar Type 2—alternating between major depression and hypomania
- Mixed episodes—alternating between depressive and manic states in the same episode

Manic Episode

- Feeling unusually "high," euphoric, or irritable for at least 1 week
- Needing little sleep; great amount of energy
- Talking fast; others can't follow
- Racing thoughts
- Easily distracted
- Inflated feeling of power, greatness, or importance
- Reckless behavior (e.g., with money, sex, drugs)

> **CLINICAL PEARL**
>
> **Rage and Bipolar Disorder**
>
> Children with bipolar disorder mania often exhibit rage instead of or along with the symptoms just listed.

Nursing Interventions

- Frequently assess child for symptoms of depression or mania.
- Encourage participation in individual and group therapy as tolerated/appropriate.
- Keep child safe.
- Watch for boundary violations.
- Aid patient in the performance of activities of daily living (ADLs).
- Administer sleep aids as needed
- Administer mood-stabilizing medications, such as lithium, Abilify (aripiprazole), and Lamictal (Lamotrigine), as needed.
- Administer antipsychotic medications such as Geodon (ziprasidone), Risperdal (risperidone), Seroquel (Quetiapine), and Zyprexa (Olanzapine) during manic periods as needed.

> **Medication**
>
> **XR and ER Medications**
>
> Be cautious with medication orders containing "XR or ER." These medications are extended release and are NOT the same as medications without those labels.

Lithium

- The primary mood stabilizer used for bipolar disorder
- Mechanism of action: unknown
- Body can't distinguish between lithium and salt
- Increased salt intake = decreased lithium uptake
- Facilitates reuptake of norepinephrine and serotonin (leaving less in the synapses)
- Blood levels: 0.5–1.2 mEq/L
- Side effects: GI upset, weight gain, polyuria, polydipsia
- Contraindicated in those with cardiac disease
- Caution in those on diuretics
- Signs of lithium toxicity
  - *Runny nose*
  - *Coughing*
  - *Chest congestion*
  - *Fever*
  - *GI upset*
  - *Blurred vision*
  - *Ringing in the ears*

> **Medication**
>
> **Medications for Pediatric Bipolar Disorder and Behavior Disorders**
>
> Depakote (Divalproex sodium) and Catapres (clonidine) are used off-label for pediatric bipolar disorder and behavior disorders.

Nursing Interventions

Nursing interventions for the child taking mood stabilizers include:

- Provide patient and family medication education.
- Emphasize compliance.
- Draw blood levels as ordered.
- Assess for symptoms of depression and mania.
- Assess suicidality.

ANXIETY DISORDERS

- The most frequent psychiatric disorders in children
- Separation anxiety is common in young children.
- Test- or school-related anxiety is common in older children.

CLINICAL PEARL

Expressions of Anxiety

Young children may not be able to verbally express anxiety. Instead, they may complain of physical symptoms such as headache or stomachache, nausea, or flatulence.

Risk Factors for Chronic Anxiety

Chronic anxiety is associated with:

- Decreased immune functioning
- Cardiovascular disease
- Diabetes
- GI issues
- Depression
- Forgetfulness
- Decreased attention span

Nursing Interventions

Nursing interventions for the child with an anxiety-based disorder:

- Stay with patient during extreme anxiety.
- Consult with key school personnel such as teachers and administrators.
- Maintain a calm, relaxed approach.
- Decrease environmental stimuli.
- Encourage verbalization of feelings.
- Encourage physical activity.
- Teach relaxation techniques.
- Teach problem-solving strategies.
- Give positive feedback and support.
- Provide psychoeducation.
- Provide cognitive-behavioral interventions.
- Hypnosis is an option.
- Administer anxiolytic medications as ordered.
- Nursing interventions for the child taking anxiolytic medications:
  - *Provide patient and family medication education.*
  - *Monitor for compliance.*
  - *Assess for sedation, addiction, and **suicidality**.*

OBSESSIVE-COMPULSIVE DISORDER (OCD)

- Severe obsessions (unwanted, reoccurring thoughts) and/or compulsions (repetitive behaviors) that interfere with quality of life
- Obsessions create anxiety, and compulsions are performed to reduce anxiety.

Medication

Anxiolytic Medications

Most **anxiolytic** medications are addicting, such as benzodiazepines. These medications may be used in a crisis situation with children but not for long-term management of an anxiety-based disorder. Vistaril (hydroxyzine) and Benadryl (diphenhydramine) are commonly used for acute anxiety in children. Buspar (buspirone) is a long-acting anxiolytic medication that is nonaddicting and nonsedating and is a better choice for treating an anxiety-based disorder. In addition, SSRIs have helped relieve chronic anxiety in children.

- A common obsession is fear of contamination, which may result in compulsive hand washing.
- Common compulsions include washing self or objects, cleaning, checking, counting, repeating actions, ordering, making confessions, and requesting assurances.
- OCD affects about 2% of the child and adolescent population (APA, 2000).
- There seems to be a genetic component.
- Children with OCD are highly somatic.
- OCD is often comorbid with personality disorders, autism, and Tourette's syndrome.
- The child may experience dissociation (a breakdown in integrated functions of memory, consciousness, perception of self, environment, or sensory and motor behavior) or depersonalization (loss of sense of personality).

Nursing Interventions

- Do not interrupt the ritual, as this will make the child more anxious.
- Thought stopping—child becomes aware of the thoughts and tries to stop them
- Relaxation techniques
- Cue cards

PHOBIA

Phobia is characterized by excessive anxiety brought on by exposure to a specific feared object or situation, often leading to avoidance behavior.

- It involves a sense of dread so intense that the individual will do everything to avoid the source of the fear.
- Common phobias in children include fear of the dark, spiders, enclosed places, heights, and social situations.

Nursing Interventions

- Provide support.
- Refer for cognitive-behavioral or exposure therapy as needed if the phobia is interfering with home/school.

PANIC DISORDER

Panic disorder is characterized by episodes of an overwhelming sense of dread/doom.

- These episodes are called "panic attacks."
- Children often report a feeling of dizziness and faintness as well as rapid heart rate and sweating during these episodes.
- Attacks may occur frequently or a child may experience an isolated attack during a period of extreme stress.

Nursing Interventions

Nursing interventions for the child experiencing a panic attack include:

- Stay with the child.
- Reassure him or her that you will not leave.
- Give clear directions.
- Assist patient to an environment with minimal stimulation.
- Walk with the patient.
- Administer prn anxiolytic medications.

POST-TRAUMATIC STRESS DISORDER

Children may develop post-traumatic stress disorder (PTSD) following a traumatic event, including hospitalization for a medical condition.

- Experiencing any element that was present during the initial trauma (e.g., the time of day, an article of clothing, a smell or sound) can trigger a flashback.
- The flashback is the limbic system of the brain reminding the prefrontal cortex not to allow a repeat of the initial trauma.
- Research shows that administering a dose of Inderal (proponolol) right after a trauma decreases the risk of PTSD.

> **CLINICAL PEARL**
>
> **Flashbacks**
>
> Do not attempt to interact with a patient who is experiencing a flashback. If you touch or talk to the patient, you could become a part of the flashback and could be in physical danger.

Nursing Interventions

Nursing interventions for the child with PTSD include:

- Provide support.
- Encourage patient to express feelings.
- Refer patient for psychotherapy.
- The child may need an anxiolytic medication after a flashback or on a long-term basis.

DISSOCIATIVE DISORDERS

- Failure to integrate identity, memory, and consciousness
- Usually found in children with a history of horrific abuse
- Is often described as overuse of a defense mechanism.
- Patients will report periods of loss of consciousness (i.e., "blackout periods" with no memory).
- Loss of memory/consciousness is a means of escaping from the current reality.
- Dissociating is easy for children, who already have magical thinking and an ability to develop and implement made-up friends and situations.

Types of Dissociative Disorders

- Dissociative amnesia—inability to recall
- Dissociative fugue—unexpected travel away from home
- Depersonalization disorder—being detached from one's body
- Dissociative identity disorder (formerly known as multiple personality disorder)—having more than one personality
- Dissociative disorder not otherwise specified—does not fit the diagnostic criteria for any of the disorders, as described by the DSM

DISRUPTIVE DISORDERS IN CHILDREN

- ADHD, oppositional defiant disorder (ODD), and conduct disorder belong in the group of disruptive behavior disorders. These disorders are characterized by significant and persistent behavior problems.
- Also referred to as externalizing disorders due to the characteristic "acting out" behaviors associated with the disorders.
- These disorders are most common in school-age males, but can present in females as well.
- Children with these disorders are at high risk for physical injury as a result of fighting and impulsive behaviors. Adolescents are at high risk for sexually transmitted infections and/or pregnancy resulting from promiscuity.

ATTENTION DEFICIT-HYPERACTIVITY DISORDER (ADHD)

- ADHD is characterized by three core symptoms—inattention, hyperactivity, and impulsivity—that are pervasive and inappropriate for the child's developmental level (APA, 2000). Symptoms present both at school and at home.
- Children can present as predominantly hyperactive, predominantly inattentive, or combined.
- The inattentive subtype is very difficult to diagnose because the child does not display the hyperactivity most often attributed to the disorder.

- Children who are predominantly inattentive appear to not listen when spoken to, have difficulty following through and completing tasks that require sustained mental effort, frequently lose items necessary for task completion, and are easily distractible and appear forgetful.
- Children who are predominantly hyperactive may be squirmy or fidgety, run or climb inappropriately, talk excessively, interrupt, or have difficulty waiting.
- Discipline is frequently an issue because parents have difficulty managing their child's disruptive behaviors.
- These children often show a narrow range of emotions.
- They have difficulty sequencing information.
- They may have slow information processing.
- Symptoms often interfere with ability to complete tasks at home and school.

Nursing Interventions

Nursing interventions for the child with ADHD include:

- Individual and family therapy
- Behavior management
- Provide emotional support.
- Promote self-esteem.
- Pharmacology

CLINICAL PEARL

Medication for ADHD

Medications used to reduce the symptoms of ADHD have a street value. Children who are not responding to treatment may not be taking the pills. Instead, the child or caregiver may be selling the medication.

Medications

The most common medications used to treat ADHD are:

- Ritalin (methylphenidate)
- Adderall XR (amphetamines mixed with salts)
- Concerta (methylphenidate)—long acting
- Vyvanse (lisdexamfetamine dimesylate)
- Daytrana transdermal patch—apply patch 2 hours before effects expected. Leave on for 9 hours. The patch will remain effective for an additional 2 hours. Not a good option for noncompliant children/families (Deglin, Vallerand, & Sanofski, 2011).
- Strattera (atomoxetine HCl)—doses must be tapered up and down.
- Tenex or Intuniv (guanfacine)—these are not stimulants.

Medication

Strattera

Strattera has been associated with increased suicidality in adolescents. Frequently assess children taking Strattera for suicidal ideation.

Nursing Considerations

Nursing considerations when administering medications for ADHD:

- Children may experience a decreased appetite and rapid weight loss.
- Other side effects include insomnia, increase in tics and/or compulsive behaviors, and/or psychotic reactions.
- ADHD medications should be given every day regardless of whether school is in session.

School-Based Interventions

School-based interventions for the child with ADHD (**Figure 14-2**):

- Have child sit near teacher.
- Assign a peer helper.
- Create a daily schedule.
- Review previously taught material.
- Do not time assignments or tests.
- Break assignments into shorter pieces.
- Give shorter assignments.
- Give directions one at a time.
- Decrease environmental distractions.
- Give the child periodic "errands" to run, such as picking up mail in the office or taking a book to the library.
- Allow the child to keep a set of books at school and a second set at home.
- Color code folders per subject.
- Help the child to organize his or her locker and desk.

OPPOSITIONAL DEFIANT DISORDER (ODD)

- Characterized by a persistent pattern of disobedience, argumentativeness, angry outbursts, low tolerance for frustration, and tendency to blame others for misfortunes (APA, 2000).

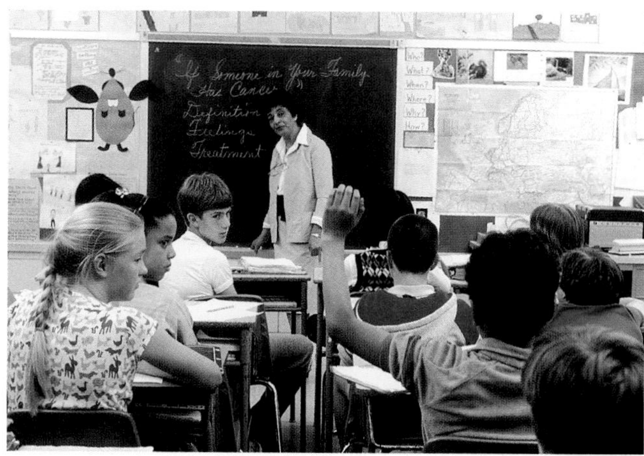

Figure 14-2 School-based interventions for the child with ADHD. *(From the National Cancer Institute. Photographer, Michael Anderson.)*

- Of children with ADHD, 40% to 60% also have symptoms of ODD (Biederman et al., 2007).
- Children have trouble with peer and social relationships and are often in conflict with adults.

Nursing Interventions

Nursing interventions for the child with ODD include:

- Consistent consequences
- Target a few behaviors at a time.
- Positive reinforcement w/activities
- Do not show emotional reactions to behavior.
- Social skills training
- Caregiver training to manage behaviors

CONDUCT DISORDER (CD)

- Childhood-onset type: at least one symptom prior to age 10
- Adolescent-onset type: at least 3 symptoms after age 10
- Characterized by *serious* violations of social norms, and includes aggressive behaviors, destruction of property, and cruelty to animals
- Children often engage in lying, larceny, theft, assault, and truancy from school.
- More prevalent in boys than girls.
- Most frequent disorder found among children residing in mental health facilities.
- Anxiety disorders and substance use/abuse are common in children with CD.
- Children generally present with a history of developmental delays, ADHD, and ODD.
- Adolescents are often hostile, sarcastic, defensive, and provocative toward others.

Nursing Interventions

Nursing interventions for the child with CD include:

- Give positive, specific feedback for desirable behavior.
- Allow for natural consequences of actions.
- Academic support
- Social skills training
- Limit the use of group therapy, as the group often reinforces negative behaviors.
- Individual therapy
- Caregiver support
- Medications such as antipsychotics (e.g., haloperidol and low-dose risperidone), mood stabilizers (e.g., lithium carbonate), and Depakote.

CRITICAL COMPONENT

Difference Between ODD and CD

The key difference between oppositional defiance disorder (ODD) and conduct disorder (CD) is that children with ODD feel remorseful when they break the rules or hurt someone and children with CD do not because they lack empathy.

IMPULSE-CONTROL DISORDERS

KLEPTOMANIA

- Failure to resist the urge to steal things
- Tension prior to theft
- Pleasure and relief after the theft
- Unknown/unrecognized motives

Nursing Interventions

Nursing interventions for the child with kleptomania include:

- Psychotherapy
- Aversion therapy
- SSRIs

PYROMANIA

- Intentional fire-setting on more than one occasion
- Tension prior to the act
- Excessive interest in or attraction to fire
- Pleasure/gratification after the fire is set and while watching the fire
- Unknown/unrecognized motives

Nursing Interventions

Nursing care for the child experiencing pyromania includes:

- Behavior modification
- Psychotherapy

INTERMITTENT EXPLOSIVE DISORDER

- Several occurrences of a failure to resist aggressive impulses that result in assaults or destruction of property
- The aggression is considered out of proportion to the perceived precipitants

Nursing Interventions

Nursing interventions for the child experiencing intermittent explosive disorder include:

- Cognitive-behavioral therapy
- SSRIs
- Antipsychotic medications such as Zyprexa (olanzapine) and Risperdal (risperidone)

SCHIZOPHRENIA

- Childhood (or early-onset) schizophrenia is characterized by delusions or hallucinations, disorganized speech or behavior, and marked impairment in social and/or school functioning.
- Childhood schizophrenia is much rarer than later-onset, or adult, schizophrenia. It is a chronic illness with periods of exacerbation and remission.

- Patients with this disorder often need lifelong medication management.

Causes of Childhood Schizophrenia

- Genetic
- Biochemical differences in the brain, particularly with increased dopamine and/or cortisol reuptake
- Increased stress levels
- Smoking marijuana laced with "wet" (formaldehyde)
- FOAD hypothesis—**f**etal **o**rigins of **a**dult **d**iseases. Child may develop schizophrenia due to in-uterine conditions.

> CLINICAL PEARL
>
> **Rule of Thirds**
>
> One-third of patients experiencing symptoms get better.
> One-third of patients experiencing symptoms stay the same.
> One-third of patients experiencing symptoms get worse.

Related Disorders

- Schizoaffective disorder
- Depression with psychotic features
- Mania with psychotic features
- Psychosis NOS

Risk Factors for Other Disorders

Patients with schizophrenia have an increased risk for:

- Cardiovascular disorders
- Depression and other dementias
- Substance abuse
- Cigarette smoking

Symptoms of Schizophrenia in Children

- Symptoms appear as inappropriate affect, loss of interest or pleasure, disturbances in sleep and concentration, and loss of appetite.
- Delays are common in social and cognitive functioning, linguistic and motor skills, and attentional and perceptual behaviors.
- These symptoms can be summarized with the acronym SLEPT; the patient with schizophrenia may experience alterations in:
  - *S—social behavior*
  - *L—language*
  - *E—emotions*
  - *P—perceptions*
  - *T—thinking*

Effects of Schizophrenia on Thought Processes and Content

- Loose association—thoughts are poorly related; thoughts are disorganized.
- Autism—patient develops and retreats into a private world.
- Slow or inhibited flow of thought—patient has difficulty expressing feelings.
- Rapid thinking
- **Perseveration**—getting stuck on something
- Circumstantial—excessive or irrelevant detail
- **Tangential**—patient digresses in the conversation and never reaches the goal.

Sensory and Perceptual Disturbances

- Hallucinations—sensory disturbances
- Delusions—perceptual disturbances rather than impairment in brain function
- Fixed false beliefs
- Cannot be validated in reality
- Exaggerated defense mechanisms
- Compensation for feelings of little worth
- The three phases to hearing voices are startling (person is disturbed by the voices), organization (coping), and stabilization (acceptance and integration of the voice into the life experience).

> CRITICAL COMPONENT
>
> **Hallucinations**
>
> The more elaborate the description of a hallucination is, the less likely it is that the hallucination is real/truthful. Patients with schizophrenia see shadows and lights. They hear noises and muffled voices. Children sometimes have difficulty distinguishing between reality and their imagination. Children who have been abused often see or hear the abuser.

- Children with schizophrenia may be hospitalized for:
  - *Initial diagnosis*
  - *Stabilization on meds*
  - *Patient safety*
  - *Inappropriate behavior*
  - *Inability to take care of basis needs*

Nursing Interventions

Nursing interventions for the child with schizophrenia:

- Safety
- Help with ADLs
- Encouragement to eat/drink
- Medications for sleep
- Psychotherapy
- Reality testing
- Social skills training
- Behavior modification
- Family education
- Referral to an outpatient provider for ongoing therapy and medication evaluation
- Medication education

Antipsychotic Medications

- Work by blocking dopamine receptors to prohibit uptake in the synapses
- Have a risk of weight gain; administering glucophage along with the medication will decrease this risk.
- Can have severe side effects, such as extrapyramidal symptoms (EPS). EPS can occur after a one-time use of an antipsychotic medication or after prolonged use, depending on the medication. Types of EPS include:
  - *Akathesia—motor restlessness*
  - *Dystonia—muscle tone impairment*
  - *Akinesia—muscular paralysis*
  - *Pseudoparkinson-like symptoms—tremors*
  - *Tardive dyskinesia—involuntary muscle movements*

> **Medication**
>
> **Extrapyramidal Symptoms**
>
> Children experiencing EPS often complain that the tongue feels thick, the neck is stiff, or the eyes keep looking up to the ceiling. EPS can also cause the throat to swell, causing shortness of breath.

- Medications to relieve EPS include Cogentin (benzatropine) and Benadryl (diphenhydramine). The first is used for issues of increased motor movement such as akathesia, parkinsonism, and tardive dyskinesia. The latter is used for decreased motor issues such as dystonia and akinesia.

Haldol (Haloperidol)

- Pill or intramuscular (IM)
- IM version is given z-track
- Haloperidol decanoate—long acting; given monthly as an injection.
- High risk of EPS
- Used across the life span
- Used to relieve symptoms that may lead to aggression
- Often given with ativan (syringe compatible)

Zyprexa (Olanzapine)

- Pill or IM
- Zyprexia Zydis is a sublingual (SL) form of Zyprexia
- Low risk of EPS
- Watch for orthostatic hypotension
- Zydis—SL form

Risperdal (risperidone)

- Pill
- Risperdal Consta: long-acting version; give every 2 weeks.
- Few side effects
- No risk of EPS
- Watch for orthostatic hypotension.

Seroquel (quetiapine)

- Pill
- May prolong the QT interval (get a baseline electrocardiogram [ECG] and follow-up ECGs)
- May cause sedation
- Useful for sleep or anxiety in low doses
- Little risk of EPS

Geodon (ziprasidone)

- Pill or IM
- May prolong the QT interval (get a baseline EKG and follow-up EKGs)
- Also helps with depression and anxiety (blocks reuptake of dopamine, serotonin, and norepinephrine)
- Few side effects
- Little risk of EPS
- Titrate up to a therapeutic range

Clozaril (clozapine)

- Blocks reuptake of dopamine and serotonin
- Gold standard for treatment of schizophrenia, yet used as a last resort
- Risk of seizures
- May cause sialorrhea (excessive salivation)
- Serious side effect: agranulocytosis (low absolute neutrophil count)
- Regular blood draws are required.
- Clozaril protocols:
  - *If baseline white blood cell count (WBC) <3500, don't start med.*
  - *Monitor WBC weekly for first 6 months, then biweekly.*
  - *Discontinue med if WBC <3,000 OR absolute neutrophil count is <1500.*

Other Side Effects of Antipsychotic Medications

Neuroleptic Malignant Syndrome

- Life-threatening, neurological disorder most often caused by an adverse reaction to antipsychotic meds
- Can be summarized with the acronym "FEVER"
  - *F—Fever*
  - *E—Encephalopathy*
  - *V—Vitals unstable*
  - *E—Elevated enzymes (elevated CPK)*
  - *R—Rigidity of muscles*
- Nursing interventions for the patient experiencing neuroleptic malignant syndrome:
  - *Stop use of the drug.*
  - *Provide supportive care to relieve symptoms.*

Metabolic Syndrome

- Onset of insulin-resistant diabetes
- Lipid abnormalities
- Hypertension
- Abdominal obesity
- Hypotension

Nursing Interventions for Metabolic Syndrome

- Monitor blood pressure.
- Monitor blood glucose level.
- Monitor weight.
- Monitor lipid levels.

Nursing Interventions for the Child Taking an Antipsychotic Medication

- Provide patient and family education regarding effects and side effects.
- Emphasize importance of continuing medications.
- Monitor vital signs, weight, and ECG.
- Monitor for symptoms of EPS, neuroleptic malignant syndrome, and metabolic syndrome.

PERVASIVE DEVELOPMENTAL DISORDERS

- Pervasive developmental disorders are thought to have multiple causes, including genetic, biochemical, and environmental factors.
- Characterized by severe and pervasive developmental impairment in social skills, communication, or the presence of stereotyped behaviors or activities (APA, 2000). Includes autism, Asperger's disorder, pervasive developmental disorder not otherwise specified (PDD NOS), Rhett syndrome, and childhood disintegrative disorder. These first three disorders (autism, Asperger's disorder, and PDD NOS) are considered autism spectrum disorders (ASDs).
- ASDs are increasing at rates of 10% to 17% per year and are considered the fastest growing pediatric disability (Centers for Disease Control and Prevention [CDC], 2007).
- Assessments for these disorders include examining the physical, psychological, and social contexts of the child.

AUTISM

- Diagnosed using DSM criteria. Autistic children are more likely to be born to moms 35 and older and born breech.
- Deficits are usually apparent by age 18 months, with the disorder diagnosed prior to age 3.
- Genetic mutations relating to autism have been discovered.
- Parents report concerns about child's interactions with others, language, or play.
- Examples of issues include: does not talk or babble by age 1, does not respond to name, does not seem to be able to hear, has violent tantrums, makes odd movements, does not smile, has poor eye contact, prefers to be alone, lines objects up, displays **obsessions/compulsions**, or shows unusual attachment to an object. For a complete list, see http://www.nichd.nih.gov/publications/pubs/upload/autism_overview_2005.pdf#page=3.
- Essential features include abnormal and impaired social interaction and communication, and restricted behaviors and interests.
- Screening tools include:
  - *The Checklist of Autism in Toddlers (CHAT)*
  - *The Modified Checklist of Autism in Toddlers (M-CHAT)*
  - *The Screening Tool for Autism in Two-Year-Olds (STAT)*
  - *The Social Communication Questionnaire (SCQ) for children age 4 and above*

Nursing Interventions

- Early intervention
- Familial involvement in treatment
- Individual and family therapy
- Highly structured settings
- Social skills training
- Enhance communication skills.
- Behavior modification
- Enhance cognitive skills.
- Support and enhance academic and vocational readiness skills.
- May need medication for OCD.

ASPERGER'S DISORDER

- Milder form of autism
- Generally diagnosed around ages 3 to 4
- Characterized by impairment in the use of typical nonverbal behaviors such as eye contact and facial expressions, failure to develop developmentally appropriate peer relationships, and lack of social and emotional relationships or enjoyment that results in deficits in social, occupational, or school functioning (APA, 2000).
- Symptoms include stereotypical movements, restricted areas of interests, social difficulties, and communication deficits (although less severe than with autism).

Nursing Interventions

- Early intervention
- Highly structured setting
- Individual and family therapy
- Enhancement of social skills
- Enhancement of communication skills
- Behavior modification
- Psychopharmacology for co-occurring anxiety, depression, and/or obsessions/compulsions

PERVASIVE DEVELOPMENTAL DISORDER NOS

- Also known as "atypical autism"
- Milder than autism and Asperger's
- May be considered "subclinical"
- Has some impairments in social and communication skills
- May have some routines or OCD
- Does not meet the diagnostic criteria for autism or Asperger's as set forth in the DSM

Nursing Interventions

- Early intervention
- Highly structured setting
- Individual and family therapy
- Enhancement of social skills
- Enhancement of communication skills
- Behavior modification as needed

SENSORY PROCESSING DISORDER

- Children with an autism spectrum disorder often have a sensory processing disorder.
- These children are highly sensitive to sensory stimuli. Lights seem extra bright, noises seem extra loud, and even mild tactile stimulation seems like a big push or shove.

Nursing Interventions

- Early intervention
- Individual and family therapy
- Short periods of exposure to increased stimuli to build tolerance, such as using:
  - *Massagers*
  - *Vibrating toothbrush*
  - *Aromatherapy*
  - *Weighted vests*
  - *Crafts involving clay, seeds, sand, soft pom-poms, or any other materials that are stimulating to touch*
  - *Lava lamp*
  - *Toys that encourage motion, such as a rocking horse or trampoline*

RHETT'S DISORDER

Rhett's disorder is considered a pervasive developmental disorder with psychiatric and neurologic components.

- Females are more likely to have the disorder than males, as it is an X-linked dominant gene mutation.
- A key protein needed for brain development is not made in children with Rhett's disorder.
- Child usually has nonsignificant prenatal and perinatal development followed by normal growth and development until age 5 months.
- After age 5 months, the child experiences a decrease in head circumference followed by loss of motor skills, social engagement, and language skills (Jedele, 2007).
- Symptoms include:
  - *Impaired cognitive functioning*
  - *Inability to generate language or movement*
  - *May have difficulty breathing on own*
  - *May experience seizures*
  - *Repetitive hand washing or hand wringing*
- Phases of the disease include:
  - *Stage one, early onset (6–18 months): Poor eye contact, loss of interest in toys, slowed head growth, and hand wringing*
  - *Stage two, rapid deterioration (1–4 years): Loss of language and movement milestones, irritability, difficulty sleeping, slowed head growth, breathing problems, and hand wringing*
  - *Stage three, plateau (2–10 years): Increased motor problems and the development of seizures*
  - *Stage four, deterioration of motor skills (after age 10): Decreased motor skills, muscle rigidity, and the development of scoliosis*

Nursing Interventions

- Individual and family therapy
- Refer for physical therapy/occupational therapy (PT/OT).
- Maintain respiratory equipment.
- Place on seizure precautions.
- Help with ADLs.
- Enhance communication skills.

CHILD DISINTEGRATIVE DISORDER

- Characterized by a marked regression in functioning (social skills, language, play, motor skills) after a period of at least 2 years of normal development (APA, 2000). Onset is usually sudden, but can lose skills gradually.
- More common in males and typically diagnosed between the ages of 3 and 4
- As symptoms progress, children are likely to be mute and have severe mental retardation.
- Common symptoms include disturbances in breathing, fixed and rigid hands, bruxism, social withdrawal and cognitive impairment, growth retardation, impaired sleep patterns from early infancy, loss of locomotion, loss of bowel/bladder control, and lack of language.

Nursing Interventions

- Individual and family therapy
- Refer for PT/OT
- Help with ADLs
- Enhance communication skills.
- Develop and maintain bowel and bladder evacuation plan/equipment.
- Behavior modification, including the implementation of a positive reward system
- May need antipsychotic medications to control aggressive behavior

EATING DISORDERS

Risk Factors

- Caucasian
- Middle class to upper class
- Adolescents to 20s
- Can cause physical and psychological debilitation

- Genetic factor
- Some neurochemical factors have been linked, but are not completely clear.
- Low self-esteem
- Conflicts over identity, role development, and body image
- Fears concerning sexuality
- Parental overemphasis or excessive worrying
- Overly close mother–daughter relationship
- Sexual abuse

Signs and Symptoms

- Focus on dieting
- Skipping meals
- Going to bathroom after eating
- Diet pills
- Laxatives
- Excessive exercise
- Extreme calorie counting

CLINICAL PEARL

Screening for Eating Disorders

Screen for eating disorders using the SCOFF tool (Morgan, Reid, & Lacey, 1999):

1. Do you make yourself **s**ick because you feel uncomfortably full?
2. Do you worry that you've lost **c**ontrol over what you eat?
3. Have you lost **o**ver 10 lbs in the last 3 months?
4. Do you believe that you're **f**at?
5. Would you say that **f**ood dominates your life?

ANOREXIA NERVOSA

- Self-starvation
- Person relentlessly pursues thinness
- Preoccupation with body and body image
- Despite extreme thinness, person thinks he or she is fat due to a distorted body image
- Diagnosed when a person drops to less than 85% of ideal body weight (Bulik, Reba, Siega-Riz, & Reichborn-Kjennerud, 2005)
- Onset is usually in early adolescence but can occur at any age.
- Often found in females more than males
- Chronic condition with relapses characterized by significant weight loss
- Often continue to be preoccupied with food
- Of those affected, 10% to 25% go on to develop bulimia nervosa (Bulik et al., 2005).
- Poor outcome is related to initial lower minimum weight, presence of purging, and later age of onset.

Complications

- Malnutrition
- Muscle wasting
- Dehydration
- Electrolyte imbalances
- Cardiac dysrhythmia
- Increased risk of infection

Nursing Interventions

- Monitor eating.
- Administer nutrition via nasogastric tube if ordered.
- Correct malnutrition.
- Resolve underlying psychological dysfunction.
- Encourage participation in psychotherapy.
- Weight restoration within 10% of normal.
- Monitor bathroom behavior.
- Administer SSRIs as prescribed.
- Administer Provigil (modafinil) as ordered off-label to stimulate the appetite. However, it may prolong the QT interval, so a baseline and follow-up ECGs are recommended.

BULIMIA NERVOSA

- Bulimia nervosa is characterized by recurrent episodes of binge eating with or without purging.
- Generally not life threatening
- Usually child is of normal weight
- There are few outward signs; behavior usually occurs in secret. Therefore, behavior may go undetected for years.

Signs and Symptoms

- Sneaking food
- Making excuses to use the bathroom after meals
- Eating large amounts of food on the spur of the moment
- Taking laxatives, vomiting, and/or overexercising to "purge" food
- Extreme concern with body weight and image
- Enamel on teeth begins to wear away, causing cavities
- May see "Russell's sign"—teeth marks on the knuckles from self-inducing vomiting

Nursing Interventions

- Stabilize and normalize eating patterns through nutritional counseling.
- Restructure dysfunctional thoughts and attitudes through individual therapy.
- Assess for comorbid depression, suicide, deliberate self-harm, and other impulsive behaviors such as shoplifting, overspending, or engaging in casual sexual encounters.
- Administer SSRIs as ordered.

COMPULSIVE OVEREATING

- Binge-eating disorder
- Characterized by an addiction to food
- May have episodes of uncontrolled eating or binging

- Continues to eat even after becoming uncomfortably full
- Usually feels guilt/depressed afterward
- Does not purge

EATING DISORDER NOS

- Does not meet criteria for a disorder but has one or more symptoms

SUBSTANCE-RELATED DISORDERS

Definitions of Substance Use

- Use—drinks alcohol; swallows, smokes, sniffs, or injects substance(s)
- Dependence—use despite adverse consequences; person feels "normal" only when on the drug
- Tolerance—the need for increasing amounts of a substance to achieve the same effects
- Abuse—use for purposes of intoxication or for treatment beyond intended use
- Addiction—psychological and behavioral dependence (**Figure 14-3**)
- Withdrawal—physical signs/symptoms that occur when the addictive substance is reduced/withheld
- Co-dependency—stress-related preoccupation with an addicted person's life, leading to extreme dependence on that person

Signs and Symptoms

- Frequent absenteeism from school, work, or extracurricular activities
- Frequent injuries/accidents
- Drowsiness
- Slurred speech

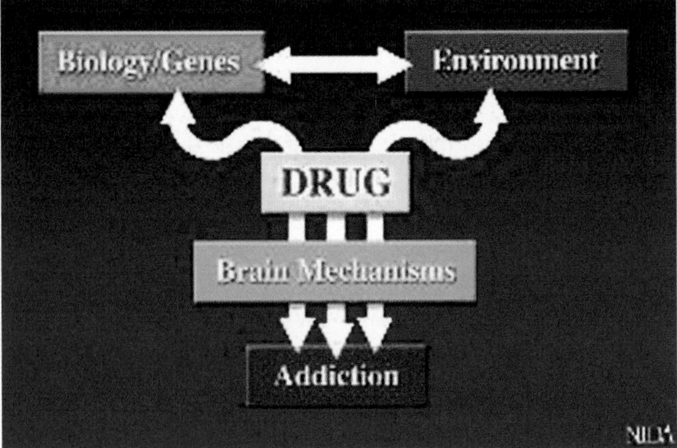

Figure 14–3 Addiction—psychological and behavioral dependence. *(From the National Institute on Drug Abuse. [2010, August].* Drugs, brains, and behavior: The science of addiction. *Retrieved from http://www.drugabuse.gov/publications/science-addiction/drugs-brain.)*

- Inattention to appearance
- Isolation
- Frequent "secretive" disappearances
- Tremors
- Flushed face
- Watery/red eyes
- Odor
- High number of physical complaints
- Missing medications/alcohol

Assessment

> **CLINICAL PEARL**
>
> **CAGE Questionnaire**
>
> Assessing alcohol or substance use/abuse using the CAGE questionnaire:
>
> 1. Have you ever felt that you should **c**ut down on your drinking/substance use?
> 2. Have people **a**nnoyed you by criticizing your drinking/substance use?
> 3. Have you ever felt bad or **g**uilty about your drinking/substance use?
> 4. Have you ever had an **e**ye-opener in the morning to steady your nerves or to get rid of a hangover?
>
> Answers:
>
> - Two yes responses is suggestive of a disorder.
> - Three or more yes responses is diagnostic of a disorder (Ewing, 1984).

- Interview tips
  - *Be aware of risk of denial/minimizing.*
  - *Ask about peer and family use.*

> **CRITICAL COMPONENT**
>
> **Peer and Family Substance Use/Abuse**
>
> If a peer or family member uses/abuses alcohol or drugs, a child is more likely to do so as well, so always ask about peer and family use/abuse.

- Be nonjudgmental.
- Do not be manipulated.
- Confront when you have to.
- Set limits.
- Provide option to verify interview data by urine, blood, or hair testing **(Table 14-1)**.
- Drug withdrawal symptoms and severity depend on:
  - *Type of drug used*
  - *Amount of drug used*
  - *Duration of drug use*
  - *Preexisting psychopathology*

Nursing Interventions

- Discuss natural consequences of substance use.
- Provide substance/medication education.

TABLE 14–1 PERIOD OF TIME AFTER INGESTION DRUG CAN BE DETECTED IN URINE

Drug Detection Period
Heroin: 2–4 days
Morphine: 2–4 days
Demerol: 2–4 days
Methadone: 2–4 days
Fetanyl: Less than 1 hour
Barbiturates: 12 hours to 3 weeks
Benzodiazepines: Up to 1 week
Amphetamines: 2–4 days
Cocaine: 2–4 days
Marijuana: 3 days to less than 1 month
PCP: 1 day to 1 month

- Offer hope for long-term recovery.
- Encourage Alcoholics Anonymous/Narcotics Anonymous attendance.
- Encourage family therapy.
- Develop a nonuse contract with the patient.
- Encourage independence in ADLs.
- Administer medications and monitor side effects.
- Provide quiet environment.
- Assess vitals, especially heart rate and blood pressure.
- Group therapy (**Figure 14-4**)

ALCOHOL

Alcohol Withdrawal

- Alcohol is metabolized rapidly (**Table 14-2**).
- Withdrawal is short term but can be severe.

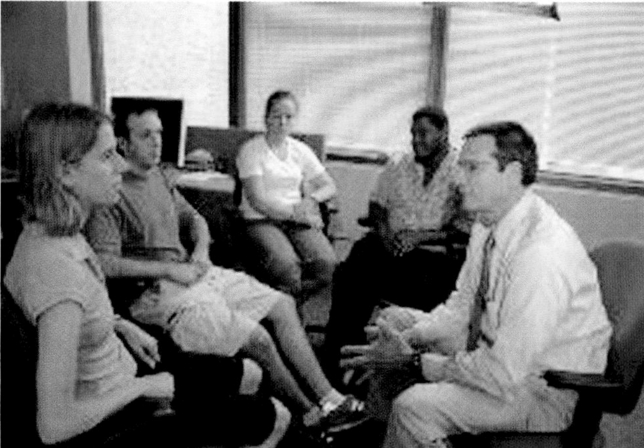

Figure 14–4 When working with children experiencing drug addiction, the nurse may recommend a group therapy setting. *(From National Institutes of Health.)*

TABLE 14–2 BLOOD ALCOHOL LEVELS AND EFFECTS

0.05%: thought, judgment, and restraint are affected
0.1%: voluntary motor actions become clumsy
0.2%: entire motor area of the brain becomes depressed; emotional behavior affected
0.4–0.5%: coma

- Symptoms begin hours after cessation of drinking.
- Symptoms peak in 2 to 3 days.
- Symptoms subside in 4 to 5 days.
- Delirium tremens (DTs)—the most severe type of alcohol withdrawal
  - *Occur within 1 week of cessation or severe reduction in alcohol use*
  - *May lead to visual and/or tactile hallucinations*
  - *Patient may be disoriented.*
  - *Patient may report* ***delusions*** *and agitated behavior.*
  - *Patient may be frightened and anxious.*
  - *Patient is at risk for grand mal seizures.*

Nursing Interventions

- Individual and group therapy
- Assessment for the use of other substances
- Encourage attendance at Alcoholics Anonymous meetings.
- Maintain a quiet environment.
- Monitor vital signs. Watch especially for increased heart rate and blood pressure.
- Monitor for seizures.
- Monitor for confusion and reports of hallucinations/delusions.
- Administer long-acting sedative hypnotics such as Librium, Valium, Phenobarbital, or Ativan as ordered. These medications will be prescribed by a protocol using the CIWA score:
  - *Clinical Institute Withdrawal Assessment for Alcohol (CIWA-Ar)*
  - *Validated 10-item assessment tool that can be used to quantify the severity of alcohol withdrawal syndrome, and to monitor and medicate patients going through withdrawal*
  - *Scores of 8 points or fewer correspond to mild withdrawal.*
  - *Scores of 9 to 15 points correspond to moderate withdrawal.*
  - *Scores of greater than 15 points correspond to severe withdrawal and an increased risk of delirium tremens and seizures.*
  - *Medication decisions are based on CIWA score.*

MARIJUANA (CANNIBIS)

- Stimulates dopamine pathways
- Causes euphoria, perception of slowed time, dry mouth, increased appetite, anxiety, suspiciousness
- All senses are enhanced with use

- Patient may have red eyes.
- Patient may develop "amotivational syndrome," a lack of motivation to complete ADLs/tasks because of the THC found in marijuana.
- Marijuana may be laced with another substance, such as formaldehyde ("wet") or cocaine.
- Withdrawal is not as intense as that of alcohol or cocaine but can last 1 to 3 weeks.

Nursing Interventions

- Individual and group therapy
- Assessment for the use of other substances
- Maintain a quiet environment.
- Administer anxiolytics for anxiety, as needed.

HALLUCINOGENS (LSD, PCP)

- Block reuptake of serotonin
- These are considered psychedelic drugs that may cause hallucinations, suicidal and homicidal thoughts, and the experience of all of the senses "running together."
- Use of these substances can cause respiratory arrest, coma, seizure, and death.
- Patient may experience flashbacks of "bad trips" at unpredictable times years later.
- These substances are usually used sporadically in children and they do not necessarily become addicted to them or need to go through withdrawal. Instead, care is focused on the child who has used the substance and is actively having problems.

Nursing interventions for the child high from LSD or PCP include:

- Individual and group therapy
- Maintain a safe environment.
- Assess for the use of other substances.
- Reality test
- Administer a sedative.
- Provide education on the effects of the drug once the patient clears.

COCAINE/CRACK COCAINE

- Children are using cocaine as a powder or in the rock preparation known as crack cocaine. Male adolescents have been known to put cocaine powder on the penis for use as a sexual aid to increase the pleasure experienced during intercourse.
- Cocaine decreases the reuptake of dopamine.
- Use of the drug causes hunger suppression, euphoria, relief of fatigue, decreased anxiety, and increased self-esteem.
- Use may lead to personality changes, irritability, disturbed concentration, compulsive behavior, and insomnia.
- Withdrawal from cocaine is rarely life threatening.
- Symptoms of acute withdrawal include intense craving, agitation, depression, poor appetite, and insomnia; symptoms last 4 to 10 days.
- Symptoms of chronic withdrawal include fatigue, depression, anhedonia (lack of pleasure), mood disturbance, and cravings.

Nursing Interventions

Nursing interventions for the child withdrawing from cocaine include:

- Individual and group therapy
- Assess for the use of other substances.
- Monitor vital signs, especially heart rate and blood pressure.
- Administer anxiolytics, antidepressants, antipsychotics, and dopamine agonists (amantidine, bromocriptine) as ordered.

OPIATES

- Examples include opium, heroin, morphine, Demerol, Dilaudid, Darvon, Percocet, codeine, and oxycontin.
- Increase the release of dopamine
- Effects resemble those of alcohol
- Patient experiences decreased sex drive and decreased hunger, thirst, and pain.
- Highly addictive
- Can be taken as a pill or crushed into powder and inhaled or injected

Opioid Withdrawal

- Rarely life threatening
- Symptoms vary based on last use of the substance:
  - *8–12 hours after last use: tearing, yawning, runny nose*
  - *12–24 hours after last use: insomnia, poor appetite, abdominal cramping, tremors*
  - *48–72 hours after last use: all of the above plus depression, diarrhea, goose pimples, bone pain, muscle spasm*
- Clinical Institute Narcotic Assessment Scale (CINA) is used to make medication decisions
  - *11 symptoms*
  - *The higher the score, the more severe the symptoms.*

Nursing Interventions

Nursing interventions for the child withdrawing from opioids include:

- Individual and group therapy
- Refer to Narcotics Anonymous (NA).
- Assess for the use of other substances.
- Monitor vital signs, especially heart rate and blood pressure.
- Use CINA tool as needed.

- Administer an opiate substitute as ordered, such as Methadone, tramadol, or Suboxone (buprenorphine), to suppress withdrawal symptoms and decrease cravings.
- Administer clonidine for increased heart rate, bentyl for stomach cramps, anxiolytics for anxiety, and analgesics for pain, as needed.

BENZODIAZEPINES

- Examples include Ativan, Xanax, Restoril, Librium, and Klonopin.
- Symptoms of withdrawal include anxiety, restlessness, insomnia, and palpitations.
- Symptoms are assessed using the CIWA-B.
- Medication decisions are based on CIWA-B score.

Nursing Interventions

Nursing interventions for the child withdrawing from benzodiazepines include:

- Individual and family therapy
- Assess for use of other substances.
- Refer to NA.
- Monitor vital signs, especially heart rate.
- Administer Phenobarbital as ordered based on CIWA-B score.

NICOTINE

- Toxic and addictive
- Toxicity: 60 mg is fatal; 1 cigarette = ½ mg.
- Use can lead to cerebral vascular disease, cancer, and respiratory diseases.
- Dependence develops quickly.
- Increases blood pressure and peristalsis
- Constricts blood vessels; decreases appetite
- Stimulates the pleasure center (hypothalamus)
- Acute symptoms of withdrawal include anxiety, irritability, increased appetite, restlessness, increased blood pressure and heart rate, headaches, and fluid retention.
- Chronic symptoms of withdrawal include cravings, mood swings, agitation, inability to concentrate, and poor attention span.

Nursing Interventions

Nursing interventions for the child withdrawing from nicotine include:

- Assess for the use of other substances.
- Administer nicotine replacements as ordered, such as gum or a patch.
- Administer anti-craving agents such as buproprion (Zyban, Wellbutrin).
- May suggest alternative therapies such as hypnosis, acupuncture, or aversion therapy

CAFFEINE

- Found in coffee, tea, cola, chocolate, and caffeine drinks/shots/pills
- Often not seen as harmful by children
- Increased alertness and verbal and physical performance
- Stimulates cardiac muscle
- Can lead to diuresis, ulcers, and psychological dependence
- Withdrawal symptoms include anxiety, agitation, restlessness, irritability, muscle twitching, rambling thoughts and speech, headache, irritability, and depression

Nursing Interventions

Nursing interventions for the child withdrawing from caffeine include:

- Provide support and encouragement.
- Educate about the ill effects of caffeine.
- Assess for the use of other substances.

INHALANTS

- Examples include glue, gasoline, and anything in a can with a propellant, such as compressed air used to clean off computer keyboards.
- Slang terms include sniffing, huffing, and bagging.
- These substances quickly cross the blood–brain barrier.
- Children may develop mouth ulcers, confusion, headaches, and GI issues.
- Butthash—children are defecating into containers and inhaling the gases days later in a practice commonly referred to as "butthash." The pediatric nurse should deter patients from engaging in this practice, which is just as dangerous as inhaling other substances such as gasoline.

Nursing Interventions

Nursing interventions for the child using inhalants include:

- Individual and family therapy
- Assess for the use of other substances.
- Educate about the ill effects of inhalants (**Figure 14-5**).
- Address any acute medical conditions caused by the inhalant.

PRESCRIPTION DRUG ABUSE

- Prescription drug abuse among children is on the rise.
- Drugs are stolen from family members or obtained through friends or the Internet.
- Children often view these drugs as safer than street drugs.

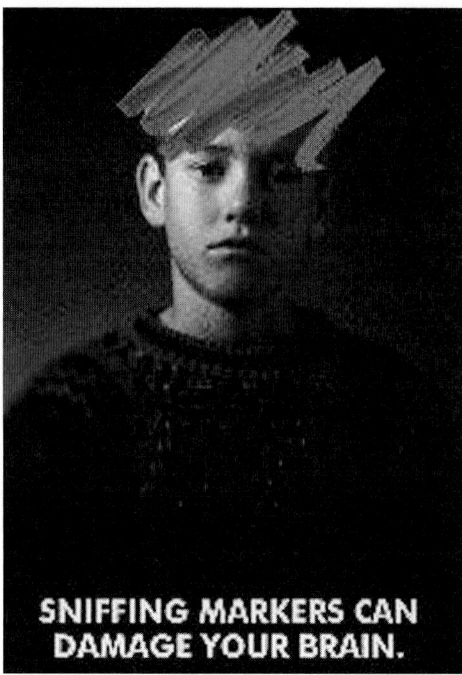

Figure 14–5 Educate children and families about the ill effects of inhalants. *(From Sniffing Markers Destroys Your Brain, reproduced with permission of the National Inhalant Prevention Coalition, 1991.)*

Nursing Interventions

Nursing interventions for the child abusing prescription drugs include:

- Individual and family therapy
- Group therapy specifically for prescription drug abusers
- Assess for the use of other substances.
- Refer for inpatient or outpatient withdrawal management.

OTHER ADDICTIONS

- Texting
- Sexting
- Gambling
- Internet surfing
- Chatting online through social networking sites
- Video games

Nursing Interventions

Nursing interventions for the child exhibiting an addiction listed above:

- Individual and family therapy
- Group therapy
- Involvement in a support group specifically for the issue, such as Gamblers Anonymous
- Administration of anxiolytic and antidepressant medications as prescribed

Warning Signs of Relapse

- Being around other users
- Severe craving
- Stop attending AA/NA
- Not expressing feelings
- Major emotional crisis

DUAL DIAGNOSIS

Dual diagnosis is having a primary mental health disorder with a co-occurring substance issue. These cases often require initial inpatient treatment with ongoing outpatient support. Interventions are aimed at addressing both mental health and addiction.

CHILDHOOD ABUSE

Risk factors for abuse and neglect include substance abuse, high levels of stress, unstable interpersonal relationships, and/or lack of social support. The experience of child abuse and neglect places a child at greater risk for developing psychiatric disorders later in life. Nurses are required by law to report any suspected abuse or neglect to child protective agencies.

- Childhood sexual abuse is broadly defined as any sexual activity with a child where consent is not, or cannot, be given (Myers et al., 2002).
- Evaluation should be done in a safe, supportive environment.
- Assessment includes questions about unwanted physical or sexual contact, photography, and/or secrecy surrounding the incident(s).
- Signs of sexual abuse include bruises, bleeding of genitals and/or rectum, sexually transmitted infections, enuresis or encopresis, sexual acting out with peers, re-traumatizing self by putting objects into body orifices, somatic complaints, sleep difficulties, and/or withdrawal.
- Signs of physical abuse include bruises or lacerations, especially on areas that are not exposed by clothing; marks from objects such as belts, ropes, hands, or cords; bite marks from adults; bald spots on hair; aggression and/or fear toward, or withdrawal from, adults; indiscriminant seeking of affection; and defensive reactions when questioned about injuries.
- Abuse can also be verbal, such as calling the child names or demeaning him or her in front of others.
- Munchausen syndrome by proxy is when the caregiver, usually the mother, attempts to make the child appear ill. The caregiver may put blood in the child's urine, stool, or vomitus, or report made-up symptoms to health-care providers. The child may be admitted to the hospital for diagnostic tests. If so, the child should be put in a room with a camera so that the caregiver's actions can be monitored.
- Recommended treatments for abuse victims include stabilization of the physical condition, individual and

family therapies, removal from the home and/or offender, and assessment for future psychiatric disorders related to the abuse (e.g., depression, anxiety, and PTSD).

RESOURCES FOR THE NURSE

American Academy of Child and Adolescent Psychiatry (www.aacap.org for practice guidelines and resource centers)
American Psychiatric Nurses Association
American Psychological Association
FDA information for pediatrics (www.fda.gov/cder/pediatric)
Journal of Child and Adolescent Psychiatric Nursing
National Alliance on Mental Illness
National Guideline Clearinghouse (www.guideline.gov)
National Institute of Mental Health

■ ■ ■ Review Questions ■ ■ ■

1. Which of the following has been identified as a current trend in pediatric psychiatry?
A. More children are dealing with anger issues.
B. An influx of providers specializing in pediatric psychiatry has led to an increase in care for children with mental disorders.
C. Children committing self-harm has decreased as seen in practice.
D. Clinical drug trials continue to be prohibited from using pediatric participants.

2. Which of the following are symptoms of dopamine deficiency?
A. Panic and phobias
B. Anxiety and compulsions
C. Food cravings and bulimia
D. Depressed mood and obsessions
E. Increased irritability and aggression

3. Known risk factors for children developing mental disorders include which of the following?
A. Physical problems
B. Low birth weight
C. Multigenerational poverty
D. Both a and b
E. All of the above

4. An 11-year-old female patient is admitted after her mother found she was cutting herself at home. The nurse is assessing the girl for suicidality. Which of the following would the nurse include in her admission assessment?
A. Ask the child if she has a plan to hurt herself.
B. Inquire if the child has access to pills or a weapon.
C. Include only the patient in obtaining the initial assessment, as the child may not provide accurate responses in the presence of the mother.
D. Both a and b are correct choices.

5. A 9-year-old male patient is receiving a mental health assessment and has scored a 75 on the Children's Global Assessment Scale (C-GAS) from Axis V of the *Diagnostic and Statistical Manual of Mental Disorders* (DSM-IV). The nurse understands which of the following to be true about the C-GAS tool?
A. The tool has an interrater reliability of 90%.
B. The tool is used to assist clinicians in determining how well an individual is functioning in everyday life.
C. A score of 50 or above is of concern and indicates a low level of functioning.
D. The lower the score, the higher the level of functioning the individual has in managing daily life.

6. A nurse is working with an 8-year-old boy who has just been diagnosed with a learning disability. The nurse includes which of the following in the educational plan for the boy and his family?
A. Being patient with the child
B. Assessing how the child learns best
C. Assessing the learning needs of the child
D. Seeking an individualized education plan (IEP) as needed
E. All of the above

7. A school nurse is working in an elementary school and has been asked to assist in the evaluation of a child with a suspected learning disability. The nurse understands which of the following to be true about learning disabilities (LDs)?
A. LDs may be developed because the child's mother smoked cigarettes during the pregnancy.
B. LDs may be caused by children watching more than 2 hours of television daily.
C. Children with learning disabilities are often of average or above-average intelligence.
D. Both a and c are correct.

8. A 12-year-old male patient has been admitted to a psychiatric inpatient unit and has become combative, attempting to punch the nursing staff. The nurse is anticipating applying restraints to the patient. The nurse considers which of the following safety precautions when considering applying restraints?
A. Contraindications include physical health issues and history of prior abuse.
B. Restraints should be used as a first-line intervention to prevent the child and staff from getting injured.
C. The patient should be checked for any injury every 30 minutes.
D. The restraints should be applied with the child's arms above his head to prevent the child from getting out of the restraints.

9. The adoptive parents of a 4-year-old girl have sought help because the child has been withdrawn. The nurse is educating the parents. Which of the following would be an appropriate statement by the nurse about reactive attachment disorder?
A. "The disorder doesn't manifest until after age 5; therefore she needs to be evaluated for some other mental health disorder."
B. "Children at risk are those who have been abused or neglected, or were adopted."

C. "She should be enrolled in a preschool program as soon as possible to assist her with socialization."
D. "When she throws a temper tantrum, you need to give in to her to develop a relationship of trust and support."

10. Which of the following is true about attachment disorders?
A. The mother alone plays an exclusive role in childhood attachment.
B. Disrupted attachments only occur when a caregiver does not respond to the infant.
C. The quality of the parent–child relationship is the cornerstone of future interpersonal relationships.
D. A child who is identified as having an attachment disorder can easily overcome this disorder by adulthood.

References

AHRQ. (2011). *Databases and related tools from the healthcare cost and utilization project (HCUP)* (AHRQ Publication No. 10-P009-EF). Retrieved from http://www.ahrq.gov/data/hcup/datahcup.htm

American Academy of Child and Adolescent Psychiatry (AACAP). (2007). Practice parameter for the assessment and treatment of children and adolescents with depressive disorders. *Journal of the American Academy of Child & Adolescent Psychiatry, 46*, 1503–1526. Retrieved from http://www.ncbi.nlm.nih.gov/pubmed/9785729

American Psychological Association (APA). (2000). *The diagnostic and statistical manual of mental disorders–text revision* (4th ed.). Washington, DC: Author.

Azeem, M., Aujla, A., Rammerth, M., Binsfeld, G., & Jones, R. (2011). Effectiveness of six core strategies based on trauma informed care in reducing seclusions and restraints at a child and adolescent psychiatric hospital. *Journal of Child & Adolescent Psychiatric Nursing, 24*, 11–15. doi: 10.1111/j.1744-6171.2010.00262.x

Biederman, J., Spencer, T., Newcorn, J., Gao, H., Milton, D., Feldman, P., & Witte, M. (2007). Effect of comorbid symptoms of oppositional defiant disorder on responses to atomoxetine in children with ADHD: A meta-analysis of controlled clinical trial data. *Psychopharmacology, 190*, 31–41. Retrieved from http://www.ncbi.nlm.nih.gov/pubmed/17093981

Bulik, C., Reba, L., Siega-Riz, A., & Reichborn-Kjennerud, T. (2005). Anorexia nervosa: Definition, epidemiology and cycle of risk. *International Journal of Eating Disorders, 37*, S2–S9. Retrieved from http://www.ncbi.nlm.nih.gov/pubmed/ 15852310

Centers for Disease Control and Prevention (CDC). (2007). Prevalence of autism spectrum disorders—autism and developmental disabilities monitoring network, six sites, United States, 2000. *Morbidity and Mortality Weekly Report, 56*, 1–11. Retrieved from http://www.cdc.gov/mmwr/preview/mmwrhtml/ss5601a1.htm

David-Ferndon, C., & Kaslow, N. J. (2008). Evidence-based psychosocial treatments for child and adolescent depression. *Journal of Clinical Child & Adolescent Psychology, 37*, 62–104. Retrieved from http://www.ncbi.nlm.nih.gov/pubmed/18444054

Deglin, J., Vallerand, A., & Sanofski, A. (2011). *Davis' drug guide for nurses* (12th ed.). Philadelphia: F.A. Davis.

Ewing, J. A. (1984). Detecting alcoholism: The CAGE questionnaire. *Journal of the American Medical Association, 252*, 1905–1907. doi: 10.1001/jama.252.14.1905

Grisso, T. (2004). *Double jeopardy: Adolescent offenders with mental disorders*. Chicago, IL: University of Chicago Press.

Harlow, H., Harlow, M., & Suomi, S. (1971). From thought to therapy: Lessons from a private laboratory. *American Scientist, 59*, 538–549. Retrieved from http://www.ncbi.nlm.nih.gov/pubmed/5004085

Jedele, K. (2007). The overlapping spectrum of Rhett and Angleman syndromes: A clinical review. *Seminars in Pediatric Neurology, 14*, 108–117. doi: 10.1016/j.spen.2007.07.002

McNeish, D., & Newman, T. (2002). Involving children and young people in decision making. In D. McNeish, T. Newman, & H. Roberts (Eds.), *What works for children? Effective services for children and families*. Milton Keynes, UK: Open University Press.

Morgan, J. F., Reid, F., & Lacey, J. H. (1999). *The SCOFF questionnaire: Assessment of a new screening tool for eating disorders*. Retrieved from http://www.bmj.com/content/319/7223/1467.full

Myers, J., Berliner, L., Briere, J., Hendrix, C., Jenny, C., & Reid, T. (Eds.). (2002). *The APSAC handbook of child maltreatment* (2nd ed.). Thousand Oaks, CA: Sage Publications.

Newman, T., & McDaniel, B. (2005). Getting research into practice: Healing damaged attachment processes in infancy. *Child Care in Practice, 11*, 81–90. doi: 10.1080/1357527052000342635

Peplau, H. (1989). Therapeutic nurse-patient interaction. In A. O'Toole & S. Welt (Eds.), *Interpersonal theory in nursing practice: Selected works of Hildegard E. Peplau* (pp. 192–204). New York: Sage.

U.S. Department of Health and Human Services. (1999). *Mental health: A report of the Surgeon General—executive summary*. Retrieved from http://www.surgeongeneral.gov/library/mentalhealth/summary.html

Verrier, N. (1993). *The primal wound: Understanding the adopted child*. Baltimore, MD: Gateway Press.

Winters, K. (2008). *Adolescent brain development and drug abuse*. Retrieved from www.mentorfoundation.org

15 Gastrointestinal Disorders

Judith D. McLeod, DNP, RN, CPNP

OBJECTIVES

- ☐ Define key terms.
- ☐ Identify the components of an abdominal examination.
- ☐ Identify the important questions to ask when taking a history about GI problems.
- ☐ Identify and describe gastrointestinal disease that is associated with the esophagus:
  - ☐ Tracheoesophageal fistula
- ☐ Identify and describe gastrointestinal diseases that present with abdominal pain:
  - ☐ Celiac disease
  - ☐ Appendicitis
  - ☐ Inguinal hernia
  - ☐ Inflammatory bowel disease, including Crohn's disease and ulcerative colitis
  - ☐ Irritable bowel syndrome
  - ☐ Peptic ulcer disease
- ☐ Identify and describe gastrointestinal disorders associated with regurgitation or vomiting:
  - ☐ Gastroesophageal reflux
  - ☐ Pyloric stenosis
  - ☐ Intestinal obstruction, including volvulus and intussusception
  - ☐ Gastroenteritis
- ☐ Identify and describe gastrointestinal disorders associated with constipation:
  - ☐ Functional constipation
  - ☐ Hirschsprung's disease
- ☐ Identify and describe gastrointestinal problems manifested by an anterior abdominal wall defect:
  - ☐ Omphalocele
  - ☐ Gastroschisis
- ☐ Identify and describe gastrointestinal disorders associated with the liver, pancreas, or gall bladder:
  - ☐ Neonatal jaundice
  - ☐ Biliary atresia
  - ☐ Hepatitis
  - ☐ Fatty liver disease
  - ☐ Gall bladder disease
- ☐ Identify and describe gastrointestinal disorders associated with nutritional problems:
  - ☐ Obesity

KEY TERMS

- Tracheoesophageal fistula
- Celiac disease
- Diarrhea
- Vomiting
- Appendicitis
- Inguinal hernia
- Crohn's disease
- Ulcerative colitis
- Irritable bowel syndrome
- Regurgitation
- Gastroesophageal reflux (GER)
- Pyloric stenosis
- Volvulus
- Intussusception
- Necrotizing enterocolitis (NEC)
- Gastroenteritis
- Constipation
- Encopresis
- Hirschsprung's disease
- Omphalocele
- Gastroschisis
- Biliary atresia
- Cholecystitis
- Hepatitis

Don't have time to read this chapter? Want to reinforce your reading? Need to review for a test? Listen to this chapter on DavisPlus at davispl.us/rudd1.

ANATOMY AND PHYSIOLOGY

The gastrointestinal (GI) system encompasses the area from the mouth to the anus and includes the organs responsible for digestion and elimination. The organs in this system include (**Figure 15-1**):

- Esophagus
- Stomach
- Small and large intestines
- Liver, gallbladder, and associated bile ducts
- Pancreas

Disruption of functions or disorders in the GI system may cause problems with the child's nutritional status. Children with disordered nutrition may be seen by a gastroenterologist for treatment.

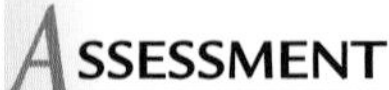

ASSESSMENT

History

- Important initial questions:
  - *What is the problem?*
  - *How long has the child had this problem?*

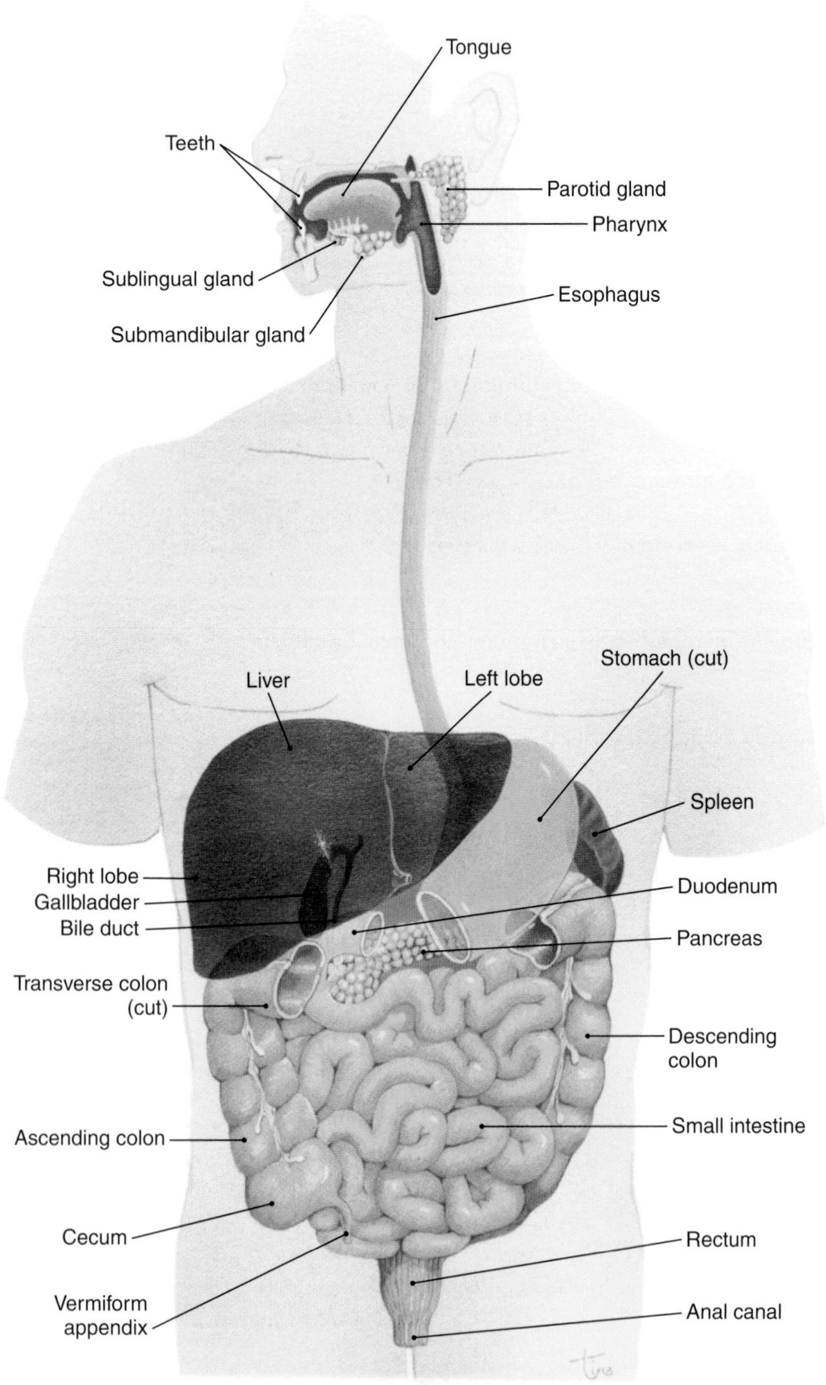

Figure 15-1 Digestive system.

- *Has there been weight loss?*
- *History of any previous illness?*
- Symptoms:
  - *Is the child having abdominal pain?*
    - How often does the pain occur?
    - Where is the pain located?
    - Does anything help the pain?
    - Does the pain improve with eating?
    - Does the pain improve with defecating?
    - Does anything make it worse?
  - *What is the normal stool pattern?*
    - Does the child defecate every day?
    - Is the stool large? Small? Hard? Watery?
    - Does the child have a ritual before stooling?
    - Does the child go to the toilet willingly?
    - Does the child hide before stooling?
    - Does the stool block the toilet after the child defecates?
  - *Does the child have diarrhea?*
    - How often is the diarrhea?
    - Is it bloody?
    - Is there pain associated with the diarrhea?
    - Does the patient have cramping or bloating?
    - What has been done to treat the diarrhea?
  - *Does the patient have vomiting?*
    - How often is the vomiting?
    - Are there symptoms associated with the vomiting?
    - Nausea? Cramping? Abdominal pain? Headache?
    - Does the child feel better after vomiting?
    - What has been done for the vomiting?
  - *What does the child normally eat?*
    - Is there a change in the eating pattern?
    - Is an infant refusing the breast or bottle?
- Review the family history, especially for history of GI problems. Complete a genogram with at least three generations to show patterns of illness, if possible.
- Review the social history:
  - *Any problems at home*
  - *Any new stressors*

Physical Examination

The Abdominal Examination

Inspection

- What to look at first
  - *Interaction of child with family*
  - *Body positions and movements*
    - Climbing up and down from the table
    - Can the child jump down from the table?
- Abdomen changes in size and shape with growth
  - *Prominent in newborn*
  - *Flatter in older children*
  - *Abnormal findings*
    - Marked distension causes shiny appearance caused by air, fluid, or solid tissue enlargement
    - Scaphoid or very flat in newborn
    - "Missing" portions of GI tract may change appearance (Greydanus, Feinberg, Patel, & Homnick, 2008)
- Children may need distraction during the exam.
  - *Children may need to be examined as much as possible while on the parent's lap.*
  - *Infants may need to suck on a pacifier or can breastfeed.*
  - *Toddlers may be reluctant to leave parent—distraction with light, toy, or other means may be effective.*
  - *Preschoolers may want to know what is happening and ask questions; they want to know how their bodies work.*
  - *School-aged children and adolescents may be more cooperative, but need an explanation of what will happen next.*

Auscultation

- Listening with the stethoscope
  - *Bowel sounds are sounds of normal peristalsis.*
  - *In newborn, air enters stomach with first cry and reaches the rectum in 3 to 4 hours.*
  - *Bowel sounds are recorded as present or absent.*
  - *Increase in sounds (frequency and volume) with eating*
  - *No diagnosis on just bowel sounds*
  - *Abnormal bowel sounds*
    - Hyperactive—may indicate gastroenteritis or lactose intolerance
    - High-pitched, loud, tinkling rushes with obstructive process
    - Absence after 5 minutes indicates a paralytic ileus (Greydanus et al., 2008)
  - *Auscultation of the infant's abdomen is easier if the baby is sucking and is quiet.*
  - *Preschoolers and school-age children may want to listen with the stethoscope after the assessment; this will increase their cooperation.*

CLINICAL PEARL

Auscultation Before Palpation

Always perform auscultation of the abdomen before you do palpation. Palpation will change the quality of the bowel sounds and therefore may change the assessment (Greydanus et al., 2008).

Percussion

- Assesses distension, liver and spleen size
  - *Tympanic sound shows gaseous area, dull sound with fluid*

Palpation

- How to perform the exam
  - *Child should be relaxed, supine, arms at side, knees flexed.*
  - *Warm palm if possible; rest entire palm on abdomen*
  - *Gentle flexion of hand; avoid tickling and poking*
  - *Light palpation to decrease pain*
  - *Having the child place his or her hand on top of the examiner's will allow the child to feel some control during the exam.*
  - *The abdomen is divided into four quadrants; check each quadrant.*
  - *Check for hernia.*

- *Examine perianal region for fissures, fistula, or skin tags.*
- *Digital exam may be done to assess anal sphincter tone*
- Note any of the following
  - *Site and severity of pain with any muscle guarding*
  - *Localized tenderness with involuntary guarding, a sign of peritoneal irritation*
  - *Check flank on each side for pain.*

GASTROINTESTINAL PROBLEMS MANIFESTED IN THE ESOPHAGUS

TRACHEOESOPHAGEAL FISTULA

Assessment

Clinical Presentation

- History of polyhydramnios while in utero
- Inability to handle secretions—baby may have an overabundance of secretions
- Cyanosis with feeding
- Resistance with passage of a feeding tube
- Associated with syndromes that may have skeletal, anorectal, or limb abnormalities
- Continual choking with feedings after passage of a feeding tube will need further investigation for possible H-type fistula (Wyllie & Hyams, 2006).
  - *Five types of* ***tracheoesophageal fistulas:***
    - Most common configuration (86%) is esophageal atresia with distal tracheoesophageal fistula: Proximal esophagus ends blindly in upper mediastinum; distal esophagus is connected to the tracheobronchial tree.
    - Second most common type (8%) is isolated esophageal atresia with no tracheoesophageal fistula: Has small stomach, gasless abdomen.
    - The third most common type (4%) is H- or N-type tracheoesophageal fistula with no esophageal atresia.
    - The fourth type (1%) is esophageal atresia with both a proximal and distal tracheoesophageal fistula.
    - The fifth type (1%) is esophageal atresia with a proximal tracheoesophageal fistula. (Wyllie & Hyams, 2006)

Diagnostic Tests

- Coiling of feeding tube is noted on x-ray.
- Bowel gas pattern may be abnormal.
- Ultrasound of renal system
- Echocardiogram
- A contrast evaluation for fistula may be performed.

Nursing Interventions

Emergency Care

- Prevention of aspiration is important.
- Tube should be placed in proximal pouch until surgery.
- IV access with fluids and antibiotics
- Supine position with head elevated

Acute Hospital Care

- Surgical repair is indicated.
- Prepare patient for surgery.
- Witness informed consent.
- IV support after surgery
- Chest tube care
- Continued antibiotics
- Frequent suctioning
- Elevate head of bed 30 to 45 degrees.
- Tube feedings start 2 to 3 days after surgery.
- Acid suppression therapy after surgery to promote healing
- If no leak 5 to 7 days after surgery, start oral feedings.
- Chest tube out with start of oral feedings
- Most babies do well, without complications.

Chronic Care

- Leak of the surgical site requires continued IV therapy and chest tube.
- Leaks usually close spontaneously.
- Stricture may occur, which may require dilation of the stricture over 3 to 6 months.
- Reoccurrence of fistula formation may require more surgery for repair.

Complementary and Alternative Therapies

- Requires a surgical repair; no alternative therapy is used.

Caregiver Education

Emergency Care

- Explain need for IV fluids.
- Provide information about the diagnostic tests.
- Preoperative teaching for the caregiver is essential.
- Provide reassurance to caregivers as needed.

Acute Hospital Care

- Explain postoperative procedures.
- Provide emotional support.
- Nonnutritive sucking with a pacifier should be encouraged before oral feeding begins.
- Caregiver may assist with oral feeding once child has improved.
- Encourage caregiver to hold infant if stable; if unable to hold baby, then touching and stroking should be encouraged.
- Teach about signs to observe for at home on discharge.

Chronic Care

- Caregiver will need instruction on observing for and treating gastroesophageal reflux (see information on gastroesophageal reflux for treatment information).

- Caregiver should be taught baby feeding cues and signs of desire for interaction, as well as disengagement cues.
- Caregiver will need to keep all follow-up appointments.
- Caregiver will need to observe for and report any pulmonary difficulties.

GASTROINTESTINAL PROBLEMS MANIFESTED BY ABDOMINAL PAIN

CELIAC DISEASE

Assessment

Clinical Presentation

See **Figure 15-2** for the clinical presentation of **celiac disease**.

- *Abdominal bloating*
- ***Diarrhea***
- ***Vomiting***
- *Weight loss—may appear very skinny in the extremities but with a normal-appearing face.*
- *Flatulence*
- *Foul-smelling stools*
- *Delayed growth and development, including short stature, delayed puberty*
- *Dental enamel defects in the teeth.*
- *Dermatitis herpetiformis—blistering, pruritic skin rash on elbows, buttocks, or knees*
    - More common in adults
    - Does not occur in all cases
- *Severe form*
    - Iron deficiency anemia
    - B_{12} deficiency
    - Osteopenia or osteoporosis due to calcium malabsorption (Amerine, 2006)

> **CLINICAL PEARL**
>
> **Celiac Disease**
>
> Celiac disease is recognized as a genetic disorder, occurring in 1 in 133 people. In patients with a first-degree relative—parent, sibling, or child—the rate is 1 in 22 people (Fasano et al., 2003).
>
> Celiac disease may also occur in conjunction with other diseases, including diabetes, autoimmune thyroid disease, autoimmune liver disease, rheumatoid arthritis, systemic lupus erythematosus, and Sjogren's disease. It is recommended that any patient diagnosed with these diseases also be tested for celiac disease. A gluten-free diet used by a diabetic with concurrent celiac disease will result in a decrease in insulin needs (Amerine, 2006).

Diagnostic Studies

- Blood:
    - *Complete blood count (CBC) with differential*
    - *Anti-tissue transglutamase antibodies*
    - *Total immunoglobulin A (IgA)*
    - *IgA antiendomysial antibodies*

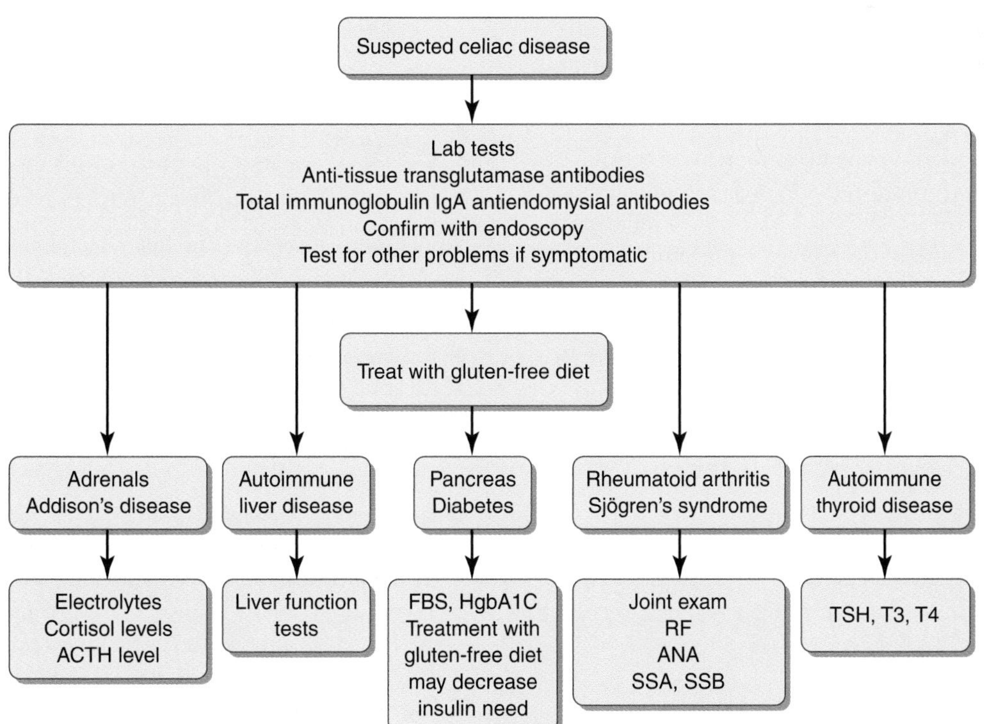

Figure 15-2 Diseases that can be associated with a diagnosis of celiac disease.

- *Vitamin B_{12} level, ferritin, total iron binding capacity, folate*
- *Stool for occult blood, fat,* Helicobacter pylori *antigen (Amerine, 2006)*

- Endoscopy and tissue biopsy for definitive diagnosis

Nursing Interventions

Emergency Care

- May require IV hydration for vomiting or diarrhea

Acute Hospital Care

- Prepare patient for endoscopy exam.
- Patient should not start gluten-free diet before endoscopy exam.
- Explain procedure to patient and family.
- Work with dietitian to teach patient and family about gluten-free diet before discharge.

Chronic Care

- Teach patient and family about gluten-free diet.
  - *Refer family to www.celiac.org for information on disease and diet.*
- Refer patient and caregivers to a support group for the disease.
- Alternative therapies:
  - *Gluten-free diet is the definitive therapy and does not require medication.*

Caregiver Education

Emergency Care

- Recognize celiac crisis—with extreme vomiting and diarrhea.
- Required IV therapy and electrolyte replacement
- Once on a gluten-free diet, most patients will not require emergency care.
- Failure to respond to the diet may indicate another underlying disease or failure to avoid gluten.

Acute Hospital Care

- Caregivers and patient will need to learn components of a gluten-free diet.
- Referral to a dietitian
- Discuss food likes and dislikes and teach family how to read labels for gluten.
- Information from www.celiac.org about diet and support groups

Chronic Care

- Monitoring adherence to the gluten-free diet by the patient is important.
- Many gluten-free products are available, so it is important to read labels.
- Provide a list of area stores that carry gluten-free products if available.
- Follow-up on a regular basis with the gastroenterologist is essential.
- Participation in a support group either in person or online is helpful.
- Encourage child's participation in camps and outings with other children with celiac disease.
- Have caregivers and other family members screened also.

CULTURAL AWARENESS: The Impact of Cultural Dietary Traditions on Illness

Food plays a part in many cultural traditions. Holidays are a time when families come together and have many traditional dishes served. When a child is diagnosed with a gastrointestinal problem that affects food intake, it is important to talk with the family members about how this will affect them in their food preparation as well as their daily lives. The child may not be able to eat some traditional dishes due to gluten intolerance or intestinal pain, and the family and care providers both need to be sensitive to this issue.

For instance, the holiday turkey with the traditionally made stuffing may not be appropriate for the child with gluten intolerance, and this diet restriction needs to be explained to all family members so they are not offended when the child does not eat this food. Many cultures use wheat in food products such as tortillas or noodles, and families need to be aware of the problems these foods could cause a child. As well, diseases such as celiac disease may make it more difficult to participate in religious ceremonies such as Communion, as Communion wafers contain wheat. Discussing this problem with church leaders may help to find solutions, such as low-gluten wafers or Communion with just wine (Amerine, 2006). Awareness of the impact of culture should be one factor that is kept in mind when teaching families about changes in the diet (see Chapter 4 for further details).

APPENDICITIS

Assessment

Clinical Presentation

Appendicitis may have the following clinical presentation.

- Initial pain in the periumbilical area that moves to the right lower quadrant of the abdomen (**Figure 15-3**)
- Low-grade fever
- May be nauseated and have vomiting—not taking oral intake
- Usually does not have stool, but may present with diarrhea or pelvic pain
- Usually lays with knees bent
- Rebound pain with exam in right lower quadrant
  - *Pain in right side when press on left and release suddenly*
  - *Pain after internal rotation of flexed thigh*
  - *Pain on passive extension of right hip*
  - *Pain in right lower quadrant when jumping and landing on the heels (Garfunkel, Kaczorowski, & Christy, 2007)*

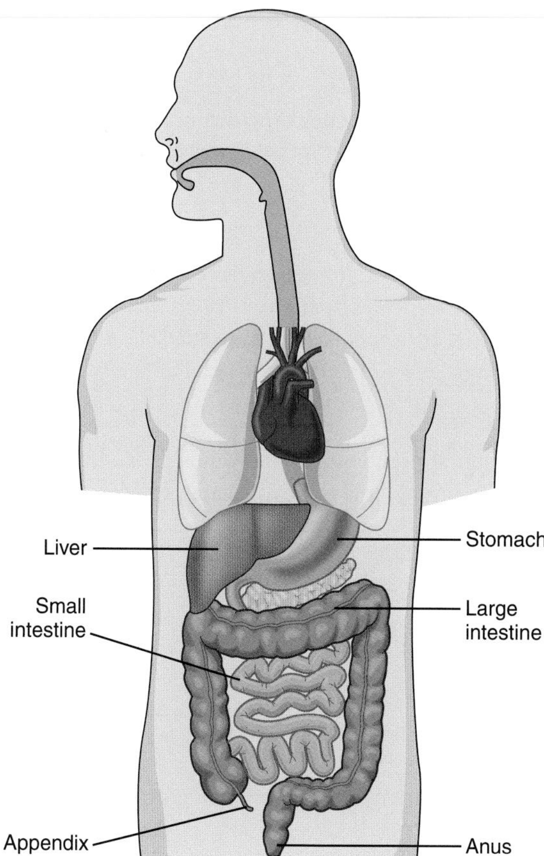

Figure 15-3 The appendix is a fingerlike pouch attached to the large intestine in the lower right area of the abdomen.

- Pain for several days with sudden resolution but an ill-looking child may indicate perforation of the appendix.

Diagnostic Testing

- CBC with differential—will sometimes show elevation and a left shift
- Urinalysis
- Ultrasound
- Computerized tomography (CT) scan
  - *Usually ordered after consultation with a surgeon*

Nursing Interventions

Emergency Care

- Patient will be NPO.
- Monitor vital signs.
- Assist with diagnostic tests, including ultrasound and CT.
- Assist with positioning patient in position of comfort.
- Administer IV fluids as ordered.
- Explain tests to patient and family.
- Prepare patient for surgery, including any teaching that may be required.

Acute Hospital Care

- Monitor vital signs.
- Maintain IV therapy and then advance diet as tolerated.
- Assess pain with appropriate pain scale (FACES for young child, scale of 1–10 for older child) and administer pain medication as ordered.
- Encourage ambulation.
- Monitor incisional sites.
- Provide discharge instructions to patient and caregiver.

Chronic Hospital Care

- If the appendix is ruptured, the patient may have a prolonged hospital stay.
- Administer IV therapy as ordered.
- Monitor vital signs.
- Monitor lab tests.
- Monitor drainage and change dressings as needed.
- Assess for pain and administer medication as needed.
- Most acute appendicitis is now treated by laparoscopic removal.
- Nonsurgical treatment
  - *Used occasionally if patient is not well enough to undergo surgery*
  - *Includes IV antibiotics*
  - *Liquid or soft diet until the infection subsides*

Caregiver Education

Emergency Care

- Provide information about the diagnostic tests.
- Preoperative teaching for the caregiver and patient is essential.

Acute Hospital

- Instruct caregiver about medication administration for pain and antibiotics.
- Encourage caregiver to assist patient with ambulation as needed.
- Encourage child and caregiver to report pain and assist with medication or nonpharmacologic methods of relief, such as massage, distraction, music, and aromatherapy.
- Teach caregiver and patient signs of infection—redness in incision, fever, unrelieved pain.
- Provide discharge instructions and follow-up care.

Chronic Care

- Instruct patient and caregivers to limit lifting and physical activity for several weeks.
- Teach patient and caregiver importance of medication administration after ruptured appendix.
- Teach caregiver and patient signs of infection—redness in incision, fever, unrelieved pain.
- Teach patient and caregiver need to keep follow-up appointment.

INGUINAL HERNIA

Assessment

Clinical Presentation

Inguinal hernia may have the following clinical presentation.

- Lump in the groin, commonly on the right side
- May have a history of intermittent pain and swelling in the groin
- Feeling of weakness or pressure in the groin
- A burning, gurgling feeling at the bulge
- Patient with a hydrocele should be checked for inguinal hernia
- With incarceration—increase in pain, fever, tachycardia, bilious vomiting, and no stooling
- With strangulation—erythema and edema over a tender groin mass

Diagnostic Testing

- Palpation of the hernia on exam
  - *Patient will be upright and cough or bear down, which causes the hernia to extrude and be felt during manual exam.*
    - Reduction of the hernia during exam
  - *Transillumination of the hydrocele to rule out hernia—no intervention needed if only hydrocele.*
  - *Report of caregiver of lump seen in groin area*

Nursing Interventions

Emergency Care

- Start IV fluids.
- Prepare patient for surgery.
- Witness informed consent.
- Provide reassurance to caregivers as needed.

Acute Care

- May be performed on an outpatient basis if no incarceration
- Start IV fluids if not emergent.
- Answer questions and provide reassurance for caregivers.
- Provide appropriate pain medication postoperatively.
- Nonnutritive sucking for infants
- Care of suture line—keep clean and dry.
  - *In infants and toddlers who are not toilet trained, frequent diaper change*
  - *Assess circulation on the side of the surgical incision.*

Chronic Care

- Once repaired, the patient should not have additional problems with that side.
- Opposite side, if not repaired, will need periodic examination.
- Umbilical hernias may also occur, but are not repaired in newborns. They usually spontaneously close at 1 year.
- In older children, may need repair later

Caregiver Education

Emergency Care

- Provide information about the diagnostic tests.
- Preoperative teaching for the caregiver and patient is essential.

Acute Care

- Teach caregiver care of surgical site.
- Encourage feeding of patient as tolerated.
- Administer pain medication as needed.
- Note importance of keeping scheduled appointments.

Chronic Care

- Caregivers should observe opposite side for hernia.
- Report any problems to health-care provider.

INFLAMMATORY BOWEL DISEASE

CROHN'S DISEASE

Assessment

Clinical Presentation

Crohn's disease may have the following presentation.

- Abdominal pain
  - *Often presents in the right lower quadrant* **(Figure 15-4)**
  - *May mimic appendicitis*
- Fever
- Diarrhea (possibly bloody)
- Nausea and vomiting
- Anorexia
- Weight loss and fatigue
- Anemia
- Delayed growth and development
- Oral aphthous ulcers
- Intestinal blockage

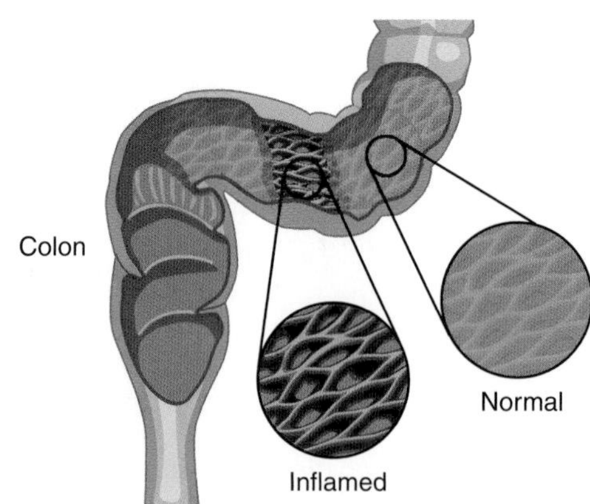

Figure 15–4 In Crohn's disease, portions of the digestive tract become inflamed. The diseased lining of the digestive tract becomes swollen and scarred.

- Fistula formation
- Periods of exacerbation and remission
- May be mild with minimal symptoms to severe with fulminant disease (Askey, 2008)

Diagnostic Testing

- CBC, electrolytes, liver enzymes, sedimentation rate, C reactive protein (CRP)
- Serum calcium and phosphorus, zinc, magnesium
- Total protein and albumin
- Urinalysis
- Stool for occult blood and white blood cells, ova, and parasites
- Stool culture
- Inflammatory bowel disease (IBD) lab panel
- Upper GI series with small bowel follow-up
- Ultrasound
- CT scan
- Colonoscopy with tissue biopsy
- Ophthalmic exam

Nursing Interventions

Emergency Care

- Periods of abdominal pain with bleeding require immediate treatment
- IV therapy
- High-dose corticosteroids

Acute Care

- May require IV therapy for hydration
- Corticosteroid therapy to induce remission
- Antibiotics may be used
- Tacrolimus or cyclosporine
- Start infliximab therapy.
- May require surgery

Chronic Care

- Drug therapy
  - *Mesalamine*
  - *Antibiotics*
  - *Immunosuppressives such as azathioprine, 6-mercaptopurine, or methotrexate*
  - *Infliximab therapy (tumor necrosis factor [TNF] blocker)—maintenance dosing every 6 to 8 weeks*
- Nutritional supplementation may be necessary.
- Surgery if medication does not control the symptoms (Askey, 2008)

Complementary and Alternative Therapies

- Probiotics—not well studied (Land & Martin, 2008)

Caregiver Education

Emergency Care

- Caregivers need to bring patient in for treatment with signs of bleeding or pain.

Acute Care

- Caregivers and patient need education about medications.
- Discuss concerns with caregiver and patient.
- Discuss feelings with child or adolescent about having a chronic disease.
- Work with child and adolescent on diet—discuss dietary likes and dislikes; try to have some normalcy in diet between exacerbations.
- Teach patient and caregivers about stress reduction techniques, such as visualization, and relaxation techniques.

Chronic Care

- Review use and side effects of medications with patient and caregivers.
- Review importance of regular follow-up exams.
- Encourage patient to report if side effects of medications occur.
- Caregivers should report any illness to the gastroenterologist for possible medication adjustment.
- Refer caregiver and child to camps or other activities so that child can experience normal activities with other children with similar diseases.
- Discuss diet and how to maintain good nutrition as well as incorporate dietary preferences.
- Refer patient and caregivers to a support group.

ULCERATIVE COLITIS

Assessment

Clinical Presentation

Ulcerative colitis may have the following clinical presentation.

- Abdominal pain (**Figure 15-5**).
- Bloody diarrhea—watery with streaks of blood
- Urgency to defecate
- Anemia
- Fatigue
- Weight loss
- Loss of appetite
- Rectal bleeding
- Skin lesions
- Joint pain
- Growth failure
- Symptoms may be mild or with frequent bouts of bloody diarrhea, fever, and abdominal cramping.

Diagnostic Testing

- CBC, electrolytes, liver enzymes, sedimentation rate, CRP
- Total protein, albumin
- Serum iron, total iron binding capacity, ferritin
- Stool for occult blood and white blood cells, ova, and parasites; stool culture

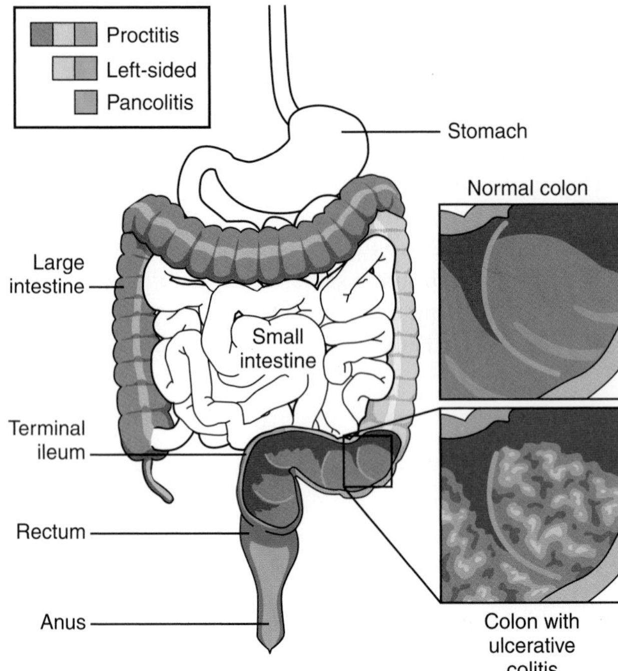

Figure 15-5 Ulcerative colitis is an inflammatory bowel disease (IBD), the general name for diseases that cause inflammation in the small intestine and colon.

- Stool for *Clostridium difficile*
- IBD lab panel
- Colonoscopy with tissue biopsy

Nursing Interventions

Emergency Care

- Periods of abdominal pain with bleeding require immediate treatment
- IV therapy
- Antibiotics

Acute Care

- May require IV therapy for hydration
- Corticosteroid therapy to induce remission
- Antibiotics may be used.
- Pain medication
- Antidiarrheals
- May require surgery

Chronic Care

- Drug therapy
  - *Aminosalicylates such as sulfasalazine or mesalamine—may be given orally, as a suppository, or as an enema.*
  - *Corticosteroids—orally, IV, enema, or suppository*
  - *Immunosuppressives such as azathioprine, 6-mercaptopurine*
  - *Cyclosporine A may be given for severe disease (Garfunkel et al., 2007).*
- Nutritional supplementation may be necessary.
- Surgery if medication does not control the symptoms

Complementary and Alternative Therapies

- Probiotics—not well studied (Land & Martin, 2008)

Caregiver Education

Emergency Care

- Caregivers need to bring patient in for treatment with signs of bleeding or pain.

Acute Care

- Caregivers and patient need education about medications.
- Discuss concerns with caregiver and patient.
- Discuss feelings with child or adolescent about having a chronic disease.
- Teach patient and caregivers about stress reduction techniques, such as visualization, and relaxation techniques.

Chronic Care

- Review use and side effects of medications with patient and caregivers.
- Review importance of regular follow-up exams.
- Encourage patient to report if side effects of medications occur.
- Report any illness to the gastroenterologist for possible medication adjustment.
- If surgical intervention, answer patient and caregiver concerns about surgery.
- Refer patient and caregivers to a support group.
- Refer caregiver and child to camps or other activities so that child can experience normal activities with other children with similar disease.

PEPTIC ULCER DISEASE

Assessment

Clinical Presentation

- Early symptoms with gastritis; may be asymptomatic (**Figure 15-6**)
  - *Recurrent abdominal pain*
  - *Nausea, vomiting, anorexia*
  - *Decrease in growth*
  - *Proceeds to crampy epigastric pain*
  - *Change in eating habits*
- Proceeds to:
  - *Chronic, recurrent abdominal pain*
  - *Episodic epigastric pain*
  - *Vomiting that is recurrent*
  - *Nocturnal awakening*
  - *Anemia*
  - *May have life-threatening GI bleeding*
  - *Perforation of the stomach or duodenum*
  - *Shock*

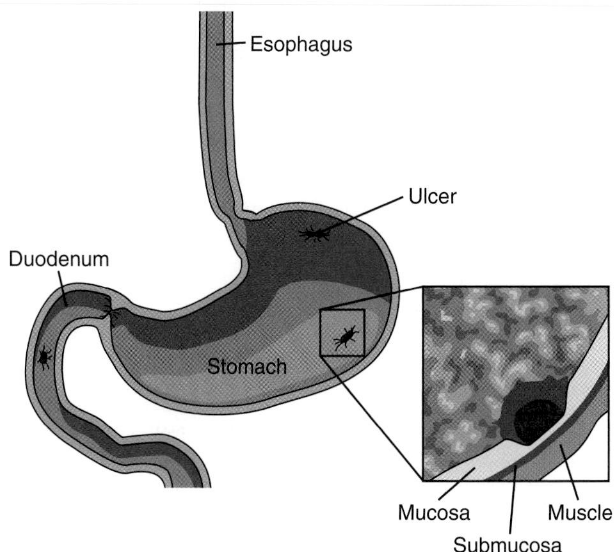

Figure 15-6 Peptic ulcers occur in the wall of the stomach and duodenum.

> **CLINICAL PEARL**
>
> **Symptoms of Peptic Ulcer**
>
> Infants may display hematemesis, melena, distention, and respiratory distress with an ulcer. Toddlers may have anorexia or vomiting. Bleeding then follows in several weeks. Preschool children have pain as the presenting symptom, which occurs on arising and is not relieved by food. Older school-aged children and adolescents will have symptoms similar to adult ulcer patients (Garfunkel et al., 2007).

Diagnostic Testing

- CBC, sedimentation rate
- *H. pylori* antibody blood test
- *H. pylori* antigen in stool
- Stool for occult blood, white blood cell count (WBC)
- Upper GI series
- Endoscopy with biopsy and *H. pylori* culture

Nursing Interventions

Emergency Care

- Patient should be seen immediately for:
  - *Sudden, persistent stomach pain*
  - *Bloody or black stools*
  - *Bloody vomit or coffee-grounds vomit*
- NPO
- IV therapy

Acute Care

- Maintain IV therapy if needed.
- Provide explanation of treatment to patient and caregiver.
- Start treatment using triple therapy.

> **Medication**
>
> **Triple Therapy**
>
> Current treatment for ulcers is usually with medication and is known as triple therapy. Triple therapy usually includes use of two antibiotics, often amoxicillin and flagyl or tetracycline or clarithromycin. Also included in the therapy is a proton pump inhibitor such as omeprazole, lansoprazole, or pantoprozole (Garfunkel et al., 2007).

Chronic Care

- Monitor medication and patient compliance.

Complementary and Alternative Therapies

- A vaccine for *H. pylori* is currently under investigation.
- Avoidance of NSAIDs
- Good hand hygiene

Caregiver Education

Emergency Care

- Caregivers should be taught to recognize signs of serious disease, including bloody vomit or stools and severe pain.
- Instruct caregivers about therapy and diagnostic tests to be performed.

Acute Care

- Assist caregiver and patient with therapy.
- Explain importance of medication compliance (**Table 15-1**).
- Teach caregiver possible medication side effects.
- Reassure caregiver and patient when stress occurs.
- Teach stress reduction techniques to child and caregiver.

Chronic Care

- Teach importance of completing therapy.
- Teach importance of follow-up care.
- Teach side effects of medication to report if they occur.
- Teach stress reduction techniques such as relaxation.
- Teach avoidance of food that may aggravate condition.
- Encourage normal activity and sleep habits.

IRRITABLE BOWEL SYNDROME

Assessment

Clinical Presentation

Irritable bowel syndrome may have the following clinical presentation.

- Cramping
- Bloating
- Diarrhea

TABLE 15–1 COMMON MEDICATIONS USED IN GASTROINTESTINAL DISEASE

Drug	Uses	Dosage	Possible Side Effects or Warnings
Omeprazole	GERD, acid-related stomach and esophageal problems, stomach and intestinal ulcers	1 mg/kg/day divided doses bid If >20 kg, give 20 mg daily	Long-term exposure may increase risk of gastric tumors Can cause palpitations, change in heart rate, nausea, flatulence, discolored stools, fever, or URI symptoms Elevated liver function tests, fatigue, dizziness, headaches and myalgias, leg pain, hematuria or glycosuria Do not crush or chew if enteric coated Can open and sprinkle in applesauce; do not chew when taking; should be administered immediately
Lansoprazole	GERD, acid-related stomach and esophageal problems, stomach and intestinal ulcers	0.5–1.5 mg/kg <10 kg 7.5 mg once daily 10–20 kg 15 mg once daily >20 kg 30 mg once daily For GERD 15 mg once daily up to 8 weeks	Can cause nausea, flatulence, discolored stools, elevated serum transaminase, fatigue, dizziness, headaches, and some cardiovascular symptoms, including hypotension Can be opened and sprinkled in applesauce, pudding, cottage cheese, or strained pears to administer to small children
Pantoprazole	GERD, acid-related stomach and esophageal problems, stomach and intestinal ulcers	40 mg once daily	Nausea, vomiting, diarrhea, headache May cause vitamin B_{12} deficiency, weakness, sore tongue, tingling of hands and feet with longer-term use (over 3 years) Tablets should not be split or crushed May not be appropriate for children who cannot swallow tablets
Ranitidine	Histamine H2 antagonist, treatment of ulcers	Newborns: 2 mg/kg/day divided doses every 12 hours 1 mo–16 yrs, ulcer treatment: 2–4 mg/kg day divided twice daily with maximum of 300 mg/day Maintenance: 1 mo–16 yrs, ulcer treatment: 2–4 mg/kg day divided twice daily with maximum of 150 mg/day GERD: 4–10 mg/kg/day divided into twice daily dose, maximum 300 mg/day Over age 16: 300 mg at bedtime for ulcers, for GERD 150 mg twice daily	The 150-mg effervescent tablet can be dissolved in 6–8 ounces of water for administration The 25-mg effervescent tablet must be dissolved in at least 1 teaspoon of water If administering to a child, use a dose-measuring device Peppermint-flavored oral syrup for young children Can cause dizziness and sedation, constipation, nausea and vomiting, hepatitis, myalgia, tachycardia or bradycardia, gynecomastia
Metoclopramide (Reglan)	Prokinetic for gastroesophageal reflux—accelerates gastric emptying and intestinal transit without increasing secretions	<6 years: 0.1mg/kg 6–14 yrs: 2.5–5 mg Children over: 14–10 mg For GERD, neonates, infants and children: 0.4/0.8 mg/kg/day in 4 divided doses 30 minutes before meals	Can cause tardive dyskinesia with chronic use (lip smacking, impaired movement of the fingers, rapid eye movements, and tongue protrusion—not usually reversible) Can cause drowsiness and restlessness, constipation, diarrhea, gynecomastia, urinary frequency Use in caution with newborn due to possibility of increasing hyperbilirubinemia

TABLE 15–1 COMMON MEDICATIONS USED IN GASTROINTESTINAL DISEASE—cont'd

Drug	Uses	Dosage	Possible Side Effects or Warnings
Cimetedine	Histamine of H2 blocker used for ulcer treatment and GERD	Neonates: 5–10 mg/kg/day every 8–12 hours Infants: 10–20 mg/kg/day every 6–12 hours Children: 20–40 mg/kg/day every 6 hours	Bradycardia, tachycardia, dizziness, headache, drowsiness, rash, gynecomastia, diarrhea, nausea, vomiting, ALT, AST elevation, myalgias, elevated serum creatinine, possible relationship with pneumonia May interfere with metabolism of other medications
Famotidine	Histamine of H2 blocker used for ulcer treatment and GERD	Neonates and infants <3 months, GERD: 0.5 mg/kg/once daily Infants >3 months to 1 year, GERD: 0.5 mg/kg/twice daily Children 1–12 years, ulcer: 0.5 mg/kg/day at bedtime or twice daily (max 40 mg/day) Children 1–12 years, GERD: 1 mg/kg/day twice daily (max 80 mg/day) Children over 12, ulcer: 20 mg twice daily Children over 12, GERD: 20 mg twice daily for 6 weeks	Contains phenylalanine—use in caution with phenylketonuria (PKU) Can cause bradycardia, tachycardia, dizziness, headache, seizures (patients with renal impairment), drowsiness, acne, rash, dry skin, diarrhea, nausea, vomiting, flatulence, dry mouth, thrombocytopenia ALT, AST elevation, cholestatic jaundice, arthralgias, muscle cramps, elevated serum creatinine and BUN, bronchospasm
Polyethylene glycol 3350 without electrolytes	Treatment of chronic constipation	Children >6 months: 0.5–1.5 gm/kg daily (initial dose 0.5 gm/kg and titrate to effect) Fecal impaction, >3 years: 1–1.5 gm/kg/daily for 3 days (maximum dose 100 gm/day) Administer in 4–8 ounces of fluid	Patient needs to be evaluated for bowel obstruction before use Can cause urticaria, abdominal bloating, cramping, diarrhea, flatulence
Lactulose	Treatment of chronic constipation	1 mL/kg bid qd-bid (max 60 mL/day) May take up to 48 hours to see effect	Can cause flatulence, abdominal discomfort, diarrhea, nausea Oral antibiotics and antacids that are not absorbed may interfere with action of drug Should not be used with children on special diet low in galactose Use special dosing device for administration of smaller doses May be given in 4 ounces of water, fruit juice, or milk
Mineral oil	Laxative, lubricant—decreases water absorption and softens stool	Children 5–11 years: 5–15 mL once daily for 1 week Children >12: 15–45 mL; may give in divided doses Can be given rectally as a enema	Nausea, vomiting, abdominal cramps, anal seepage Lipid pneumonitis if aspirated Can decrease the absorption of fat-soluble vitamins, carotene, calcium, and phosphorus May administer with meals if emulsified (better tasting)

Continued

TABLE 15–1 COMMON MEDICATIONS USED IN GASTROINTESTINAL DISEASE—cont'd

Drug	Uses	Dosage	Possible Side Effects or Warnings
Docusate sodium Senokots or Senna preparation	Laxative, stimulant; short-term treatment of constipation	Infant 1 month to 2 years: 1.25–2.5 mL (syrup) at bedtime not to exceed 5 mL Children 2–5 yrs: 2.5–3.75 mL at bedtime or ½ to 1 tablet po at hs Children 6–12 yrs: 5–7.5 mL at bedtime Tablets: 2 tablets at bedtime	Syrup can be mixed with juice, milk, or ice cream Can cause abdominal cramping, diarrhea, nausea and vomiting, and diarrhea; can have bitter taste Discolors feces and urine
Bisacodyl	Laxative, stimulant	Children 3–12 yrs: 5–10 mg in a single dose, oral Children >12 yrs: 5–15 mg day in a single dose Rectal Children <2 yrs: 5 mg/day as a single dose Children 2–11 years: 5–10 mg/day in a single dose Children >12 yrs: 10 mg/day	Long-term use may be habit forming and cause laxative dependence and possible electrolyte imbalance Can cause abdominal cramping, diarrhea, nausea and vomiting, sensation of rectal burning, and diarrhea May interact with antacids to cause delayed-release tablets to release sooner than in the small intestine, causing gastric irritation Do not take within 1 hour of dairy products

Source: Taketomo, C. K., Hodding, J. H., & Kraus, D. K. (2009). *Pediatric dosage handbook* (16th ed.). Hudson, OH: Lexi-Comp; Wyllie, R., & Hyams, J. (2006). Pediatric gastrointestinal and liver disease (3rd ed.). Philadelphia: Saunders Elsevier; Pediatric Lexi-Drugs Online. (2009). Retrieved from http://www.lexi.com/institutions/online.jsp?id=databases; Epocrates Online. (2011). Retrieved from http://www.epocrates.com.

- Constipation
- Change in appearance of the stool:
  - *Loose or hard*
  - *Thin or like pellets*
  - *Mucus in the stool*
- Urgency to have a bowel movement
- More common in women than men (**Figure 15-7**)
- May be associated with other functional pain syndromes (e.g., chronic fatigue, fibromyalgia)

Diagnostic Testing

- In most cases, the diagnosis is established by history.
- CBC, stool studies for ova and parasites, occult blood, WBC, stool culture
- Endoscopy if any bleeding occurs to rule out IBD

Nursing Interventions

Emergency Care

- Patient may be evaluated for pain, but pain is usually relieved by having stool.

Acute Care

- Stress the need to eat small meals and avoid trigger foods.
- Monitor medication administration and effects.

Chronic Care

- Dietary changes—removing trigger foods such as fatty foods, dairy, carbonated beverages, and caffeine
- Diary of symptoms, bowel habits, and diet
- Increase in high-fiber foods
- Eating several small meals
- Fiber supplements

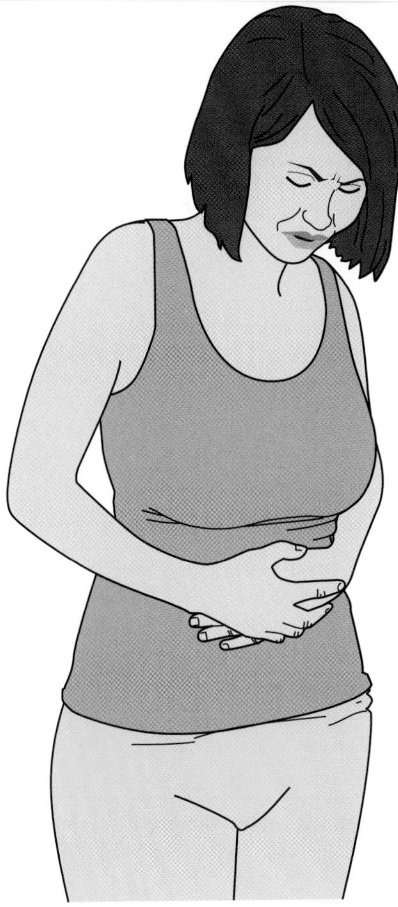

Figure 15-7 Girls with IBS often have more symptoms during their menstrual periods. Stress does not cause IBS, but it can make your symptoms worse.

- Laxatives such as Miralax to relieve constipation
- Imodium to relieve diarrhea

Complementary and Alternative Therapies

- Probiotics may be helpful for some patients but are not well studied.

Caregiver Education

Emergency Care

- Emergency care may not be needed. Caregiver should know to have patient evaluated for unusual symptoms.

Acute Care

- Teach caregiver and patient importance of using medication for symptom management.
- Teach caregiver and patient use of diet and foods to avoid.

Chronic Care

- Review food diary with patient and caregiver to identify triggers.
- Review use of medication for symptoms.
- Teach use of diet—have child or adolescent help with planning meals and food selection (**Table 15-2**).
- Teach patient and caregiver stress reduction techniques.

Complementary and Alternative Therapies

- Some use of probiotics
- Fish oil capsules

GASTROINTESTINAL PROBLEMS MANIFESTED BY VOMITING

CRITICAL COMPONENT

Regurgitation by Infants

All babies spit up, some babies more than others. Approximately 40% of 4-month-olds regurgitate, approximately 20% to the extent that caregivers seeks assistance (Orenstein, Bauman, DiLorenzo, & Hassell, 2007). One problem with **regurgitation** is estimating the amount the patient is spitting up. Caregivers may be taught to describe the regurgitation by how much is on a diaper—dime sized, quarter sized, or covering the entire diaper. The vomiting may also be described as dribbling out of the nose, vomiting down the caregiver's leg or through the patient's nose, or so forceful that the vomitus goes several feet. The color of the emesis may be useful. Colors include milk colored and curdled milk or bilious in nature. Accurate description will help identify the problem causing the regurgitation or vomiting.

GASTROESOPHAGEAL REFLUX DISEASE

Assessment

Clinical Presentation

Gastroesophageal reflux (GER) may have the following clinical presentation.

- With reflux, eating is unpleasant and hurts.
- May see large amount of fluid with recurrent vomiting
- Silent type, where milk comes just into the esophagus, causing burning, coughing, and choking
- Slow weight gain or no weight gain due to association of eating with pain
- Excessive irritability and crying, especially after meals
- Arching during or after meals
- Children may have a chronic cough.

TABLE 15–2 GASTROINTESTINAL OR OTHER PROBLEMS THAT MAY REQUIRE A SPECIAL DIET	
CELIAC DISEASE	Gluten-free diet (avoid, wheat, barley, and rye) Can eat oats but need to be careful of cross-contamination from gluten containing-products Important to teach caregiver and child to read labels Child can learn to help plan meals with gluten-free foods Need to be on diet for life
IRRITABLE BOWEL SYNDROME	Avoid trigger foods—caffeine, citrus, nuts, carbonated beverages, fatty foods, dairy Have child keep diet diary Discuss and teach diet choices Increase fiber in diet Increase fluid intake Encourage use of daily probiotics, either in capsule or by eating yogurt with probiotics
PHENYLKETONURIA	Low-phenylalanine diet—special formula for infants Restrict high-phenylalanine carbohydrates Supplements—children can assist in preparation of supplements Supplement may be put in juice or prepared as a frozen drink Need to read labels on food Need to continue diet for life
CROHN'S DISEASE	Nutritional therapy—inclusion of probiotics and fish oil; may need enteral therapy if severe Avoid irritating foods—fried foods, carbonated beverages Decrease intake of high-fiber food during inflammation Use small, frequent meals Low-fat intake—may need emulsified fat Need vitamin supplements Increased caloric and protein needs
LACTOSE OR MILK INTOLERANCE	Avoid milk and milk products, including cheese and ice cream, and products containing whey and casein
CONSTIPATION	Avoid constipating food such as bananas, excessive milk, pasta Needs increase in fresh fruit, vegetables, whole grains, and fiber
GLYCOGEN STORAGE DISEASE	May need continuous feeding through a gastrostomy tube Frequent feedings in the daytime Cornstarch slurry at bedtime Monitoring of glucose
GALL BLADDER DISEASE	Avoid foods containing fat and cream-based soups
SHORT BOWEL SYNDROME	Will usually require parenteral nutrition at first with move to enteral nutrition Need vitamin supplementation With very short colon: No lipid restriction High-dose antimotility agent Soluble fiber to slow gastric emptying Oral hydration solution with high sodium

TABLE 15–2 GASTROINTESTINAL OR OTHER PROBLEMS THAT MAY REQUIRE A SPECIAL DIET—cont'd

	Small bowel reminant: Lipid restriction Low-dose antimotility agent Soluble fiber Oral rehydration solution with low sodium
FAILURE TO THRIVE	Utilize a high-calorie formula such as Neocate or Pediasure Regular meals and frequent snacks Fortify milk by adding 1 cup nonfat dry milk powder to a quart of milk; use in cooking as well as for drinking Add additional margarine or cheese to food Use instant breakfast in whole milk Watch infant or child for satiety cues

Source: Burns, C. E., Dunn, A. M., Brady, M. A., Starr, N. B., & Blosser, C. G. (2009). *Pediatric primary care* (pp. 211-216). St. Louis: Saunders; Gluten free diet. (2009). Retrieved from http://www.celiac.org; Wyllie, R., & Hyams, J. (2006). Pediatric gastrointestinal and liver disease (3rd ed., pp. 534-535). Philadelphia: Saunders Elsevier.

- May develop chronic episodes of pneumonia
- Older children may have pain in the epigastric area.
  - *Mid-sternal discomfort*
  - *Sleep interruption*
  - *Persistent throat soreness not associated with any infectious disease (Bhatia & Parrish, 2009; Wyllie & Hyams, 2006)*

CLINICAL PEARL

Sandifer's Syndrome

Sandifer's syndrome is characterized by sudden arching of the head, neck, and upper trunk during feeding due to reflux. The head is twisted side to side continuously and the upper trunk is bent to one side so the head points to the floor. The patient may be very irritable during this time. Improvement of the reflux may appear with this posturing. Successful treatment with medication, such as Ranitidine or Omeprazole, will cause this behavior to stop (Kabakus & Kurt, 2006).

Diagnostic Testing

- Weight, length, head circumference
- Stool for occult blood
- Chest x-ray for respiratory symptoms
- pH probe
- Esophagram
- Gastric emptying study in older child
- In some cases, endoscopy may be used.

Nursing Interventions

Emergency Care

- If baby chokes and stops breathing, initiate cardiopulmonary resuscitation (CPR).

Acute Hospital Care

- Monitor intake and output.
- Monitor weight.
- Prepare infant for pH probe or other diagnostic tests.
- Assess mother's feeding style if breastfeeding; rule out overactive letdown with excessive milk.
- Administer medication as ordered.
  - *Ranitidine*
  - *Reglan may be indicated for infants.*
  - *Proton pump inhibitors—Lanpranzole, Omeprazole (may be opened and sprinkled on food)*
- May be treated with Nissen fundoplication, if severe (Wyllie & Hyams, 2006)
- If surgery is indicated, provide preoperative teaching to the caregivers.
- Give support postoperatively.
  - *Monitor intake and output, including nasogastric tube secretions.*
  - *Gradual increase in feedings*

Chronic Hospital Care

- Positioning is important in infants.
- Avoidance of food that may trigger symptoms
- Administration of medication

Chronic Home Care

- May continue to breastfeed; help correct overactive letdown if present; baby may breastfeed in upright position.
- Teach caregivers positioning.
- Teach importance of medication administration.
- Teach caregivers how to thicken feedings, if needed.

- In older children, teach avoidance of food that may trigger symptoms—fatty foods, acidic foods (citrus juices, carbonated beverages, tomato products).
- Reduction in weight in older children who are obese

Caregiver Education

Emergency Care

- Teach caregiver to recognize symptoms of reflux and intervene immediately.
- Initiate CPR if reflux causes baby to stop breathing.

Acute Hospital Care

- Caregivers need to learn to administer medication as required.
- Assist caregivers with feedings.
- Teach caregivers to recognized symptoms.

Chronic Home Care

- Small, frequent feedings
  - *May continue to breastfeed; help correct overactive letdown if present; baby may breastfeed in upright position.*
  - *Frequent burping*
- Change formula to protein hydrolyzed formula if bottle feeding.
- Frequent burping during feeding
- Upright positioning during and after feeding
- Avoid placing patient in car seat or carrier after feeding.
- Folded blanket in the well of the car seat to extend hips
- Administration of medication 30 minutes before morning feeding
- For older children
  - *No eating or drinking 2 hours before bedtime*
  - *Avoidance of caffeine, chocolate, spicy foods, fatty foods, acidic foods, and carbonated beverages*
  - *Avoidance of exposure to cigarette smoke*
  - *Weight loss if the child is obese*
- Medication administration before breakfast by 30 minutes

Complementary and Alternative Therapies

- A low-fiber diet may help reduce reflux.

PYLORIC STENOSIS

Assessment

Clinical Presentation

Pyloric stenosis may have the following clinical presentation.

- Found more in boys than girls (4:1); higher incidence if mother had disease (Wyllie & Hyams, 2006)
- Forceful, progressive, nonbilious vomiting after each feeding
- Onset of vomiting from the first week of life to as late as 5 months of age
- Vomiting becomes projectile over time.
- Observation of peristaltic waves from left to right before vomiting occurs
- Eventual dehydration with decrease in serum chloride
- Poor weight gain
- Failure to thrive
- Jaundice in 2% to 5% of cases

Diagnostic Testing

- Palpation of pyloric mass in the mid-epigastrium (olive sign)
- Ultrasound visualization of pyloric thickening
- Upper GI series
- CBC with electrolytes
- Liver function tests, including bilirubin total and direct

Nursing Interventions

Emergency Care

- Patient will need to be NPO.
- Provide patient with pacifier for comfort.
- Provide IV therapy with isotonic solution and added electrolytes as needed.
- Teach caregivers about diagnostic tests to be performed.

Acute Hospital Care

- Prepare patient for surgical correction.
- Teach caregivers about surgery to be performed and answer questions.
- Provide emotional support to caregivers.
- Provide breastfeeding mother with electric pump for pumping and storage.
- Give appropriate pain medication postoperatively.
- Monitor incisional site for infection.
- Fold diapers low to avoid incisional area.
- Monitor intake and output.
- Daily weight
- Advance diet as ordered; small amounts of fluid frequently.
- Important to burp patient after feeding to decrease air in stomach

Chronic Hospital Care

- Patient may continue to vomit postoperatively due to edema.
- Monitor intake and output.
- Provide caregiver reassurance.
- Assist with diagnostic tests as needed.
- In most cases, the surgery alleviates the problem.

Complementary and Alternative Therapies

- No current alternative therapy

Caregiver Education

Emergency Care

- Bring patient to the hospital or clinic for evaluation.

Acute Hospital Care

- Assist with feeding as needed.
- Reassure caregivers about their ability to care for the patient.

Chronic Home Care

- Report continuation of vomiting if present.
- Advance diet as advised.
- Remind caregivers about keeping regular appointments and starting or continuing immunizations.

> **Clinical Reasoning**
>
> **Projectile Vomiting**
>
> Sammy comes to clinic with his caregivers. He is 5 weeks old today, and the caregivers are concerned because he has started to vomit all of his feedings. They state the vomiting is very forceful. They are wondering if they should be concerned.
>
> 1. What would you look for on an exam of this baby?
> 2. What tests might be performed?
> 3. What would you tell the caregivers about the treatment for this baby?

INTESTINAL OBSTRUCTION

> **CLINICAL PEARL**
>
> **Bilious Vomiting**
>
> Bilious vomiting in an infant is a surgical emergency until proven otherwise (Garfunkel et al., 2007). Malrotation (Figure 15-8) occurs when the small or large intestines are not positioned in the abdominal cavity in the correct position. When either the small or large intestines are twisted or malpositioned they carry with them the bands, vascular vessels, and ligaments that supply these organs. The symptom of bile in the emesis of an infant is therefore an ominous sign until proven otherwise.

VOLVULUS

Assessment

Clinical Presentation

Volvulus may have the following clinical presentation.

- Most often occurs in the first 6 months (**Figure 15-9**)
- Intense crying and pain
- Pulling up of the legs
- Abdominal distension
- Vomiting, usually bilious
- Tachycardia and tachypnea

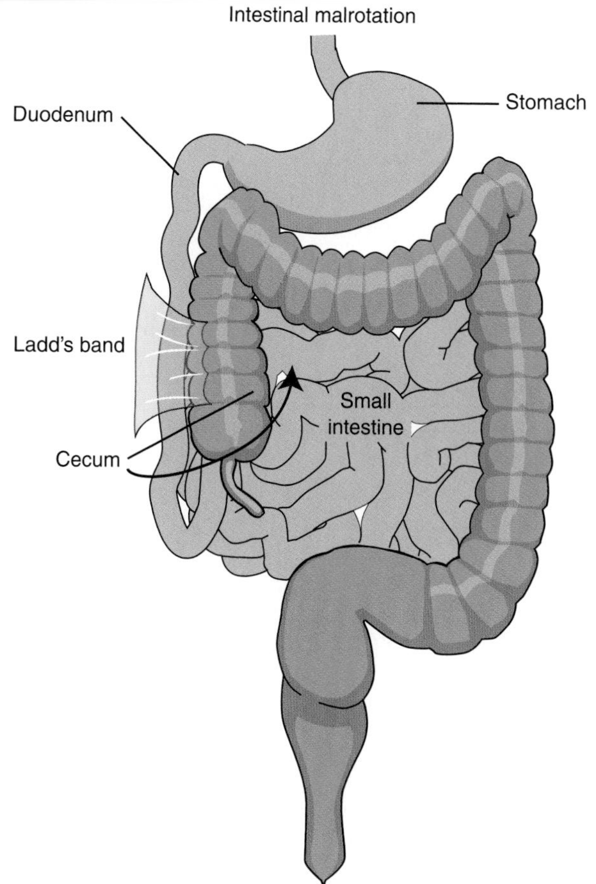

Figure 15-8 In malrotation, the cecum is not positioned correctly. The tissue that normally holds it in place may cross over and block part of the small bowel.

Diagnostic Testing

- Upper gastrointestinal series
- CBC with electrolytes

Nursing Interventions

Emergency Care

- Surgical emergency
- Patient needs counterclockwise rotation to restore normal perfusion.
- With significant damage may need resection

Acute Hospital Care

- Keep patient NPO.
- Establish IV therapy.
- Insert nasogastric tube.
- Maintain record of intake and output.
- Prepare patient for surgery.
- Provide patient with pacifier.
- Provide emotional support for caregiver.
- Provide pain relief after surgery—use Neonatal Pain Scale for infants.
- Monitor incisional area.

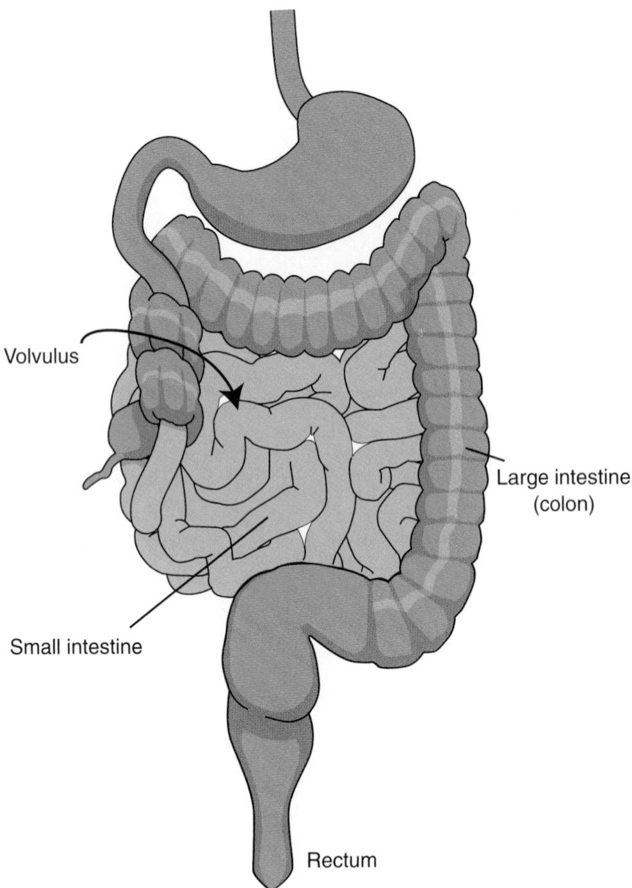

Figure 15-9 In volvulus, a portion of the intestine twists around itself.

- Monitor nasogastric (NG) tube.
- With return of bowel sounds, start feedings

Chronic Care

- Maintain record of intake and output.
- Once patient is maintaining good intake, he or she will be discharged.

Caregiver Education

Emergency Care

- Explain procedures to caregivers.
- Answer caregiver questions as needed.
- Encourage caregiver to hold and rock patient.

Acute Care

- Explain procedures to caregiver.
- Encourage caregiver to hold patient, either postprocedure or postoperatively.
- Encourage caregiver to participate in oral feedings.
- Encourage nonnutritive sucking before oral feedings.

Chronic Care

- Teach caregivers signs of infection or complications.
- Teach caregivers importance of follow-up appointments.

INTUSSUSCEPTION

Assessment

Clinical Presentation

Intussusception may have the following clinical presentation.

- May be caused by Meckel's diverticulum, polyp, or enlargement of lymph tissue
- Sudden drawing up of legs and crying with possible vomiting, then symptom free
- Pain will occur in regular intervals, every 15 to 20 minutes.
- Vomiting will contain bile.
  - *After 12 hours, develop currant-jelly stools*
  - *Increased abdominal distension*
- As problem progresses
  - *Fever*
  - *Peritoneal irritation with tenderness and guarding*
  - *Tachycardia*
  - *Elevated WBC (Wyllie & Hyams, 2006)*

Diagnostic Testing

- Ultrasound
- CBC with differential
- Barium enema

Nursing Interventions

Emergency Care

- Begin IV therapy.

Acute Care

- Prepare patient for ultrasound.
- Keep patient NPO.
- Establish IV therapy.
- Maintain record of intake and output.
- Provide patient with pacifier.
- Reduction may be done with barium enema, air insufflation, or water-soluble solution.
  - *Keep patient NPO.*
  - *Reintroduce to regular feeding gradually.*
- Surgical reduction
  - *Maintain nasogastric tube.*
  - *Maintain IV therapy.*
  - *Provide pain medication as needed.*
  - *When bowel sounds return, start gradual oral feedings.*

Chronic Care

- Maintain record of intake and output.
- Once patient is maintaining good intake, he or she will be discharged.

Caregiver Education

Emergency Care

- Explain procedures to caregivers.
- Answer caregiver questions as needed.

Acute Care

- Encourage caregiver to hold and rock patient.
- Explain procedures to caregiver.
- Encourage caregiver to hold patient, either postprocedure or postoperatively.
- Encourage caregiver to participate in oral feedings.

Chronic Care

- Teach caregivers signs of infection or complications.
- Teach caregivers importance of follow-up appointments.

> CLINICAL PEARL
>
> **Atresia and Stenosis**
>
> Atresia, or complete obstruction of the lumen of the gut, and stenosis, which is an incomplete obstruction, can occur in the midgut, which is the duodenum, jejunum, and ileum. Atresia occurs more often than stenosis. These conditions present with bilious vomiting and abdominal distension, failure to pass meconium, and jaundice (Wyllie & Hyams, 2006).

NECROTIZING ENTEROCOLITIS

Assessment

Clinical Presentation

Necrotizing enterocolitis (NEC) may have the following clinical presentation.

- Happens in premature infants, especially after infection or ischemic incident
- Tense, distended abdomen
- Large residual greater than 2 mL
- Stool positive for occult blood
- Increased periods of apnea
- Decreased blood pressure
- Poor temperature stability

Diagnostic Testing

- CBC, CRP
- Stool for occult blood
- Abdominal x-ray
- Increase in abdominal girth measurement

Nursing Interventions

Emergency Care

- Stop feedings to rest GI tract.
- Maintain IV therapy.

Acute Care

- Maintain and monitor IV therapy.
- Monitor total parenteral nutrition (TPN).
- Administer antibiotic therapy.
- If surgical intervention is required, prepare patient for surgery.
  - *Monitor IV therapy postoperatively.*
  - *Maintain NG tube.*
  - *Monitor operative site.*
- If patient develops short bowel syndrome:
  - *Start TPN.*
  - *Start enteral feedings early with continuous feedings.*
  - *Monitor stool output to advance feedings.*
  - *Monitor lab as appropriate.*
  - *If ostomy present, consult with ostomy nurse.*

Chronic Care

- After symptoms subside, restart feeding gradually, preferably with breast milk.
- Baby with short bowel syndrome may require long-term parenteral nutrition.
- The goal of therapy for short bowel syndrome is to advance to enteral feedings.
- If liver failure occurs, child may need liver transplant.

Caregiver Education

Emergency Care

- Explain procedures to caregivers.
- Answer caregiver questions as needed.

Acute Care

- Explain procedures to caregiver.
- Encourage caregiver to hold patient, either postprocedure or postoperatively.
- Encourage caregiver to participate in oral feedings.
- Encourage nonnutritive sucking with pacifier.
- Have caregiver provide breast milk if possible; provide breast pump for use as needed.

Chronic Care

- Teach caregivers signs of infection or complications.
- Teach caregivers importance of follow-up appointments.
- If patient has short bowel syndrome:
  - *Teach caregiver administration of enteral feedings.*
  - *Avoid hypertonic liquids (e.g., Kool-aid, juices, soda; Garfunkel et al., 2007).*
  - *Start patient on solids at normal developmental age, with meats first if possible.*
  - *Discuss long-term parenteral nutrition with caregiver if small bowel is less than 40 cm.*
- Teach caregiver signs of infection and complications.

GASTROINTESTINAL PROBLEMS MANIFESTED BY DIARRHEA

GASTROENTERITIS

Assessment

Clinical Presentation

Gastroenteritis may have the following clinical presentation.

- Watery diarrhea
- Abdominal cramping

- Vomiting
- Headache
- May have fever and chills
- Signs of dehydration—depressed fontanels, lack of tears, poor skin turgor, lethargy
- Symptoms last from 1 to 2 days up to 10 days

Diagnostic Testing

- Usually diagnosed by symptoms and exam
- May do stool for culture, ova and parasites (O&P), WBC
- Blood work—CBC and electrolytes if patient appears dehydrated

Nursing Interventions

Emergency Care

- Stools with blood or pus, temperature above 102.5
- If the patient is dehydrated, IV therapy needs to be instituted.
- Patient may require additional electrolytes in the IV if there is an imbalance.

> **CLINICAL PEARL**
>
> **Signs of Dehydration**
>
> Signs of dehydration include excessive thirst, dry mouth, little or no urine or dark urine, decreased tears, severe weakness or lethargy, and dizziness or lightheadedness. If children have any of these symptoms, caregivers should notify a health-care provider for further instructions about treatment (National Digestive Diseases Information Clearinghouse, 2011).

Acute Care

- If severe diarrhea or vomiting, may institute IV therapy
- Antibiotics may be administered if stool culture is positive.
- If patient is not dehydrated, care may be given at home.
- Withhold fluids for 2 to 3 hours.
- Start with 1 tablespoon of fluid every 15 minutes for 1 hour, then 1 ounce of fluid.
- Every ½ hour—Pedialyte, water, popsicles, and ginger ale
- After several hours of retaining fluid, may have clear broth and several saltines
- If patient starts to vomit, then stop fluids and start over.
- If only diarrhea, provide brief period of rest from intake, then start fluids.
- Moisturize lips with Vaseline.
- Allow pacifier for infants for nonnutritive sucking.
- Keep perineal area clean and dry between diarrhea episodes.

Chronic Care

- Second 24 hours should use the bland or BRAT diet (bananas, rice cereal, applesauce, and toast). (**Figure 15-10**)
- Reintroduce the patient's regular diet after 48 hours.

Caregiver Education

Emergency Care

- Caregiver should bring patient to clinic or hospital if there are any of the following symptoms:
  - *Prolonged vomiting*
  - *No urination for 8 to 12 hours*
  - *Depressed fontanel*
  - *Dry mucous membranes*
  - *Lethargy*

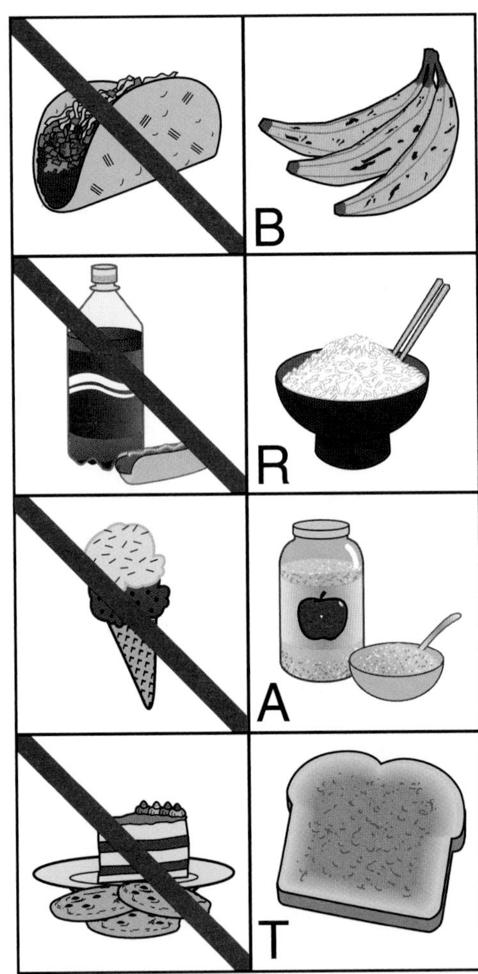

Figure 15-10 Treatment for diarrhea. As you feel better, begin eating soft, bland food, such as bananas, plain rice, boiled potatoes, toast, crackers, cooked carrots, and baked chicken without the skin or fat. Children can eat bananas, rice, applesauce, and toast (sometimes called the BRAT diet).

Acute Care

- Instruct caregivers on how to give fluids for recovery.
- Instruct caregivers not to give any antidiarrheals such as Imodium or Peptobismol.

Chronic Care

- Teach caregivers not to give unlimited fluid.
- Remind caregivers to advance diet back to a regular diet after 48 hours.

Promoting Safety

Hand Hygiene

Gastrointestinal illness can be spread by handling items, especially food, after using the bathroom. Diarrheal illnesses can be especially contagious. Good hand hygiene is essential when caring for children with these illnesses or any time stool needs to be collected for the lab. Practicing good hand hygiene is important, as well as teaching good hand hygiene to caregivers and children.

GASTROINTESTINAL PROBLEMS MANIFESTED BY CONSTIPATION

FUNCTIONAL CONSTIPATION

Assessment

Clinical Presentation

Functional **constipation** may have the following clinical presentation.

- Infrequent stools that are usually hard and may be small and pebble like or large in size, two or less times a week
- Complaints of pain with stooling
- Leaking of stool between bowel movements (**encopresis**)
- Holding behaviors with stooling (hiding, dancing movements, squeezing buttocks together)
- Impaction—inability to stool with abdominal pain and sometimes vomiting
- History should cover general stooling habits.
- On physical exam, stool may be palpated in the colon.
- Assessment for anal wink and exam of anus for fissures on rectal exam

Diagnostic Testing

- Occult blood
- Flat plate of abdomen
- Barium enema (unprepped)—helps to rule out Hirschsprung's disease
- Colonic transport exam (done infrequently)
- Anorectal manometry

Nursing Interventions

Emergency Care

- Impaction, accompanied by vomiting, may need admission for disimpaction.
- Child may need IV fluids.
- Enemas or oral electrolyte solutions may be used for disimpaction.

Acute Care

- If disimpaction is needed but child is not in acute distress, child may be treated at home with high-dose Polyethylene glycol with close follow-up monitoring.
- Child may be admitted to the hospital if disimpaction does not work at home or child becomes worse with similar treatment as above.
- Family will need to understand importance of using medication as directed.

Chronic Home Care

- Medications, including:
  - *Polyethylene glycol 3350 without electrolytes (Miralax or Glycolax)*
  - *Mineral oil*
  - *Lactulose*
  - *Short-term therapy with Senna (Senokots)*
  - *Ducolax also may be used for short-term therapy.*
  - *Enemas may be helpful on a short-term basis.*
- Behavior modification
  - *Regular times for stooling, usually after meals for 5 to 10 minutes*
  - *Daily record of stools and medication*
  - *Reward chart for success*
- Increase in exercise
- Increase in fluid intake
- Dietary improvement, including increased fiber
- Elimination of cow's milk protein may help.
- Biofeedback therapy
- Follow-up visits are important for weaning of medication

Caregiver Education

Emergency Care

- If the child starts to vomit or has severe abdominal pain, caregiver should bring the child for immediate evaluation.

Acute Care

- Education of caregiver and child about procedures
- Education of caregiver and child about medication
- On discharge, caregiver and child need to know importance of continuing medication regularly.

Chronic Care

- Regular use of medication

Medication

Treating Constipation

Regular medication administration is important in treating constipation. Oral laxatives have become the mainstay of treatment.

Polyethylene glycol 3350 without electrolytes (Miralax or Glycolax) is the commonly used medication, as it is well tolerated and easily administered. The dose is adjusted according to the child's need, but may start at 17 g (1 capful) in 8 ounces of water once or twice daily. Fluid volume may be adjusted for the child's age. Most children do not taste the medication.

Mineral oil is another alternative. Most caregivers do not like to administer mineral oil because the child complains of the taste and the mineral oil can leak from the rectum onto the underwear in high doses. Mineral oil is given as 1–4 mL/kg/day. Many health-care providers give mineral oil as 1 tablespoon per year of age.

Lactulose is usually administered to infants. One of the side effects is an increase in gassiness. It can be very effective in this population, especially with premature infants with constipation due to immaturity of the GI tract.

The dose is 1–2 mL/kg/day.

Occasional use of Senna or Biscodyl may be necessary in those children with severe constipation and encopresis after disimpaction. These medications are considered short-term adjunct therapy only.

Caregivers need to understand the importance of complying with therapy and using the medication as prescribed, including during periods of weaning from the medication (Wyllie & Hyams, 2006).

- Discuss behavior modification with caregiver and child.
  - *Child should sit on toilet for set time and not get up until he or she has bowel movement or time is up (5–10 minutes at least, depending on child's age).*
  - *Child should sit on toilet after meals.*
  - *Record of stools and medication should be kept.*
  - *Use of reward chart*
  - *Participation of child is important for success in the therapy.*
  - *Reward should be privilege such as extra TV or video game time; child should be part of selecting reward.*
  - *No food rewards*
- Change in diet
  - *Increase of fruits and vegetables*
  - *Increase of fluids*
    - Increase fiber in diet—for ages 1–3 need 19 g; age 4–8, 25 g; ages 9–13, 26 g for girls, 31 g for boys; ages 14–18, 29 g for girls, 38 g for boys (Gidding et al., 2006). Some health-care providers start with increased fiber in the diet as age in years +5 equals grams of fiber needed in the diet daily (Tobias, Mason, Lutkenhoff, Stoops, & Ferguson, 2008). This can be used to start increase in fiber intake to work toward dietary recommendations.

Complementary and Alternative Therapies

- Dietary therapy alone may be helpful for mild constipation.
- Use of probiotics may be helpful. Study about their use is ongoing.

HIRSCHSPRUNG'S DISEASE

Assessment

Clinical Presentation

Hirschsprung's disease may have the following clinical presentation.

Failure to pass meconium in the first 24 hours of life with increased abdominal distension (**Figure 15-11**)

- Constipation from birth
- No bowel movement more than once a week
- Ribbon-like or watery stools
- Thin child with protuberant abdomen
- Vomiting
- Poor weight gain

Diagnostic Testing

- Empty rectum on digital examination
- Abdominal x-ray (KUB)

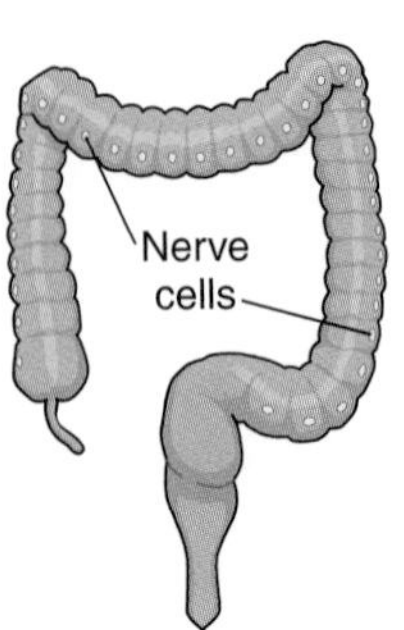

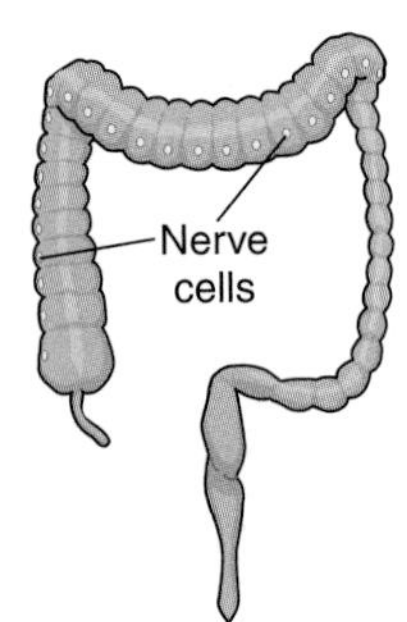

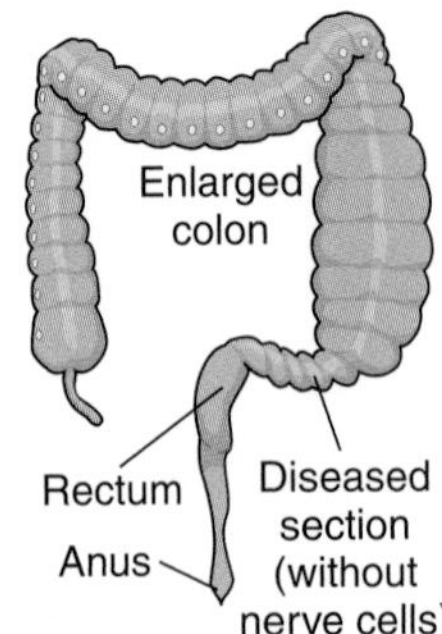

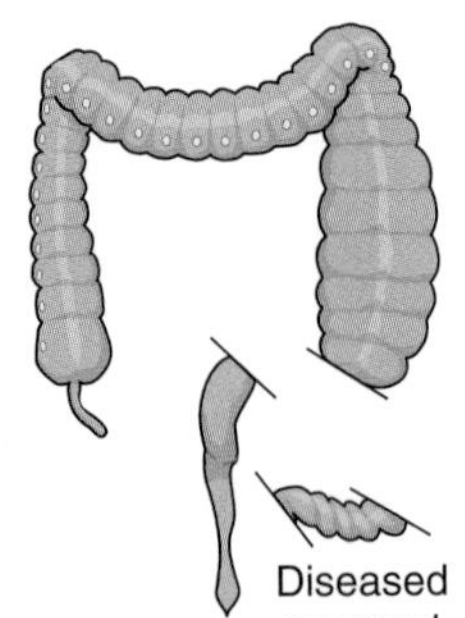

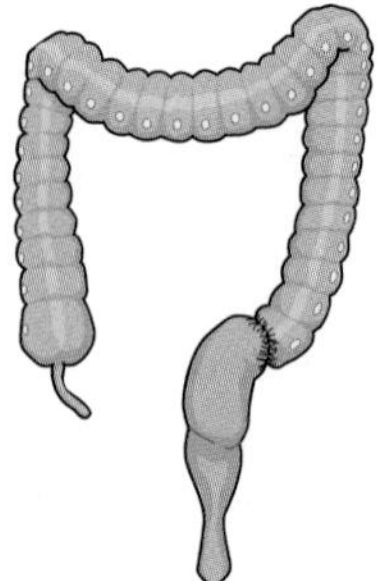

Figure 15-11 Hirschsprung's disease, or HD, is a disease of the large intestine. The large intestine is also sometimes called the colon. The word *bowel* can refer to the large and small intestines. HD usually occurs in children. It causes constipation, which means that bowel movements are difficult. Some children with HD can't have bowel movements at all. The stool creates a blockage in the intestine.

- Barium enema (unprepped)
- Rectal biopsy (definitive test for diagnosis)
- Anorectal manometry—more accurate for short or ultra-short segments

Nursing Interventions

Emergency Care

- Establish IV therapy for fluid and electrolyte balance.
- Antibiotic therapy as needed

Acute Care

- If not an emergency, caregiver may administer enemas before admission for surgery.
- Caregiver will need instruction in giving enema.
- Prepare child for surgery.
  - *May need enema to evacuate colon*
  - *Provide emotional support for caregiver.*
- If surgical intervention is required, prepare patient for surgery.
  - *Monitor IV therapy postoperatively.*
  - *Maintain NG tube.*
  - *Monitor operative site.*
  - *Administer antibiotics.*
- Observe for complications such as enterocolitis (watery diarrhea, abdominal distension, and fever).
  - *Treat with IV fluids.*
  - *Warm saline irrigation of rectum*
  - *Antibiotic therapy*
- Advance feedings as tolerated if no complication.

Chronic Care

- Monitor for complications, such as chronic constipation or impaction.
- Refer to gastroenterologist for follow-up.
- Observe stools for normal pattern and consistency.

Caregiver Education

Emergency Care

- Explain procedures to caregivers.
- Answer caregiver questions as needed.
- Teach parent signs of enterocolitis and impaction that need immediate intervention.

Acute Care

- Explain procedures to caregiver.
- Encourage caregiver to hold patient, either postprocedure or postoperatively.
- Encourage caregiver to participate in oral feedings.
- Have caregiver provide breast milk if possible; provide breast pump for use.

Chronic Care

- Teach caregivers signs of infection or complications.
- Teach caregivers importance of keeping follow-up appointments.
- Child may be having difficulty with passing stools or leaking, due to tight anus and pull-through surgery.
  - *Caregiver needs to monitor stooling and be alert for problems.*
- Teach caregiver that child may be a fussy eater at first; it is important to deemphasize mealtime stress.
- Treatment for older child may be the same as for chronic constipation; child needs to be active participant in treatment.
- Genetic counseling may be recommended.

GASTROINTESTINAL PROBLEMS MANIFESTED BY ANTERIOR ABDOMINAL WALL DEFECT

OMPHALOCELE AND GASTROSCHISIS

Assessment

Clinical Presentation

- Malrotation is present in both defects.
  - ***Omphalocele***
    - Stomach and intestines on the outside of the abdomen contained within a sac made of amnion, peritoneum, and Wharton's jelly.
    - Defect varies from 4 to 12 cm.
    - In large defects, the liver, spleen, gonads, and bladder may also be contained in the sac.
    - Sac may rupture in utero
    - Commonly associated with anomalies (Wyllie & Hyams, 2006)
  - ***Gastroschisis***
    - Opening on the right side of the umbilical cord
    - Stomach and small and large intestine are involved but rarely the liver
    - Intestine may be at risk for vascular compromise—matted with exudate
    - Normally developed abdominal musculature
    - Unusual to have other anomalies (Wyllie & Hyams, 2006)

Diagnostic Testing

- Elevated maternal triple screen AFP
- Usually diagnosed on prenatal ultrasound
  - *Serial ultrasounds are recommended.*
- Amniocentesis is recommended.

Nursing Interventions

Emergency Care

- Decision on type of delivery
  - *Many babies delivered by cesarean section*
- Immediate resuscitation after delivery
  - *Orogastric insertion*
  - *Intravenous insertion*
  - *Respiratory support if necessary*
- Wrap and support defect to prevent fluid loss and hypothermia

Acute Care

- Support fluid needs.
- Closure of the defect by surgical means
  - *May be done in stages*
- Orogastric tube to decompress intestines
- Parenteral nutrition
- IV antibiotics
- Support nonnutritive sucking needs—infant may need pacifier.
- Observe surgical site for possible infection.
- Observe for defecation.
- Gradual resumption of feeding when ileus resolves, with breast milk or predigested formula

Chronic Care

- May have TPN for several months
- Slow increase in oral feedings
- Close monitoring of growth
- Teach importance of follow-up visits.

Caregiver Education

Emergency Care

- Explain procedures to caregivers.
- Answer caregiver questions as needed.

Acute Care

- Explain procedures to caregiver.
- Encourage caregiver to hold patient postoperatively, if possible.
- Encourage caregiver to participate in nonnutritive sucking.
- Have caregiver provide breast milk if possible; provide breast pump for use as needed.
- Have caregiver participate in oral feeding when feedings are started.

Chronic Care

- Teach caregivers signs of infection or complications.
- Teach caregivers importance of follow-up appointments.
- Teach caregivers that child may be a fussy eater at first; it is important to deemphasize mealtime stress.

GASTROINTESTINAL PROBLEMS MANIFESTED BY LIVER, PANCREATIC, OR GALL BLADDER INVOLVEMENT

NEONATAL JAUNDICE

Assessment

Clinical Presentation

- Elevation of the bilirubin above normal
- Concern if jaundice develops before 24 hours
- Higher risk in preterm infants
- At higher levels of jaundice
  - *Lethargy*
  - *Poor feeding*
  - *May have signs of infection*
- Bilirubin encephalopathy (kernicterus)—may occur with severe jaundice; preventable
  - *Opisthotonic posturing*
  - *Hypotonia or hypertonia*
  - *High-pitched cry*
  - *Seizures*
  - *Poor sucking (Maisels, 2005a, 2005b, 2005c)*

Diagnostic Testing

- Transcutaneous bilimeter assessment—screening test
- Bilirubin total and direct
- CBC
- Reticulocyte count
- Urinalysis (UA) and urine culture if suspect infection
- Blood type and RH, Coombs
- Test for G6PD
- CRP and blood culture if signs of infection
- With elevated direct bilirubin, may need additional testing, including liver function tests, gamma GT, alpha-1 antitrypsin, TSH, and cortisol.
- May also need ultrasound of gall bladder with elevated direct bilirubin

Nursing Interventions

Emergency Care

- Bilirubin results above 20 mg/dL may need admission to the neonatal intensive care unit or hospital if outpatient for phototherapy.
- Bilirubin results above 25mg/dL may require exchange transfusion.

Acute Care

- Newborns should be assessed for jaundice before discharge.
  - *Visual assessment is not always accurate.*
  - *Transcutaneous bilimeter reading*
- Mothers should be encouraged to feed frequently; provide lactation support.
- Importance of early follow-up after discharge should be taught to caregivers.
- Jaundice in the first 24 hours requires intervention.
  - *Close follow-up with repeat testing is necessary.*
  - *Phototherapy with Biliblanket.*
- If level is high, may need additional interventions with fluids and phototherapy lights
  - *May require IV fluids*
  - *Phototherapy—eyes will be patched.*
  - *Oral fluids—mom may continue to breastfeed if baby is feeding well.*
- Prepare for exchange transfusion if level is high.
  - *Blood will be used, either typed or O negative.*
  - *Patient will need close monitoring during and after procedure.*
- Patient may continue on Biliblanket after discharge.

Chronic Care

- May require follow-up appointment to follow bilirubin levels
- If jaundice develops after first week, may interrupt breastfeeding for 12 to 24 hours to reduce level; done infrequently.
- Baby with elevated bilirubin that has a persistent direct component may need further testing to determine cause.

Complementary and Alternative Therapies

- Although once used as a therapy, indirect sunlight does not affect bilirubin levels.

Caregiver Education

Emergency Care

- Caregiver should be taught to return to the hospital or clinic for blood tests if baby becomes jaundiced into the legs.
- Caregiver should also bring in patient if baby is feeding poorly or is very sleepy.

Acute Care

- Caregiver should feed patient frequently by breastfeeding or with formula.
- Time under the phototherapy lights or on the Biliblanket should be maximized if possible; feeding without removing the Biliblanket is essential.
- Importance of follow-up visits and labs

Chronic Care

- Patient may need frequent follow-up after discharge to follow bilirubin levels.
  - *Caregivers need to know to do follow-up tests and keep appointments.*
- Patients with problems that develop from bilirubin will need chronic care.
  - *Although rare, bilirubin encephalopathy is a neurological problem that requires long-term care.*

BILIARY ATRESIA

Assessment

Clinical Presentation

Biliary atresia may have the following clinical presentation.

- Significant jaundice at 2 weeks of age (**Figure 15-12**)
- Rise in the direct bilirubin (usually greater than 20% of the total value of bilirubin)
- Poor absorption of fat and the fat-soluble vitamins (A, D, E, and K)
- Dark urine
- Light-colored stools—after 2 months, may be pale, gray, or white
- Enlarged liver (Wyllie & Hyams, 2006)

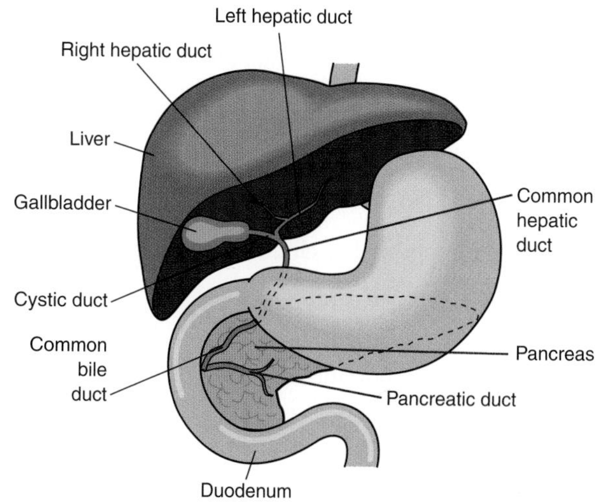

Figure 15–12 Biliary system.

Diagnostic Testing

- Liver function tests—AST is normal early, then elevated
- Bilirubin, total and direct
- Alkaline phosphatase (elevated)
- Calcium level
- Ultrasound of the abdomen and liver
- Liver scan
- Liver biopsy

Nursing Interventions

Emergency Care

- Stabilize patient with IV fluids.
- Prepare patient for diagnostic tests as needed.
- Explain tests to caregivers and provide reassurance as needed.

Acute Care

- IV fluids
- Low-fat, high-protein diet
- Administration of vitamins A, D, and K
- Surgery
  - *After surgery, care of NG tube*
  - *Pain medication as needed*
  - *Administer antibiotics as ordered to prevent infection.*
  - *Encourage nonnutritive sucking with pacifier.*
  - *Care of the incisional site*
  - *Check abdominal girth size daily.*
  - *With return of bowel function, diet to advance as tolerated from oral fluids*
  - *Description of stools, including color*

Chronic Care

- Low-fat, high-protein diet
- Parenteral nutrition

Complementary and Alternative Therapies

- If initial surgery is not successful, then liver transplant may be indicated.

Caregiver Education

Emergency Care

- Bring child to hospital or clinic for care if prolonged jaundice or pale, gray, or white stools.

Acute Care

- Teach caregiver importance of diet.
- Answer questions about NG tube.
- Teach caregiver dressing change as needed.
- Caregiver to assist with nonnutritive sucking

Chronic Care

- Teach caregiver about diet and maintenance of diet if needed.
- Stress with caregiver the importance of follow-up visits.
- Review possible signs of infection or problems to be reported.
- If liver transplant will occur, then refer to transplant team for teaching.
- Discuss caregiver concerns and provide emotional support.

FATTY LIVER DISEASE

Assessment

Clinical Presentation

- Becoming more prevalent in the adolescent population due to obesity
- May be diagnosed even earlier as increase in obesity occurs
- May be asymptomatic
- Fatigue
- Right upper quadrant pain
- Usually, but not always, overweight
- Signs of insulin resistance—acanthosis nigricans or menstrual irregularities
- Minimal to no alcohol consumption (less than 2 drinks daily/male or 1 drink or less/female) (Leaf, 2008)
- Hepatomegaly (50%)
- May be associated with the following
  - *Diabetes*
  - *Familial lipodystrophies*
  - *Polycystic ovary syndrome*
  - *Celiac disease*
  - *Profound weight loss*
  - *Total parenteral nutrition*
  - *Wilson disease (Leaf, 2008)*

Diagnostic Testing

- Liver function tests
  - *Hepatitis B and C testing*
  - *Fasting iron*
  - *Antinuclear Antibody (ANA)*
  - *Antismooth muscle antibody*
  - *Antimitochrondial antibody*
  - *Ceruloplasmin levels*
  - *Serum protein electrophoresis*
  - *Glucose*
  - *Triglycerides*
  - *Ultrasound*
  - *Liver biopsy in later stages (Leaf, 2008)*

Nursing Interventions

Emergency Care

- As this is a longer-term diagnosis, may not need emergency treatment
- Would need immediate care for acute liver failure

Acute Care

- Assist with lifestyle modification.
  - *Use group-based sessions.*
  - *Increased physical activity*
  - *Dietary modification for weight loss (prevent rapid weight loss)*

Chronic Care

- Lifestyle modification
- Pharmacologic therapy
  - *Vitamins A and E*
  - *Metformin (Leaf, 2008)*

Caregiver Education

Emergency Care

- Caregiver to recognize signs of diabetic coma
- Acute abdominal pain should be assessed immediately.

Acute Care

- Teach ways to modify lifestyle.
  - *Discuss dieting and avoidance of fad diets.*
  - *Discuss exercise options, including increasing activity and decreasing screen time.*
- Help family find an appropriate support group.
- Discuss feelings of child or adolescent about disease; provide emotional support.

Chronic Care

- Teach family importance of taking medications.
- Teach family importance of keeping follow-up appointments.
- Review lifestyle changes and diet modification with child or adolescent on a regular basis and modify as needed.

CYSTIC FIBROSIS

Assessment

Clinical Presentation

- Pulmonary manifestations (covered in the respiratory chapter)

- Effect on the pancreatic exocrine gland function—15% with normal gland function
  - *Failure to thrive*
  - *Chronic diarrhea*
  - *Respiratory symptoms*
- First manifestation may be meconium ileus (15%)
  - *Lack of passage of meconium for 48 hours*
  - *Diagnosed by barium enema*
- Rectal prolapse
- Steatorrhea
- Pancreatitis
- Diabetes mellitus
- May have slow or poor growth and nutrition (Wyllie & Hyams, 2006)

Diagnostic Testing

- Sweat chloride test
- Chromosome analysis
- 72-hour fecal fat test

Nursing Interventions

Emergency Care

- Recognize signs of intestinal obstruction with meconium ileus.
- Recognize and treat signs of pancreatitis if they occur.
- Explain care and tests for diagnosis to caregivers.

Acute Care

- Assist with treatment as needed.
- Support nutrition; support breastfeeding if mom desires to breastfeed.
- Administer medication as needed.
  - *Includes pancreatic enzymes and fat-soluble vitamins* (**Table 15-3**)
- Teach caregivers reason for medication and importance of use.

Chronic Care

- Measure and monitor growth.
- Teach family proper use of medications, including supplemental enzyme therapy.
  - *Enzymes should be taken before eating and with all meals and snacks.*
  - *Enzymes should not be skipped.*
  - *Enzymes work for about 1 hour after eating. Higher dose may be needed for foods high in fat (e.g., fast food).*
  - *For infants and young children, enzymes should be mixed with a soft acidic food such as applesauce, not with any milk-based food such as yogurt.*

TABLE 15–3 PANCREATIC ENZYMES AND OTHER MEDICATIONS USED TO TREAT CYSTIC FIBROSIS

PANCREATIC ENZYMES	Creon Pancrease, Pancrease MT, Pancrecarb (should not be given if allergic to pigs or pork), Ultrase, Ultrase MT, Viokase	Given before meals and snacks and may be opened for administration Young children can have it sprinkled in applesauce Helps to digest carbohydrate, protein, and fat and promote nutrient absorption, which will help increase weight
VITAMIN A	0–1 years: 1500 IU 1–3 years: 5000 IU 4–8 years: 500 to 10,000 IU Older than 8 years: 10,000 IU	Given as a supplement Also may be absorbed some from food such as orange-colored fruits and vegetables and dark green vegetables Take with pancreatic enzymes for better absorption
PROBIOTICS	*Lactobacillus rhamnosus* GG capsules or in some yogurt	Reduces intestinal inflammation, reduces respiratory infection
VITAMIN D	Infants: 400 IU Children need 400–800 IU day with cystic fibrosis due to poor fat absorption	Will need supplement Some in foods—milk, salmon, tuna with oil, sardines, fortified cereal Take with pancreatic enzymes for better absorption
VITAMIN E	0–1 years: 40–450 IU 1–3 years: 80–150 IU 4–8 years: 100–200 IU Older than 8: 200–400 IU	Is an antioxidant Used in the production of red blood cells Helps with intestinal health and protects against infection in lung lining Found in nuts, vegetable oil, wheat germ oil, olives, corn, leafy green vegetables, fortified cereal Take with pancreatic enzymes for better absorption

Source: Cystic Fibrosis Foundation. (2005). Retrieved from http://www.cff.org; National Institute of Health, Office of Dietary Supplements. (2008). Fact sheets.

- *Enzymes should not be mixed in food ahead of time and should not be refrigerated.*
- *If the child is on a tube feeding, the enzyme should be taken by mouth before the tube feeding.*

- Encourage proper nutrition.
  - *Teach child foods that may be eaten without taking enzymes, including fruits, juice, soft drinks or sports drinks, tea, lollipops, fruit snacks, jelly beans, gum, and popsicles or freezer pops.*
  - *Child may require gastrostomy tube if failure to thrive occurs.*
- Stress importance of regular immunizations.

Caregiver Education

Emergency Care

- Explain procedures and answer caregiver questions.

Acute Care

- Address caregiver concerns.
- Stress importance of maintaining medication regimen.
- Stress importance of nutrition.

Chronic Care

- Address caregiver concerns.
- Stress importance of maintaining medication regimen.
- Stress importance of nutrition.
- Review immunizations needed at each visit.
- Encourage caregiver to visit www.cff.org for more information about cystic fibrosis.
- Encourage caregivers to allow child to attend camp or other activities with other children with cystic fibrosis.
- Caregivers may need genetic counseling.

> **CLINICAL PEARL**
>
> **Symptoms of Cystic Fibrosis**
>
> Cystic fibrosis may be manifested by mainly respiratory or mainly gastrointestinal symptoms, or a combination of both. Although it usually occurs in Caucasians, it may also be seen in African American and Native American populations (Garfunkel et al., 2007).

CHOLECYSTITIS AND GALLSTONES

Assessment

Clinical Presentation (**Figure 15-13**)

Cholecystitis and gallstones may have the following clinical presentation.

- Jaundice in infants
- Fever
- Right upper quadrant pain with vomiting (older children and adolescents)

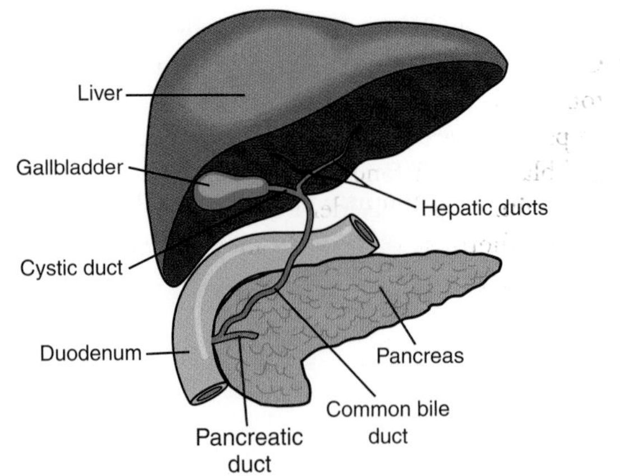

Figure 15-13 The gallbladder and the ducts that carry bile and other digestive enzymes from the liver, gallbladder, and pancreas to the small intestine are called the biliary system.

Diagnostic Testing

- Localized tenderness to palpation
- CBC
- Bilirubin
- Alkaline phosphatase and gamma GT
- Amylase
- Urinalysis
- Liver function tests
- Plain film radiograph
- Ultrasound

Nursing Interventions

Emergency Care

- Vomiting and pain may require immediate hospitalization.
- Start IV fluids.
- Patient should be NPO.
- Endoscopic retrograde cholangiopancreatography (ERCP) may be performed to remove gallstones from the bile duct.

Acute Care

- Continue IV therapy.
- Analgesic medication as appropriate
- Administer antibiotics if ordered for persistent fever.
- Prepare patient for surgery.
  - *Surgery usually performed laproscopically*
- Monitor patient postoperatively for any complications.
  - *Analgesics as appropriate*
  - *Advance diet as tolerated; monitor intake and output.*
  - *Monitor incisional sites.*
- Caregivers will need teaching about signs of infection, pain relief, and incisional site care.

Chronic Care

- Surgery usually corrects problems.

Complementary and Alternative Therapies

- Gallstones in infancy do not need removal unless symptomatic, as gallstones usually resolve spontaneously.
- In patients with Crohn's disease who need a functioning gall bladder, gallstones may be removed from the bile duct without gall bladder removal.
- Laser lithotripsy is currently an experimental therapy.
- Enteral feedings for patients on TPN

Caregiver Education

Emergency Care

- Bring patient to the hospital or clinic for evaluation.

Acute Hospital Care

- Assist with feeding as needed.
- Reassure caregivers about their ability to care for the patient.
- Teach caregivers care of incisional site.
- Teach caregivers about pain relief.

Chronic Home Care

- Advance diet as tolerated.
- Observe for signs of infection.
- Administer pain mediation as needed.
- Remind caregivers about keeping regular appointments and starting or continuing immunizations.

HEPATITIS

Assessment

Clinical Presentation

Hepatitis may have the following clinical presentation.

- Hepatitis A is caused by oral–fecal contamination, either through contamination of food or the environment.
- Hepatitis B and C are caused by exposure to infected blood or blood products or through sexual contact. Hepatitis B may be spread during delivery.
- Hepatitis A, B, and C may be asymptomatic.
- May have any or all of the following symptoms:
  - *Jaundice, including icteric sclera*
  - *Abdominal pain*
  - *Malaise*
  - *Loss of appetite*
  - *Low-grade fever*
  - *Dark urine and light-colored stools*
  - *Hepatospenomegaly*
  - *Petechiae, ecchymosis, spider angiomas*

Diagnostic Testing

- Liver function tests, including Alanine Aminotransferase (ALT)
- Serologic tests
  - *Hepatitis A—anti-HAV-IgM: Confirms diagnosis of recent acute infection.*
  - *Hepatitis A—anti-HAV-total: Predominantly IgG, confirms previous exposure to hepatitis A, recovery, and immunity; does not distinguish recent from past infection.*
  - *Hepatitis B—HB surface antigen (HBsAg): If positive, earliest indicator of active infection. It is also present in chronic disease or carrier state. Does not become positive after immunization.*
  - *HB surface antibody (anti-HBsAg): Presence without HBsAg indicates recovery from infection, and immunity from previous exposure or vaccine.*
  - *HB Be antigen (HBeAg): In blood only when virus is present, and can be passed to others; monitors treatment. Useful to determine resolution of infection or presence of carrier state (persistence after 20 weeks indicates chronic or carrier state).Presence in HBsAg-positive mom indicates 90% chance of infant acquiring infection.*
  - *AntiHBc-total: First antibody to appear after appearance of HBsAg. The presence with HBsAg and absence of anti-HBsAg indicates chronic infection.*
  - *AntiHBc-IgM: Earliest specific antibody. May be the only serologic marker after HBsAg and HBeAG subside. Can differentiate acute from chronic infection.*
  - *Anti-HBe: Appears after HBeAg disappears; detectable for years. Indicates decreasing infectivity and good prognosis for recovery from acute infection. Presence with anti-HBc and absence of HBsAb and anti-HBs indicates recent acute infection.*
  - *HBV-DNA (PCR): Indicates active infection; the most sensitive and specific assay for early diagnosis; may be detected when all other markers are negative. Measures HBV replication.*
  - *Hepatitis C—anti-HCV test for antibody: Indicates infection, past or present, but does not differentiate. Confirmation of positive test with HCV RIBA. HCV RNA assay (viral load) now being used more because of better sensitivity. Viral genotyping may also be used (Wallach, 2007).*
- Ultrasound
- Liver biopsy

Nursing Interventions

Emergency Care

- Sudden onset of symptoms of liver failure may cause caregivers to bring patient for assessment.
- Development of ascites in a chronic patient may require hospitalization for supportive care.

Acute Care

- Hepatitis A is passed by the oral–fecal route, so good hand hygiene and Standard Precautions are essential.
- Prevention of needle sticks
- Balanced diet that prevents dehydration
- Bedrest
- Antiviral therapy for hepatitis C
- Supportive care, including monitoring for complications
- If patient remains in good health, no restrictions on activity.

- With hepatitis A, child should not return to day care until virus has cleared.
- Therapy will be related to the severity of disease. Careful monitoring and follow-up are essential.
- Family members should be vaccinated for hepatitis A and hepatitis B.
- Children who are not infected should complete immunizations for hepatitis (**Figure 15-14**).

Complementary and Alternative Therapies

- Infants should receive hepatitis B series of immunizations at birth and 2, 4, and 6 months.
- All mothers should be tested for hepatitis B during pregnancy.
- Infants of hepatitis B–positive mothers should receive the HBIG vaccine at birth as well.

Caregiver Education

Emergency Care

- Bring patient to hospital or clinic for evaluation.

Acute Care

- Help patient to maintain bedrest; encourage quiet activities for entertainment.
- Teach elements of proper nutrition to maintain calories and hydration.
- Teach importance of medication regimen.

Chronic Care

- Teach importance of maintaining follow-up visits as scheduled.
- Teach importance of proper immunization for all family members.

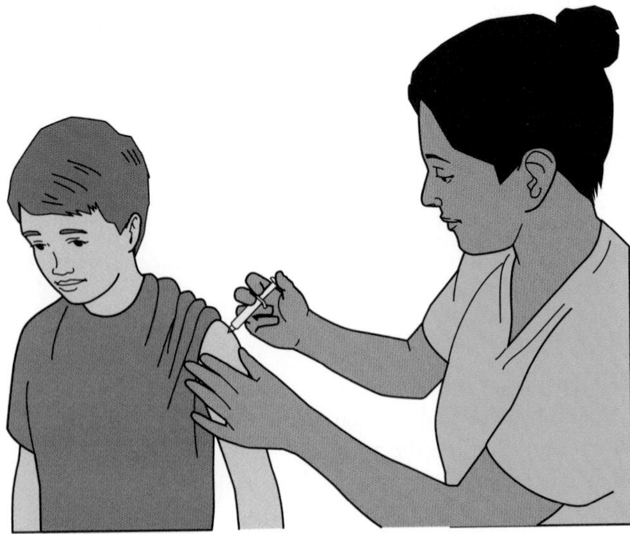

Figure 15-14 Vaccines protect you from getting hepatitis A.

- Teach caregivers to help child avoid medications that can cause liver damage.
- Always wash hands after using the toilet and before fixing food.
- Gloves are indicated for anyone handling another's stool.

Evidence-Based Practice Research: Decrease in Incidence of Hepatitis A

Koslap-Petraco, M., Shub, M., & Judelsohn, R. (2008). Hepatitis A: Disease burden and current childhood vaccination strategies in the United States. *Journal of Pediatric Health Care, 22,* 3–9. doi: 10.1016/j.pedhc.2006.12.011

Hepatitis A has shown a decrease in incidence due to immunization strategies. Originally, vaccination was done in selected states with high rates of hepatitis A, but hepatitis A has now increased in states with lower risk, and universal immunization is now recommended for all children starting at age 1. It has been shown that children are a reservoir for hepatitis A, and immunization would reduce this risk to the elderly as well as healthy adults.

1. Why should immunization be used for hepatitis A?
2. At what age should children be vaccinated?

GASTROINTESTINAL PROBLEMS MANIFESTED BY NUTRITIONAL CHANGES

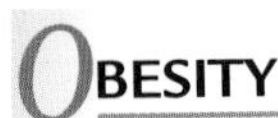

OBESITY

Assessment

Clinical Presentation

- Body mass index (BMI) >95% is considered obese.
- BMI of 85% to 94% is considered overweight.
- Adiposity rebound at a young age
- Knee pain
- Abdominal pain
- Daytime somnolence
- Polycystic ovary disease
- Menstrual irregularities
- Acne
- Hirsutism
- Infertility
- May have associated problems
  - *Diabetes—glycosuria*
  - *Acanthosis nigricans*
  - *Fatty liver disease*
  - *Heart disease*
  - *Hypertension*
  - *Hyperlipidemia*
  - *Obstructive sleep apnea*
  - *Gallbladder disease*
  - *Slipped capital femoral epiphysis*

Diagnostic Testing

- Height, weight, BMI at each visit
- CBC
- Lipid profile
- Fasting glucose
- Liver function tests
- Thyroid Stimulating Hormone (TSH), a.m. (morning) cortisol
- Height and weight measurements
- BMI = weight in kilograms divided by the height in meters squared (kg/m^2)
  - *Most commonly used measure*
- Skinfold thickness—calipers measure subcutaneous fat from several areas and compare to controls
- Bioelectric impedance analysis
- Ultrasound
- Sleep study (Garfunkel et al., 2007)

Nursing Interventions

Emergency Care

- Symptoms of heart disease, uncontrolled hypertension, or diabetes with blood sugar not well controlled may require hospitalization.
- Hip or leg pain should have immediate evaluation.

Acute Care

- Stabilize any conditions.
- Encourage caregivers to not overfeed in infancy.

Chronic Care

- Program for patient needs to be individualized.
- Nutrition assessment
  - *Referral to nutrition*
  - *Change in diet*
  - *Discuss speed of eating.*
  - *Discuss caregiver effect on eating.*
  - *Encourage patient to not skip meals.*
  - *Encourage increase and change in physical activity.*
- Decrease screen time (television or video games) to 2 hours a day or less.
- No eating in front of the TV
- Change daily routine to increase activity.
- Behavior modification
  - *Small gradual changes over time*
  - *Positive reinforcement for changes*
  - *Provide some choice.*
- Family involvement
  - *Family needs to be involved in plan.*
  - *Need education concerning short- and long-term consequences of obesity*
  - *Promote positive parenting skills; consistent messages.*
  - *Provide healthy meals and snacks.*
- Support groups
- Medication
  - *Only for patient 16 or older*
  - *Orlistat—needs close supervision if used*
- Surgical intervention—bariatric surgery
  - *May be a consideration for late adolescent patient*
  - *Must meet stringent criteria*

CLINICAL PEARL

Smoking for Weight Control

Adolescents may use smoking as a weight control strategy. Asking about this during history taking is important, as well as counseling the adolescent about risks with smoking (Garfunkel et al., 2007).

Caregiver Education

Emergency Care

- Signs of complications such as uncontrolled diabetes and heart disease should be taught to the caregiver and patient.

Acute Care

- Caregiver should be taught short- and long-term consequences of obesity.
- Caregiver needs to know importance of not overfeeding.
- Importance of healthy diet and activity should be emphasized, with input from family.
- Discuss with caregiver and child feelings about food and mealtimes.

Chronic Care

- Obesity is a chronic condition that requires caregiver assistance for success with weight loss.
- Teach importance of diet—use resources such as California Food Guide (2008; see **Table 15-4**).
- Teach importance of regular exercise.
- Teach importance of reduction in sedentary behavior.
- Assist parent with learning positive parenting techniques.
- Encourage participation in support group.
- Reinforce importance of follow-up visits.

TABLE 15–4 RESOURCES FOR DIGESTIVE DISORDERS

This directory lists various organizations involved in digestive diseases–related activities for patients.

American Celiac Disease Alliance (ACDA)
2504 Duxbury Place
Alexandria, VA 22308
Phone: 703-622-3331
E-mail: info@americanceliac.org
Internet: www.americanceliac.org
Publications: *Celiac Disease: A Hidden Epidemic* and *Gluten-Free Diet: A Comprehensive Resource Guide* (books); *Gluten-Free Living* (magazine).

American Celiac Society—Dietary Support Coalition
Annette & James Bentley
P.O. Box 23455
New Orleans, LA 70183-0455
Phone: 504-737-3293
E-mail: info@americanceliacsociety.org
Internet: www.americanceliacsociety.org
Publications: Newsletter—*Whooo's Report. Call a Friend With Celiac Sprue.*

American College of Gastroenterology (ACG)
P.O. Box 342260
Bethesda, MD 20827-2260
Phone: 301-263-9000
Internet: www.acg.gi.org
Publications: Journals—*American Journal of Gastroenterology* and *Nature Clinical Practice Gastroenterology & Hepatology.*

American Gastroenterological Association (AGA)
National Office
4930 Del Ray Avenue
Bethesda, MD 20814
Phone: 301-654-2055
Fax: 301-654-5920
E-mail: member@gastro.org
Internet: www.gastro.org
Publications: Journals—*Gastroenterology* and *Clinical Perspectives in Gastroenterology*; weekly newsletter—*GI Practice Management News*; reports—*Legislative Report* and *Burden of Diseases Report*; membership magazine—*AGA Digest.*

American Liver Foundation (ALF)
75 Maiden Lane, Suite 603
New York, NY 10038-4810
Phone: 1-800-GO-LIVER (465-4837),
1-888-4HEP-USA (443-7872), or 212-668-1000
Fax: 212-483-8179
E-mail: info@liverfoundation.org
Internet: www.liverfoundation.org

ARPKD/CHF Alliance
Autosomal Recessive Polycystic Kidney Disease & Congenital Hepatic Fibrosis Alliance
P.O. Box 70
Kirkwood, PA 17536
Phone: 717-529-5555
Fax: 1-800-807-9110
E-mail: info@arpkd.org
Internet: www.arpkd.org

Association of Gastrointestinal Motility Disorders, Inc. (AGMD)
(formerly American Society of Adults with Pseudo-Obstruction, Inc.)
AGMD International Corporate Headquarters
12 Roberts Drive
Bedford, MA 01730
Phone: 781-275-1300
Fax: 781-275-1304
E-mail: digestive.motility@gmail.com
Internet: www.agmd-gimotility.org
Publications: Member publications—*AGMD Beacon* and *AGMD Search and Research.*

Celiac Disease Foundation (CDF)
13251 Ventura Boulevard, #1
Studio City, CA 91604
Phone: 818-990-2354
Fax: 818-990-2379
E-mail: cdf@celiac.org
Internet: www.celiac.org
Publications: Quarterly newsletter—*Guidelines for a Gluten-Free Lifestyle;* brochures.

TABLE 15–4 RESOURCES FOR DIGESTIVE DISORDERS—cont'd

Celiac Sprue Association/USA Inc.

P.O. Box 31700

Omaha, NE 68131-0700

Phone: 1-877-CSA-4CSA

Fax: 402-643-4108

E-mail: celiacs@csaceliacs.org

Internet: www.csaceliacs.org

Crohn's & Colitis Foundation of America (CCFA)

386 Park Avenue South, 17th floor

New York, NY 10016

Phone: 1-800-932-2423 or 212-685-3440

Fax: 212-779-4098

E-mail: info@ccfa.org

Internet: www.ccfa.org

Cyclic Vomiting Syndrome Association (CVSA)

CVSA USA/Canada

3585 Cedar Hill Road, NW

Canal Winchester, OH 43110

Phone: 614-837-2586

Fax: 614-837-2586

E-mail: waitesd@cvsaonline.org

Internet: www.cvsaonline.org

Publications: Member newsletter—*Code V.*

Digestive Disease National Coalition

507 Capitol Court NE, Suite 200

Washington, DC 20002

Phone: 202-544-7497

Fax: 202-546-7105

Internet: www.ddnc.org

Gastro-Intestinal Research Foundation

70 East Lake Street, Suite 1015

Chicago, IL 60601-5907

Phone: 312-332-1350

Fax: 312-332-4757

E-mail: girf@earthlink.net

Internet: www.girf.org

Publications: Several newsletters; patient education pamphlet—*Issues in Women's Gastrointestinal Health.*

Gluten Intolerance Group of North America (GIG)

31214 124th Ave SE

Auburn, WA 98092

Phone: 253-833-6655

Fax: 253-833-6675

E-mail: info@gluten.net

Internet: www.gluten.net

Publications: Member newsletter—*GIG Newsletter.*

Hepatitis B Coalition

Immunization Action Coalition

1573 Selby Avenue, Suite 234

St. Paul, MN 55104

Phone: 651-647-9009

Fax: 651-647-9131

E-mail: admin@immunize.org

Internet: www.immunize.org and www.vaccineinformation.org

Publications: Semiannual publications—*NEEDLE TIPS, Vaccinate Adults,* and *Vaccinate Women.*

Hepatitis B Foundation

3805 Old Easton Road

Doylestown, PA 18902

Phone: 215-489-4900

Fax: 215-489-4313

E-mail: info@hepb.org

Internet: www.hepb.org

Publications: Newsletters—*B Informed, B Connected,* and *B News You Can Use;* brochures—*The Hepatitis B Foundation Cause for a Cure, Someone You Know Has Hepatitis B, Protect Yourself and Those You Love Against HBV, What Hepatitis B Carriers Should Know,* and *The First Loving Act—Vaccination;* fact sheets—*Advice to Parents of Children With HBV* and *Hot Sheet.*

Hepatitis Foundation International (HFI)

504 Blick Drive

Silver Spring, MD 20904-2901

Phone: 1-800-891-0707 or 301-622-4200

Fax: 301-622-4702

E-mail: hfi@comcast.net

Internet: www.hepfi.org

Continued

TABLE 15–4 RESOURCES FOR DIGESTIVE DISORDERS—cont'd

International Foundation for Functional Gastrointestinal Disorders (IFFGD) Inc.

P.O. Box 170864

Milwaukee, WI 53217-8076

Phone: 1-888-964-2001 or 414-964-1799

Fax: 414-964-7176

E-mail: iffgd@iffgd.org

Internet: www.iffgd.org

Publications: Quarterly newsletters—*Participate, Digestive Health Matters,* and *Digestive Health in Children.*

National Foundation for Celiac Awareness

P.O. Box 544

Ambler, PA 19002

Phone: 215-325-1306

Fax: 215-283-2335

E-mail: info@celiaccentral.org

Internet: www.celiaccentral.org

Publications: Books—*Celiac Sprue, A Guide Through the Medicine Cabinet; Gluten-Free Diet: A Comprehensive Resource Guide; Triumph Dining; NFCA Gluten-Free Resource Guide.*

Oley Foundation for Home Parenteral and Enteral Nutrition (HomePEN)

214 Hun Memorial, MC-28

Albany Medical Center

Albany, NY 12208-3478

Phone: 1-800-776-OLEY (6539) or 518-262-5079 (outside U.S.)

Fax: 518-262-5528

E-mail: info@oley.org

Internet: www.oley.org

Pediatric/Adolescent Gastroesophageal Reflux Association Inc. (PAGER)

P.O. Box 486

Buckeystown, MD 21717-0486

Phone: 301-601-9541

Fax: 630-982-6418

E-mail: gergroup@aol.com

Internet: www.reflux.org

Pull-thru Network

2312 Savoy Street

Hoover, AL 35226-1528

Phone: 205-978-2930

E-mail: info@pullthrunetwork.org

Internet: www.pullthrunetwork.org/

Publications: Quarterly publication—*Pull-thru Network News;* free brochure—*Anorectal Malformations—A Parent's Guide.*

Reach Out for Youth with Ileitis and Colitis Inc.

84 Northgate Circle

Melville, NY 11747

Phone: 631-293-3102

Fax: 631-293-3102

E-mail: reachoutforyouth@reachoutforyouth.org

Internet: www.reachoutforyouth.org

TEF-VATER International

15301 Grey Fox Road

Upper Marlboro, MD 20772

Phone: 301-952-6837

Fax: 301-952-9152

E-mail: info@tefvater.org

Internet: www.tefvater.org

Publications: Newsletter—*Inside Connections.*

United Ostomy Associations of America, Inc.

P.O. Box 66

Fairview, TN 37062-0066

Phone: 1-800-826-0826 or 949-660-8624

Fax: 949-660-9262

E-mail: info@uoaa.org

Internet: www.uoaa.org

Publications: Journal—*Ostomy Quarterly.*

Weight-control Information Network (WIN)

1 WIN Way

Bethesda, MD 20892-3665

Phone: 1-877-946-4627 or 202-828-1025

Fax: 202-828-1028

E-mail: win@info.niddk.nih.gov

Internet: www.win.niddk.nih.gov

Publications: Quarterly newsletter—*WIN Notes.*

TABLE 15–4 RESOURCES FOR DIGESTIVE DISORDERS—cont'd

National Digestive Diseases Information Clearinghouse 2 Information Way Bethesda, MD 20892-3570 Phone: 1-800-891-5389 TTY: 1-866-569-1162 Fax: 703-738-4929 E-mail: nddic@info.niddk.nih.gov Internet: www.digestive.niddk.nih.gov The National Digestive Diseases Information Clearinghouse (NDDIC) is a service of the National Institute of Diabetes and Digestive and Kidney Diseases (NIDDK). The NIDDK	is part of the National Institutes of Health of the U.S. Department of Health and Human Services. Established in 1980, the Clearinghouse provides information about digestive diseases to people with digestive disorders and to their families, health-care professionals, and the public. The NDDIC answers inquiries, develops and distributes publications, and works closely with professional and patient organizations and government agencies to coordinate resources about digestive diseases. Its publications are not copyrighted. The Clearinghouse encourages users of its publications to duplicate and distribute as many copies as desired.

Adapted from: Mullin, G.E., Integrative Gastroenterology. Directory of Digestive Diseases Organizations for Patients. Oxford, 2011.
National Digestive Diseases Information Clearinghouse (NDDIC). Directory of Digestive Diseases Organization. http://digestive.niddk.nih.gov/resources/Directory_Digestive_Diseases_Orgs_508.pdf

Review Questions

1. What are two questions that should be asked while taking a history?
- A. What is the problem? What are your symptoms?
- B. Where do you live? What type of insurance do you have?
- C. Where does it hurt? Can you tell me your name?
- D. What did you eat for breakfast? What type of insurance do you have?

2. List the four steps in doing an abdominal exam in the correct order of examination.
- A. Auscultation, percussion, palpation, inspection
- B. Inspection, percussion, palpation, auscultation
- C. Inspection, auscultation, percussion, palpation
- D. Inspection, auscultation, palpation, percussion

3. What symptoms might lead a health-care provider to suspect a tracheoesophageal fistula?
- A. Excessive vomiting of stomach contents
- B. Excessive gaseous distention of the abdomen
- C. Excessive respiratory distress without gaseous distention
- D. Excessive oral secretions and cyanosis with feedings

4. What is the current treatment for celiac disease, and why should families read food labels?
- A. Patients with celiac disease require a high-carbohydrate, low-fat diet.
- B. Patients with celiac disease require a low-carbohydrate, high-fat diet.
- C. Patients with celiac disease require a low-gluten diet.
- D. Patients with celiac disease require a gluten-free diet.

5. Where will the pain be identified in a patient with appendicitis?
- A. Rebound pain in right lower quadrant
- B. Sharp, intense pain in the left lower quadrant with rebound tenderness
- C. Dull pain in the right lower quadrant
- D. Pain on external rotation of the right hip

6. What does bilious vomiting in an infant indicate?
- A. The infant probably just has an upset stomach.
- B. The infant ingested too much protein.
- C. The infant is experiencing a surgical emergency.
- D. The infant was overfed.

7. What treatment should be recommended for a patient with gastroenteritis?
- A. Continue feeding normal formula as tolerated.
- B. Withhold fluids for 2 to 3 hours and feed Pedialyte® as tolerated.
- C. Continue feeding water as tolerated.
- D. Make the infant NPO for 8 hours.

8. What symptoms might be present in a patient with pyloric stenosis?
- A. Emesis that starts after 1 month of age
- B. Emesis that occurs as drips and dribbles all day long
- C. Emesis that is projectile, starting during the first week of life and progressing over time
- D. Emesis that starts at 5 months of age and mainly results in gastroesophageal reflux

9. If a patient does not have a meconium stool in the first 24 hours, what might be the suspected diagnosis?
- A. Malrotation
- B. Hirschsprung's disease
- C. Volvulus
- D. Appendicitis

10. What laboratory tests might be done for a patient with jaundice?
   A. Total bilirubin levels and creatinine clearance level
   B. Total bilirubin levels, CBC, Coombs test
   C. CBC, CRP, and blood urea nitrogen levels
   D. Total bilirubin levels, CBC, and T3 levels

References

Amerine, E. (2006). Celiac disease goes against the grain. *Nursing*, 36, 46–48.

Askey, B. (2008). Your role in managing Crohn's disease. *The Clinical Advisor, 11,* 25–30.

Bhatia, J., & Parrish, A. (2009). GERD or not GERD: The fussy infant. *Journal of Perinatology, 29,* S7–S11.

Burns, C. E., Dunn, A. M., Brady, M. A., Starr, N. B., & Blosser, C. G. (2009). *Pediatric primary care.* St. Louis, MO: Saunders.

California Food Guide. (2008). Sacramento, CA: California Department of Health Care Services and California Department of Public Health. Retrieved from http://www.cafoodguide.ca.gov

Cystic Fibrosis Foundation. (2005). Retrieved from http://www.cff.org.

Epocrates Online. (2011). Retrieved from http://www.epocrates.com.

Fasano, A., Berti, I., Gerarduzzi, T., Colletti, R., Drago, S., Elitsur, Y, . . . & Horvath, K., (2003). Prevalence of celiac disease in at-risk and not-at-risk groups in the United States. *Archives of Internal Medicine, 163,* 286–292.

Garfunkel, L., Kaczorowski, J., & Christy, C. (2007). *Pediatric clinical advisor instant diagnosis and treatment.* St Louis, MO: Mosby.

Gidding, S. S., Dennison, B. A., Birch, L. L., Daniels, S. R., Gilman, M. W., Lichtenstein, A. H., . . . Van Horn, L. (2006). Dietary recommendations for children and adolescents: A guide for practitioners. *Pediatrics, 117,* 544–559. doi: 10.1542/peds.2005-2374

Greydanus, D., Feinberg, A., Patel, D., & Homnick, D. (2008). *The pediatric diagnostic examination.* New York: McGraw Hill.

Kabakus, N., & Kurt, A. (2006). Sandifer syndrome: A continuing problem of misdiagnosis. *Pediatrics International, 48,* 622–625. doi: 10.1111/j.1442-200x.2006.02280x

Koslap-Petraco, M., Shub, M., & Judelsohn, R. (2008). Hepatitis A: Disease burden and current childhood vaccination strategies in the United States. *Journal of Pediatric Health Care, 22,* 3–9. doi: 10.1016/j.pedhc.2006.12.011

Land, M., & Martin, M. (2008). Probiotics: Hype or helpful? *Contemporary Pediatrics, 25,* 34–42.

Leaf, D. (2008) Nonalcoholic fatty liver disease: Update on evaluation and treatment. *Consultant, 48,* 916–919.

Maisels, M. J. (2005a). Jaundice in a newborn: Answers to questions about a common clinical problem. *Contemporary Pediatrics, 22,* 34–40.

Maisels, M. J. (2005b). Jaundice in a newborn: How to head off an urgent problem. *Contemporary Pediatrics, 22,* 41–54.

Maisels, M. J. (2005c). Treating acute bilirubin encephalopathy—before it's too late. *Contemporary Pediatrics, 22,* 57–72.

National Digestive Diseases Information Clearinghouse. (2011). *Viral gastroenteritis* (NIH Publication No. 11–5103). Bethesda, MD: National Institutes of Health. Retrieved from http://digestive.niddk.nih.gov/ddiseases/pubs/viralgastroenteritis/index.aspx

National Institute of Health, Office of Dietary Supplements. (2008). Fact sheets. Retrieved from http://ods.od.nih.gov/factsheets/list-all/

Orenstein, S., Bauman, N., DiLorenzo, C., & Hassell, E. (2007). Issues in diagnosis and management of pediatric GERD. *Contemporary Pediatrics Supplement, 24,* Retrieved from http://www.modernmedicine.com/modernmedicine/

Pediatric Lexi-Drugs Online. (2009). Retrieved from http://www.lexi.com/institutions/online.jsp?id=databases

Taketomo, C. K., Hodding, J. H., & Kraus, D. K. (2009). *Pediatric dosage handbook* (16th ed.). Hudson, OH: Lexi-Comp

Tobias, N., Mason, D., Lutkenhoff, Stoops, M., & Ferguson, D. (2008). Management principles of organic causes of childhood constipation. *Journal of Pediatric Health Care 22,* 12–23.

Wallach, J. (2007). Interpretation of diagnostic tests (8th ed.). Philadelphia: Lippincott Williams and Wilkins.

Wyllie, R., & Hyams, J. (2006). *Pediatric gastrointestinal and liver disease* (3rd ed.). Philadelphia: Saunders Elsevier.

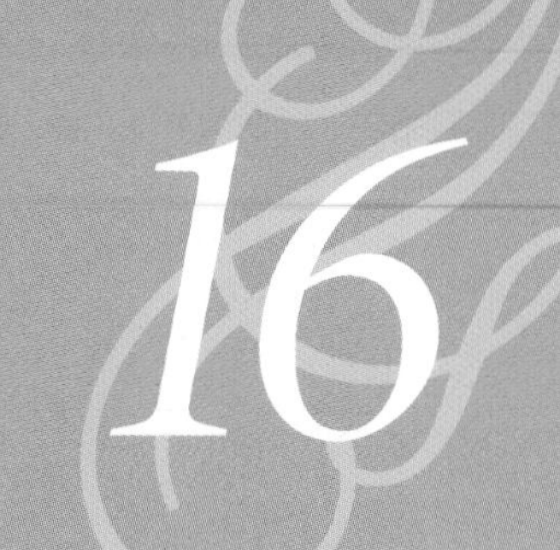

Renal Disorders

Bonnie Kitchen, MNS(c), RN, PNP, ACPNP

OBJECTIVES

- ☐ Define key terms.
- ☐ Review, comprehend, and apply the basic pathophysiology of selected renal disorders.
- ☐ Understand and recognize normal and abnormal values of common laboratory findings in selected renal disorders.
- ☐ Accurately distinguish between selected renal disorders based on clinical presentation.
- ☐ Safely perform nursing interventions on selected renal disorders while in the acute hospital setting.
- ☐ Educate family and patient regarding home therapies for selected renal disorders.

KEY TERMS

- End-stage renal disease
- Renal failure
- Henoch–Schönlein purpura
- Acute kidney injury
- Urinary tract infection (UTI)
- Vesicoureteral reflux (VUR)
- Nephrotic syndrome
- Acute postinfectious glomerulonephritis (APIGN)
- Hemolytic uremic syndrome (HUS)

ANATOMY AND PHYSIOLOGY

- The two kidneys are located in the retroperitoneal space on each side of the vertebra slightly above the umbilicus (**Figure 16-1**).
- The renal arteries supply the kidney with blood flow.
- The right kidney is slightly lower than the left kidney.
- Each kidney contains 1 million nephrons.
  - *The nephron contains a glomerulus, a tubule, and collecting duct.*
  - *Nephrons filter harmful products from the blood.*
  - *Normal renal function is not completely matured until approximately 2 years of age (Kher, Schnaper, & Makker, 2007) (**Table 16-1**).*
- Each renal pelvis extends to form a ureter.
- Each ureter drains into the urinary bladder.
- The urinary bladder collects urine, which is excreted via the urethra.
- The normal urethra has one-way valves allowing drainage and prevention of retrograde reflux of urine.

CRITICAL COMPONENT

End-Stage Renal Disease and Pediatric Developmental Abnormalities

Developmental abnormalities account for 30% to 50% of all cases of **end-stage renal disease** in children (Kher et al., 2007).

ASSESSMENT

General History

- Associated symptoms
- Alleviating factors
- Preceding illnesses
- Past medical history
- Hospitalizations

Don't have time to read this chapter? Want to reinforce your reading? Need to review for a test? Listen to this chapter on DavisPlus at davispl.us/rudd1.

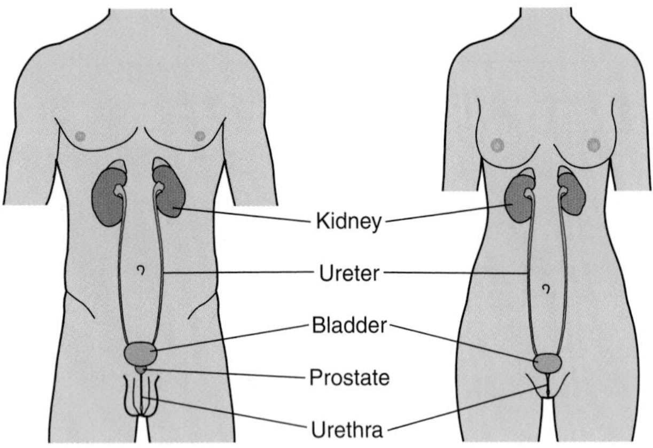

Figure 16-1 Urinary tract system.

TABLE 16-1 SELECTED NORMAL LABORATORY VALUES

Urinalysis
Specific gravity: 1.001-1.035
pH: 5.0-8.5
Protein: Negative
Glucose: Negative
Ketones: Negative
Bilirubin: Negative
Blood: Negative
Nitrite: Negative
Leukocyte esterase: Negative
Serum Electrolytes
Sodium: 135-145 mEq/liter
Potassium: 3.5-5.0 mEq/liter
Chloride: 98-107 mEq/liter
Carbon dioxide: 22-28 mEq/liter
Blood urea nitrogen (BUN): 8-20 mg/deciliter
Creatinine: 0.6-1.2
Complete Blood Count
White blood cells: 5,000-10,000 cells/microliter
Red blood cells: 4.6-4.8 million/uL
Hemoglobin: Male 13.6-17.5 gram/deciliter; female 12.0-15.5 gram/deciliter
Hematocrit: Male 39-49%; female 35-45%
Platelets: 150,000-350,000(Custer & Rau, 2009)

Adapted from Custer & Rau (2009).

- Use of indwelling catheters, as the use of catheters increase the risk for infection by contamination
- Recent or current medication usage
  - *Nephrotoxic medications affect the kidney by altering renal blood flow, causing acute tubular vnecrosis, intratubular obstruction, or a hypersensitivity reaction.*
  - *Common nephrotoxic drugs include aminoglycosides, amphotericin B, vancomycin, nonsteroidal anti-inflammatories, heavy metals, and ACE inhibitors (Webb & Postlethwaite, 2003).*
- History of fractures with minimal trauma
  - *Osteoporosis is a common finding in chronic renal diseases.*
- History of growth retardation, frequent infections
- History of urological anomalies
- History of previous surgeries, sexual activity
  - *Sexual activity is a risk factor, although the mechanism remains unclear.*

Family History

- Recurrent urinary tract infections
- Chronic kidney disease, renal anomalies
- Deafness
- Metabolic disorders
- Immune disorders
- Renal calculi
- Thyroid disturbances
- Gout
- Family members needing dialysis
- Family members with growth retardation

Dietary History

- Protein intake
  - *A high-protein diet may worsen kidney disease*
- Fluid intake
  - *Fluid restriction is an important component of many renal disorders.*
  - *Poor fluid intake or dehydration may lead to an acute renal failure.*
- Calories per kilogram per day
- Special dietary needs
  - *A ketogenic diet increases the risk of nephrolithiasis.*
  - *High-oxalate foods may increase the risk of nephrolithiasis.*
- History of failure to thrive
  - *Many renal disorders manifest in infancy with failure to thrive.*

Physical Examination

General Assessment

- Ill appearing—a child who has the appearance of not feeling well, but stable
- Toxic appearance—a child who has the appearance of not feeling well and not stable
- Well appearing—a child with a healthy appearance

Pulmonary System

- Alterations in breath sounds, cough, shortness of breath, and rapid respiratory rate should be investigated further, as these symptoms may indicate fluid overload of a renal origin.
- Pulse oximetry reading of less than 93% should be further investigated.

CRITICAL COMPONENT

Fluid Balance

A major function of the renal system is to regulate fluid balance. Fluid accumulation from poor glomerular filtration and urinary excretion can lead to pulmonary edema.

Cardiovascular System

- Kidney function is crucial to the hemodynamic status of the human body, as its major function is to maintain fluid balance, maintain electrolyte balance, and excrete waste products (Kliegman, Behrman, Jenson, & Stanton, 2007).
  - *Decreased pulses in lower extremities can indicate decreased blood pressure and poor perfusion from a renal origin.*
  - *A capillary refill of less than 4 seconds indicates poor perfusion.*
- Blood pressure
  - *An elevated blood pressure can indicate glomerulonephritis, acute or chronic* ***renal failure****, renal artery stenosis, or dysplastic kidney (Delaune & Ladner, 2002).*

CLINICAL PEARL

Blood Pressure Cuff

Blood pressure needs to be taken with a cuff of the appropriate size for an accurate reading. The blood pressure cuff should encircle the arm without overlapping. A narrow cuff may give a false high reading, and a cuff that is too large may give a false low reading (Delaune & Ladner, 2002).

- Pulses should be assessed for bounding, which can indicate fluid overload.
- Heart sounds
- Extremity temperature (extremities should be the same temperature as the core to sensation)

Gastrointestinal System

- Chronic kidney disease is associated with anorexia, constipation, and failure to thrive.
  - *Palpable stool in abdomen indicates constipation.*
  - *Diarrhea can indicate a urinary tract infection in infants (Kliegman et al., 2007).*
  - *Vomiting can indicate a urinary tract infection in children.*
  - *Weight loss or failure to thrive should be investigated for a urinary tract infection or renal disease.*
  - *Weight gain may reflect extracellular fluid collection and should be investigated for renal disease.*
  - *Abdominal pain*
    - Abdominal pain can be a hallmark symptom in urinary tract infections in older children (Kliegman et al., 2007).
- Organomegaly, such as enlarged kidneys, can indicate a congenital anomaly or dysplastic kidneys.

Genitourinary System

- Anatomical abnormalities such as pulmonary hypoplasia, VATER/VACTERL syndrome, or Turner syndrome can be associated with renal disease (Kliegman et al., 2007).
  - *Pulmonary hypoplasia is a congenital disorder that usually occurs in association with another intrauterine disorder that causes abnormal lung development.*
  - *VATER/VACTERL syndrome is a complex syndrome of multiple congenital anomalies, including vertebral, anorectal, cardiac, tracheal, esophageal, renal, and radial bone anomalies.*
  - *Turner's syndrome is a genetic condition resulting from a complete or partial absence of the second X chromosome (see Chapter 17 for an in-depth review).*
- Circumcision
  - *Uncircumcised males have a higher incidence of urinary tract infections (Kher et al., 2007).*
- Suprapubic tenderness
  - *Can be associated with a urinary tract infection or an enlarged bladder from posterior urethral valves*
- Frothy urine
  - *Can be associated with proteinuria*
- Urine color
  - *Hematuria causes urine to be tea colored, cola colored, or red.*
  - *Red urine can be caused by nephritis, medications, food dyes, or blood and should be further investigated (Kliegman et al., 2007).*
- A poor or weak urine stream can be associated with the posterior urethral valves and secondary vesicoureteral reflux.
- Intake and output
  - *Fluid maintenance requirements arise from the basal metabolism.*
  - *Based on the Holliday-Segar method, 100 mL fluid will be needed for each 100 calories metabolized.*
  - *Approximately 50% to 65% of this fluid is needed for kidney filtration, and subsequently urinary losses. The remaining 35% is required for skin, respiratory tract, and stool losses, or insensible losses. These fluid needs are reduced in children with renal disease based on their renal function.*

CLINICAL PEARL

Fluid Needs

Fluid needs per kilogram for 24-hour period (with normally functioning kidneys)

Weight	Fluid Needs
0–10 kg	100 mL per kg
11–20 kg	50 mL per kg
21 kg and above	20 mL per kg

From Custer & Rau (2009).

Dermatologic System

- Rash
  - *Palpable purpura on the posterior surface of the extremities is a sign of* ***Henoch–Schönlein purpura*** *(Zaidi et al.,2008). Palpable purpura can be described as a raised, port-wine-colored, nonblanching rash* ***(Figure 16-2)****.*
- Sticky or dry mucosal moisture indicates dehydration.
  - *Severe dehydration can lead to* ***acute kidney injury****.*

Neurologic System

- Hearing acuity/loss and/or physical ear anomalies
  - *Embryonic development of the auditory and renal systems occurs at the same time, and the two systems may have associated anomalies.*
- Pain is always pathological until proven otherwise.
  - *Can be indicative of infection, necrosis, or organomegaly*

Musculoskeletal System

- Appropriate linear growth and appropriate weight gain
  - *Many renal disorders present with poor weight gain, growth retardation, and failure to thrive. Growth hormone is decreased in chronic renal diseases.*
- Muscle cramping may indicate electrolyte disturbances such as hypokalemia, hyponatremia, and hypocalcemia.
- Bone pain and fractures may be caused from osteodystrophy/osteopenia of chronic renal disease. Osteopenia is secondary to hypocalcemia, which arises from the inability of the kidney to convert vitamin D into the active form (Kliegman et al., 2007).

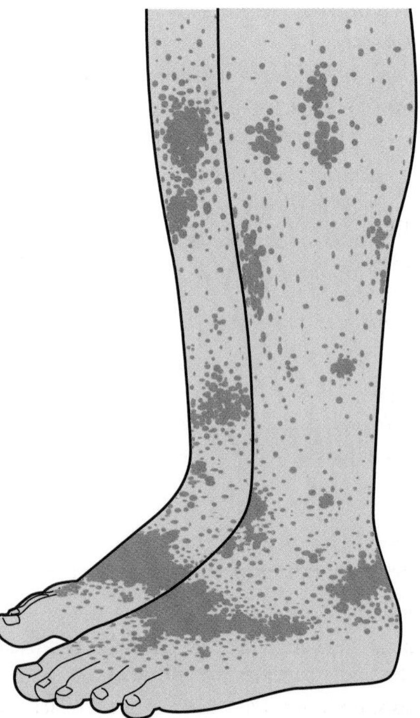

Figure 16–2 Palpable purpura in the lower extremities.

- Costovertebral tenderness is associated with urinary tract infections in older children.
- Weakness and malaise may be secondary from anemia of chronic kidney failure and poor nutritional intake.

> **CRITICAL COMPONENT**
>
> **Socioeconomic Factors in Growth and Development**
>
> Many chronic and acute illnesses can compromise the growth and development of children. Socioeconomic issues compromise the vast majority of poor growth and development.
>
> 1. How does the nurse obtain an accurate history to differentiate between socioeconomic problems versus those of pathologic conditions?
> 2. What are red flags that would indicate more than socioeconomic components of poor growth and development?

Lymphatic System

- Periorbital edema
- Facial edema
- Ascites (excessive buildup of fluid in the abdominal cavity)
- Scrotal edema
- Sacral edema
- Dependent edema
  - *Edema can be caused by decreased circulating protein (hypoalbuminemia). Nephrotic syndrome is characterized by proteinuria and hypoalbuminemia resulting in edema (Kliegman et al., 2007).*

> **CLINICAL PEARL**
>
> **Edema**
>
> Edema is associated with poor renal function and is often found in areas of dependence as well as large, hollow cavities.

> **CRITICAL COMPONENT**
>
> 1. How does the nurse assess edema?
> 2. What parameter is critical in assessing and quantifying edema?

Endocrine System

- Palpable thyroid
  - *A palpable thyroid may indicate hyperthyroidism, which is associated with chronic kidney disease.*

> **CRITICAL COMPONENT**
>
> Increased parathyroid activity is commonly seen in children with chronic renal disease. Explain the pathophysiology of secondary hyperparathyroidism and hypocalcemia.

Renal System

- Palpable kidneys
  - *Large, dysplastic kidneys may be felt on physical examination.*
- Urine output
  - *Alterations in urine output can be associated with various renal diseases.*
  - *Normal urine output in children is 2 cc/kg/hour; 0.5 to 1.0 cc/kg/hour is acceptable in teenagers.*

DISORDERS OF THE RENAL SYSTEM

URINARY TRACT INFECTION

A **urinary tract infection (UTI)** is an infectious process that involves the urethra, bladder, ureters, renal pelvis, renal calyces, and renal parenchyma, either isolated or compromising the entire urinary tract.

- UTIs are more commonly seen in children between the ages of 2 and 6 years.
- *Escherichia coli* is the most common bacterial cause of UTIs, with other gram-negative organisms secondary (Committee on Quality Improvement, 1999).
- Symptoms of a UTI in infants and young children do not mimic the typical urinary symptoms in adults and may be as subtle as fever alone.
- If left untreated, urinary tract infections can lead to renal scarring and renal failure (Prajapati, Prajapati, & Patel, 2008).

Assessment

Clinical Presentation

- Fever (temperature above 38.3)
- Vomiting
- Abdominal pain
- Flank pain
- Back pain
- Dysuria (painful urination)
- Frequency (urinating at frequent intervals not associated with increased volume)
- Urgency (an unstoppable urge to urinate)
- Hematuria (blood in the urine)
- Jaundice (a yellow discoloration of the skin and sclera due to increased bilirubin levels)
- Poor oral intake
- Hyperthermia
- Hypothermia
- Failure to thrive (failing to have adequate growth)

CLINICAL PEARL

Children with Spina Bifida

Children with spina bifida are at increased risk for urinary tract infections due to the neurogenic bladder. A neurogenic bladder is characterized by incomplete emptying, causing urinary stasis. Clean intermittent urinary catheterization is a safe standard of care for treatment of a neurogenic bladder (Martins, Soler, Batigalia, & Moore, 2009).

Promoting Safety

The use of sterile and clean intermittent urinary catheterization is safe and decreases the number of urinary tract infections (Moore, Fader, & Getliffe, 2007).

Diagnostic Tests

- Urinalysis: nitrites, leukocyte esterase
- Urine microscopy: bacteria, white blood cells
  - *A urinalysis can be suspicious, but not diagnostic, of a urinary tract infection.*
  - *Urine nitrites are almost diagnostic of UTIs (Custer & Rau, 2009).*

CLINICAL PEARL

Prevention of Contamination in Urine Cultures

A bag urine specimen is not an appropriate collection of urine for culture. Urine cultures should be obtained by catheterization, suprapubic tap, or clean catch if the patient is toilet trained. These methods decrease secondary contamination of the urine specimen.

- Urine culture: specific bacterium (**Table 16-2**)

CLINICAL PEARL

Diagnostic Urine Culture

A urine culture is necessary to accurately diagnose and treat urinary tract infections.

CLINICAL PEARL

Urinalysis Evaluation Guidelines

The new guidelines from the American Academy of Pediatrics (AAP) report that a urinalysis suggestive of infection (pyuria and/or bacteriuria) and the presence of at least a colony count of 50,000 per milliliter in febrile infants and children under 3 years of age is considered positive (AAP, 2011).

- Renal ultrasonography: structural anomalies or vascular compromise
- Voiding cystourethrogram (VCUG): vesicoureteral reflux
  - *During this procedure, the bladder is catheterized and a radioiodinated contrast is instilled into the bladder until the bladder is full. Radiographic images are taken of the full bladder, the ureterovesical junction, the kidneys, and the urethra. The contrast is eliminated by spontaneous voiding or catheter drainage.*

CLINICAL PEARL

Voiding Cystourethrogram (VCUG)

A VCUG is no longer recommended to be performed routinely after the first febrile UTI. A VCUG is indicated if the renal ultrasound reveals hydronephrosis, renal scarring, or other abnormalities that would suggest vesicoureteral reflux (AAP, 2011).

TABLE 16–2 URINE CULTURE AND DIAGNOSTIC CRITERIA FOR A URINARY TRACT INFECTION

COLLECTION METHOD	Clean Catch	Urethral Catheterization	Suprapubic Aspiration
COLONY COUNT	>100,000 colony count of a single organism	>10,000 colony count of a single organism	>1,000 colony count of gram-positive organisms and any number of gram-negative organisms

Adapted from Custer & Rau (2009).

- DTc-dimercaptosuccinic acid scan (DMSA): renal scarring (AAP position statement, 1999)
  - *A radiopharmaceutical agent is infused intravenously, filtered by the glomeruli, and excreted in the urine. During the filtration phase, imaging is done to evaluate the renal parenchyma as well as the anatomic structures of the urinary system.*

Nursing Interventions

Emergency Care

- Stabilization of circulatory status by delivering 20-cc/kg intravenous fluid bolus of normal saline
- Immediate administration of broad-spectrum intravenous antibiotics
  - *Ceftriaxone 50–75 mg/kg/day divided twice daily intravenously*
  - *Cefotaxime 100–200 mg/kg/day divided every 6–8 hours daily intravenously*

CLINICAL PEARL

Guidelines for Infants Under 2 Months Old

Any infant less than 2 months of age with a urinary tract infection needs a septic workup, hospitalization, and the administration of intravenous antibiotics until cultures and sensitivities have been completed.

Acute Hospital Care

- Broad-spectrum antibiotics should be started immediately after obtaining an appropriate urine specimen for culture.
- Antibiotics should be tailored to an appropriate intravenous or oral medication as soon as susceptibilities on culture are known.
  - *Amoxicillin 25–50 mg/kg/day divided every 8–12 hours daily orally*
  - *Co-Trimoxazole 8–10 mg/kg/day divided every 12 hours daily orally (Custer & Rau, 2009)*
- Ensure appropriate diagnostic testing is performed.
- Strictly monitor vital signs, with emphasis on temperature and blood pressure.
- Understand family values and cultural practices and incorporate into the hospital plan of care, if possible.

Chronic Hospital Care

- Urinary tract infections are the number one hospital-acquired infection.
  - *Good hand hygiene*
  - *Aseptic technique*
  - *Avoidance of indwelling Foley catheters*

Promoting Safety

When inserting urinary catheters, sterile technique is essential to decrease the introduction of a secondary, or nosocomial, infection.

Chronic Home Care

- Complete antibiotic course in its entirety (7–14 days).
- Educate family and patient on the importance of follow-up testing.
- Educate family and patient on prophylactic antibiotics if prescribed.
  - *Co-Trimoxazole 2 mg/kg/day as a single dose or 5 mg/kg twice weekly 8–10 mg/kg/day divided every 12 hours*
  - *Amoxicillin 10 mg/kg/day as a single dose orally*
  - *Nitrofurantoin 1–2 mg/kg/day as a single dose daily orally*
  - *Cephalexin 10 mg/kg/day as a single dose orally*
  - *Ampicillin 20 mg/kg/day as a single dose orally (Field & Mattoo, 2010)*
- Encourage liquid intake appropriate for age and weight.
- Promote regular voiding.
- Avoid perineal irritants.
- Correct constipation.
  - *High-fiber diet*
  - *Postprandial stooling attempts*

Complementary and Alternative Therapies

- Cranberry juice has been used for prevention of urinary tract infection; however, there is no evidence-based data to support this practice.

Caregiver Education

Emergency Care

- Seek medical attention immediately for fever in infants less than 3 months of age.

Acute Hospital Care

- Include family's participation in daily care of the hospitalized child.
- Educate family and patient on medication administration, route, reason, and side effects.
- Use aseptic technique to prevent hospital-acquired infections.

Chronic Home Care

- Educate family and patient on home medication administration and side effects.
- Educate family and patient on importance of follow-up studies.
- Educate family and patient on any home procedures (in and out catheterization).

Complementary and Alternative Therapies

- Educate families and patients on reliable sources of information when researching alternative therapies.
- High-fiber diet and ample water intake may help constipation.
- Avoid tight clothing and diapers to prevent local irritation.
- Avoid the use of bubble baths or essential oils in baths to prevent local irritation.
- Encourage adults to practice postcoital urination to decrease chance of urinary tract infections.

> CLINICAL PEARL
>
> **Chronic UTIs**
>
> Repetitive urinary tract infections can cause permanent renal damage. Febrile illnesses should be investigated with a urinalysis and culture in a child with a previous urinary tract infection.

> **Promoting Safety**
>
> Any prepubescent child with repetitive urinary tract infections without a known etiology should be considered for sexual abuse.

VESICOURETERAL REFLUX

Vesicoureteral reflux (VUR) is an anatomical abnormality that allows the retrograde flow of urine from the bladder into the ureters (**Table 16-3**).

- VUR is the most common congenital anomaly affecting the urinary tract in children.
- VUR and urinary stasis increase children's risk for urinary tract infections and renal scarring, which could lead to end-stage renal disease.
- VUR may be secondary to posterior urethral valves.

Assessment

Clinical Presentation

- Frequent urinary tract infections
- Suprapubic pain
- Urinary incontinence
- Family history of vesicoureteral reflux
- Enlarged bladder

Diagnostic Tests

- Urinalysis
- Urine culture
- Postvoiding catheterization: residual urine present
- Renal ultrasound: evidence of hydronephrosis
- Voiding cystourethrogram: gradation of VUR
- DTc-dimercaptosuccinic acid (DMSA) scan: detection of renal scarring

> CLINICAL PEARL
>
> **Vesicoureteral Reflux (VUR)**
>
> Young children and infants should have a diagnostic investigation for VUR with the first proven urinary tract infection by VCUG radiography (Field & Mattoo, 2010).

> **CRITICAL COMPONENT**
>
> **Testing a Sibling for VUR**
>
> A sibling of a child with VUR who has never had a urinary tract infection is encouraged to have a voiding cystourethrogram. The family asks if this is a necessary test.
>
> 1. Explain to the family the rationale for this invasive procedure.

Nursing Interventions

Emergency Care

- Prepare for dialysis if renal failure is present.

Acute Hospital Care

- Appropriate administration of antimicrobials if urinary tract infection is present
- Ensure appropriate diagnostic testing performed efficiently
- Postoperative care if surgical correction is performed
- Strict monitoring of vital signs, with emphasis on blood pressure
- Understand family values and cultural practices and incorporate into the hospital plan of care, if possible.

Chronic Hospital Care

- Accurate administration of medications if a urinary tract infection is present
  - *Ceftriaxone 50–75 mg/kg/day divided twice daily intravenously*
  - *Cefotaxime 100–200 mg/kg/day divided every 6–8 hours intravenously daily*

TABLE 16–3 DIFFERENT STAGES OF VESICOURETERAL REFLUX

Grade I	Grade II	Grade III	Grade IV	Grade V
Ureter only	Ureter, pelvis, calyces; no dilation, normal calyceal fornices	Mild or moderate dilatation and/or tortuosity of ureter; mild or moderate dilatation of the pelvis; but no or slight blunting of the fornices	Moderate dilatation and/or tortuosity of the renal pelvis and calyces; complete obliteration of sharp angle of fornices; but maintenance of papillary impressions in the majority of calyces	Gross dilatation and tortuosity of ureter; gross dilatation of renal pelvis and calyces; papillary impressions are no longer visible in majority of calyces

Reproduced with permission by Elsevier Mosby from Custer, J., & Rau, R. (2009). *The Harriet Lane handbook* (18th ed.).Philadelphia: Elsevier Mosby.

- *Co-Trimoxazole 8–10 mg/kg/day divided every 12 hours daily orally*
- *Amoxicillin 25–50 mg/kg/day divided every 8–12 hours daily orally (Custer & Rau, 2009)*

- Postoperative care if surgical correction is performed

Evidence-Based Practice Research: Prophylactic Antibiotics for VUR

Pennesi, M., Travan, L., Peratoner, L., Bordugo, A., Cattaneo, A., Ronfani, L., Ventura, A. (2008). Is antibiotic prophylaxis in children with vesicoureteral reflux effective in preventing pyelonephritis and renal scars? A randomized, controlled trial. *Pediatrics, 121,* 1489–1494. doi: 10.1542/peds.2007-2652

Current studies are under way to evaluate prophylactic antibiotic use in children with VUR and the need for routine radiographic studies with the first urinary tract infection, such as the randomized intervention for children with vesicoureteral reflux sponsored by the National Institute of Diabetes and Digestive and Kidney Diseases.

Source: Retrieved from http://kidney.niddk.nih.gov/about/Research_Updates/UrologicDiseasesFall07/3.htm

- Magnetic resonance imaging has recently been used to evaluate VUR with similar or superior sensitivity to DMSA scintigraphy (Lim, 2009).

Caregiver Education

Acute Hospital Care

- Educate family and patient on diagnostic tests.
- Educate family and patient on medication (reason, route, length of therapy, side effects).

Chronic Home Care

- Educate family and patient on medical therapy and compliance.
- Educate family and patient on medication (reason, route, length of therapy, side effects).
- Educate family and patient on need for follow-up diagnostic testing.
- Educate family that siblings are at higher risk for vesicoureteral reflux and may need screening.

CLINICAL PEARL

Surgical Intervention and VUR

Most cases of VUR resolve with time; however, some forms may require surgical intervention (Kliegman et al., 2007).

NEPHROLITHIASIS (RENAL CALCULI)

Nephrolithiasis, or kidney stones, is a clinical condition where urinary crystals coalesce and form growing renal calculi.

- Other metabolic diseases, the use of loop diuretics, urinary tract infections, or congenital anomalies of the urinary tract may increase the chance of stone formation (Reddy & Minevich, 2007).
- Nephrolithiasis is also a complication of metabolic disorders such as cystic fibrosis and inflammatory bowel disease as well as urinary tract infections. Some metabolic

disorders have deficiencies or excesses that promote stone formation (Cameron, Sakhaee, & Moe, 2005).

Assessment

Clinical Presentation

- Colic-type abdominal, flank, or back pain
- Hematuria
- Urinary tract infection
- Poor feeding
- Acute renal failure if single kidney is present and obstructed
- Nausea and vomiting

Diagnostic Testing

- Urinalysis: hematuria or casts
- Abdominal radiograph: calcium calculi
- Ultrasonography: calculi, obstruction, or hydronephrosis
- Computed tomography: calculus
- Laboratory analysis of renal calculus
- 24-hour urine collection

> **Evidence-Based Practice Research: Computed Tomography to Diagnose Kidney Stones**
>
> Kher, K. K., Schnaper, H. W., & Makker, S. P. (Eds.). (2007). *Clinical pediatric nephrology* (2nd ed.). Abingdon, UK: Informa Healthcare.
>
> Computed tomography has a high sensitivity and specificity for imaging stones and is considered the gold standard radiographic evaluation for nephrolithiasis.

Nursing Interventions

Emergency Care

- Adequate fluid intake; intravenous fluids should be at 1.5–2 times the maintenance rate.
- Pain control with narcotic and non-narcotic medication
  - *Morphine 0.1–0.2 mg/kg/dose every 2–4 hours intravenously*
  - *Oxycodone 0.05–0.15 mg/kg/dose every 4–6 hours orally*
  - *Acetaminophen 10–15 mg/kg/dose every 4 hours orally (Custer & Rau, 2009)*
- Accurate urinary output recording
- Monitor for urinary obstruction.
  - *Assist in percutaneous nephrostomy placement.*
- Monitor for renal failure.

> **CLINICAL PEARL**
>
> **Children with Renal Calculi and One Kidney**
>
> Children with a single kidney and calculi with signs of acute renal failure are a surgical emergency.

Acute Hospital Care

- Provide adequate fluid intake (intravenous and oral).
- Strain urine for stone collection.
- Obtain laboratory studies appropriately and accurately.
- Provide pain control with narcotic and non-narcotic medication.
- Strictly monitor vital signs.
- Prepare family and patient for possible stone removal by open or closed surgical intervention.
- Prepare family and patient for possible extracorporeal shock-wave lithotripsy.
- Understand family values and cultural practices and incorporate into the hospital plan of care, if possible.

Caregiver Education

Emergency Care

- Educate family and patient on presenting signs of nephrolithiasis, obstruction, and renal failure.

Acute Hospital Care

- Educate family and patient on diagnostic studies, medications, invasive treatment, and pain control measures.
- Educate family and patient on how to strain urine.
- Educate family and patient on surgical procedures.

Chronic Hospital Care

- Educate family and patient on ongoing management.
- Educate family and patient on how to strain urine.
- Educate family and patient on medication administration (**Table 16-4**).
  - *Furosemide 1–6 mg/kg/dose every 12–24 hours orally*
  - *Spironolactone 1–3 mg/kg/day divided every 1–4 times daily orally*
  - *Oxycodone 0.05–0.15 mg/kg/dose every 4–6 hours orally*
- Educate family and patient on fluid intake and dietary modifications.

Chronic Home Care

- Educate family and patient on how to strain urine.
- Educate family and patient on appropriate nutritional requirements based on age.
- Educate family and patient on appropriate nutritional restrictions.
- Educate family and patient on appropriate fluid requirements based on age.
- Educate family and patient on home medications if ordered.
  - *Thiazide diuretics may be beneficial in the treatment of certain types of kidney stones.*
- Complete course of antimicrobial therapy if urinary tract infection is present
  - *Amoxicillin 25–50 mg/kg/day divided every 8–12 hours daily orally*
  - *Co-Trimoxazole 8–10 mg/kg/day divided every 12 hours daily orally (Custer & Rau, 2009)*
- Educate family and patient on importance of metabolic testing

> **CLINICAL PEARL**
>
> **Ketogenic Diets and Risk for Kidney Stones**
>
> Children on a ketogenic diet (high fat, low carbohydrate, adequate protein) for seizure control are at higher risk for developing kidney stones, for unknown reasons. Taking daily doses of potassium citrate can decrease the occurrence and increase the age of onset (Vining, 2008).

TABLE 16–4 COMMONLY USED DIURETICS

Drug	Dosage	Side Effects	Administration Options
Furosemide	1–6 mg/kg/dose every 12–24 hours	Orthostatic hypotension, vertigo, photo sensitivity, electrolyte disturbances, nephrocalcinosis	Oral tablets or liquid
Furosemide	0.5–2 mg/kg/dose every 6–12 hours	Orthostatic hypotension, vertigo, photo sensitivity, electrolyte disturbances, nephrocalcinosis	Intravenous injection
Metolazone	0.2–0.4 mg/kg/24hr ÷ daily to twice daily	Orthostatic hypotension, syncope, vertigo, muscle cramps, electrolyte imbalances	Oral tablets; compounded liquid suspension
Bumetanide	0.015–0.1 mg/kg/dose once daily to every other day	Orthostatic hypotension, syncope, vertigo, muscle cramps, electrolyte imbalances	Oral tablets; intravenous injection
Spironolactone	1–3.3 mg/kg/24 hours ÷ daily to four times daily	Lethargy, confusion, electrolyte disturbances, weakness, decreased renal function	Oral tablets; compounded liquid suspension

From Custer & Rau (2009).

Complementary and Alternative Therapies

- Low-oxalate diet
  - *Oxalates are chemicals found in plant food that can increase stone formation in some people.*
- Avoidance of high protein intake
- Avoidance of fast foods and artificially flavored/sweetened drinks

CRITICAL COMPONENT

Vegetarian Diet and Prevention of Kidney Stones

In obtaining a dietary history on a child with kidney stones, the nurse discovers the family is vegetarian.

1. List foods high in oxalate.
2. Give better choices of foods within the vegetarian dietary culture.

NEPHROTIC SYNDROME

- **Nephrotic syndrome** is characterized by a combination of clinical manifestations, including massive proteinuria, hypoalbuminemia, edema, and hyperlipidemia of unknown etiology (**Figure 16-3**). Macromolecules are filtered in the glomeruli, allowing albumin to cross the capillary wall. The loss of protein in the urine changes the oncotic pressure within the intravascular space, causing intravascular depletion of volume and extracellular edema.
- The peak incidence is seen in children between 2 and 5 years of age.

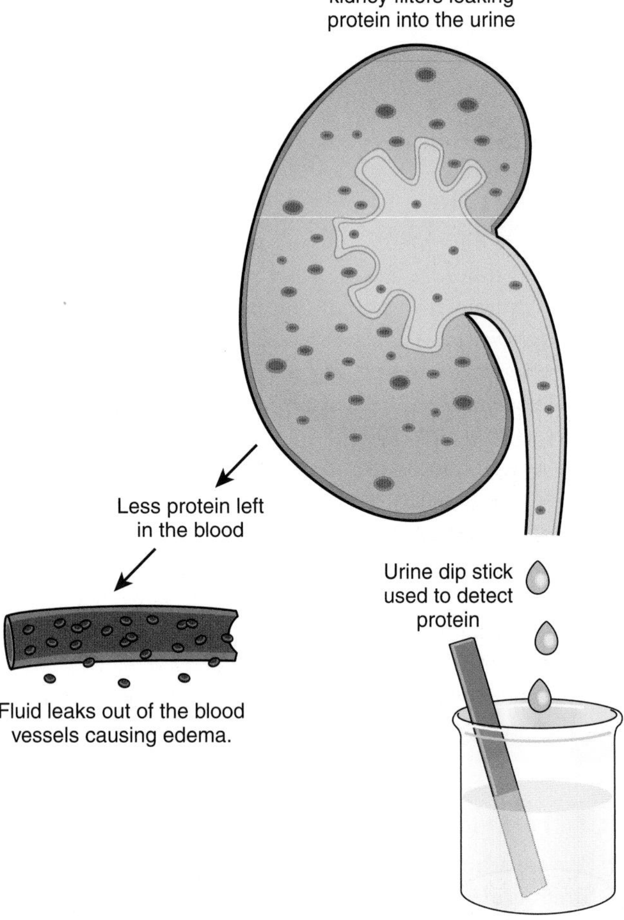

Figure 16–3 Nephrotic syndrome.

- Nephrotic syndrome is the most common type of kidney disease in children.
- The types of nephrotic syndrome are minimal change disease, focal segmental glomerulosclerosis, membranoproliferative glomerulonephritis, and mesangial proliferative glomerulonephritis.
- Nephrotic syndrome often occurs after an upper respiratory tract infection.
- Edema is gravity dependent and occurs gradually.
- Decreased circulating volume is often present despite increased extracellular fluid volume, causing tachycardia, oliguria, and orthostatic hypotension.
- Possible complications of nephrotic syndrome include peritonitis, pulmonary embolism, acute renal failure, and malnutrition.

Assessment

Clinical Presentation

- Edema (most notable around eyes, scrotal/sacral, ascites, and pretibial)
- Weight gain (tight clothing, umbilical hernia, protruding abdomen)
- Decreased urine output
- Anorexia
- Easily fatigued
- Hypertension

CRITICAL COMPONENT

Weight Gain and Nephrotic Syndrome

A 2-year-old child is admitted with a new diagnosis of nephrotic syndrome. The mother notes that the child has had a 5-pound weight gain in the past 3 weeks. She asks the nurse the reason for the weight gain and swelling. How will the nurse explain this so that the mother will understand?

Diagnostic Testing

- Urinalysis: heavy proteinuria (greater than 50 mg/kg/day), +/– microscopic hematuria
- Serum protein: less than 2.5 gM/dL
- Electrolytes: hyponatremia is occasionally seen.
- Compliments: +/– decreased C3 and C4
- Urea, creatinine: usually normal at presentation
- Serum cholesterol, low-density lipoproteins: grossly increased
- Serum calcium: reduced
- Ionized calcium: normal (Webb & Postlethwaite, 2003)
- Renal ultrasound: to detect possible structural anomalies
- Chest radiograph: to detect possible pleural effusion

Nursing Interventions

Emergency Care

- Oxygen delivery for respiratory distress
- Computerized tomography to evaluate for pulmonary emboli
- Preparation for drainage of pleural effusion
- Administration of intravenous fluids at 20-cc/k bolus of normal saline for hemodynamic instability
- Administration of intravenous diuretics for fluid overload
  - *Furosemide 0.5–2 mg/kg/dose every 6–12 hours intravenously (Custer & Rau, 2009)*
- Administration of intravenous antibiotics for peritonitis
  - *Cefotaxime 100–200 mg/kg/day divided every 6–8 hours daily (Custer & Rau, 2009)*

CLINICAL PEARL

Thrombus Formation

Children with nephrotic syndrome are at high risk for spontaneous peritonitis and thrombus formation (Kher et al., 2007). *Streptococcus pneumonia* peritonitis is the most common infection in nephrotic syndrome. The reason for this is both immunosuppression from the high-dose steroids and the lowered function of the innate immune system. A combination of increased platelet aggregation, increased procoagulant factors, and increased loss of coagulation inhibitors in the urine are all thought to increase the risk for thrombus formation.

Acute Hospital Care

- Initiate corticosteroid therapy.
  - *Prednisone 2 mg/kg/day with a maximum of 60 mg daily (Custer & Rau, 2009)*

CLINICAL PEARL

Comorbidities and Corticosteroid Therapy

The child with comorbidities such as diabetes still requires high-dose corticosteroids. Secondary complications such as hyperglycemia are individually managed.

- Initiate diuretic therapy
  - *Furosemide 1–6 mg/kg/dose every 12–24 hours orally*
  - *Furosemide 1–4 mg/kg/dose every 12–24 hours orally (infants) (Custer & Rau, 2009)*
- Intravenous albumin infusion
  - *25% albumin 0.5–1 g/kg/dose over 30–120 minutes intravenously every 1–2 days (Custer & Rau, 2009)*
- Ensure nutritional consult to correct malnutrition and maintain appropriate fluid restriction.
- Strict monitoring of daily weight
- Strict monitoring of intake and output
- Monitoring of abdominal girth
- Monitoring of vital signs, with emphasis on heart rate and blood pressure
- Encourage ambulation and physical activity to prevent stasis complications.
- Understand family values and cultural practices and incorporate into the hospital plan of care, if possible.

CRITICAL COMPONENT

Shortness of Breath

A child with nephrotic syndrome is complaining of shortness of breath. The child should be evaluated for what condition(s)?

Chronic Hospital Care

- Monitor daily laboratory studies.
- Administer vaccinations appropriately.
  - *Prevnar annually (pneumococcal vaccination)*
- Prevent skin breakdown.
- Prevent infection with good hand washing and limitation of sick contacts.
- Provide patient/family emotional support.
- Placement of PPD before immunosuppressive therapy

Chronic Home Care

- Provide instructions on medication administration and side effects.
- Provide appropriate supplies for home blood pressure monitoring.
- Provide appropriate supplies for urine chemistry checks.
- Provide written material regarding diet and fluid restriction.

Caregiver Education

Emergency Care

- Educate family and patient on signs of pulmonary emboli and respiratory distress.
- Educate family and patient on signs of peritonitis.

Acute Hospital Care

- Educate family and patient on medication administration and side effects.
- Educate family and patient on therapeutic treatments.

Chronic Hospital Care

- Educate family and patient on disease process and side effects.
- Educate family and patient on adherence to nutritional needs and fluid restriction.
- Educate family and patient on daily blood pressure monitoring and parameters.
- Educate family and patient on monitoring daily weight.
- Educate family and patient on activities to prevent venous stasis.

Chronic Home Care

- Daily monitoring of blood pressure and weight
- Daily monitoring of urine for proteinuria
- Compliance with nutritional requirements and fluid restriction
- Compliance with daily medication administration
- Knowledge of disease pathology and possible emergencies
- Knowledge of patient's immunosuppressive state and ways to minimize infection
- Knowledge of yearly vaccinations
- Provide information on local psychosocial support systems or agencies.

ACUTE POSTINFECTIOUS GLOMERULONEPHRITIS

Acute postinfectious glomerulonephritis (APIGN) is an inflammation of the glomeruli in response to a preceding illness, most commonly a streptococcal upper respiratory or skin infection, and is clinically apparent 1 to 3 weeks after the acute infection (**Figure 16-4**).

- APIGN usually affects children 2 to 12 years of age. Most cases of APIGN resolve spontaneously without chronic kidney disease (Ilyas & Tolaymat, 2008).
- The peak ages of APIGN are 2 to 15 years.

Assessment

Clinical Presentation

- Painless hematuria; may be tea colored, cola colored, or bright red
- Proteinuria
- Oliguria
- Hypertension
- Edema
- Anorexia
- Antecedent upper respiratory or skin infection
- Arthralgias
- Pulmonary edema
- Abdominal pain
- Malaise
- Impaired renal function

Diagnostic Testing

- Serum urea and creatinine: elevated
- Serum protein: decreased
- Serum white blood cell count: elevated
- Erythrocyte sedimentation rate: elevated
  - *Reflective of systemic inflammatory process*
- Serum complement (C3): decreased
- Serum complement (C4): normal
  - *The complement system is triggered with an infectious agent causing a decrease in C3 in APIGN.*
- Urinalysis: hematuria, proteinuria, red blood cell casts, hyaline casts
- Anitstreptolysin O, anti-DNase B, Streptozyme: +/– positive
  - *Reflective of previous streptococcal infection*
- Renal biopsy: may be necessary in some cases
- Throat culture: +/– beta hemolytic streptococcus

Nursing Interventions

Emergency Care

- Hemodialysis for renal failure
- Antihypertensive management
  - *Nifedipine 0.25–0.5 mg/kg/dose every 4–6 hours orally or sublingually (Custer & Rau, 2009)*

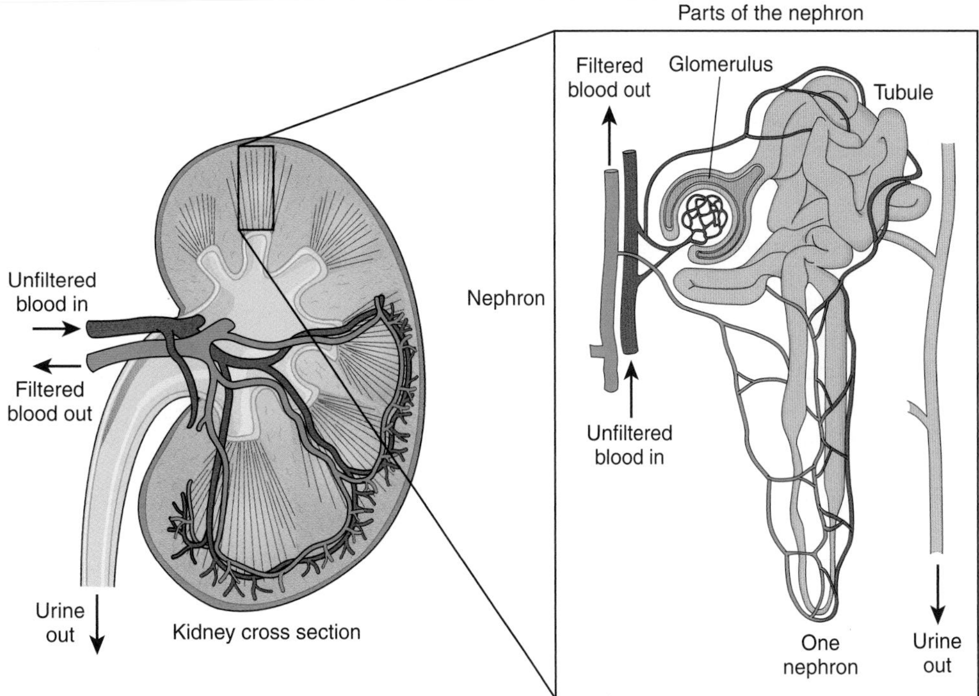

Figure 16-4 Nephron and glomeruli.

- *Administration of sodium polystyrene sulfonate for hyperkalemia*
- *Seizure control for hypertensive encephalopathy*
- *Lorazepam 0.05–0.1 mg/kg/dose every 15 minutes intravenously (Custer & Rau, 2009)*

Acute Hospital Care

- Antibiotics to eradicate the offending organism if present
  - *Cefotaxime 100–200 mg/kg/day divided every 6–8 hours daily*
  - *Ceftriaxone 50–75 mg/kg/day divided twice daily intravenously (Custer & Rau, 2009)*
- Strict monitoring of vital signs, with emphasis on blood pressure
- Strict monitoring of intake and output
- Strict monitoring of daily weight
- Administration of diuretics
  - *Furosemide 1–6 mg/kg/dose every 12–24 hours orally (Custer & Rau, 2009)*
- Monitoring and correction of electrolyte imbalances
- Understand family values and cultural practices and incorporate into the hospital plan of care, if possible.

Chronic Hospital Care

- Nutritional consult for no-added-salt diet and fluid requirements
- Assess neurological status for cerebral complications.
- Renal replacement therapy if required
- Activities as tolerated

Chronic Home Care

- Provide appropriate home blood pressure monitoring equipment.
- Provide written dietary instructions.
- Provide psychosocial support.

Caregiver Education

Emergency Care

- Educate family and patient on blood pressure elevations and appropriate intervention.
- Educate family and patient on seizure precautions.
- Educate family and patient on signs of hyperkalemia.

CLINICAL PEARL

Children with Hyperkalemia

Any child with hyperkalemia should have an emergent electrocardiogram to evaluate for life-threatening rhythm changes.

CRITICAL COMPONENT

What electrocardiogram changes are associated with hyperkalemia?

Acute Hospital Care

- Educate family and patient on medication administration and side effects.
- Educate family and patient on pathology of disease.
- Educate family and patient on reason and necessity for testing.
- Educate family and patient on dialysis.

Chronic Hospital Care

- Educate family and patient on dietary restrictions and fluid restrictions.
- Educate family and patient on home medication administration and side effects.
- Educate family and patient on accurate intake and output monitoring.
- Educate family and patient on accurate daily weights.

Chronic Home Care

- Educate family and patient on daily monitoring of weight.
- Educate family and patient on daily blood pressure monitoring.
- Educate family and patient on importance of follow-up appointments.
- Educate family and patient on infection prevention.
- Provide family and patient information on local psychosocial support groups.

HENOCH–SCHÖNLEIN PURPURA

Henoch–Schönlein purpura (HSP) is the most common multisystem vasculitic disorder of children, classified by a tetrad of symptoms—rash, arthralgias, abdominal pain, and renal disease.

- In most cases HSP is a self-limiting disorder, with 90% of children having a full recovery.
- HSP is most often seen in the fall and winter months and frequently follows an antecedent upper respiratory tract infection.
- Intussusception is a common emergent condition seen in children with HSP. This is thought to be from the intestinal edema and hemorrhage (Betz & Snowden, 2005).

Assessment

Clinical Presentation

- Colicky abdominal pain
  - *May represent intussusception*
- Palpable purpura most prominent in dependent areas
- Nonmigratory arthritis/arthralgia located mostly in the knees, ankles, elbows, and wrists
- Edema of face, lips, dorsum of hands and feet, scrotum
- Occult or gastrointestinal bleeding
- Microscopic hematuria
- Proteinuria
- Anorexia
- Malaise
- Erythema nodosum (red or purple subcutaneous nodules found in the pretibial area)

Diagnostic Testing

- Complete blood count: anemia with evidence of hemolysis, thrombocytosis, leukocytosis
- Erythrocyte sedimentation rate: elevated
- C-reactive protein: elevated
- Coagulation studies: normal
- Urinalysis: proteinuria and hematuria
- Stool occult blood: positive
- Abdominal ultrasound to evaluate for intussusceptions
- Skin biopsy can be definitive diagnostic test
- Renal biopsy: IgA deposits
  - *Increased IgA is a histologic confirmation of HSP.*

Nursing Interventions

Emergency Care

- If intussusception is present, this is a surgical emergency. The patient should be prepared for immediate transport to the operating room.
- If renal failure is present, emergent hemodialysis may be necessary. The patient should be prepared for surgical placement of a hemodialysis catheter.
- Family support for emergent procedures
- Family consent for emergent procedures

> CLINICAL PEARL
>
> **Colic and Intussusception**
>
> Any child with colicky abdominal pain and hematochezia should be evaluated for intussusception.

Acute Hospital Care

- Intravenous fluid hydration with an isotonic fluid at 20-cc/kg bolus if hemodynamically unstable
- Fluid restriction to insensible losses if oliguric or anuric
- Strict monitoring of vital signs, with emphasis on blood pressure
- Accurate measuring of daily weights
- Pain control with pharmacologic analgesics, avoiding nonsteroidal anti-inflammatory medications
  - *Acetaminophen 15 mg/kg/dose every 4 hours orally*
  - *Oxycodone 0.05–0.15 mg/kg/dose every 4–6 hours orally*
  - *Morphine 0.1–0.2 mg/kg/dose every 2–4 hours intravenously (Custer & Rau, 2009)*
- Pain control with nonpharmacologic measures, such as positioning, distraction, therapeutic play
- Skin care to prevent breakdown from edema and rash
- Accurate monitoring for abdominal pain
- Accurate monitoring for occult blood in stool
- Understand family values and cultural practices and incorporate into the hospital plan of care, if possible.

Chronic Hospital Care

- Administer antihypertensive medications.
  - *Nifedipine 0.25–0.5 mg/kg/dose every 4–6 hours orally or sublingually*
  - *Enalapril 0.1 mg/kg/day divided 1–2 times daily orally (Custer & Rau, 2009)*
- Administration of corticosteroids
  - *Prednisone 2 mg/kg/day with a maximum of 60 mg daily orally (Custer & Rau, 2009)*

Evidence-Based Practice Research: Corticosteroid Use

Retrieved from: http://www.kidney.org/professionals/kdoqi/guidelines_pedbone/guide17.htm (KDOQI, 2005).

Studies do not support the use of corticosteroids, and their use is controversial. Multiple studies both confirm and deny the increase in clinical condition. The use of corticosteroids can lead to depression of growth in children with chronic kidney disease and therefore practitioners are cautioned to use the lowest dose of corticosteroids to maintain kidney function.

- Accurate blood pressure monitoring
- Accurate recording of daily weights
- Accurate recording of intake and output

Chronic Home Care

- Provide equipment for and educate family and patient about home blood pressure monitoring device and parameters.
- Provide family and patient with urine chemistry strips for hematuria and proteinuria.
- Educate family and patient on medication administration and side effects.
- Educate family and patient on possibility of relapse in condition.

Caregiver Education

Emergency Care

- Educate family and patient on need for surgical intervention.
- Educate family and patient on need for hemodialysis.
- Psychosocial support

Acute Hospital Care

- Educate family and patient on medication administration and side effects.
- Incorporate family and patient in assessing need for analgesia.
- Educate family and patient on temporary status of rash.
- Educate family and patient on strict monitoring of vital signs, with emphasis on blood pressure.

Chronic Hospital Care

- Educate family and patient on medication administration and side effects.
- Educate family and patient on careful monitoring of intake and output.

Chronic Home Care

Educate the family and patient on:

- home blood pressure monitoring and parameters of acceptable blood pressures
- monitoring for hematuria/proteinuria
- importance of follow-up
- the fact that HSP has recurrences and when to seek medical attention
- medication administration and side effects

HEMOLYTIC UREMIC SYNDROME

Hemolytic uremic syndrome (HUS) is a disease of unknown etiology, but consists of a triad of symptoms—microangiopathic hemolytic anemia, thrombocytopenia, and acute renal failure (Fiorno, Raffaelli, & Adam, 2006). HUS is diagnosed based on clinical findings and consistent laboratory studies.

- HUS is the most significant complication of infection by *Escherichia coli*, usually serotype O157:H7; however *Streptococcus pneumoniae*, shigella, and salmonella have been implicated in HUS (Kher et al., 2007).
- HUS develops approximately 2 to 14 days after onset of diarrhea.
- HUS typically occurs in children less than 5 years of age and seems to have a seasonal occurrence between summer and fall.

Assessment

Clinical Presentation

- Hematochezia (bloody diarrhea)
- Pallor
- Oliguria or anuria
- Hypertension
- Bruising, purpura, and/or petechiae
- Jaundice
- Edema
- Irritability
- Anorexia
- Seizures

Diagnostic Testing

- Urinalysis: hematuria, proteinuria, cellular casts
- Complete blood count: anemia, thrombocytopenia, mild leukocytosis
- Peripheral smear: schistocytosis, helmet cells
- Reticulocyte count: elevated
- Lactate dehydrogenase (LDH): elevated
  - *This is due to the increased hemolysis of blood cells.*
- Coombs' test: Negative
- Prothrombin and partial thromboplastin: normal
- Blood urea nitrogen (BUN): elevated
- Creatinine: elevated
- Electrolytes: hyperkalemia, hyponatremia, hypocalcemia, hyperphosphatemia
- ANION gap: elevated with metabolic acidosis
- Total bilirubin: elevated

Nursing Interventions

Emergency Care

- Prepare family and patient for possible hemodialysis.
- Prepare family and patient for possible blood transfusion.
- Administer antiepileptic medications for seizure control.
  - *Lorazepam 0.05–0.1 mg/kg/dose every 15 minutes intravenously*
  - *Fosphenytoin 10–20 mg PE/kg intravenously for loading dose*
  - *Fosphenytoin 4–6 mg/kg/day intravenously for maintenance (Custer & Rau, 2009)*
- Obtain appropriate consent for emergency procedures.

Acute Hospital Care

- Provide intravenous fluid hydration using isotonic fluid, paying careful attention to intake and output.
- Transfuse slowly with packed red blood cells as indicated.
- Monitor weight at least once daily.
- Accurately report intake and output.
- Assess meticulously for edema.
- Assess for mental status changes.
- Administer analgesics if necessary, avoiding nonsteroidal anti-inflammatory medications.
  - *Acetaminophen 15 mg/kg/dose every 4 hours orally*
  - *Oxycodone 0.05–0.15 mg/kg/dose every 4–6 hours orally*
  - *Morphine 0.1–0.2 mg/kg/dose every 2–4 hours intravenously (Custer & Rau, 2009)*
- Administer antihypertensives as ordered
  - *Nifedipine 0.25–0.5 mg/kg/dose every 4–6 hours orally or sublingually*
  - *Enalapril 0.1 mg/kg/day divided 1–2 times daily orally (Custer & Rau, 2009)*
- Strict monitoring of vital signs, with emphasis on blood pressure
- Provide family and patient education regarding pathology and procedures.
- Provide family and patient psychosocial support.
- Understand family values and cultural practices and incorporate into the hospital plan of care, if possible.

Chronic Hospital Care

- Monitor fluid and electrolyte status.
- Provide high-calorie, high-carbohydrate, no-added-salt, low-potassium diet.
- Provide enteral feeding if oral intake is inadequate.
- Monitor daily weight.
- Provide skin care for peritoneal or hemodialysis catheter site.
- Provide skin care for possible breakdown related to edema and decreased perfusion.

Chronic Home Care

- Provide home blood pressure monitoring device.
- Educate family and patient on appropriate medication administration and side effects.
- Educate family and patient on nutritional restrictions.
- Provide follow-up appointment dates/times.
- Educate family and patient on monitoring parameters (Siegler & Oakes, 2005).

Complementary and Alternative Therapy

- Plasma exchange may be done in the acute phase.

Caregiver Education

Emergency Care

- Educate family and patient on emergent procedures.

Acute Hospital Care

- Educate family and patient on possible complications of HUS.
- Educate family and patient on medication administration and side effects.
- Educate family and patient on need for accurate intake and output recording.
- Educate family and patient on dietary restrictions.
- Instruct family and patient on appropriate skin care.

Chronic Hospital Care

- Provide information regarding dietary restrictions.
- Educate family and patient on signs of fluid overload.
- Provide instructions on enteral or parenteral nutrition, if needed.
- Educate family and patient on how to provide skin care.

Chronic Home Care

- Educate family and patient on blood pressure monitoring and parameters.
- Instruct family and patient on importance of follow-up care.
- Instruct family and patient on dietary restrictions.
- Instruct family and patient on nonsteroidal medications and avoiding their use.
- Educate family and patient on avoiding the use of antidiarrheals and antibiotics with gastroenteritis-type illnesses.

ACUTE KIDNEY INJURY

Acute kidney injury (AKI), previously known as acute renal failure, is an abrupt cessation of renal function, leading to an inability of the kidney to clear the blood of urea and the inability to regulate fluid and electrolyte balance (Andreoli, 2008).

- AKI is the result of poor renal perfusion or injury; in children this is caused by ischemia, toxicity, nephropathy, and sepsis.
- Volume depletion is still the most common cause of AKI in pediatrics.
- AKI is usually reversible; however, some progress to end-stage renal failure, and the prognosis is dependent on the underlying pathology (Bunchman, 2008).

- Renal replacement therapy (dialysis) is the mainstay of treatment.
  - *Hemodialysis is effective in the acute setting for critically ill patients with fluid overload, intoxication/ingestion, and hyperkalemia. Hemodialysis uses a machine whereby the blood flows through a series of components that act as a filter. In this manner toxins and waste products are removed.*
  - *Peritoneal dialysis is used with chronic renal failure and is delivered intraperitoneally. The peritoneal cavity is filled with a dialysate fluid and retained for a specific length of time, or cycled throughout a time frame. At the end of the time period the fluid is removed via gravity drainage. The dialysate acts as a filter by osmosis, removing toxins and waste products from the body.*
  - *Both hemodialysis and peritoneal dialysis require extensive specialized nursing training.*

Assessment

Clinical Presentation

- History of fluid loss (vomiting, diarrhea, blood loss, burns)
- History of taking nephrotoxic agents (aminoglycosides, intravenous contrast, and nonsteroidal anti-inflammatory medications are common nephrotoxic agents)
- Oliguria/anuria
- Hypertension
- Changes in level of consciousness
- Anemia
- Seizures
- Edema

Diagnostic Testing

- BUN: markedly elevated
- Creatinine: markedly elevated
- Electrolyte: hyperkalemia, hyponatremia, metabolic acidosis
- CBC: anemia
- Urinalysis: may be normal; proteinuria, hematuria
- Stool and blood cultures: identification of an organism for cause and appropriate treatment
- Renal ultrasound: normal or large kidneys
- Electrocardiogram: possible arrhythmias from electrolyte imbalance

Nursing Interventions

Emergency Care

- Intravenous fluid resuscitation with an isotonic fluid if hemodynamically unstable

CLINICAL PEARL

Renal Failure and IV Fluids

Regardless of the degree of renal failure, shock from intravenous depletion must be promptly corrected with intravenous fluid resuscitation.

- Fluid removal with dialysis (peritoneal or hemodialysis) if fluid overload is present
- Prepare family and patient for possible hemodialysis.
- Obtain appropriate consent for emergency procedures.
- Seizure control
  - *Lorazepam 0.05–0.1 mg/kg/dose every 15 minutes intravenously*
  - *Fosphenytoin 10–20 mg PE/kg intravenously for loading dose*
  - *Fosphenytoin 4–6 mg/kg/day intravenously for maintenance (Custer & Rau, 2009)*

CRITICAL COMPONENT

Seizures and Renal Failure

A child presents to the emergency department and is having seizure activity. The child has a past medical history of renal failure. In addition to giving intravenous antiepileptic medications, what other clinical findings are you interested in?

Acute Hospital Care

- Preparation for renal replacement therapy
  - *Peritoneal dialysis*
  - *Hemodialysis*
- Accurate fluid replacement of insensible losses (400 mL/m^2/24 hours)
- Accurate replacement of fluid losses from diarrhea, vomiting, urine production
- Recognition and correction of life-threatening electrolyte imbalances
- Obtaining electrocardiography with electrolyte imbalances
- Accurate administration of antihypertensive medications
  - *Nifedipine 0.25–0.5 mg/kg/dose every 4–6 hours orally or sublingually (Custer & Rau, 2009)*
- Accurate monitoring of vital signs, with emphasis on blood pressure
- Accurate monitoring of intake, output, and weight daily
- Monitoring proper nutritional intake
- Understand family values and cultural practices and incorporate into the hospital plan of care, if possible.

Chronic Hospital Care

- Monitor fluid and electrolyte status.
- Provide adequate calorie through no-added-salt, low-potassium, low-phosphate diet, without fluid excess.
- Provide enteral or parenteral feeding if oral intake is inadequate.
- Monitor daily weight.
- Provide skin care for peritoneal or hemodialysis catheter site.
- Provide skin care for possible breakdown related to edema and decreased perfusion.

Chronic Home Care

- Educate family and patient on home dialysis, if needed.
- Provide home blood pressure monitoring device.

- Educate family and patient on appropriate medication administration and side effects.
- Educate family and patient on nutritional restrictions.
  - *Avoid high-protein diet.*
  - *Appropriate fluid restriction*
  - *Decreased-potassium diet*
  - *Decreased-phosphorus diet*
- Provide follow-up appointment dates/times.
- Educate family and patient on monitoring parameters.

Caregiver Education

Emergency Care

- Educate family and patient on emergent procedures.

Acute Hospital Care

- Educate family and patient on possible complications of AKI.
- Educate family and patient on medication administration and side effects.
- Educate family and patient on need for accurate intake and output recording.
- Educate family and patient on dietary restrictions.
- Instruct family and patient on appropriate skin care.

Chronic Hospital Care

- Provide information regarding dietary restrictions.
- Educate family and patient on signs of fluid overload.
- Provide instructions on enteral or parenteral nutrition, if needed.
- Educate family and patient on how to provide skin care.

Chronic Home Care

- Educate family and patient on blood pressure monitoring and parameters.
- Instruct family and patient on importance of follow-up care.
- Instruct family and patient on dietary restrictions.
- Instruct family and patient on nonsteroidal medications and to avoid their use.

GENITOURINARY ANOMALIES

CRYPTORCHIDISM

Undescended testis is the most common birth disorder of sexual differentiation in males (Kliegman et al., 2007). Thirty percent of premature infant males have undescended testis.

Cryptorchidism is more commonly bilateral (25%) (Thomas, Duffy, & Rickwood, 2008) and most cases resolve spontaneously.

Classification:

Abdominal: nonpalpable

Peeping: abdominal but can be pushed into the upper part of the inguinal canal

Gliding: can be pushed into the scrotum but immediately retracts

Ectopic: perineal or superficial inguinal pouch

Assessment

Clinical Presentation

- Asymmetrical scrotum
- Small-appearing scrotum
- No palpable testis in scrotum

Nursing Interventions

Acute Hospital Care

- If found in newborn care, refer to pediatrician or pediatric urologist
- Consider the possibility of virilization from congenital adrenal hyperplasia in babies with bilateral undescended testes
- If outpatient admission for orchiopexy:
  - *Pain control*
  - *Discharge education*
  - *Follow-up appointment arranged*

Chronic Home Care

- Routine follow-up with pediatrician to track testis descent
- Surgical correction to be done between 6 and 15 months

Complementary and Alternative Therapies

- Hormonal treatment is infrequently used.
  - *Intranasal luteinizing hormone 6 times daily for 3 weeks*
  - *Human chorionic gonadotropin IM 1–2 times weekly for 3 weeks*

> **CLINICAL PEARL — Cryptorchidism and Testicular Cancer**
>
> Men with a history of cryptorchidism are at increased risk for testicular cancer (Thomas et al., 2008).

BLADDER EXSTROPHY

Occurs rarely, 1 in 35,000–40,000 live births (Kliegman et al., 2007). There is a male-to-female ratio of 2:1.

Assessment

Clinical Presentation

- Visible bladder below the umbilicus (Thomas et al., 2008)
- Short, thick penile shaft
- Genitalia may or may not be easily recognizable.
- Usually healthy baby without other anomalies

Nursing Interventions

Acute Hospital Care

- Protect the bladder mucosa with a film wrap to keep the mucosa moist.

> **CLINICAL PEARL**
> **Avoiding Gauze and Petroleum Products**
> Avoid gauze or petroleum products, as these may cause significant mucosal inflammation (Kliegman et al., 2007)

- Prompt surgical correction of the defect
- Transfer to pediatric center with pediatric urology

Chronic Home Care

- Routine follow-up with pediatric urologist

HYPOSPADIAS

A hypospadias is a urethral opening on the ventral surface of the penis (Kliegman et al., 2007). One in 250 male newborns is born with this condition. It is usually an isolated anomaly.

Assessment

Clinical Presentation

- Urethral meatus on the glans penis (glanular), coronal, subcoronal, midpenile, penoscrotal, scrotal, or perianal area (Kliegman et al., 2007)
- Ventral curvature of the penis
- Hooded foreskin (Thomas et al., 2008)
- May have undescended testis
- May have inguinal hernia

Nursing Interventions

Acute Hospital Care

- Avoid circumcision in the newborn period.
- Surgical repair between 6 and 12 months of age
- Transfer to pediatric urologist

Chronic Home Care

- Routine follow-up with pediatric urologist

Review Questions

1. A 4-month-old male infant is admitted with a febrile illness and a urine culture is ordered. The most appropriate way to obtain a urine specimen for culture is
A. voiding midstream collection.
B. bag specimen collection.
C. transurethral catheterization.
D. saturated cotton ball collection from the diaper.

2. A 3-year-old African American male is admitted with facial edema, proteinuria, hypertension, and hypoalbuminemia. Based on these findings, the likely diagnosis is
A. acute postinfectious glomerulonephritis.
B. nephrotic syndrome.
C. hepatorenal syndrome.
D. end-stage renal disease.

3. The appropriate medical treatment for the patient in question 2 is
A. Ceftriaxone 50 mg/kg/day intravenously.
B. Prednisone 2 mg/kg/ day orally.
C. 20 mL/kg intravenous crystalloid intravenous fluids.
D. 5 mL/kg blood transfusion intravenously.

4. A 10-year-old Caucasian male is admitted for acute postinfectious glomerulonephritis (APIGN). His family asks you if not taking all his medications for a preceding streptococcal pharyngitis caused this illness. The nurse's best response is to
A. explain that not finishing a complete course of antibiotics is not directly related to acquiring APIGN.
B. note that APIGN has nothing to do with preceding illnesses.
C. explain that by not finishing the complete course of antibiotics, the child was placed at greater risk for acquiring APIGN.
D. explain that the reason for completing a full course of antibiotics is to prevent APIGN.

5. A 4-year-old child is admitted with Henoch–Schönlein purpura. His blood pressure is 154/87, his urine output is 0.2 cc/k/h over the past 12 hours, and he appears edematous. The nurse recognizes which of the following?
A. Elevated blood pressure related to his abdominal pain
B. Hemodynamic instability related to his gastrointestinal losses
C. Acute renal failure related to vasculitis
D. Normal course for Henoch–Schönlein purpura

6. A 4-year-old child with Henoch–Schönlein purpura is being discharged. The discharge education should include
A. accurate blood pressure monitoring.
B. a low-phosphorus diet as tolerated.
C. instructions on pneumonia as a complication.
D. follow-up routine complete blood count checks with primary care provider.

7. Which of the following is NOT a characteristic of hemolytic uremic syndrome?
A. Thrombocytopenia
B. Hemolytic anemia
C. Hypertension
D. Acute renal failure

8. The most common preceding pathogen in hemolytic uremic syndrome is
A. *Streptococcus pneumoniae.*
B. beta-hemolytic streptococcus.
C. *Escherichia coli* 0157:H7.
D. *Salmonella typhi.*

9. A 2-year-old male has his first urinary tract infection. After completion of 2 days of intravenous antibiotics, he is switched to an oral antibiotic. In explaining the discharge education, the nurse should stress the importance of
  A. proper nutrition.
  B. completion of entire course of antibiotics.
  C. adequate hydration.
  D. avoiding sick contacts while finishing antibiotics.

10. The appropriate studies for the 2-year-old male with his first urinary tract infection are
  A. ultrasound of the kidneys and bladder.
  B. CT scan of the abdomen and pelvis.
  C. MRI of the abdomen and pelvis.
  D. acute abdominal series x-rays.

References

American Academy of Pediatrics, Committee on Quality Improvement, Subcommittee on Urinary Tract Infection. Practice parameter: the diagnosis, treatment, and evaluation of the initial urinary tract infection in febrile infants and young children. (published corrections appear in *Pediatrics*: 1999;103(5, pt 1): 1052; 1999;104(1, pt 1):118; and 2000;105(1, pt 1): 141). *Pediatrics*. 1999;103(4, pt 1):843-852.

American Academy of Pediatrics Clinical Practice Guideline. (2011). Urinary tract infection: Clinical Practice Guideline for the Diagnosis and Management of the Initial UTI in Febrile Infants and Children 2 to 24 months. *Pediatrics, 128*, 595–610. doi: 10.1542/peds. 2011-1330.

Andreoli, S. P. (2008). Management of acute kidney injury in children: A guide for pediatricians. *Pediatric Drugs, 10*, 379–390. doi: 10.2165/0148581-200810060-00005

Betz, C. L., & Sowden, L. A. (2008). *Mosby's pediatric nursing reference* (6th ed.). St. Louis, MO: Mosby.

Bunchman, T. (2008). Treatment of acute kidney injury in children: From conservative management to renal replacement therapy. *Nature Clinical Practice Nephrology, 4*, 510–514. doi: 10.1038/ncpneph0924

Cameron, M. A., Sakhaee, K., & Moe, O. W. (2005). Nephrolithiasis in children. *Pediatric Nephrology, 20*, 1587–1592. doi: 10.1007/s00467-005-1883-z

Committee on Quality Improvement. (1999). Practice parameter: The diagnosis, treatment and evaluation of the initial urinary tract infection in febrile infants and young children. *Pediatrics, 103*, 843–852. Retrieved from http://pednephrology.stanford.edu

Custer, J., & Rau, R. (2009). *The Harriet Lane handbook* (18th ed.). Philadelphia: Elsevier Mosby.

Delaune, S., & Ladner, P. (2002). *Fundamentals of nursing standards and practice* (2nd ed.). Clifton Park, NY: Delmar.

Field, L., & Mattoo, T. (2010). *Pediatrics in Review, 31*, 451–463.

Fiorno, E. K., Raffaelli, R. M., & Adam, H. M. (2006). Hemolytic-uremic syndrome. *Pediatrics in Review, 27*, 398–399. doi: 10.1542/pir.27-10-398

Ilyas, M., & Tolaymat, A. (2008). Changing epidemiology of acute post-streptococcal glomerulonephritis in Northeast Florida: A comparative study. *Pediatric Nephrology, 23*, 1101–1106. doi: 10.1007/s00467-008-0778-1

Kidney Disease Outcomes Quality Initiatives. (2005). Clinical practice guidelines for bone metabolism and disease in children with chronic kidney disease. Retrieved from: http://www.kidney.org/professionals/kdoqi/guidelines_pedbone/guide17.htm

Kher, K. K., Schnaper, H. W., & Makker, S. P. (Eds.). (2007). *Clinical pediatric nephrology* (2nd ed.). Abingdon, UK: Informa Healthcare.

Kliegman, R., Behrman, R., Jenson, H., & Stanton, B. (2007). *Nelson textbook of pediatrics* (18th ed.). Philadelphia: Saunders.

Lim, R. (2009). Vesicoureteral reflux and urinary tract infection: Evolving practices and current controversies in pediatric imaging. *American Journal of Roentgenology, 192*, 1197–1208. doi: 10.2214/AJR.08.2187

Martins, G., Soler, Z., Batigalia, F., & Moore, K. (2009). Clean intermittent catheterization educational booklet directed to caregivers of children with neurogenic bladder dysfunction. *Journal of Wound Ostomy Continence Nursing, 36*, 545–549. doi: 10.1097/WON.0b013e3181b41301

Moore, K. N., Fader, M., & Getliffe, K. (2007). Long-term bladder management by intermittent catheterisation in adults and children. *Cochrane Database of Systematic Reviews, 4*. doi: 10.1002/14651858.CD006008

Pennesi, M., Travan, L., Peratoner, L., Bordugo, A., Cattaneo, A., Ronfani, L., & Ventura, A. (2008). Is antibiotic prophylaxis in children with vesicoureteral reflux effective in preventing pyelonephritis and renal scars? A randomized, controlled trial. *Pediatrics, 121*, 1489–1494. doi: 10.1542/peds.2007-2652

Prajapati, B. S., Prajapati, R. B., & Patel, P. S. (2008). Advances in management of urinary tract infections. *Indian Journal of Pediatrics, 75*, 809–814. doi: 10.1007/s12098-008-0152-0

Reddy, P. P., & Minevich, E. (2007). Renal calculus disease. *The Kelalis-King-Belman textbook of clinical pediatric urology* (5th ed.). Abingdon, UK: Informa Healthcare.

Siegler, R., & Oakes, R. (2005). Hemolytic uremic syndrome; pathogenesis, treatment, and outcome. *Current Opinion in Pediatrics, 17*, 200–204. doi: 10.1097/01.mop.0000152997.66070.e9

Thomas, D., Duffy, P., & Rickwood, A. (Eds.). (2008). *Essentials of paediatric urology* (2nd ed.). London, UK: Informa Healthcare.

Vining, E. (2008). Long-term health consequences of epilepsy diet treatments. *Epilepsia, 49*, 27–29. doi: 10.1111/j.1528-1167.2008.01828.x

Webb, N. J., & Postlethwaite, R. J. (Eds.). (2003). *Clinical pediatric nephrology* (3rd ed.). New York: Oxford University Press.

Zaidi, M., Singh, N., Kamran, M., Ansai, N., Nasr, S. H., & Acharya, A. (2008). Acute onset of hematuria and proteinuria associated with multiorgan involvement of the heart, liver, pancreas, kidneys, and skin in a patient with Henoch-Schönlein purpura. *Kidney International, 73*, 502–508. doi: 10.1038/sj.ki.5002662

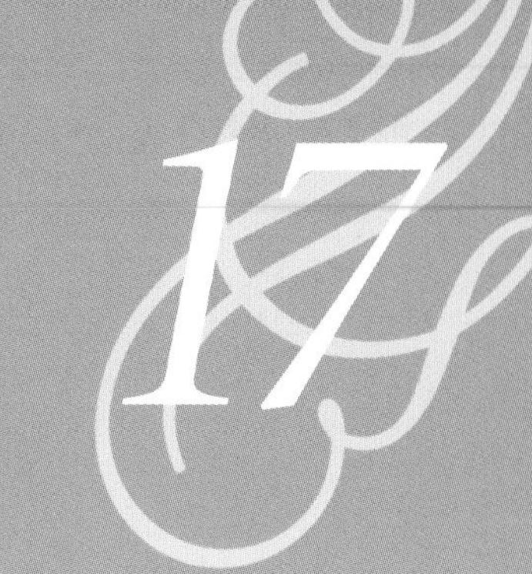

17 Endocrine Disorders

Kelly J. Betts, MSN Ed, RN

OBJECTIVES

- ☐ Define key terms.
- ☐ Identify the anatomy and physiology of the endocrine system.
- ☐ Identify areas of focus for performing an age-appropriate endocrine assessment.
- ☐ Identify clinical manifestations of various endocrine disorders.
- ☐ Recognize diagnostic and laboratory findings of patients with endocrine disorders.
- ☐ Describe nursing interventions for the emergency care of patients with endocrine disorders.
- ☐ Describe nursing interventions for the acute and chronic care of the patient with endocrine disorders.
- ☐ Integrate home-care concepts into nursing interventions for the patient with an endocrine disorder.
- ☐ Identify possible alternative therapy interventions for patients with endocrine disorders.
- ☐ Develop a family teaching plan that will optimize therapy outcomes for patients with endocrine disorders.
- ☐ Utilize critical thinking concepts to evaluate care of the patient with an endocrine disorder.

KEY TERMS

- Hormone
- Positive feedback
- Negative feedback
- Pituitary gland
- Growth charts
- Body mass index (BMI)
- Premature thelarche
- Growth velocity
- Premature adrenarche
- Goiter
- Thyroid storm
- Ambiguous genitalia
- Polydipsia
- Polyuria
- Polyphagia
- Diabetic ketoacidosis
- Acanthosis nigricans

ANATOMY AND PHYSIOLOGY

- The endocrine system regulates growth and development; energy use and storage; levels of glucose, fluid, and sodium in the bloodstream; sexual development; and the child's response to stress (Ward & Hisley, 2009).
- Comprised of organs that produce and secrete hormones (**Figure 17-1**)
- **Hormones** are chemicals produced by the endocrine glands and circulated in the bloodstream to another part of the body. They activate or inhibit cells in the target organs, and act as messengers.
- Two types of hormones
  - *Protein hormone from amino acids*
  - *Steroid hormones from fat*
- **Positive feedback**—when hormone levels fall, the hypothalamus secretes releasing hormone that stimulates the pituitary gland to release stimulating hormone that then affects the target organ (**Figure 17-2**).
- **Negative feedback**—when hormone levels are too high, the hypothalamus secretes inhibitory hormones that stimulate the pituitary gland to release inhibitory factors.

Glands of the Endocrine System

Hypothalamus

- Located at the base of the brain
- Sends messages from the autonomic nervous system to the target organs (Ward & Hisley, 2009)
- Instructs the master gland (**pituitary gland**) through the secretion of releasing or inhibitory hormones
  - *Thyroid-releasing hormone (TRH)*
  - *Corticotropin-releasing hormone (CRH)*
  - *Luteinizing-hormone-releasing hormone (LHRH)*

Don't have time to read this chapter? Want to reinforce your reading? Need to review for a test? Listen to this chapter on DavisPlus at davispl.us/rudd1.

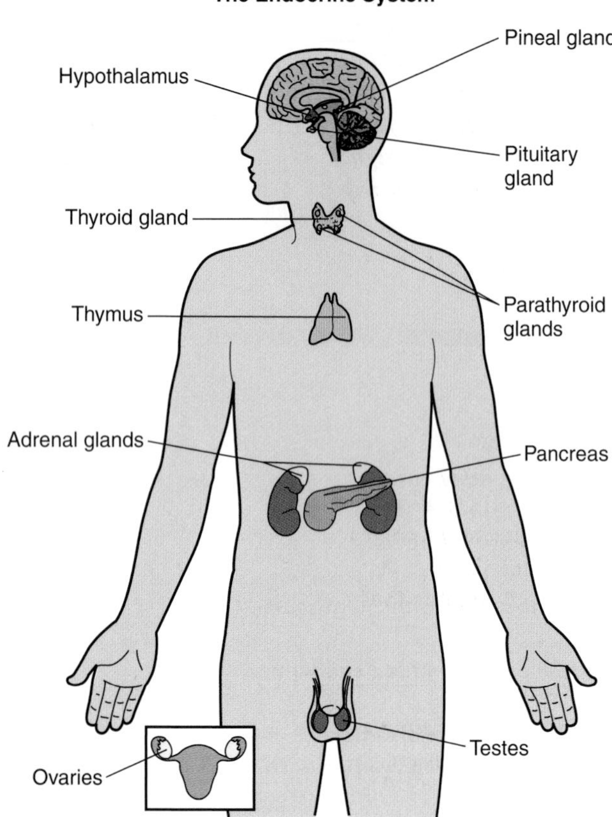

Figure 17–1 The endocrine system.

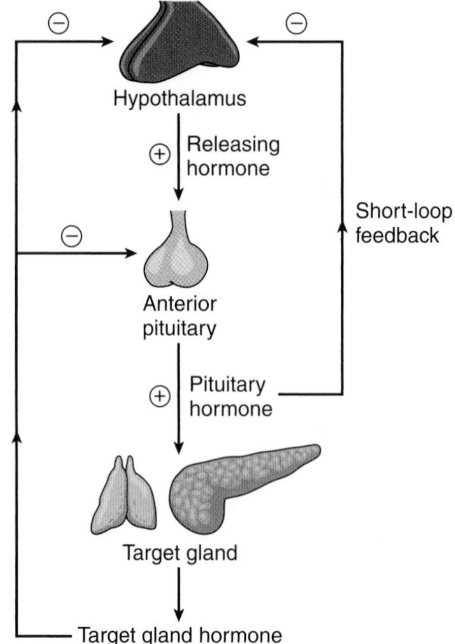

Figure 17–2 Feedback system from the pituitary to the target glands.

- *Growth-hormone-releasing hormone (GHRH)*
- *Somatostatin—stimulates the pituitary gland to stop the release of growth hormone*

Pituitary Gland (Hypophysis)

- Master gland
- Located beneath the hypothalamus in the base of the brain
- Controls other glands through stimulating hormones or inhibitory factors that turn the target glands on or off
- Two main lobes
  - *Anterior lobe (adenohypophysis)—secretes the following:*
    - Growth hormone (GH)—stimulates growth of cells; stimulates protein synthesis and prevents protein breakdown
    - Thyroid-stimulating hormone—stimulates the thyroid glands to make thyroid hormones
    - Adrenocorticotrophic hormone (ACTH)—stimulates the cortex of the adrenal glands to make cortisone
    - Prolactin—stimulates milk production in the mammary glands of females
    - Follicle-stimulating hormone (FSH)—stimulates the ovaries to develop eggs within the follicles of the ovaries
    - Luteinizing hormone (LH)—stimulates the follicles in the ovaries to rupture and release the egg and corpus luteum production in females; stimulates testosterone production in males
    - Melanocyte-stimulating hormone (MSH)—stimulates melanin synthesis and release from skin and hair
  - *Posterior lobe (neurohypophysis)—secretes the following:*
    - Antidiuretic hormone (ADH) (Vasopressin)—stimulates the kidneys to absorb and conserve water, increasing blood volume
    - Oxytocin (Pitocin)—stimulates smooth muscle contraction, milk letdown reflex, and the expulsion of the fetus and placenta

Pineal Body

- Located in the middle of the brain
- Stimulated by light exposure through the optic nerve
- Secretes the hormone melatonin
- Regulates wake–sleep cycles, circadian rhythms

Thymus

- Located in the anterior ventral aspect of chest at the base of the heart
- Atrophies with age
- Responsible for cellular immunity

Thyroid Gland

- Two lobes in anterior neck region below the larynx
- Produce T3 and T4 in response to TSH from pituitary gland
  - *T3—tri-iodothyronine active*
  - *T4—tyroxine*
- Responsible for synthesis of protein and cholesterol, glucose metabolism, heat production, growth and development, and metabolism
- Calcitonin—stimulates bone construction, thereby inhibiting calcium release from the bones and decreasing calcium blood levels

Parathyroid Glands

- Four glands, two on each side of thyroid gland
- Produce parathyroid hormone
  - *Increases calcium concentration in the bloodstream by stimulating the osteoclasts in the bone to release calcium*
  - *Increases serum calcium levels by increasing the absorption of calcium from the gastrointestinal tract; increases calcium reabsorption in the kidneys*
  - *Increases phosphate release from bones increasing blood levels; inhibits phosphate reabsorption in kidneys so that more phosphate is excreted*

Adrenal Glands

- Located on top of the kidneys
- Two parts: cortex and medulla
  - *Cortex produces steroids, hormones made from cholesterol*
    - Glucocortiocoids—mainly cortisone, which increases blood sugar, decreases inflammation, and aids in stress reduction
    - Mineralocorticoids (Aldosterone)—secreted in response to renin-angiotensin to conserve water as well as retain sodium
  - *Medulla*
    - Adrenaline (epinephrine)—fight-or-flight response; increases heart rate, respiratory rate; dilates pupils; increases utilization of glucose; suppresses digestion and immune system
    - Norepinephrine—fight-or-flight response (same as above)
    - Dopamine—increases blood pressure

Pancreas

- Has both exocrine (with ducts) and endocrine function
  - *Exocrine—secretes amylase, lipase, trypsin for small intestine digestion*
  - *Endocrine—islet of Langerhans*
    - Beta cells secrete insulin, which forces glucose into the cells and stimulates glycogen formation; independent of pituitary control; stimulated by the ingestion of glucose.
    - Alpha cells work in the opposite manner as insulin; they break down glycogen in liver to increase blood sugar.

Sex Glands (Gonads)

Testes

- Testes—produce androgens, mainly testosterone, in interstitial cells when stimulated by FSH and LH
  - *Testosterone produces secondary sex characteristics in males, sperm formation, and sex drive.*

Ovaries and Uterus

- Ovaries—produce estrogen and follicle cells
  - *Estrogen produces secondary sex characteristics in females and mammary development.*
  - *Follicle cells produce corpus luteum (meaning "yellow body"), which makes the hormone progesterone after the egg leaves the follicle.*
    - Progesterone maintains pregnancy by relaxing the uterus and stimulates milk production in the mammary glands.
- Ovaries and uterus while pregnant:
  - *Produce relaxin, which is a hormone that relaxes the cervix, vagina, and ligaments around the birth canal in preparation for the delivery of a fetus*
  - *Human chorionic gonadotropin (HCG) hormone is produced during pregnancy by the developing embryo; it inhibits immune response to the developing fetus.*

ASSESSMENT

General History

Prenatal/Birth History

- Prenatal care
- Type of delivery
- Estimate of gestational age
- Complications of pregnancy or delivery
- Substance abuse
- Neonatal complications

Hospitalizations

- Overnight stays
- Surgeries—type and recovery time
- Accidents or injuries

Current Medications

- Prescribed
- Over the counter (OTC)
- Dietary supplements
- Alternative/natural remedies

Allergies

- Medications
- Seasonal
- Foods/other

Immunizations

- Current/missed doses/due dates

Family History

- Endocrine disorders
- Extreme short stature
- Parental heights/sibling heights
- History of other chronic disease

Developmental History

- Age of developmental milestones
- School performance
- History of behavioral problems

Nutrition

- Type of infant feeding (breast or formula)
- Types of food preferred
- Diet history—2 to 3 days
- Eating patterns
- Type/frequency of fast-food consumption

- Amount of milk consumed per day
- Any eating-related vomiting/gastrointestinal (GI) distress
- Problems with chewing, swallowing, eating, or drinking

Activities

- Daily activities—type, quantity, how often
- Physical activity in school/team sports
- Number of TV/computer/video game hours per day

Physical Examination

Review of Systems

- Basic head-to-toe physical assessment of normal versus abnormal findings

Weight

- Infant weight without diaper on infant scale
- Minimal clothing for other children
- Scales should be calibrated for accuracy before weighing

Height

- Supine measurement for infants until age 24 months
- Children over 24 months should be measured using a stadiometer (scales with measuring arms not recommended).
- While using a stadiometer, take the child's shoes off and make sure the child is standing with feet together, heels against the wall, and standing straight with the hands down to the side. Girls with ponytails should take their hair down (Lipman, Euler, Markowitz, & Ratcliffe, 2009).

Head Circumference

- Obtained using a measuring tape until age 36 months unless otherwise indicated by physician
- Level of fontanels should be assessed in infants.

Vital Signs

- See vital sign parameters in Chapter 7.

Tanner Stage of Puberty

- Refer to Tanner Staging Chart in Chapter 10.
- Assess for signs of ambiguous genitalia and abnormal advancement in puberty (Horner, 2007).

Height and Weight

- Careful and accurate plotting of height, weight, and head circumference on **growth chart** (Lipman et al., 2009)
- Body surface area (BSA; refer to Chapter 10)
- Mid-parental height (MPH)/target height (TH)
  - *Mother's height (inches) × father's height (inches) divided by 2 = Mid-parental height. To get the target height, add 2.5 inches for boys and subtract 2.5 inches for girls.*
- **Body mass index (BMI)** (Ball, Bindler, & Cowen, 2010):

$$\frac{\text{(Weight in kg)}}{\text{(Height in cm divided by 100)}^2} \text{ OR } \frac{\text{(Weight in kg)}}{\text{(Height in meters)}^2}$$

- Height velocity
  - *Number of centimeters (cm) or inches (in) growth per year*

Skin

- Assess skin for any unusual areas of skin discoloration or areas of increased skin pigmentation.

Body Odor

- Assess for unusual smells (e.g., musty, cheesy, sweet).

Neck

- Assess neck for the presence of any enlarged areas, nodules, or glands.

Muscles

- Assess strength and muscle tone. Note excess fat accumulation or decrease in muscle mass.

Facial Characteristics

- Assess the face for any unusual facial features such as a protuberant tongue, bulging of the eyes, excessive hair growth, or excessive roundness of the face.

HYPOPITUITARISM (GROWTH HORMONE DEFICIENCY)

Assessment

Clinical Presentation

- Delayed growth <2 inches (3–4 cm) per year
- Consistent declination of growth measurements on the growth chart over a period of time
- In infants, delayed closure of the anterior fontanel
- Delayed dental eruption
- Greater weight-to-height ratio with increased abdominal fat
- Decreased muscle mass
- Cherubic-like appearance or appears to be younger than actual age
- Delayed puberty during the adolescent period
- High-pitched voice

Promoting Safety

Frequent or recurrent hypoglycemia, prolonged jaundice, and small penis/testes in the neonatal period may indicate the possibility of congenital hypopituitarism. Infants with this condition are started on growth hormone replacement therapy immediately to help regulate blood sugar levels. This type of neonatal hypoglycemia can be fatal if not treated immediately upon diagnosis. These infants undergo further testing to find out if there are other pituitary hormone deficiencies that need to be treated (Ward & Hisley, 2009).

Diagnostic Testing

- Thorough review of growth plots on a growth chart to determine the rate of growth per year; special attention is given to those children whose growth is less than the 3rd percentile.
- Biological parental heights are calculated to determine the mid-parental height of the parents or the average. This is used as an estimate only.
- Bone age x-ray of the left hand and wrist—this determines the actual age of the bones in comparison to the child's actual (chronological) age. If the bone age is > 2 SD scores below normal, further evaluation is done (Alt et al., 2003).
- Magnetic resonance imaging (MRI) of the head, with a focus on the pituitary gland, to look for any abnormalities of the gland or absence of the gland
- Baseline blood tests such as cortisol, complete blood count (CBC), and electrolytes
- Provocative growth hormone testing—this test utilizes certain medications that stimulate the pituitary gland to make growth hormone (Ball et al. 2010).

CRITICAL COMPONENT

Growth Hormone Secretion

It is important to remember that growth hormone is secreted in pulsatile spurts during a 24-hour period and is not constant. A single lab measurement of growth hormone is not indicative of growth hormone deficiency.

- Insulin-like growth factor 1 (IGF-1) and insulin-like growth factor binding protein 3 (IGFBP3) to test for growth hormone deficiency
- Karyotype in girls to rule out Turner syndrome
- Thyroid function test to detect hypothyroidism
- ACTH and cortisol levels to detect if patient has any other hormone deficiencies
- Urine creatinine, pH, specific gravity, blood urea nitrogen (BUN), and electrolytes to detect possibility of short stature being caused by chronic renal failure
- CBC and sedimentation rate to rule out any inflammatory bowel disease
- Antigliadin antibodies to screen for celiac disease

Evidence-Based Practice Research: Accurate Measurement of Height

Lipman, T. H., Hench, K. D., Benyi, T., Delaune, J., Gilluly, K. A., Johnson, L., . . . Weber, C. (2004). A multicentre randomized controlled trial of an intervention to improve the accuracy of linear growth measurement. *Archives of Disease in Childhood, 89,* 342–346. doi: 10.1136/adc.2003.030072

Accurate height measurements are crucial to obtaining accurate height progression on a growth chart. The child should be measured with his or her shoes off and a measuring device known as a stadiometer should be used for accurate measurements. Children should be measured at every well- and sick-child visit to the pediatrician or family practitioner. Height should also be documented on an age-appropriate growth chart so that trends in growth can be assessed.

Nursing Interventions

- Careful measurement and documentation of growth on the child's age- and sex-appropriate growth chart, noting any declining trends in the child's growth patterns over a 6-month to 1-year period
- Assess for any psychosocial clues that the child or parents are having trouble dealing with the child's stature.
- Educate the patient and parents regarding the disease process of growth hormone deficiency (GHD), including the causes, diagnostic testing methods, and medical treatments available.
- Educate the family regarding the medications administered for the treatment of GHD and the potential side effects of the medication.
- Growth hormone replacement therapy is a medical regimen that is administered in the home setting. Follow-up with the endocrinologist every 3 to 4 months is crucial for assessing response to therapy.

Caregiver Education

- Provide detailed instructions regarding the administration of growth hormone replacement therapy.
- Provide the parents with educational and online resources and support groups.
  - *The Human Growth Foundation (http://www.hgfound.org)*
  - *The Magic Foundation (http://www.magicfoundation.org)*
- Stress the importance of medication compliance and clinic follow-up appointments with the endocrinologist every 3 to 4 months to ensure patient is responding to therapy.
- Educate the parent regarding the side effects of Somatropin and when to contact the physician with concerns.

Medication

Growth Hormone Replacement Therapy

Growth hormone replacement therapy consists of the child receiving daily subcutaneous injections of manufactured growth hormone called Somatropin. As with many medications, several manufacturers have developed growth hormone with different trade names. Some of these names include Genotropin®, Nutropin®, Humatrope®, TevTropin®, and Norditropin®. These derivatives of growth hormone lack one amino acid in being identical to human growth hormone. Somatropin is dosed differently depending on the manufacturer, but recommended doses start at 0.3 mg/kg/week. As with insulin, growth hormone is available in vials that have to be reconstituted, pen devices that contain cartridges, and needleless injection devices. Some of the side effects include achiness in the joints and muscles, particularly the knees, ankles, and wrists, and headache. If side effects occur, the physician may decrease the starting dose and increase the dose slowly until the side effects resolve (Deglin & Vallerand, 2007).

HYPERPITUITARISM (GROWTH HORMONE EXCESS)

Assessment

Clinical Presentation

- The excess secretion of growth hormone from the pituitary gland causes excessive growth rates in children; however, the condition is rare.
- If the patient has precocious puberty in conjunction with hyperpituitarism, the cause may be related to a tumor on or near the hypothalamus or pituitary gland.
- Once the closure of the epiphyseal plates occurs and hyperpituitarism continues, overgrowth of the bones occurs. This is referred to as acromegaly.
- Enlargement of the hands and feet and coarseness of facial features, including the forehead, nose, lips, tongue, and jaw, are common. Other symptoms may include generalized muscle weakness and pain in the muscles and joints

Diagnostic Testing

- Early identification is essential. Monitoring growth charts for excessive growth spurts or consistent growth above the 95th percentile is warranted. It should also be noted that an estimated mid-parental height that is greater than 2 standard deviation (SD) scores above normal should be monitored.
- IGF-1 levels will be elevated with hyperpituitarism.
- Radiological testing such as a bone age x-ray will depict advancement of bone growth.
- An MRI may be necessary to evaluate the hypothalamus and pituitary gland to rule out a growth-hormone-producing or other type of tumor.

Nursing Interventions

- Nursing care should focus on accurate assessment of growth trends by carefully documenting height and weight on the appropriate growth chart.
- Physical assessment is important to evaluate for early physical signs of excess bone growth characteristics and other features of gigantism.
- Evaluation of laboratory values indicative of hyperpituitary function is essential.
- If surgery is indicated for the patient, preoperative and postoperative nursing interventions such as neurological assessment, vital signs, wound assessment, and dressing care and assessment for potential complications are important.
- Follow-up home-care may be indicated depending on the status of the patient after surgical intervention. The nurse should take responsibility to refer the patient/family to a home-care provider.

Caregiver Education

- Focus on educating patients and families about the disorder, treatment options, psychosocial support, and surgical preparation if indicated.
- Patient and family education regarding home medications such as somatostatin analogs, dopamine agonists, and GH receptor antagonist.
- Promotion of medication compliance
- Focus on long-term complications of noncompliance, such as hypertension, cardiomegaly, subsequent cardiovascular disease, diabetes mellitus, osteoarthritis, sleep apnea, and early death.

DIABETES INSIPIDUS

- Antidiuretic hormone (ADH) is stored in the posterior pituitary gland.
- Insufficient production of ADH
- ADH acts on kidneys to restore water and control the amount of urine that is excreted by the kidneys.
- Two forms:
  - *Central (or neurogenic) diabetes insipidus (DI)—the production of ADH is insufficient.*
  - *Nephrogenic diabetes insipidus—occurs when the kidneys fail to respond to appropriate levels of ADH.*
  - *Both forms of DI can have an abrupt onset and have similar manifestations.*

Assessment

Clinical Presentation

- Central (neurogenic) DI:
  - *Polyuria, polydipsia, enuresis*
  - *Getting up to drink water throughout the night*
  - *Irritability in infants that can only be relieved by giving water instead of formula or breast milk*
  - *Constipation, fever, dehydration, and hypernatremia*
- Nephrogenic DI:
  - *Polyuria, polydipsia*
  - *Hypernatremia in the neonatal period*
  - *Dilute urine, vomiting, dehydration*
  - *Fever and possible changes in mental status*

CRITICAL COMPONENT

Dehydration

Dehydration is a critical effect of diabetes insipidus in children. Severe dehydration can occur very quickly in infants and smaller children, thus the need to increase fluids as soon as possible during exacerbation. The nurse must be able to recognize signs and symptoms of dehydration, such as dry mucous membranes, sunken fontanel in infants, tachycardia, decreased tears when crying, and decreased skin turgor. Severe dehydration can lead to hypovolemic shock. The administration of IV fluids is essential to treat severe dehydration, especially when the child can't tolerate liquid intake (Suddaby & Mowery, 2007).

Diagnostic Testing

- 24-hour urine collection for daily output
- Serum sodium is elevated (greater than 150–170 mEq/L) (Ward & Hisley, 2009).
- Urine osmolality is decreased (less than 300 mOsm/L).
- Urine specific gravity is decreased (less than 1.005).
- Urine-to-serum osmolarity ratio is less than 1 (Ball et al., 2010)

Evidence-Based Practice Research: Water Deprivation Test

Alt, P., Babler, E. K., Betts, K. J., Carney, P. H. , Courtney, J. A., Flores, B. M. . . . Worley, D. D. (2003). *Clinical handbook of pediatric endocrinology*. St. Louis, MO: Quality Medical Publishing.

Styne, D. M. (2004). *Core handbook in pediatrics: Pediatric endocrinology*. Philadelphia: Lippincott Williams & Wilkins.

Water deprivation testing is performed to diagnosis diabetes insipidus. The patient is under direct supervision by the nurse while the nurse carefully monitors vital signs and weight. Urine and blood are collected early in the day and tested for osmolarity and electrolytes. Then the child is deprived from intake of water until significant dehydration occurs. The child is weighed every 2 hours until 2% to 5% of body weight is lost. Urine specific gravity is monitored every hour. This test is stopped once the urine specific gravity reaches 1.014 or higher. The testing should never last more than 4 hours for an infant and 7 hours for a child. During the test, vital signs are carefully monitored for signs of hypotension and fever.

Nursing Interventions

- Recognition of the differences between central (neurogenic) and nephrogenic DI is essential in order to assess and make decisions regarding the appropriate nursing care of the patient.
- Acute hospital care includes nursing responsibility related to the diagnostic water deprivation test, such as vital signs, getting weights, collecting blood and urine samples, and careful assessment for signs and symptoms of dehydration.
- The nurse is responsible for administration and education regarding the use of medications to treat the two types of DI.
- Accurate intake and output should be monitored at all times.

Caregiver Education

- Emergency care involves teaching the parents about the signs and symptoms of dehydration and the need to take the child to the hospital for intravenous fluid replacement.
- During the initial states of exacerbation, it is important to teach the parents and child to increase fluids until the medication begins to take effect.
- Chronic home care involves teaching the parents of the child with DI the importance of medication compliance and the correct way to administer the medications, as DI is a lifelong condition that will require long-term use of medications for treatment.
- It is also important for the nurse to educate the parents regarding the importance of making the child's school aware of the condition so that appropriate care can be provided at school.
- The parents should provide the child with an emergency alert bracelet and the bracelet should be worn at all times by the infant or child.

Medication

Types of Diabetes Insipidus Medications

Central DI medications include Vasopressin analogs such as DDAVP. This medication is usually given intranasal, but can be given orally or SQ. Diuretics may also be used to treat central DI to decrease urine volume as much as 75% (Ward & Hisley, 2009). The medications used to treat nephrogenic DI are diuretics, such as Midamor. Midamor is potassium sparing. In addition to diuretics, nonsteriodal prostaglandins such as Indocin may be used.

CRITICAL COMPONENT

Vasopressin

Vasopressin (DDAVP) cannot effectively treat nephrogenic DI because the kidney is unresponsive to the mechanism of action of the drug, thus making it very important to diagnosis the correct type of diabetes insipidus.

CLINICAL PEARL

Intranasal Medications

Tips regarding the administration of intranasal medications:

- Have the child blow his or her nose before the administration of the medication.
- In infants, clear the nose with a bulb syringe before administering the medication.
- Positioning when the child or infant is given the medication can enhance the absorption of the medication.
- Infants and children with colds or severe congestion should receive an alternate route of the medication, as this congestion interferes with its absorption.

SYNDROME OF INAPPROPRIATE ANTIDIURETIC HORMONE (SIADH)

- Excessive amounts of ADH are produced.
- The kidneys are unable to conserve appropriate amounts of water.
- The body retains water, leading to water intoxication, hyponatremia, and cellular edema.

Assessment

Clinical Presentation

- SIADH is very closely associated with children who have encountered infections of the central nervous system (CNS) or intrathoracic disease, and may occur in postoperative patients.
- The signs and symptoms may have varying degrees of seriousness.
- Excessive SIADH may include nausea, vomiting, seizures, and personality changes such as irritability, combativeness, hallucinations, and confusion, leading to stupor and coma (Ward & Hisley, 2009).
- Other signs may include increased blood pressure, neck vein distension, crackles heard on lung examination, weight gain with no external visible edema, decreased urine output despite a high urine specific gravity, and low sodium levels.

Diagnostic Testing

- Serum laboratory levels are monitored and diagnosis is confirmed when the laboratory levels present the following results:
  - *High urine osmolarity (>1200 Osmol/kg)*
  - *High urine specific gravity (>1.030)*
  - *Low serum osmolarity (<275 mOsmol/kg)*
  - *Low serum sodium (<125 mEq/L)*
  - *Decreased BUN (<10mg/dL)*
  - *Decreased hematocrit*

Nursing Interventions

- Fluid restriction is essential for a child with SIADH. The fluid restriction protocol may begin with restricting 75% of fluid maintenance and decreasing the fluids to half of maintenance if there is no improvement in 4 to 6 hours.
- Emergency management of severe SIADH may include the administration of a hypertonic sodium chloride solution, especially if hyponatremia is severe and neurological disease is present.
- If adrenal insufficiency is present, corticosteroids will be administered according to stress dosing protocols.
- Very detailed intake and output must be monitored by the nurse. All routes of fluid administration must be accounted for. Careful attention must be paid to those children old enough to reach water fountains or toilets.
- Strict diaper weights must be obtained in infants.
- Medications should be given during the meal so that additional fluid intake is not needed when administering medications.
- Irrigate all feeding tubes with normal saline as opposed to water to prevent the pulling of sodium from the body.
- A diet high in sodium and protein should be encouraged.
- Neurological assessment is crucial for patients with SIADH, as decreased sodium levels can cause altered level of consciousness (LOC) that may lead to seizures.
- Seizure precautions at the bedside should be employed and documented on the patient's chart.

Caregiver Education

- Emergency patient/family education should consist of teaching how to recognize the signs and symptoms of sodium depletion, such as weight gain, altered LOC, confusion, complaints of headache, and irritability. The parents should be taught to take the child to the emergency room or call for emergency assistance.
- Education regarding the importance of fluid balance is essential. The child and parents/family should be taught to carefully assess intake and output, such as fluid restriction, using diaper weights, and urinals or "toilet hats" to monitor output. Careful consideration must be taken to teach patients and family about hidden water in food sources such as popsicles. Encouraging a diet high in sodium and protein is also indicated.
- Encourage the patient to wear a medical alert bracelet.

> **CRITICAL COMPONENT**
>
> **Low Sodium and Risk for Seizure**
>
> Low sodium levels less than 125 mEq/L may cause seizure activity in children with SIADH. Sodium levels should be as near to normal as possible; this is the primary goal of treatment. The pediatric nurse must be very thorough in keeping accurate track of intake, output, and daily weights of the child (Ward & Hisley, 2009).

PRECOCIOUS PUBERTY

- Early pubertal development in girls <8 and boys <9
- Caused by premature release and secretion of gonadotropin hormones from the pituitary gland
- Three classes of precocious puberty (**Table 17-1**):
  - *Complete or true precocious puberty*
  - *Incomplete precocious puberty*
  - *Other conditions*

Assessment

Clinical Presentation

- Presence of breast development (Tanner Stage 2 or greater) for girls <8 years
- Presence of testicular development (Tanner Stage 2 or greater) for boys <9 years
- Scrotum is reddened and thinner
- Tanner Stage 2 pubic hair or greater
- Vaginal mucosa pink and thicker
- Sebaceous activity on face; acne
- Café au lait spots, presence of bone lesions on x-ray—McCune–Albright syndrome may be suspected.

TABLE 17.1 CLASSIFICATION OF SEXUAL PRECOCITY

True Precocious Puberty, Complete	Incomplete Precocious Puberty	Precocious Puberty Caused by Other Conditions
Caused by premature activation of gonadotrophic hormones from the hypothalamic–pituitary feedback system **Examples:** Familial or constitutional central precocious puberty Central nervous system tumors such as craniopharyngiomas, hamartoma, and hypothalamic astrocytoma Idiopathic precocious puberty	Caused by ovarian or adrenal secretion of, or ingestion of, estrogen (Styne, 2004); in this case the serum gonadotropins will be suppressed and serum estradiol levels will be elevated **Examples:** ***Boys*** Gonadotropin-releasing tumors Increased androgen secretion from the adrenal gland or testis, such as in congenital adrenal hyperplasia Leydig cell adenoma Familial testotoxicosis (sex-limited autosomal dominant disorder) ***Girls*** Ovarian cyst Estrogen-secreting ovarian or adrenal tumor Peutz-Jeghers syndrome ***Both Sexes*** McCune–Albright syndrome Hypothyroidism Iatrogenic or exogenous exposure to estrogens in foods, drugs, or cosmetics	May be caused by condition that directly affects the central nervous system **Examples:** Encephalitis Static encephalopathy Brain abscess Hydrocephalus Head trauma Arachnoid cyst Myelomeningocele Vascular lesions Cranial irradiation

From Alt et al. (2003)

- Advanced bone age
- Increased height velocity
- GnRH stimulation testing results with increased LH response >10 IU/L (Alt et al., 2003)
- Leuprolide acetate stimulation test results with LH levels greater than 8 IU/L (Alt et al., 2003)

Diagnostic Testing

- Serum studies include: luteinizing hormones, estradiol, FSH, and testosterone
- Provocative stimulation testing: GnRH stimulation testing and leuprolide acetate stimulation testing
- Radiologic studies such as bone age x-ray and MRI

CRITICAL COMPONENT

Symptoms of Precocious Puberty

There are other variations in pubertal development that may lead the health-care professional to suspect precocious puberty. These variations are usually benign and do not progress into full sexual pubertal development, but must be evaluated frequently to make a definitive diagnosis. These variations are:

- **Premature thelarche**
  - Isolated breast development that occurs earlier than normal
  - Most common <2 years and >6 years
  - No increased **growth velocity**
  - May have unilateral/bilateral breast development with areolae maturation
  - No other signs of puberty present
- **Premature adrenarche**
  - Early development of pubic hair in girls <8 years and boys <9 years
  - No increase in growth velocity
  - Tanner 2 or greater pubic hair
  - May also be accompanied by axillary hair, body odor, mild acne, and oily skin
  - May also be seen as a result of girls born prematurely
  - Testis 3 cc or less by Tanner Stage
- Adolescent gynecomastia of boys
  - Glandular enlargement >0.5 cm of the male breast tissue
  - Most common between the ages of 13 to 14 years, but usually resolved by age 17 years
  - May be caused by high estrogen-to-testosterone ratio

CLINICAL PEARL

Tanner Staging Assessment

Tanner staging assessment is a critical step in assessing the child with advanced pubertal development. Refer to Chapter 10 for information regarding Tanner staging assessment.

Nursing Interventions

- Early identification and treatment are essential.
- Careful monitoring of height velocity is necessary to determine if treatment methods are providing effective hormone suppression.
- Carefully assess sexual characteristics (Tanner staging) at each visit.
- Administer a gonadotropin-releasing hormone analogue (GnRHa) to stop the progression of pubertal development and suppress the release of gonadotropin hormones monthly.
- If GnRHa is given intramuscularly, assess injection sites for signs of sterile abscess.
- Perform psychological assessment of the child's response to the advanced pubertal development to determine if psychological referral is indicated.

Caregiver Education

- Provide education about the condition and treatment options prescribed.
- Teach parents the importance of dressing the child age appropriately despite advances in sexual characteristics.
- Encourage the importance of medication compliance, as not using the medication directly as prescribed may cause elevation of gonadotrophic hormones and advancement of sexual characteristics and height velocity.
- Discuss with the parents the need to talk about issues of sexuality at an earlier age than normal. Protective guidance measures should be offered, as children with precocious puberty may be at risk for sexual advances by older children, teens, or adults.
- Educate parents that medication should suppress the child's moodiness and emotional lability.
- Educate parents that use of GnRHa will not cause infertility problems later in life and that once the child is at an age where puberty is appropriate, the medication can be discontinued and spontaneous puberty will appear normally.

HYPOTHYROIDISM

- Caused by underactive thyroid gland
- Three thyroid hormones:
  - *T4—thyroxine*
  - *T3—tri-iodothyronine*
  - *TRH—thyroid-stimulating hormone*

Medication

Lupron

Leuprolide acetate (Lupron Depot Pediatric) is the most common medication utilized for treating true central precocious puberty in children. The dose is weight based. It is important to note that this medication is also used to treat adults for other causes, and it is crucial when ordering this medication to make sure that the child receives the pediatric formulation. Beginning doses start at 3.75 mg and are increased based on weight to a maximum dose of 15 mg. This medication can be given IM or SQ. The medication should be given as directed or the child may experience an increase of hormone levels that will cause progression of the signs of puberty (Deglin & Vallerand, 2007).

- Two types of hypothyroidism:
  - *Congenital*
  - *Acquired*

CONGENITAL HYPOTHYROIDISM

Assessment

Clinical Presentation

- Most infants are born asymptomatic.
- Of affected infants, 10% have symptoms that develop within weeks to months after birth.
- Symptoms may include: hypotonia, lethargy, open posterior fontanel, open cranial sutures, umbilical hernia, prolonged jaundice, pallor, enlarged tongue, hoarse cry, constipation, dry skin, respiratory difficulties, poor weight gain, generalized edema, **goiter**, abdominal distention, and increased birth weight.

Diagnostic Testing

- Thyroid labs are part of the state mandatory newborn screening.
- In children with suspected acquired hypothyroidism, T4, TSH, and antithyroid antibodies are taken.
- Thyroid scan or ultrasound may be indicated to confirm the presence and position of the thyroid gland.
- Assessment of the infant or child's growth velocity may also indicate hypothyroidism, especially if there are extreme differences between height and weight percentiles.

Nursing Interventions

- Immediate initiation of thyroid replacement hormone is essential to prevent cognitive damage in newborns and infants.
- Follow up with newborn screening results prior to or at the first newborn visit within 1 week of age.
- Carefully assess height and weight on the growth chart to determine growth delay

- Obtain history of infant's activity level, feeding ability, frequency of feedings, and bowel habits during follow-up visits.
- Provide patient/family education regarding thyroid replacement therapy and medication administration.

Caregiver Education

- Teach parents how to administer thyroid medications by having them crush and mix the medication with a small amount of water, breast milk, formula, or baby food.
- Instruct parents to give thyroid medications at the same time each morning and not to skip or double doses.
- Instruct parents to administer medication via needleless syringe and not to put medication in bottle.
- Instruct parents that formula should be milk based and not soy based, as soy-based formulas can break down the effects of the medication.
- Reinforce the importance of medication compliance and the lifelong need for thyroid medications.
  - *Instruct parents on the potential side effects of thyroid replacement medications and instruct them to notify their physician immediately if side effects are experienced.*

ACQUIRED HYPOTHYROIDISM

- Onset in childhood or teen years
- Cause may be related to an autoimmune condition known as Hashimoto's thyroiditis
- Medications such as lithium may interfere with thyroid synthesis.

Assessment

Clinical Presentation

- Decreased appetite, thinning of the hair or hair loss, dry and cool skin, depressed tendon reflexes, bradycardia, constipation, extreme fatigue, sensitivity to cold temperatures, abnormal menstrual cycles
- Manifestations unique to children include changes or deceleration in growth velocity, weight increase, delayed bone age, delayed dentition, muscle weakness, and delayed or precocious puberty.
- School-aged children may show a decline in school performance.
- A goiter may be present.

Diagnostic Testing

- In children with suspected acquired hypothyroidism, lab results of T4, TSH, and anti-thyroid antibodies are evaluated.
  - *Thyroid scan or ultrasound may be indicated to confirm the presence and position of the thyroid gland.*
  - *Bone age x-ray to assess delayed growth*
  - *Assessment of infant or child's growth velocity may also indicate hypothyroidism, especially if there are extreme differences between height and weight percentiles.*

Nursing Interventions

- Carefully assess height and weight on the growth chart to determine growth delay and/or excessive weight gain.
- Obtain history of child's activity level, appetite, incidences of hair loss or thinning, constipation, or other symptoms of hypothyroidism.
- Obtain family history for autoimmune thyroid problems, especially in female family members.
- Provide patient education regarding thyroid replacement therapy and medication administration.

Caregiver Education

- Instruct parents to give thyroid medications at the same time each morning and not to skip or double doses.
- Instruct parents to administer medication via needleless syringe and not to put medication in bottle.
- Reinforce the importance of medication compliance and the lifelong need for thyroid medications.
- Instruct parents on the potential side effects of thyroid replacement medications and instruct them to notify their physician immediately if side effects are experienced.
- Stress the importance of follow-up physician visits every 6 months so that thyroid lab levels can be assessed. The dosage of thyroid medications depends on body weight and the dose may need to be adjusted frequently as the child grows.
- Teach parents to modify child's diet with fruit and bulk if the child is experiencing constipation.
- Teach parents about the complications related to lack of thyroid treatment, such as myxedema.

Promoting Safety

A severe complication of hypothyroidism is a condition known as myxedema. This is a life-threatening crisis. This occurs when thyroid levels are extremely low. TSH levels are critically high and T4 levels are usually undetectable. The clinical manifestations of myxedema include nonpitting edema, severe edema of the face (face will appear round), edema of the tongue, metabolic disturbances, and hypothermia. If this condition is not treated immediately, the child or infant will progress to hypoglycemia, hypotension, cardiovascular arrest, and coma (myxedema coma). This condition is rare in children but does exist in children who go untreated.

CLINICAL PEARL

Laboratory Indicators for Hypothyroidism

When evaluating laboratory results for hypothyroidism, the nurse will see the following lab indicators:

Serum T4 ↓
Serum T3 normal
Serum TSH ↑

Medication

Thyroid Hormone Replacement Therapy

DRUG: Levothyroxine sodium (Synthroid, Levoxyl, Levothroid, and others)

PREPARATIONS:

Tabs	25, 50, 75, 88, 100, 112,125, 137, 150, 175, 200, 300 μg
IV, IM	50–75% of oral dose
Injection	0.2 mg/vial, 0.5 mg/vial

DOSING RECOMMENDATIONS:

Age Range	Daily Dose (μg/kg)	Daily Dose (μg/day)	Weight Range (kg)
Children <6 months	6–10	25–50	3–9
6–12 months	6–8	37.5–75	6–12
1–5 years	4–5	75–100	9–23
6–12 years	5–6	75–100	15–55
12–18 years	2–3	75–175	30–90

From Deglin & Vallerand (2009).

HYPERTHYROIDISM

- Overproduction of thyroid hormone
- Often referred to as Graves' disease
- Occurs most frequently in teens between ages 12 and 14 years
- Tends to be familial
- Manifestation period of 6 to 12 months

Assessment

Clinical Presentation

- Elevated serum levels of T4 and T3 with low or undetectable levels of TSH
- A goiter may be present, along with exopthalmus (bulging of the eyes).
- Other symptoms may include physical restlessness, fatigue, tachycardia, high blood pressure, increased perspiration, increased appetite, weight loss, difficulty sleeping, tremor, heat intolerance, fine hair, systolic murmurs, absence of menses, and mood changes or irritability.
- **Thyroid storm** can occur if symptoms go untreated for a long period of time and become severe.
- Thyroid storm is a life-threatening condition that requires medical intervention and hospitalization.

Diagnostic Testing

- Serum T4, T4, TSH, and thyroid antibodies
- Thyroid ultrasound

Nursing Interventions

- Complete physical assessment, especially for those children who are referred for symptoms of attention deficit/hyperactivity disorder (ADHD) (Amer, 2005)
- A complete school history of performance and behavioral problems; history of sleep patterns and changes in mood
- Menstruation cycle history in girls
- Outpatient follow-up is recommended every 4 to 6 months until stabilized.
- The nurse must understand the administration, dosage, side effects, and nursing interventions of medications administered for hyperthyroidism.
- Radioactive iodine therapy may be indicated to decrease the production of thyroid hormone. In this case, the nurse must be familiar with patient education and outcomes related to the therapy.
- If surgery is indicated to remove an overactive nodule of the thyroid gland, the nurse must take precautions postoperatively to make sure the patient's respiratory status is stable and the environment is quiet and calm, and assess the operative site for excessive edema or excessive bleeding.
- Patients receiving a thyroidectomy will receive lifelong thyroid hormone replacement therapy to treat hypothyroidism.
- Emotional support should be provided to patients with hyperthyroidism and their families.

Caregiver Education

- Patient/family education regarding the importance of medication compliance, adverse reactions to medications, and follow-up care is essential.
- For patients who have had a thyroidectomy, teaching the importance of lifelong hormone replacement therapy is crucial.
- Parents should be encouraged to educate teachers and school personnel about the child's physical and emotional instability during the treatment period.
- Emergency care involves teaching the patient/family signs and symptoms of thyroid storm and instructing them to bring the child to the hospital immediately if these symptoms occur.
- Stress the importance of a low-stress, low-pressure environment during and after hospitalization and until the child's symptoms of hyperthyroidism are decreasing.

HYPOPARATHYROIDISM

- Rare in children
- Inadequate production of PTH
- PTH may be released from parathyroid gland, but kidneys or bones do not respond to it

CRITICAL COMPONENT

Medications for Hyperthyroidism

The most common medications used to treat hyperthyroidism are antithyroid medications and beta-blocking agents. The antithyroid agents help to lower the level of T4 by blocking the synthesis of T4 and T3. These medications can have toxic side effects (see chart on p. 12). Beta-blocking agents do not decrease the amount of thyroid hormone, but provide comfort for the patient who is experiencing tachycardia, restlessness, and tremors.

Side Effects of Antithyroid Medications

Mild effects: Skin rash, mild leucopenia, loss of taste, arthralgia, and loss of hair or abnormal hair pigmentation

Severe effects that can be fatal: Agranulocytosis (as evidenced by sore throat and high fever), symptoms similar to lupus, hepatitis, hepatic failure, and glomerulonephritis

CLINICAL PEARL

Laboratory Indicators for Hyperthyroidism

When evaluating laboratory results for hyperthyroidism, the nurse will see the following lab indicators:

Serum T4 ↑
Serum T3 ↑
Serum TSH ↓ (May be undetectable)

Clinical Reasoning

Mallory S. is a 15-year-old who has been diagnosed with hyperthyroidism since age 13. Mallory's hyperthyroidism has been well controlled with antithyroid medications. However, she has been missing doses of her medication due to being "too busy and forgetting" to take her medication as prescribed. Over the last 2 weeks, she has had an increased appetite, increased perspiration, and extreme fatigue, and has become very irritable and restless. She tells her mother that she is having trouble concentrating in school. She begins to have severe diarrhea and tells her mother that she feels like her heart "is racing." Mallory's mother takes her to the emergency room, where she is diagnosed with thyroid storm and hospitalized. During the hospitalization, she is placed on a beta-blocking agent.

1. As the nurse taking care of Mallory, what do you think has caused her to develop thyroid storm?
2. What nursing interventions would be appropriate in caring for Mallory?
3. What patient educational topics are warranted for Mallory and her parents?

Assessment

Clinical Presentation

- Vomiting, poor tooth development, headaches, confusion, seizures, and spasms of the face, hands, arms, and feet
- Infants may experience increased irritability, muscle rigidity, abdominal distention, and episodes of apnea or cyanosis.

Diagnostic Testing

- Serum calcium levels are low, phosphate levels are high, magnesium levels are low, and parathyroid hormone levels are low.
- Decreased bone mineral density
- Bone or soft tissue abnormalities as confirmed by x-ray or CT scans
- Evidence of prolonged QT interval confirmed by 12-lead electrocardiogram (EKG)

Nursing Interventions

- A thorough physical assessment and history should be taken to determine if the patient has experienced muscle spasms, muscle twitching, seizure activity, vomiting, or headaches.
- Thorough knowledge of medications used to treat hypoparathyroidism, such as calcium and vitamin D, is necessary.
- In the beginning phase of diagnosis, the patient may require IV calcium infusions. The nurse must frequently check the IV site for symptoms of infiltration or extravasations. Carefully check and re-check the calcium dose and dilution order and follow facility IV calcium infusion protocols.
- Once the patient's calcium has normalized, the nurse must evaluate the oral tolerance of vitamin D and calcium for 24 hours to make sure the patient is able to tolerate the medication before discharge.
- Vital signs are assessed frequently.
- Seizure precautions are exercised until calcium levels normalize.
- Cardiac telemetry may be indicated, and the nurse should carefully monitor cardiovascular status.
- Assessment for hyperreflexia of the muscles should be performed frequently while calcium levels are unstable.
- The nurse must provide dietary recommendations to the patient/family.

CLINICAL PEARL

Chvostek Sign

Assessment of hyperreflexia of the muscles can be performed by tapping on the facial nerve. If a spasm occurs in the facial muscles, then a positive Chvostek sign has occurred. This confirms that the child has muscle spasms, pain, cramping, and twitches. This is an important test for infants and small children, as they are unable to communicate pain or muscle spasms.

Caregiver Education

- Encourage dietary compliance, such as avoiding caffeine and limiting the intake of carbonated beverages.
- Encourage foods high in calcium and vitamin K.
- Instruct parents to give calcium and vitamin D with acidic substances such as orange juice or with salads that contain lemon juice in the dressing.

- Provide dietary instruction regarding alternative dietary supplements in addition to calcium and vitamin D, such as magnesium, boron, and vitamin K.
- Encourage follow-up appointment with physician to have calcium levels checked.
- Instruct family and patient regarding the need for lifelong medication therapy.

HYPERPARATHYROIDISM

- Rare in children
- Overactive parathyroid gland
- Most common in females during adolescence

Assessment

Clinical Presentation

- Signs and symptoms may include bone and joint pain, bone loss or evidence of osteoporosis, bone fractures, muscle weakness, abdominal pain, heartburn, nausea, vomiting, constipation, lack of appetite, kidney stones, excessive thirst, excessive urination, depression, anxiety, memory loss, and drowsiness or fatigue.
- Approximately 50% of patients with hyperparathyroidism do not have any symptoms, and approximately 1% of patients are undiagnosed (Ward & Hisley, 2009).

Diagnostic Testing

- Serum calcium is elevated along with elevated PTH levels.
- X-ray or bone densitometry reveals signs of bone loss.
- Renal calculi may be present in the kidneys

Nursing Interventions

- Postoperative care of the child with a parathyroidectomy focuses on maintaining the airway and breathing.
- The nurse should assess the surgical site for edema that may lead to altered respiratory status.
- Frequently assess for sign and symptoms of infection and hematoma.
- The nurse should administer IV fluids as ordered and keep track of intake and output.
- Careful monitoring of electrolytes is also important.

Caregiver Education

- Instruct parents on the sign and symptoms of infection at the operative site to monitor for once they are discharged home.
- Nutritional guidance should include food and liquids high in calcium and vitamin D, as removal of the parathyroid glands can cause the patient to be deficient in both.
- Parents should be taught the signs and symptoms of hypocalcaemia and when to alert their physician.
- Remind parents and patient that calcium and vitamin D supplements are a lifelong therapy.

CUSHING'S SYNDROME

- Overexposure to excessive amounts of cortisol hormone
- Most common causes are cortisol-producing tumor, adrenal hyperplasia, and benign adrenal tumors
- Chronic steroid use may be a causal factor.
- Very hard to diagnosis; symptoms may take up to 5 years to manifest

Assessment

Clinical Presentation

- Clinical manifestations develop slowly.
- Alkalosis related to hypokalemia and hypercalcemia
- Excessive urinary calcium excretion
- Other symptoms include weight gain, pendulous abdomen, fatigue, muscle wasting, weakness of the extremities, round "moon-shaped" face, facial flushing, fat pad located between the shoulder blades known as a buffalo hump, and pink or purple stretch marks on the abdomen, thighs, and arms.
- Psychologically, the child may experience mood changes such as depression, anxiety, irritability, and euphoria.
- Growth delay may also be seen on physical exam.
- Females may experience irregular or absent menstrual cycles.
- Excessive cortisol levels may lead to hyperglycemia, causing diabetes, high blood pressure, or arteriosclerosis.

Diagnostic Testing

- Referral to a pediatric endocrinologist is warranted.
- 24-hour urine collection for urinary free cortisol and 17-hydroxycorticosteriod (17-OHCs)
- Dexamethasone suppression test
- Saliva swabs to test cortisol levels
- Serum blood levels of glucose, cortisol, and electrolytes
- Bone scan to rule out osteoporosis
- MRI of the pituitary gland
- CT scan of the adrenal glands

Nursing Interventions

- Nursing care is dependent on the cause of the overproduction of cortisol.
- The nurse must be knowledgeable regarding the pharmaceutical treatments that inhibit the production of cortisol.
- If surgery is not possible, the nurse may have to educate the patient/family regarding the use of radiation therapy.
- Surgical intervention may be necessary to excise or remove a tumor. The nurse must provide pre- and postoperative education.
- Postoperative nursing care involves maintaining IV fluids, monitoring hydration status, providing pain control, and postoperative assessment and initiation of medications.
- Monitor serum electrolytes.

Caregiver Education

- Emergency care involves educating the patient regarding lifelong cortisol replacement therapy daily and in emergency situations.
- The patient will need to be taught stress dosing with hydrocortisone injections during times when the child is extremely ill, has a fever, is vomiting, experiences trauma, or is going in for surgery.
- The parents should be reassured that the cushingoid appearance will improve over time with treatment.
- Offer nutritional guidance for healthy food selections that will help lower the weight gained.
- Instruct the parents on the signs and symptoms of adrenal insufficiency, such as increased irritability, headache, confusion, restlessness, nausea and vomiting, diarrhea, abdominal pain, dehydration, fever, loss of appetite, and lethargy. These symptoms can be life threatening and the parents should take the child to the emergency room as soon as symptoms are identified.

CONGENITAL ADRENAL HYPERPLASIA (CAH)

- Inability to produce cortisol in the adrenal glands
- Excessive amounts of corticosteriod-releasing hormone and adrenocoricotropic hormone (ACTH)
- Hyperplasia of the adrenal gland develops.
- The end result is excessive androgen production from the adrenal glands.

Assessment

Clinical Presentation

- 21-hydroxylase deficiency is the most common cause and leads to cortisol and aldosterone deficiency (Demirci & Witchell, 2008).
- Approximately 75% of patients with CAH are salt-losing, caused by aldosterone deficiency. Approximately 25% will be non-salt-losers with simple virilization (Demirci & Witchell, 2008).
- In males, there are generally no manifestations until later in childhood. These manifestations include early development of pubic hair, enlargement of the penis, or both; advancement in growth velocity; and advanced bone age compared to the child's chronological age.
- Virilization (development of secondary sexual characteristics) occurs in females.
- The most noticeable manifestations occur with females, as at birth they will have abnormal development of the genitalia that is referred to as **ambiguous genitalia**. The clitoris may be enlarged and there may be fusion of the labial folds. These manifestations give the appearance that the female may be male; however, the internal sex organs will be normal.

Diagnostic Testing

- Genetic paternal screening is available; however, the screening may show "false positive" results. In this case, the health-care provider will need to evaluate for symptoms at birth.
- Serum 17-hydroxyprogesterone (17-OHP) will be elevated. If the levels continue to be elevated after birth, CAH is expected, as normal growth and development will decrease 17-OHP as the infant matures.
- Chromosomal analysis will be performed to determine the infant's gender in the case of ambiguous genitalia.
- In some cases, surgery of the genitalia is performed to meet the needs of the determined sex of the child.

Nursing Interventions

- Early diagnosis is the key to successful treatment. The nurse must be able to carefully assess for pre- and postnatal risk factors.
- Referral to a genetics clinic may be indicated.
- Dehydration is a complication of CAH and the nurse must assess for signs and symptoms of dehydration, electrolyte imbalance, and hypovolemic shock when the child is salt-wasting.
- Careful monitoring of cardiopulmonary status
- Frequent vital sign assessment
- Assess the parents' emotional status related to the ambiguity of the infant's genitalia. Understanding cultural and spiritual beliefs when counseling parents is important.
- Provide detailed education regarding the cause of the diagnosis, symptoms, and available treatment options.
- If the infant's gender is questionable at birth, refer to the infant as "your baby" and not "your son" or "your daughter."

CRITICAL COMPONENT

Administering Corticosteroids and Mineralocorticoids

Emergency care involves education regarding the administration of lifelong medications such as corticosteroids and mineralocorticoids. Emergency administration of corticosteroids given via injection should be taught to the parents for use when the child is in a crisis, such as febrile illness, surgery, trauma, or severe stress. The doses will need to be doubled or tripled during the period of crisis. This is referred to as "stress dosing." The most common medications administered are hydrocortisone and Florinef (Alt et al., 2003).

Caregiver Education

- Emergency care involves teaching the parents and family how to administer medications.
- Teaching the family the signs and symptoms of adrenal crisis and the performance of stress dosing is crucial.
- Instruct the parents regarding the signs and symptoms of dehydration.

- Encourage the parents to seek emotional support from CAH support groups in their area or through a national organization, such as www.congenitaladrenalhyperplasia.org.
- Educate the parents regarding future pregnancies and the importance of prenatal screening for CAH and refer them to a genetics clinic.
- Allow parents and family members to discuss their concerns, feelings, and beliefs regarding their infant's condition. Refer them to the appropriate center for psychological support; involve the social work team and offer spiritual support such as the clergy or designated chaplain for their faith.
- If surgery is indicated, provide education regarding pre- and postoperative care and let the parents know that there may be more than one surgery to correct the genitalia.

ADRENAL INSUFFICIENCY (ADDISON'S DISEASE)

- Insufficient cortisol and aldosterone production from adrenal glands
- Cause is most often unknown
- Thirty percent of cases occur from a direct attack on the adrenal gland (e.g., cancer, infections, autoimmune diseases, or chronic steroid use).

Assessment

Clinical Presentation

- Hypoglycemia, especially during stressful periods such as surgery or febrile illness
- The symptoms may be mild unless the child gets sick and are very individualized.
- Manifestations include but are not limited to: weakness, fatigue, dizziness, and rapid pulse; dark skin that appears as if the child is very tanned; black freckles; bluish-black discoloration around the nipples, scrotum, and vagina; and weight loss, dehydration, loss of appetite, intense salt cravings, nausea and vomiting, and cold intolerance.

> **CRITICAL COMPONENT**
>
> **Adrenal Insufficiency, Congenital Adrenal Hyperplasia, and Hormone Replacement**
>
> It is important to remember that children with adrenal insufficiency, as well as CAH, require lifelong hormone replacement. Children with adrenal insufficiency tend to grow poorly in height and weight, but puberty will present at a normal age despite the growth delay. These children may require growth hormone replacement therapy along with corticosteroid and mineralocorticoid replacement therapy.

Diagnostic Testing

- Low serum sodium, high potassium, and low blood sugar
- Diagnosed by assessing manifestations

> **Promoting Safety**
>
> Addisonian crisis is a life-threatening event that requires the child to receive immediate medical attention. If ignored, the child may die. The symptoms of an Addisonian crisis are sudden, penetrating pain in the lower back or legs, severe vomiting and diarrhea, dehydration, low blood pressure, and loss of consciousness (National Institute of Health [NIH], 2004). This type of crisis is very overwhelming for parents, and a detailed plan of care and patient education can help the parents be ready for an emergency if it occurs.

- Low blood pressure
- Serum cortisol level drawn around 8:00 a.m. because the levels are the highest upon arising in the morning
- Cortisol levels <3 mg/dL indicate Addison's disease. Levels between 3 and 19 mg/dL are considered suspicious and further testing is needed to confirm diagnosis.

Nursing Interventions

- Frequent lab assessment
- Administration of corticosteroids such as Solu-Cortef; this medication is given 2–3 times per day (Riepe & Sippell, 2007).
- Administer IM Solu-Cortef if the child is vomiting, nauseated, or has diarrhea and is unable to tolerate oral intake (**Table 17-2**).
- Assessment of hydration status
- Strict intake and output to avoid dehydration
- Teach the parents how to administer IM Solu-Cortef for home emergency situations.
- Careful assessment for signs and symptoms of hypovolemic shock in the severely dehydrated patient (Riepe & Sippell, 2007)
- Make sure that the child has been referred to a pediatric endocrinologist to diagnose and treat this condition.

Caregiver Education

- Emergency care involves teaching parents the signs and symptoms of adrenal crisis and how to administer IM Solu-Cortef if the child develops crises outside of the hospital (Riepe & Sippell, 2007).
- Chronic home care involves teaching the parents the importance of medication compliance and avoidance of skipping doses, as this can lead to adrenal crisis.
- The child should wear a medical alert bracelet at all times.
- Teach the parents how to "stress dose" in times when the child has fever, vomiting, diarrhea, emotional stress, trauma, or surgery.
- Teach the parents to make sure the child is well hydrated before being involved in a physical activity or sports.
- Educate school teachers and staff regarding the potential for dehydration and hypovolemic shock so that measures can be taken to provide the child with extra fluids prior to and during physical activity.

TABLE 17–2 MEDICATIONS USED TO TREAT ADRENAL DISORDERS

	Fludrocortison Acetate (Florinef)	Hydrocortisone (Solu-Cortef, Hydrocortone, Cortef)
How Supplied	0.1-mg tablets	Tablets—5, 10, 20 mg Injection—100, 250, 500, 1000 mg/vial Acetate (Hydrocortone)—25, 20 mg/ml
Dose/Route	*Addison's Disease:* 2.1 mg/daily (dose may vary from 0.1 mg 3 times/week to 0.2 mg/daily) *Salt-losing Congenital Adrenal Hyperplasia:* 0.1–0.2 mg/daily PO	*Physiological Dosing:* *PO:* 0.5–0.75 mg/kg/day or 20–25 mg/m^2/day divided every 8 hours *IM:* 0.25–0.35 mg/kg/dose or 12–15 mg/m^2/day every day ***Stress Dosing:*** 2–3 times the normal physiologic dose, depending on the severity of the illness or stress
Potential Side Effects	Hypertension, edema, cardiac enlargement, congestive heart failure, potassium loss, hypokalemia alkalosis	Hypertension, euphoria, insomnia, acne, hyperglycemia, growth suppression, immunosuppression, and adrenal suppression

Source: Deglin & Vallerand (2009).

- Encourage the child and parents to increase salt intake during the warmer months of the year to maintain adequate mineralocorticoid levels.

PHEOCHROMOCYTOMA

- Rare in children
- Usually occurs between ages 9 and 12 years
- Caused by adrenal tumor
- Excessive amounts of catecholamines are produced.

Assessment

Clinical Presentation

- Hypertension with systolic blood pressure as high as 250 mm Hg
- Typical symptoms include increased heart rate (tachycardia), headache, palpitations, dizziness, poor weight gain, nausea and vomiting, and growth failure.
- Other symptoms may include abdominal pain, profuse sweating, cool extremities, **polydipsia**, and **polyuria**.
- Pheochromocytoma may mimic the symptoms of hyperthyroidism and diabetes mellitus.

Diagnostic Testing

- 24-hour urine to assess the presence of catecholamines
- MRI or CT scan to determine the location of the tumor

Nursing Interventions

- Removal of the tumor is usually indicated.
- Preoperative administration of medications to inhibit the release of catecholamines may begin 1 to 3 weeks prior to surgery.
- If surgery is not an option, administration of medications such as alpha-adrenergic blocking agents is used to provide medical management. This medication may be combined with beta-adrenergic blocking agents to maximize the efficacy of treatment.
- Careful assessment of vital signs, especially blood pressure, is crucial.
- Blood glucose levels should be taken and assessed daily pre- and postoperatively, as blood sugar levels may be higher than normal.
- Postoperatively, the patient should be placed in a minimally stimulating environment.

CRITICAL COMPONENT

Avoid Palpating the Adrenal Glands

During the physical assessment of the patient, the nurse should avoid palpating the area of the adrenal glands where the tumor is located, as it can cause an elevated release of catecholamines, which will increase metabolism and produce a potential hypertensive crisis or tachyarrhythmias.

Caregiver Education

- Preoperative education begins with providing information regarding the cause, symptoms, and treatment options for the condition.
- If surgery is not an option, the nurse must provide thorough education regarding medications used for the treatment of the condition.
- Parents should provide a low-stress environment for the child during the pre- and postoperative periods.

DIABETES MELLITUS TYPE 1 (INSULIN-DEPENDENT DIABETES)

- Destruction of the beta cells in the pancreas
- Pancreas unable to produce insulin
- Child must have exogenous insulin to survive

Assessment

Clinical Presentation

- Polyuria, polydipsia, and **polyphagia**
- Unintentional weight loss over several days
- High glucose levels in the blood and urine
- Nausea and vomiting, excessive fatigue, abdominal pain, increased susceptibility to infections, dehydration, blurred vision, irritability, and restlessness (Halvorson, Yasuda, Carpenter, & Kaiserman, 2005)

Diagnostic Testing

- Elevated blood glucose levels >200 mg/dL
- Elevated hemoglobin A1C levels >7.0
- Decreased serum insulin levels
- Presence of serum and urine ketones
- Of affected individuals, 85% to 90% may have one or more of the following positive autoantibodies:
  - *ICA*
  - *IAA*
  - *GAD_{65}*
  - *IA-2ß (Halvorson et al., 2005)*

Nursing Interventions

- Nursing interventions should focus on the following major areas:
  - *Physical assessment*
  - *Administration of insulin (**Table 17-3**)*
    - Always double check insulin orders to make sure orders are clear and concise. When drawing up insulin, another RN must verify that the correct dosage is drawn up in the syringe.
    - Make sure that the correct strength of insulin has been ordered, as there are multiple strengths and types available.
    - Only use insulin syringes to draw up insulin doses.

TABLE 17–3 TYPES OF INSULIN USED TO TREAT DIABETES MELLITUS

Insulin Type	Onset	Peak	Duration	Availability	Dose	Route	Considerations
			SHORT-ACTING INSULIN				
Humulin R, Humulin R U-500, Novolin R	30-60 minutes	2-4 hours	5-7 hours	100 units/mL in 10-mL vials, 3-mL disposable delivery devices, 500 units/mL in 20-mL vials	SQ doses individualized per patient IV; doses start at 0.5-1.0 unit/kg/day	SQ	May be given IV to treat diabetic ketoacidosis (DKA)
			INTERMEDIATE-ACTING INSULIN				
NPH Insulin, Humulin N, Novolin NPH, Novolin N	1-2 hours	4-12 hours	18-24 hours	100 units/mL in 10-mL vials, 3-mL disposable delivery devices	0.1 unit/kg/day	SQ	Only given SQ
			LONG-ACTING INSULIN				
Insulin Determir (Levemir), **Insulin Glargine** (Lantus)	**Insulin Detemir:** 3-4 hours **Insulin Glargine:** 3-4 hours	**Insulin Detemir:** 3-14 hours **Insulin Glargine:** No peak	**Insulin Detemir:** 24 hours **Insulin Glargine:** 24 hours	**Detemir:** 100 units/mL in 10-mL vials, 3-mL cartridges or prefilled syringes **Glargine:** 100 units/mL in 10-mL vials, 3-mL cartridges or prefilled disposable pens	**Detemir:** 0.1-0.2 units/kg once daily in the a.m. or 10 units once or twice daily **Glargine:** 50-75% of daily insulin requirements once daily	SQ	Only administered SQ Only indicated for children >6 years old Glargine cannot be given in the same site as other insulin

TABLE 17-3 TYPES OF INSULIN USED TO TREAT DIABETES MELLITUS—cont'd

Insulin Type	Onset	Peak	Duration	Availability	Dose	Route	Considerations
INSULIN MIXTURES							
Insulin lispro protamine suspension/ insulin lispro solution mixtures, rDNA origin (Humalog 75/25. Humalog Mix 50/50)	15–30 minutes	2.8 hours	24 hours	100 units/mL in 10-mL vials, 3-mL disposable delivery devices	0.5–1.0 unit/ kg/day	SQ	Only Administered SQ
Insulin aspart protamine suspension/ insulin aspart solution mixtures, rDNA origin (NovoLog Mix 70/30)	15 minutes	1–4 hours	18–24 hours	100 units/mL in 10-mL vials, 3-mL disposable delivery devices	0.5–1.0 unit/ kg/day	SQ	Only administered SQ
NPH/regular insulin mixtures (Humulin 50/50, Humulin 70/30, Novolin 70/30)	30 minutes	4–8 hours	24 hours	100 units/mL in 10-mL vials, 3-mL disposable delivery devices	0.5–1.0 unit/ kg/day	SQ	Only administered SQ

Source: Deglin & Vallerand (2009).

- When using insulin pen devices, replace the pen needle with each dose and store the insulin pen in the refrigerator. Some insulin may be stored at room temperature for up to 28 days after opening. Always check the manufacturer's recommendations in the prescribing information that comes with the insulin vial or pen cartridge.
- Only regular insulin may be used intravenously during the management of **diabetic ketoacidosis**.
- Verify dose with a second RN and document dose of insulin administration in chart
- Rotate insulin injection sites with each dose (abdomen, arms, legs, buttocks).
- Assess for injection-site reactions.
- Monitor body weight daily, as weight loss or gain will indicate a possible increase or decrease in insulin dose.
- If a sliding-scale insulin regimen is ordered, the nurse must be diligent with obtaining blood glucose levels prior to meals and at bedtime in order to adjust insulin dose. Sliding scales are individualized per patient.

- Diet and nutrition education
  - *Once the diagnosis of T1DM has been made, the nurse needs to take a thorough dietary history of the patient's eating habits. The patient and parents should have a dietary consult so that the patient can be placed on a diabetic diet or be taught to count carbohydrate exchanges and adjust insulin requirements based on dietary intake.*
- Education regarding physical exercise
  - *Assessment of the child's exercise ability and regimen should be taken into account to determine the possibility for hypoglycemia during exercise and the need for pre-exercise snacks.*
  - *The child must eat an extra complex carbohydrate and protein serving at least 30 minutes to 1 hour prior to engaging in exercise or sports.*
- Education regarding differences between hypoglycemia and hyperglycemia (**Table 17-4**).
- Stress management or "sick day rules" should be established and taught to the patient, parents, family members, and teachers in order to have basic guidelines for how to manage diabetes in times of stress such as sickness, emotional stress, minor accidents, surgery, or dehydration.

TABLE 17–4 CLINICAL COMPARISON OF HYPOGLYCEMIA AND HYPERGLYCEMIA

Clinical Condition	Manifestations	Critical Nursing Actions
	HYPOGLYCEMIA	
Too much insulin for amount of food eaten	Rapid onset Irritable Nervous	• Give 15 grams of carbohydrates
Injected insulin into muscle	Shaky feeling, tremors	• Recheck blood glucose in 15 minutes
Too much activity for insulin dose	Difficult to concentrate Difficult to speak	• If blood glucose is <70 mg/dL, give another 15 grams of carbohydrates
Too much time between meals	Behavior change Confused Repeats over and over	• Recheck again in another 15 minutes
Too few carbohydrates eaten	Unconscious Seizure	• If unconscious, give IM glucagon
Illness or stress	Tachycardia Shallow breathing Pale, sweaty Hungry Headache Dizzy Vision blurry or double Photophobic Numbness or mouth or lips	
	HYPERGLYCEMIA	
Too little insulin for the food eaten	Gradual onset Lethargic Sleepy	• Give additional insulin at usual injection time
Illness or stress	Slow response Confused	• Use sliding-scale doses for specific level of blood glucose
Too many carbohydrates eaten	Breathes deeply and rapidly Skin flushed and dry	• Increase fluids
Meals too close together	Mucous membranes dry	• If ketones are elevated, give an extra insulin injection
Too many snacks	Thirsty Hungry Dehydrated	
Insulin given just under the skin	Weak Tired Headache	
Too little activity	Abdomen hurts Nausea and vomiting Vision blurry Shock	

Source: Ward, S. L., & Hisley, S. M. (2009). *Maternal-child nursing care* (revised reprint, p. 913). Philadelphia: F.A. Davis.

- Blood glucose and urine ketone monitoring
  - *Monitor blood glucose every 4 to 6 hours or as ordered by physician.*
  - *Test urine for the presence of ketones using urine ketosticks.*
  - *On follow-up clinic visits to the endocrinologist, it is important to evaluate the patient's blood sugar log for daily blood sugar trends, doses of insulin, the presence of ketones in the urine, and the presence of hypoglycemia.*
- Assessment of laboratory values
  - *Assess laboratory values such as phosphorus, magnesium, and potassium, as insulin may decrease serum levels.*
  - *Monitor hemoglobin A1C levels frequently to assess average blood glucose levels over a 9-day period. This will also help to identify if the insulin regimen is appropriate or needs to be adjusted.*
- Psychosocial support
  - *Provide psychosocial support to patient, parents, and family, taking into consideration the age-appropriate developmental needs of the patient.*
  - *Refer the patients to diabetes support organizations.*
    - American Diabetes Association: www.diabetes.org/
    - Juvenile Diabetes Foundation: www.jdrf.org/
  - *Encourage participation in diabetes education classes and diabetes support groups provided by the institution.*
  - *Make referral to social services or psychosocial counselor if indicated.*

Caregiver Education

- Patient and family education regarding the administration of insulin (**Figure 17-3, Box 17-1**)
- Patient and family education regarding stress management or "sick day rules" (Halvorson et al., 2005)

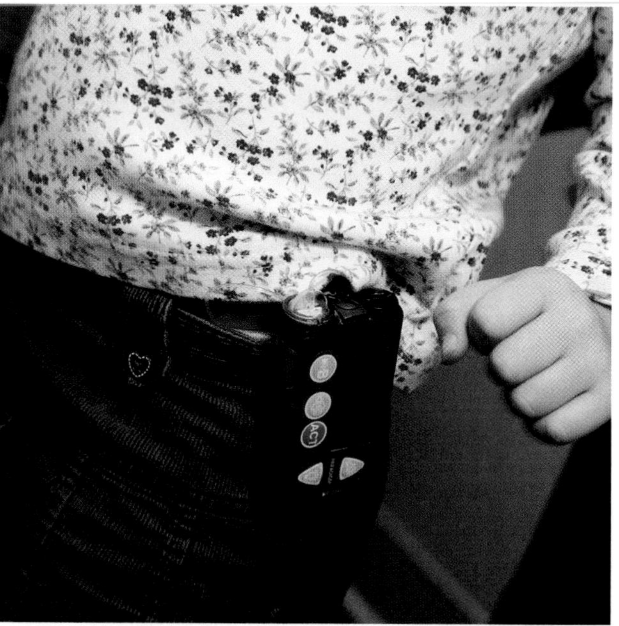

Figure 17–3 Wearing an insulin pump allows children to control the release of insulin throughout the day, more closely resembling the body's natural response.

CLINICAL PEARL

Important Things to Teach Regarding Sick Day Rules

M—Monitor blood sugar levels more frequently
D—Do not stop taking insulin
C—Check urine for ketones
B—Be careful with over-the-counter medicines
H—Have a game plan and don't hesitate to ask for help
F—Force fluids

Box 17–1 TEACHING PARENTS HOW TO INJECT INSULIN

Purpose

To teach parents how to inject insulin

Equipment

Insulin bottle from refrigerator (remove up to 1 hour before injection to allow it to warm to room temperature)
Appropriate syringe (U-30, U-50, or U-100)
Alcohol wipes
Container for the dirty, used syringe

Steps

1. Check the expiration date on the insulin bottle.
   RATIONALE: *Ensures that the insulin has not expired.*
2. Wash hands.
   RATIONALE: *Prevents the spread of bacteria.*
3. Clean rubber stopper on insulin bottle with alcohol wipe.
   RATIONALE: *Promotes asepsis.*
4. Remove syringe cap and pull air into the syringe; line up the end of the black plunger to the exact amount the insulin dose will be.
   RATIONALE: *Ensures accurate dosage of insulin to be drawn up.*
5. Put the syringe needle through the bottle rubber top and push syringe plunger so that all the air goes from the syringe into the bottle.
6. Turn the insulin bottle upside down and pull the syringe plunger so that the insulin enters the syringe until the top of the black plunger exactly lines up with the dose of insulin to be given.
7. Remove every air bubble, always checking that the dose is exact.
   RATIONALE: *Exact dosing is essential in managing the child's condition.*
8. Choose (or let the child choose) the site of the injection.
   RATIONALE: *Allowing the child to participate may help the child feel more in control of the condition.*
9. Clean the injection site with an alcohol swab.
   RATIONALE: *Alcohol will decrease the presence of microorganisms.*

Continued

Box 17–1 TEACHING PARENTS HOW TO INJECT INSULIN—cont'd

10. Pinch up the skin slightly and gently, with the syringe at a 90-degree angle (perpendicular) to the skin; with a dart-like motion, insert the needle into the skin; release the skin.
    RATIONALE: *Ensures proper medication administration.*
11. Slowly inject the dose of insulin.
12. Discard the used syringe in a hard, rigid container with a tight-fitting lid.

CLINICAL ALERT

The nurse teaches the parents to evaluate the child for the signs and symptoms of either hypo- or hyperglycemia. In understandable terms, explain these signs and symptoms to the parents so they can watch for them at home:

HYPOGLYCEMIA (LOW BLOOD SUGAR)	HYPERGLYCEMIA (HIGH BLOOD SUGAR)
Cold, pale skin (cold sweat)	Increased thirst, even if consuming a large amount of liquids
Shakiness/hand tremors	Loss of appetite, nausea/vomiting
Sudden hunger (crave salt/sweet)	Weakness, stomach pains/aches
Emotional outbursts (personality changes)	Heavy, labored breathing
Drowsiness/extremely tired	Fatigue, tired often sleepy
Pounding heartbeat/palpitations	Large amounts of sugar in urine
Nervousness/dizziness	Ketones in urine
Anxiety/irritability	Frequent urination
Headache, mental confusion, difficulty concentrating	Blurred/double vision
Numbness or tingling of lips/mouth	
Poor coordination/staggering unable to walk	
Slurred or slow speech	
Dilated, enlarged pupils	
Fainting (needs emergency treatment *NOW*)	

Teach Parents

If the child expresses that the injection is painful, the following measures can be taken to decrease the pain:

- Inject room-temperature insulin.
- Clear even the tiniest air bubbles from the syringe.
- Let the alcohol dry completely before injection.
- Tell the child to relax the muscles in the area of injection (the more tense the muscles during injection, the more painful the procedure).
- Use syringe-like dart to pierce the skin quickly.
- Do not change the needle direction during insertion or withdrawal.
- Never reuse syringes.
- Rotate sites with *each* injection (giving the insulin in the *same* place twice in one day can cause unnecessary discomfort for the child and undue stress on the tissue).

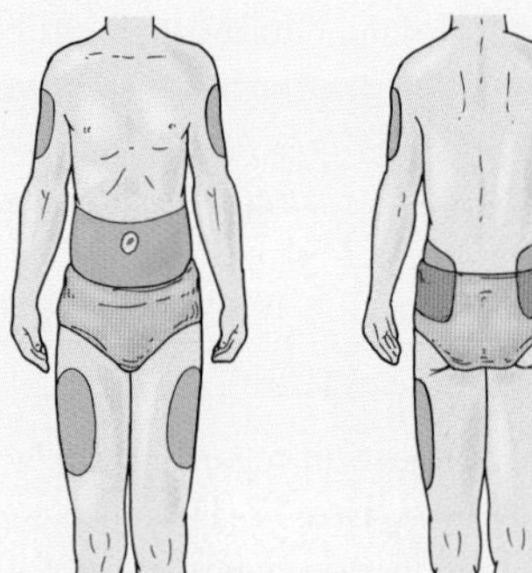

- Document exactly where each injection was given so as to avoid the same place more than once a day.
- Create and keep a Diabetes Management Notebook with the plan and a place to record daily blood sugar values as well as doses of insulin administered, including injection site.

For example:

DATE	BLOOD GLUCOSE AM	BLOOD GLUCOSE PM	INSULIN DOSE GIVEN AND TIME	INJECTION SITE	GIVEN BY
8/9/07	124		4 units Regular at 0700	right mid-arm	Mom
8/9/07		144	4 units Regular 4 units NPH 1230	left mid-thigh	Dad

Documentation

Mother gave 4 units of Regular at 0700 in right mid-arm, noted by R. Such, RN Father gave 4 units of Regular and 4 units NPH at 1230 in left mid-thigh, noted by

—R. Such, RN

Source: Ward, S. L., & Hisley, S. M. (2009). *Maternal-child nursing care: Optimizing outcomes for mothers, children, & families* (pp. 908–909). Philadelphia: F.A. Davis.

- Patient and family education regarding blood glucose monitoring (**Figure 17-4**)
  - *Patient and family should demonstrate proficiency with glucometer.*
  - *Discuss importance of monitoring blood sugar 3 to 4 times daily and keeping a blood sugar log with readings.*
    - Patient and family education regarding assessment of urine for urine ketones, especially when sick or under stress
    - Patient and family education regarding how to manage hypoglycemia
    - Preparing the patient and family for school guidance
    - Preparing teachers and school administrators regarding insulin regimen of the child, sick day rules, monitoring of blood glucose levels, signs and symptoms of hypoglycemia, and the administration of glucagon
    - Emergency doses of glucagon and glucogel should be kept at home and at school in the event that severe hypoglycemia occurs.
- Management of diabetic ketoacidosis
  - *Administer IV fluids and IV insulin as ordered.*
  - *Correct acidosis and restore acid–base balance.*
  - *Correct electrolyte imbalance by administering IV fluids with electrolytes.*
  - *Monitor laboratory values.*
  - *Frequent blood sugar checks and vital signs*
  - *Frequent assessment for signs of further complications*
  - *Assess respiratory status for signs of complications, such as Kussmaul breathing. This type of breathing is very deep and laborious and means that the patient is trying to correct the metabolic acidosis and "blow off" excess carbon dioxide (CO_2).*
  - *Frequently assess IV site, as multiple infusions of fluids, electrolytes, and insulin will increase chances of infiltration. The nurse must use an IV Y-Port to allow for multiple infusions at the same time. The nurse must also check drug compatibility before infusing multiple infusions through the same IV tubing.*

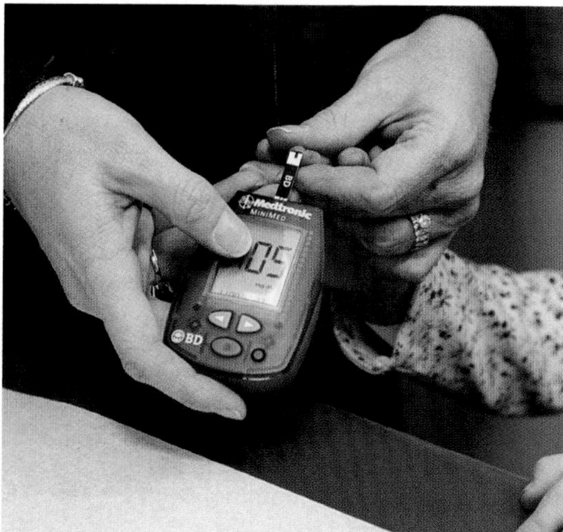

Figure 17-4 Home monitoring requires parents to perform glucose checks on the child with diabetes.

CRITICAL COMPONENT

Diabetic Ketoacidosis

Diabetic ketoacidosis (DKA) is confirmed when a glucose is >200 mg/dL, ketonuria, or ketonemia with a serum bicarbonate level of <15mEq/L. There are three levels of acidosis to consider:

0 Mild DKA—venous blood pH = 7.2–7.3
1 Moderate DKA—venous blood pH = 7.10–7.19
2 Severe DKA—venous blood pH <7.0

DKA is a complex, emergent condition that combines hyperglycemia, acidosis, and ketosis that results in severely deficient insulin levels that alter metabolism of carbohydrates, protein, and fat. Some of the precipitating factors that the nurse must assess for are as follows:

- Poor compliance with insulin regimens
- Patients entering puberty and beginning of the menstrual cycle
- Caregiver lack of competence regarding insulin management
- Insulin pump failure
- Insulin that is out of date
- Underlying illness, surgery, or trauma

CRITICAL COMPONENT

Family Teaching Guidelines: Dealing with a Hypoglycemic Crisis

How to: Recognize the signs of hypoglycemia—child is pale, sweaty, dizzy, "shaky" (tremors), confused, irritable, numb on lips or mouth, and can have an altered mental status.

Essential Information:

- Check blood glucose level.
- If blood glucose is below 70 mg/dL, rapidly give one of the following sources of carbohydrates (about 10–15 grams each), in the right amount to treat hypoglycemia:
  - ½ to ¾ cup of orange or grape juice (a juice box is good when one is away from home)
  - 2 glucose tablets or 2 doses of glucose gel
  - 2–4 pieces of hard candy
  - Gumdrops
  - 1–2 tablespoons of honey
  - 1 small box of raisins
  - 6 oz regular (not diet) soda (about half a can)
  - 2 tablespoons of cake icing
- Recheck blood glucose in 15 minutes. If reading is still below 70 mg/dL, then:
  - Give another glass of juice, etc.
  - Recheck blood glucose again after another 15 minutes.
- When blood glucose returns to at least 80 mg/dL, a more substantial snack (nonconcentrated sugar) may be given (i.e., cheese and crackers, bread and peanut butter, etc.) if the next meal is more than 30 minutes away or if a physical activity/exercise is planned.
- If the child is unconscious, glucagon should be given either subcutaneously or intramuscularly (ADA, 2007).

Source: Ward, S. L., & Hisley, S. M. (2009). *Maternal-child nursing care* (revised reprint). Philadelphia: F.A. Davis.

Promoting Safety

If the child is conscious, a 4-oz glass of orange juice will help increase blood sugar levels. When a child is severely hypoglycemic and is not able to take glucose tablets by mouth due to confusion or loss of consciousness, a dose of glucagon must be given IM or IV. In most cases the drug is administered IM in the home or school setting to reverse the effects of severe hypoglycemia. The recommended dose to administer for children <20 kg is 0.5 mg and for children >20 kg is 1.0 mg. Doses may be repeated again in 15 minutes if needed.

TYPE 2 DIABETES MELLITUS

- In type 2 diabetes mellitus (T2DM), the body becomes resistant to insulin production from the pancreas.
- Termed "adult-onset" diabetes when occurring in adulthood
- The age of onset is getting younger due to the increase in pediatric obesity in the United States.

Assessment

Clinical Presentation

- Children with T2DM usually have no symptoms and the condition is diagnosed with routine well-check visits.
- The initial symptom will be an elevated blood glucose level, or the child begins to have complications such as DKA.
- **Acanthosis nigricans** (dark pigmented areas of the skin on the back of the neck, axilla, and arms) is evidence of insulin resistance.
- Any child with a BMI over the 85th percentile for weight and age should be monitored for early signs of T2DM, as obesity is a key predisposing factor, followed by hypertension and high cholesterol levels.
- Other symptoms that might occur are gradual and may consist of a burning sensation of the feet, ankles, and legs; poor wound healing; changes in vision; and fatigue.

Diagnostic Testing

- Elevated fasting blood glucose levels >125 mg/dL
- Random blood glucose levels >200 mg/dL
- Elevated hemoglobin A1C level >7
- Oral glucose tolerance testing

Nursing Interventions

- Early assessment for risks, detection, and diagnosis is crucial.
- Obtain dietary history and refer to dietitian for dietary counseling.
- Encourage exercise and refer the parents to a physical therapist if indicated.
- Administer oral antihyperglycemics as ordered to help decrease high blood glucose levels.
- Assess for symptoms of psychosocial problems, such as altered body image, depression, and ineffective individual coping, and refer to a psychologist if needed.

CRITICAL COMPONENT

Risk Factors for Type 2 Diabetes Mellitus

In 2007, the American Diabetes Association (ADA) established guidelines for the diagnosis and treatment of obesity in children due to the increased incidence of insulin resistance and type 2 diabetes mellitus. As a result of these guidelines, it was established that if certain risk factors appear in the history of the child, then at age 10, the child should begin preliminary testing for T2DM every 2 years. Some of these risk factors are:

- BMI >85th percentile for age and weight
- Family history of T2DM
- Certain race/ethnicity groups: African American, Latino, Asian American, American Indians, and Pacific Islanders
- Signs of insulin resistance as evidenced by acanthosis nigricans
- Maternal history of gestational diabetes or diabetes

Diagnosis is confirmed when the child has a fasting glucose of >125 mg/dL or two random blood glucose readings over 200 mg/dL (Ball et al., 2010; Ward & Hisley, 2009).

Caregiver Education

- Explain to the family that treatment options include dietary compliance and exercise to help lose weight and lower glucose levels.
- Involve the entire family in the dietary and exercise education, as many patients have obese parents and siblings with pre-diabetes or T2DM. The concept of working as a team is very important because the child can't be compliant with treatment unless the family is involved and supportive of the child.
- Educate the child and family regarding the long-term effects of T2DM, such as permanent vision loss, cardiovascular disease, hypertension, high cholesterol, and orthopedic problems.
- Teach the parents how to limit sedentary play time such as playing video games and watching TV, and encourage team sports and daily exercise.
- If oral antihyperglycemics are ordered, the nurse must teach the parents and patient regarding reasons for the medication, dose, route, and frequency. Potential side effects should also be discussed.
- The patient should be taught the signs and symptoms of hypoglycemia, hyperglycemia, and DKA.

Review Questions

1. The nurse is teaching an 11-year-old girl and her parents how to administer growth hormone injections. The nurse knows that the following interventions will promote the best response to therapy. (Select all that apply)
   A. Injections given each morning
   B. Daily rotation of injection sites
   C. Strict adherence and minimal doses missed
   D. Follow-up appointments every 3 to 4 months to monitor growth progress and adjust doses

2. A 10-year-old boy is 2 days post-op following the resection of a craniopharyngeoma. You are providing care and notice that he is having enuresis, constantly drinking water, and having frequent urination. Based on the clinical manifestations, you suspect that he might be experiencing what condition?
   A. Diabetes mellitus
   B. Syndrome of inappropriate antidiuretic hormone
   C. Diabetes insipidus
   D. Acute glomerulonephritis
3. The mother of a 6-year-old Hispanic girl comes into the clinic stating that her daughter is developing breast and pubic hair and has acne on her face. On assessment, you note that the child has Tanner Stage 2 breast and pubic hair development, oily skin, and some blemishes on her chin and forehead. You suspect that based on this assessment, the child could be having precocious puberty. What lab result would the nurse expect to see in a child with precocious puberty?
   A. High LH
   B. Low LH
   C. High TSH
   D. Low FSH
4. *True or False:*
   To ensure that an infant with congenital hypothyroidism is getting the full dose of his or her thyroid replacement medication, the nurse should instruct the parents to put the medication in the infant's bottle of formula.
5. *True or False:*
   Beta blockers are frequently used in clients who have uncontrolled Graves' disease and exhibit clinical symptoms of thyroid storm.
6. *Fill-in-the-blank:*
   A 15-year-old boy is being seen in the diabetes clinic. He is obese and has dark pigmented areas on the back of his neck and axilla. The nurse knows that this condition is called _______________.
7. Glycosolated hemoglobin is an acceptable method used to
   A. diagnose diabetes mellitus.
   B. assess the control of diabetes.
   C. assess the oxygen saturation of hemoglobin.
   D. determine the insulin levels in the blood.
8. The nurse is teaching a newly diagnosed diabetic patient about the importance of exercise and physical activity. The nurse knows that prior to exercise or physical activity, the child should do which of the following?
   A. Administer an extra dose of insulin.
   B. Decrease the amount of fluids prior to exercise.
   C. Restrict exercise to noncontact sports.
   D. Eat an extra protein and complex carbohydrate snack.
9. Exopthalmos may occur in children with which of the following conditions?
   A. Hypothyroidism
   B. Hyperparathyroidism
   C. Hyperthyroidism
   D. Hypoparathyroidism
10. Infants are screened at birth for hypothyroidism because of which of the following conditions that occurs if untreated?
   A. Mental retardation
   B. ADHD
   C. Cerebral palsy
   D. Failure to thrive

References

Alt, P., Babler, E. K., Betts, K. J., Carney, P. H. , Courtney, J. A., Flores, B. M., ... Worley, D. D. (2003). *Clinical handbook of pediatric endocrinology*. St. Louis, MO: Quality Medical Publishing.

Amer, K. S. (2005). Advances in assessment, diagnosis, and treatment of hyperthyroidism in children. *Journal of Pediatric Nursing, 20*, 119–126. doi: 10.1016/j.pedn.2004.12.013

American Diabetes Association. (2009). Glucagon training for standards for school personnel: Providing emergency medical assistance to pupils with diabetes. Retrieved from: http://web.diabetes.org/Advocacy/school/glucagon.pdf

Ball, K., Bindler, K. J., & Cowen, R. C. (2010). *Child health nursing: Partnering with children and families* (2nd ed.). Upper Saddle River, NJ: Prentice Hall.

Deglin, J. H., & Vallerand, A. H. (2009). *Davis drug guide for nurses* (11th ed.). Philadelphia: F.A. Davis.

Demirci, C., & Witchell, S. F. (2008). Congenital adrenal hyperplasia. *Dermatologic Therapy, 21*, 340–353. doi: 10.1111/j.1529-8019.2008.00216.x

Halvorson, M., Yasuda, P., Carpenter, S., & Kaiserman, K. (2005). Unique challenges for pediatric patients with diabetes. *Diabetes Spectrum, 18*, 167–173. doi: 10.2337/diaspect.18.3.167

Horner, G. (2007). Genitourinary assessment: An integral part of a complete physical exam. *Journal Pediatric Health Care, 21*, 162–170. Retrieved from http://www.jpedhc.org/

Lipman, T. H., Euler, D., Markowitz, G. R., & Ratcliffe, S. J. (2009). Evaluation of linear measurement and growth plotting in an inpatient pediatric setting. *Journal Pediatric Nursing, 24*, 323–329. doi: 10.1016/j.pedn.2008.09.001

Lipman, T. H., Hench, K. D., Benyi, T., Delaune, J., Gilluly, K. A., Johnson, L., ... Weber, C. (2004). A multicentre randomized controlled trial of an intervention to improve the accuracy of linear growth measurement. *Archives of Disease in Childhood, 89*, 342_346. doi: 10.1136/adc.2003.030072

National Institute of Health. (2004). Adrenal insufficiency and Addison's disease. Retrieved from: http://www.endocrine.niddk.nih.gov/pubs/addison/addison.aspx

Riepe, F. G., & Sippell, W. G. (2007). Recent advances in diagnostic, treatment and outcome of congenital adrenal hyperplasia due to 21-hydroxylase deficiency. *Review Endocrine Metabolism Disorders, 8*, 349–363. doi: 10.1007/s11154-007-9053-1

Styne, D. M. (2004). *Core handbook in pediatrics: Pediatric endocrinology*. Philadelphia: Lippincott Williams & Wilkins.

Suddaby, B., & Mowery, B. (2007). Complications of diabetes insipidus: The significance of headache. *Pediatric Nursing, 33*, 58–59. Retrieved from http://www.ncbi.nlm.nih.gov/pubmed/17411003

Ward, S. L., & Hisley, S. M. (2009). *Maternal-child nurse care: Optimizing outcomes for mothers, children & families*. Philadelphia: F.A. Davis.

18

Reproductive and Genetic Disorders

Irene Cihon Dietz, MD, FAAP
Tina Goodpasture, RN, MSN, FNP

OBJECTIVES

- ☐ Define key terms.
- ☐ Identify the anatomy of the male and female reproductive systems.
- ☐ Discuss common pediatric reproductive health concerns.
- ☐ Describe the signs and symptoms and interventions for common sexually transmitted infections.
- ☐ Explain the human genome and its function.
- ☐ Describe errors in reproduction, including mitosis, meiosis, and their contribution to genetic disorders.
- ☐ Explain differences and similarities among autosomal dominant, recessive, and X-linked disorders.
- ☐ Describe a variety of common genetic syndromes.
- ☐ Explain the recommended age-appropriate care and pediatric surveillance for common genetic syndromes.

KEY TERMS

- Oocyte
- Fetus
- Endometrium
- Andrenarche
- Amenorrhea
- Bacterial vaginosis (BV)
- Menorrhagia
- Epididymides
- Spermatic cords
- Testicular torsion
- Inguinal hernia
- Syphilis
- Cytoplasm
- Nucleus
- Chromosome
- Deoxyribonucleic acid (DNA)
- Gene
- Allele
- Autosome
- Mitosis
- Gamete
- Recombination
- Nondisjunction
- Zygote
- Embryo
- Mosaicism
- Haploid
- Diploid
- Translocation
- Trisomy
- Deletion
- Mutation
- Autosomal dominant inheritance
- X-linked

FEMALE REPRODUCTIVE SYSTEM

ANATOMY AND PHYSIOLOGY

The female anatomy contains organs that work together for reproduction (**Figure 18-1**).

- **Ovaries**
  - *The two female organs that produce the ova (eggs) and sex hormones*
  - *Each is the size of a walnut.*
- **Ovum**
  - *The mature female reproductive cell, also known as the egg, or* **oocyte**
  - *Ova are formed within the ovaries and are released on a cyclic basis.*
  - *The development of the ovum is under hormonal control.*
- **Fallopian tube(s)**
  - *Also known as the oviduct, a muscular tube that extends from the uterus to the ovary*
  - *There are two, one for each ovary.*
  - *About 4 inches (10 cm) long*

Don't have time to read this chapter? Want to reinforce your reading? Need to review for a test? Listen to this chapter on DavisPlus at davispl.us/rudd1.

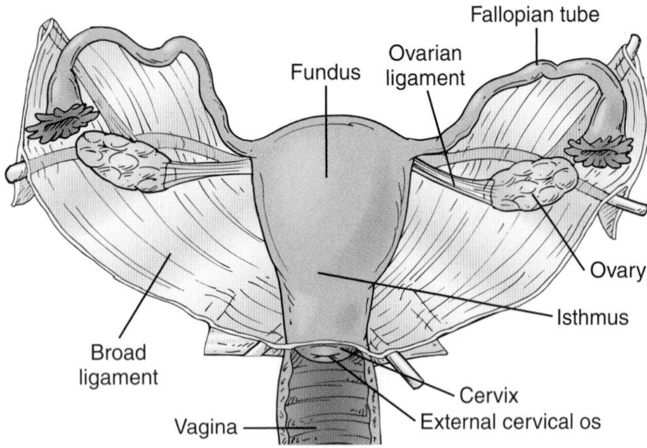

Figure 18-1 Female reproductive system.

- **Uterus (Figure 18-2)**
  - *Commonly called the womb*
  - *A pear-shaped organ in the female abdominal cavity*
  - *Holds the developing infant or* **fetus**
- **Endometrium**
  - *Layer of cells lining the uterus*
  - *Responds to hormones (estrogen and progesterone)*
  - *Shed to produce the menstrual cycle*
- **Clitoris**
  - *A small area of erectile tissue, situated below the pelvic bone and partially covered by the labia minora*
- **Vagina**
  - *Tubular area connecting external female genital tract from vulva upward to the cervix*
- **Hymen**
  - *Thin fold of skin that lies between the labia minora*
  - *Disrupted by sexual intercourse or other means of rupture*
- **Urethra**
  - *Muscular tube through which urine may exit the bladder*

Pubertal Changes in Girls

- **Adrenarche** is when the adrenal gland starts to produce sex hormones. These outward changes are characterized by the stages of puberty (**Table 18-1**).
- These staging events have been published by Marshall and Tanner (1969) and are referred to as "Tanner Stages" (see Chapter 10).

CLINICAL PEARL

Age of Pubertal Onset

The age of pubertal onset varies with genetic and environmental influences, including physiologic stress. In the United States, pubertal onset before age 8 is considered precocious, and later than 16 years is considered delayed and merits endocrine evaluation.

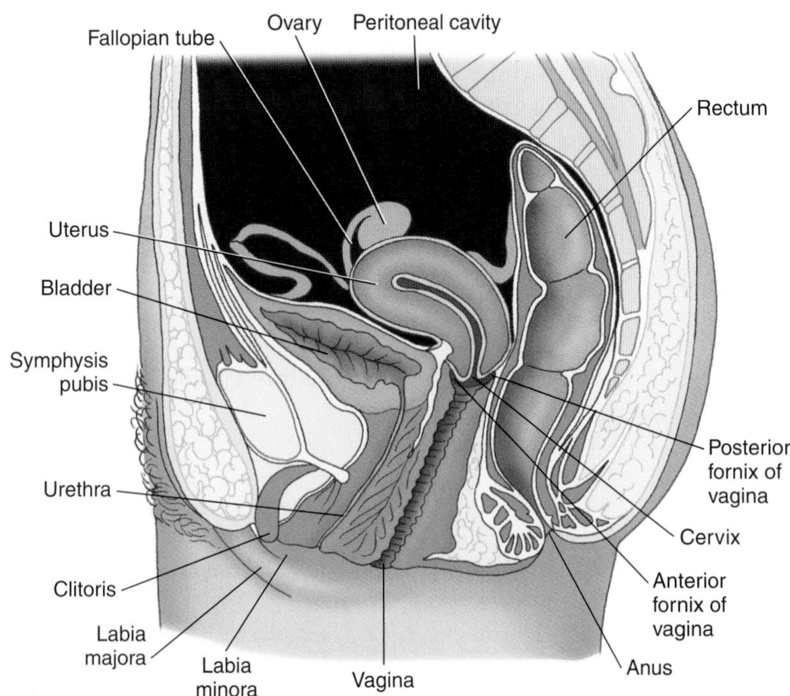

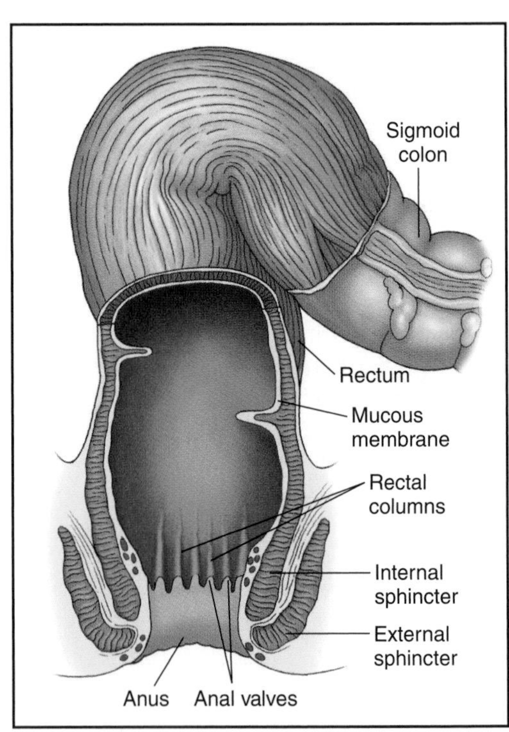

Figure 18-2 Internal female genitalia and cross-section of rectum.

TABLE 18–1	STAGES OF PUBERTY IN FEMALES
Pubarche	Appearance of pubic hair
Thelarche	Appearance of breast tissue maturation
Menarche	Onset of first menstrual period

COMMON PEDIATRIC AND ADOLESCENT PROBLEMS OF THE FEMALE GENITAL TRACT

STRADDLE INJURY

- Injury to genitals as the result of fall over a blunt object
- Commonly caused from monkey bars or bicycle
- Common in school-age children

Nursing Interventions

- May cause a hematoma—trapped blood between tissues; most do not need special treatment (Reyes Mendez, 2011)
- Avoid surgical drainage to prevent introduction of bacteria and abscess
  - *Small—size of a hen's egg: bed rest, intermittent use of ice pack with pressure for 12 to 24 hours.*
  - *Medium—size of an orange: as above, bed rest, ice for first 12–24 hours, then warm tub baths or Sitz-type soaking bath in addition.*
  - *Large—size of a grapefruit (greater than 15-cm diameter): must assess for urethral obstruction; may require suprapubic catheter.*

LACERATIONS OR SKIN TEARS

- May require examination under anesthesia to identify the source of the bleeding
  - *With labial or vulvar tears, it is best to avoid treatment by suturing and instead allow to heal by secondary intention if possible (Garcia, 2006).*
  - *Large areas need repair and exploration under anesthesia for additional vaginal injury.*
- Hymenal injuries occur most often from penetrating trauma.
  - *Penetrating injury can cause vaginal and/or internal injury; treatment varies by degree of bleeding.*

Nursing Interventions

- Evaluation for possible sexual abuse
- Area and type of injury and placement of bruising should be examined by abuse expert.

VULVOVAGINITIS

- Inflammation of the vulva and vaginal areas
- Most common complaint involving the genital area of prepubescent girls (Joishy, Ashtekar, Jain, & Gonsalves, 2005)
- Symptoms may include vaginal itching (pruritus), soreness, redness (erythema), thin vaginal discharge, or painful urination (dysuria)
- Causes may be specific or nonspecific.
- Prepubescent girls are more susceptible.
  - *Labial tissue lacks estrogen*
  - *Tissue is thinner and more susceptible to irritants*
  - *Infection and chronic masturbatory activity in small children is irritating*
  - *Vulvovaginitis may also indicate the presence of vaginal foreign body.*
  - *Of girls with a foreign body, 25% to 75% may present with odor or discharge (Laufner & Emans, 2011).*

Nursing Interventions

- Teach hygiene with front-to-back wiping after bowel movements.
- Consider using moist wipes rather than dry paper to wipe.
- Allow air flow by wearing cotton underwear. Avoid wearing tight clothing on lower body.
- Daily warm bath for 10 to 15 minutes in clear water; minimal use of gentle soap, rinsed just before getting out of tub; pat dry, or may use hair dryer distant from skin on cool or low setting

Specific Causes of Vulvovaginitis

Pinworm

- Vulvar and perianal itching usually present (Laufner & Emans, 2011; see **Figure 18-3**)

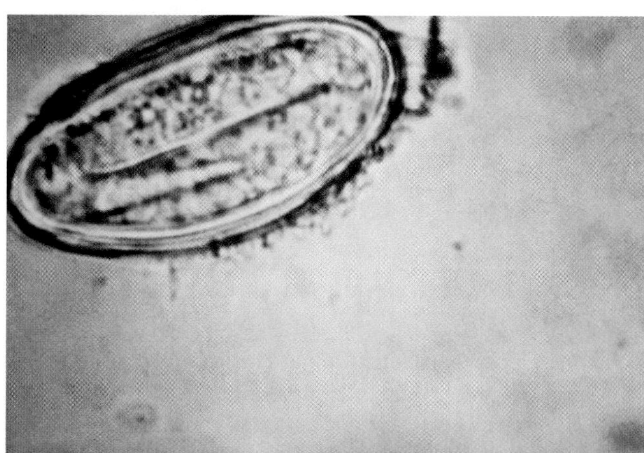

Figure 18–3 Pinworm. *(From the Centers for Disease Control and Prevention, Department of Health and Human Services. [1979]. Retrieved from http://phil.cdc.gov/Phil/details.asp 4819)*

- Tiny worms with fecal–oral spread
- Adult female worms live in gastrointestinal (GI) tract, are not shed in stool, and come out to lay eggs in warm perineal areas, mostly at night.
- "Tape test": use sticky side of tape to lift bean-shaped white eggs from area; may see white 5- to 13-mm adult worms.

Nursing Interventions

- Teach proper hand hygiene after using the bathroom and after contact with feces.
- Medications as prescribed by physician
- Avoid scratching perianal area

Vulvar Ulcers

- Also known as Lipshutz ulcers, "virginal" ulcers, "aphthous" ulcers
- Generally seen in girls ages 10 to 15 years
- Present as one or more painful ulcers >1 cm in diameter with purulent bases and raised red edges
- Nonsexually transmitted; associated with viral infections such as influenza A, Epstein–Barr virus (EBV), or cytomegalovirus? (CMV), but should also test for herpes simplex virus type 1 and type 2

Nursing Interventions

- May require a Foley catheter to urinate
- Topical antibiotic if secondary infection
- Usually heals in 1 to 3 weeks
- Pain management

Imperforate Hymen

- Congenital malformation
- May be seen at birth with white or mucoid material detained behind the area, but will reabsorb if missed
- More often presents as a bluish bulge in a teen with complaints of **amenorrhea**
- Can be associated with chronic pain in abdomen or back from retained blood within the vagina

Nursing Interventions

- Provide anticipatory guidance for the treatment of surgical repair.
- Pain management
- Reassure teen girl if body image issues are present.

ADOLESCENT VAGINAL COMPLAINTS

BACTERIAL VAGINOSIS (BV)

- The absence of inflammation is the basis for the term "vaginosis" rather than "vaginitis" (Sobal, 2011).
- **Bacterial vaginosis (BV)** is the most common cause of vaginal discharge in adolescents and women of childbearing age.
- Of affected women, 50% to 75% may have minimal symptoms, or may have fishy-smelling, thin, whitish-gray discharge (Klebanoff et al., 2004).
- Not the result of one organism but a complex change in normal vaginal organisms and increase in other organisms (**Figure 18-4**)

Nursing Interventions

- Up to one-third of cases will resolve spontaneously.
- May consider in treatment in partners for women who have sex with women or lesbians
- Presence of BV is associated with HIV acquisition as well as increased risk for preterm labor in pregnant women.
- Menstruation is the active shedding of the endometrial lining of the uterus in a cyclic fashion in response to estrogen and progesterone hormone changes (**Figure 18-5**)

> **CRITICAL COMPONENT**
>
> **Normal Menstrual Cycle**
>
> The normal menstrual cycle results from a complex feedback system involving the hypothalamus, pituitary, ovary, and uterus. The cyclic changes in the major pituitary and gonadal hormones are illustrated in Figure 18-5. Although the development of secondary sexual characteristics varies by race and geographic location, the average age of menarche in the United States is 12.3 years (Wu, Mendola, & Buck, 2002).

ABNORMAL UTERINE BLEEDING (AUB)

- Menstrual cycles are often irregular in the first months after menarche.
- The median length of the first cycle after menarche is 34 days, with 38% of cycles exceeding 40 days and 7% occurring less than 20 days apart (World Health Organization, Task Force on Adolescent Reproductive Health, 1986).

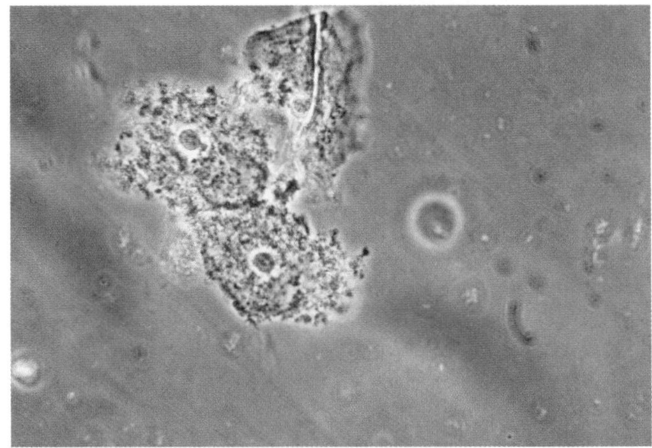

Figure 18-4 Vaginosis "clue cells" indicating a change in normal vaginal organisms. *(From the Centers for Disease Control and Prevention, Department of Health and Human Services. [1978]. Retrieved from http://phil.cdc.gov/Phil/quicksearch.asp 3719)*

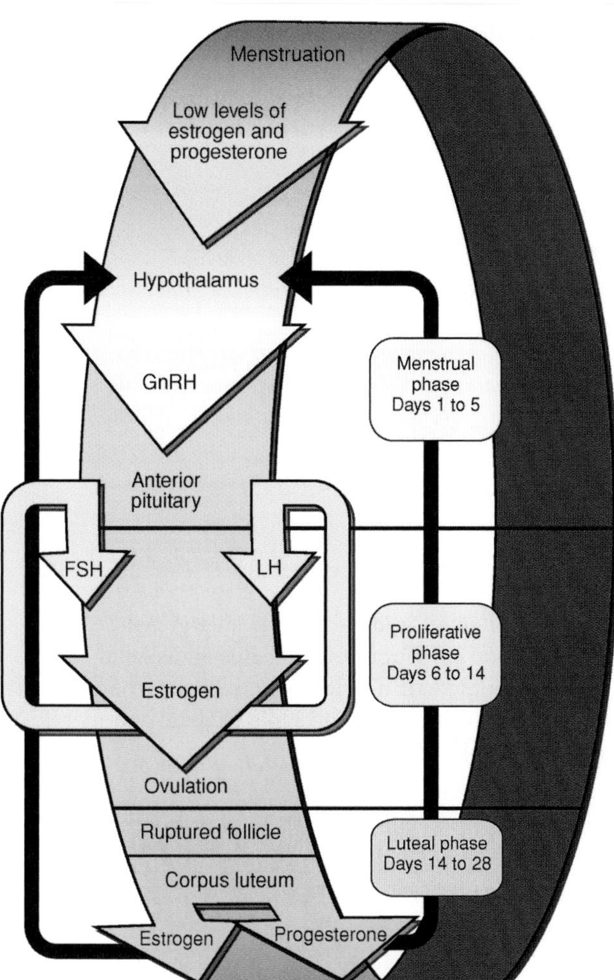

Figure 18–5 Menstrual cycle.

- Cause of most frequent gynecologic complaints
- Most cases of AUB in adolescents are caused by anovulatory cycles, where no ovum (egg) is released. This is seen most often during the first 12 to 18 months after menarche.
- Other common causes: pregnancy, infection, the use of hormonal contraceptives, stress (psychogenic or exercise induced), bleeding disorders, and endocrine disorders (e.g., hypothyroidism, polycystic ovary syndrome)

AMENORRHEA

- Absence of periods or menses

Primary Amenorrhea

- *Period has never been present*
- *The average age of menarche is 12.3 years, and 95% of females in the United States have onset of menses by 14.7 years (Anderson & Must, 2005).*
- *Girls need endocrine evaluation if no menses by 16 years.*

Nursing Interventions

- Obtain detailed physical history.
- Obtain family history of reproductive problems.

Secondary Amenorrhea

- Periods had started and then ceased at some time
- Absence of menses for more than three cycles or 6 months in women who previously had menses
  - *Etiology of secondary amenorrhea is most often pregnancy*
  - *Workup by excluding pregnancy through urine or blood pregnancy test*

Nursing Interventions

- Hormone therapy as indicated by physician
- Assess for vaginal bleeding.
- Document amount of vaginal bleeding as output.

Caregiver Education

- Teach the importance of keeping track of when the period starts and when it ends.
- Teach that hormone therapy does not prevent sexually transmitted infections.

Menorrhagia

- **Menorrhagia** is characterized by menstrual flow of excessive duration, greater than 7 days, and/or heavy volume, greater than 80 ml/cycle (DeSilva & Zurawin, 2011).
- Typically occurs at irregular intervals, indicating anovulatory (lack of ova release) cycles
- Need to also consider coagulation disorders, especially if present with very heavy first menses, or those with refractory anemia

Nursing Interventions and Caregiver Education

- Complete blood count, platelets, and iron level as indicated by physician
- Consider evaluation for von Willebrand disease
  - *The most common inherited cause of excessive bleeding*
  - *Individuals have missing or decreased function of von Willebrand Factor (important for clotting and adherence of platelets)*
- Provide education to evaluate amount of vaginal discharge.
- Encourage a well-balanced diet and food rich in iron during menses.

MALE REPRODUCTIVE SYSTEM

ANATOMY AND PHYSIOLOGY

- **Penis**
  - *Male reproductive organ* (**Figure 18-6**)
  - *Both urine and semen leave the body through the penis.*
  - *Contains the urethra and two tubular and honeycombed areas of erectile tissue*

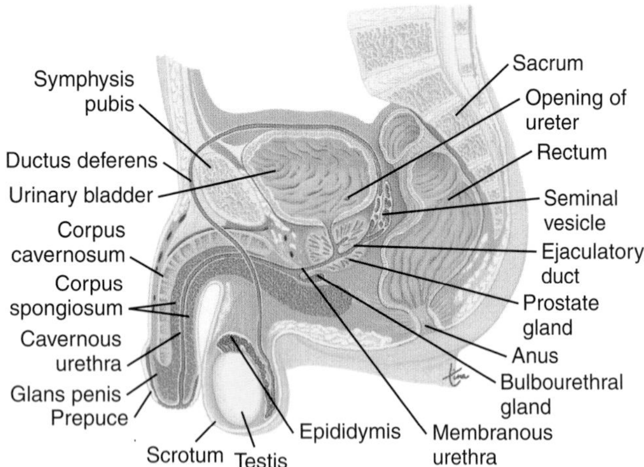

Figure 18-6 Male reproductive system.

- **Glans**
  - *External bulbous area at the end of the penis; a particularly sensitive area*
- **Prepuce**
  - *Known as the foreskin*
  - *Small area of skin that covers the glans*
  - *Removed in male circumcision*
- **Testis (testicle)**
  - *One of the male reproductive organs (plural* testicles*) or gonads*
  - *After puberty, the testes produce the male hormone testosterone and the reproductive cells (sperm).*
  - *Each is about 1.5 inches (4 cm) long in adults*
- **Sperm**
  - *The male sex cell, also known as the spermatozoon*
  - *Produced within the testicles*
  - *Ejaculated in the semen*
  - *Each sperm (and ovum) contains one-half of the normal number of chromosomes required to form a single cell*
- **Semen**
  - *Creamy discharge secreted through the penis during ejaculation*
  - *Consists of sperm and fluids secreted by the prostate gland and seminal vesicles, certain epithelial cells, and other gland secretions*
- **Spermatic cord**
  - *The cord by which the testicle is suspended within the scrotum*
  - *Encloses the vas deferens, blood vessels, and nerves that serve each testicle*
- **Epididymis**
  - *Long, coiled tube that rests on the backside of each testicle*
  - *Transports and stores sperm cells that are produced in the testes*
  - *Brings the sperm to maturity, as the sperm that emerge from the testes are immature and incapable of fertilization*
  - *Each male has two* **epididymides**.
- **Vas deferens**
  - *Also known as the sperm duct*
  - *Tube that carries mature sperm from the epididymis to the seminal vesicles (where the sperm is stored)*
- **Prostate gland**
  - *A walnut-shaped organ that is part of the male urogenital system*
  - *Lies beneath the bladder and surrounds the urethra*
  - *Produces secretions that maintain the vitality of the sperm*
- **Scrotum**
  - *The baglike structure of skin that contains the testicles, epididymides, and parts of the* **spermatic cords**
  - *The skin of the scrotum contains muscles that can raise or lower the testicles, thereby keeping them at optimum temperature for sperm reproduction*

PUBERTY IN BOYS

- Pubertal changes in boys include enlargement of the genitals, both in length of the penis and size of the testicles, pubic hair development, increased body hair, deepening of the voice, and rapid skeletal and muscle growth (**Table 18-2**).

COMMON PEDIATRIC AND ADOLESCENT PROBLEMS OF THE MALE GENITAL TRACT

CIRCUMCISION

- Surgical removal of the foreskin (**Figure 18-7**)
- Often done in infancy
- May be done for religious or cultural purposes

CULTURAL AWARENESS: The Jewish "Bris"

Jewish custom is to perform circumcision (a ritual "bris") on the eighth day of life. The child's birthday is counted as day 1. Jewish days begin at sunset, so this will influence when the eighth day is identified.

Nursing Interventions

- Provide pain management.
- Wash with soap and water.

TABLE 18-2 STAGES OF PUBERTY IN MALES

Adrenarche	Adrenal medulla area starts to produce androgens (testosterone and estrogen); typically occurs before the onset of puberty
Pubarche	Appearance of pubic hair
Gonadarche	Activation of the gonads by the pituitary hormones: follicle-stimulating hormone (FSH) and luteinizing hormone (LH)

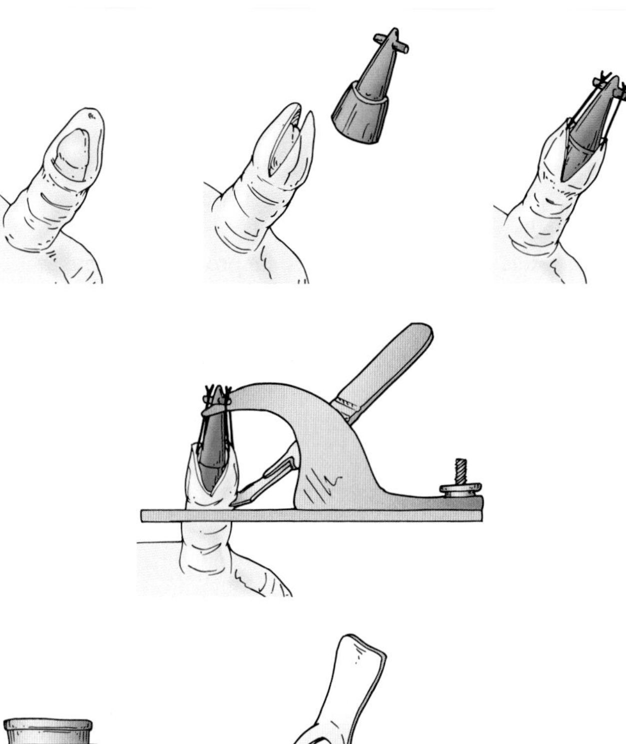
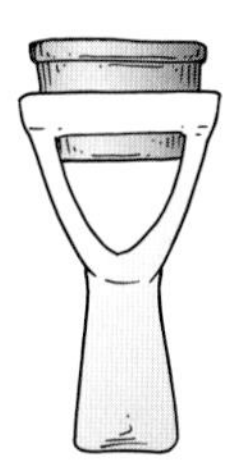
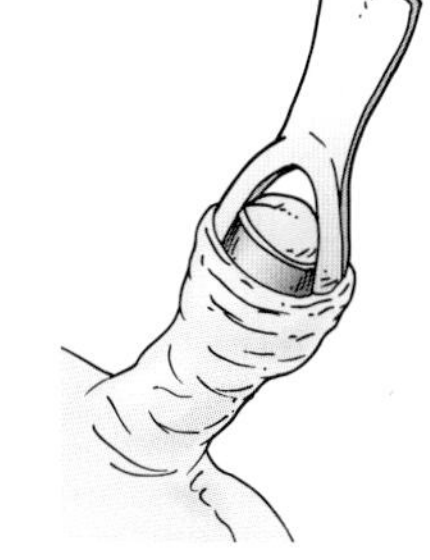
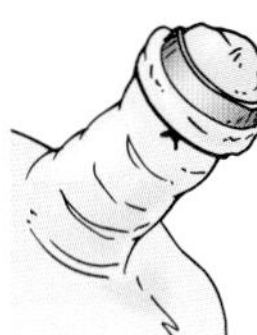

Figure 18–7 Circumcision.

- Dressing may not be necessary.
- Alert physician to excessive bleeding.

Caregiver Education

- Notify physician if oozing, swelling, or drainage noted around surgical site.
- Notify physician of fever.
- Wash with soap and water after diaper changes.
- Provide Tylenol as ordered by physician.

UNCIRCUMCISED PENIS

- By seventh grade, only about 1% of uncircumcised boys cannot retract the foreskin (Hsieh, Chang, & Chang, 2006).

Nursing Interventions

- Wash or cleanse the penis and glans as you would any other part of the body.
- The foreskin does not need to be retracted in infancy or toddler years.

Caregiver Education

- During this time caregivers should leave the foreskin alone.
- Avoid forcible retraction.
- As the foreskin naturally begins to retract, cleaning and then drying underneath the foreskin can be performed.
- Foreskin should always be pulled down to its normal position covering the glans after drying.

PHYSIOLOGIC PHIMOSIS

- Inability to retract the foreskin beyond the glans penis
- Physiologic phimosis is present in almost all newborn males.

Nursing Interventions

- School-age boys without a fully retractable foreskin and/or their parents should be counseled that there is normally a wide range of retractability.
- Reinforce proper hygiene.

Caregiver Education

- Patients and/or parents can be taught to perform gentle stretch exercises.
- As ordered by a physician, a 4- to 8-week course of topical corticosteroids may be prescribed (Zampieri, Corroppolo, Camoglio, Giacomello, & Ottolenghi, 2005).
- Council parents and child that nearly all men develop the ability to retract the foreskin by adulthood without specific treatment.

PATHOLOGIC PHIMOSIS

- Secondary nonretractability of the foreskin after retractability at an earlier age
- Irritation or bleeding from the preputial orifice
- Pain with urination (dysuria)
- Painful erection
- Chronic urinary retention with ballooning that is only resolved with manual compression

Nursing Intervention

- Pediatric urologic consultation should be sought.

PARAPHIMOSIS

- Inability to return the foreskin to its natural position once retracted, resulting in swelling and pain in the glans penis
- Medical emergency in order to avoid vascular injury to the glans

Nursing Interventions and Caregiver Education

- Educate child and caregiver that anesthesia is generally required to return foreskin and may require possible circumcision.
- Steroid may also be used as noted earlier if circumcision is not desired.

ZIPPER INJURIES

- Penile injuries related to zipper entrapment
- One of the more common genital injuries; involve penile entrapment
  - *Usually entrapment of the foreskin or redundant skin, with localized edema and pain being the most common complications; skin loss or necrosis is rare*

Nursing Interventions

- Treatment is release of the zipper.
- Most often recommend cutting the zipper's median bar with wire cutters, bone cutters, or small hacksaw
- Sedation or local pain control is recommended.

Caregiver Education

- Teach child to carefully zip pants once underwear has been pulled up.
- Do not force zip-up if difficulty noted.
- Encourage the child to ask for assistance when zipper is difficult to manage.

CRITICAL COMPONENT

Circumcision

Circumcision in the United States is most often performed for social reasons. Often this is as part of a religious rite of passage near birth, or an initiation into adulthood. Frequently it is because it is the tradition in the family, or because the majority of the boys in the neighborhood are circumcised. There is no medical reason for routine circumcision of boys. Current medical evidence also does not support circumcision as having any effect on the incidence of cancers of the penis or of the cervix (CDC, 2012).

DEVELOPMENT OF THE TESTIS

Understanding of the development and movement of the testis into the scrotum is important to understand many types of masses of the scrotum.

- The testicles develop in the male unborn infant, or fetus, in the abdomen in a position very close to that of the ovaries in the female.
- Around 10 weeks of gestational age, an outpouching through the abdominal cavity develops; ultimately this migrates down into the scrotum.
- By 12 weeks, the testicles start to migrate down through the abdominal wall to reside in the scrotum.
- The processus vaginalis forms from an outward protrusion of the peritoneum that lines the abdominal wall.
- Between the seventh and ninth months of gestation, the testes descend into the scrotum, pushing the processus vaginalis ahead, and then protrude into its cavity.
- Once this process is complete, the processus vaginalis obliterates spontaneously, usually by age 2 years.
- Many males are born with incomplete descent of the testis, and the process may be completed after birth.

CRYPTORCHIDISM (UNDESCENDED TESTIS)

- Congenital condition in which the testis fails to descend into the scrotum
- Most often the testis remains in the inguinal canal or higher up in the groin.
- May be palpated on exam

Nursing Interventions

- Refer to urology or surgery by age 2 years if undescended testicle is palpated in the groin or inguinal area.
- Anticipate ultrasound of the scrotum if the testicle is not palpated within the scrotum or canal.

Caregiver Education

- Encourage loose clothing worn on the lower body.
- Ultrasound or other tests may be needed to evaluate the current condition.

SCROTAL SWELLING

- Causes vary from benign incidental findings to medical emergencies, and by age and clinical symptoms
- Generally divided into painless versus painful swelling, or chronic versus acute changes

HYDROCELE

- A painless collection of fluid between the layers of tissue or capsule covering the testis, the tunica vaginalis
- Fluid moves through the processus vaginalis to surround the testis.
- Very common in newborns, generally resolves by 1 year of age
- Exam is of a cystic structure, and can be transilluminated (light easily passes through the area)
- May occur in older children and adolescents, both spontaneous or related to infection or trauma

Nursing Interventions and Caregiver Education

- Monitoring for resolution of fluid/swelling when under 1 year of age.
- Refer for further evaluation when over 1 year of age.

VARICOCELE

- A painless collection of dilated and tortuous veins in the plexus surrounding the spermatic cord in the scrotum
- Can be asymptomatic, or present complaining of a dull ache or fullness of the scrotum upon standing
- A palpable varicocele has the texture of a "bag of worms" and may become fuller with bearing down or in Valsalva maneuver
- May be associated with infertility—about 20% of male patients in infertility clinics have a varicocele (Skoog, Roberts, Goldstein, & Pryor, 1997).

Nursing Interventions

- No clear guidelines established for treatment of a varicocele in childhood
- Observation until teen years

Child and Caregiver Education

- Provide anticipatory guidance when aggressive surgical treatment is necessary.

TORSION (TWISTING) OF THE TESTICLE

- **Testicular torsion**, or twisting of the testicle, has the following characteristics:
  - *Painful scrotal swelling*
  - *Abrupt, severe constant pain in the scrotum, lower abdomen, and groin area; 90% with nausea and vomiting (Perron, 2006)*
  - *Peak incidence in boys 12 to 18 years; smaller group in neonatal period*
  - *Present with scrotal edema; the affected testis is tender, swollen, and slightly elevated; the testis may lie horizontally and may have a reactive hydrocele.*
  - *Intermittent torsion can present with intermittent sharp pain and swelling, and then rapid resolution.*
- Torsion of the appendix testis
  - *Twisting of a very small remnant in the upper pole of the testis, a residual appendage with no function after fetal development*

Nursing Interventions

- Provide pain management.
- Prepare for possible surgery.
- Prepare child age-appropriately for diagnostic testing.

EPIDIDYMITIS

- Inflammation of the epididymis related to infection
  - *May have diffuse swelling; may also have increased urination (frequency), painful urination (dysuria), or discharge from the urethra; sometimes fever*
  - *Testis is in normal vertical lie on exam and scrotum may be red or edematous*
  - *Chlamydia is the most common cause of epididymitis in sexually active males and is also associated with gonorrhea, but can be due to* Escherichia coli *and even some viruses.*

Nursing Interventions

- Can occur in young boys after infection with enteroviruses, adenovirus, and mycoplasma
- Associated with structural anomalies of the urinary tract in prepubertal boys
- Diagnosis by clinical exam, but Doppler ultrasound or nuclear scan considered if uncertain, as torsion needs immediate surgical referral

Child and Caregiver Education

- Prepare for diagnostic Doppler ultrasound.
- Prepare for possible surgery.
- Preparation should be explained in a developmentally appropriate manner.

ORCHITIS

- Painful inflammation/infection of the testis
- Present with scrotal swelling
- Pain
- Tenderness
- Redness and shininess of the overlying skin

Nursing Interventions

- Associated with other systemic infections
- Anticipate treatment to be based on cause of infection (viral or bacterial).

Child and Caregiver Education

- Bed rest
- Ice packs as ordered
- Nonsteroidal anti-inflammatory agents (ibuprofen) as ordered by physician
- Support of the inflamed testis
- Appropriate antibiotics as ordered by physician

PRIMARY INGUINAL HERNIA

- A hernia is a protrusion of any organ or tissue through an abnormal opening in the wall that should contain it.
- Passage of tissue into the groin area occurs in 1% to 5% percent of all newborns and 9% to 11% percent of those born prematurely (Grosfeld, 1989).
- **Inguinal hernias** occur three to four times more often in males than females, and occur bilaterally in about 10% (Skoog & Conlin, 1995; see **Figure 18-8**).
- Inguinal hernia repair is the most commonly performed surgical procedure in children.

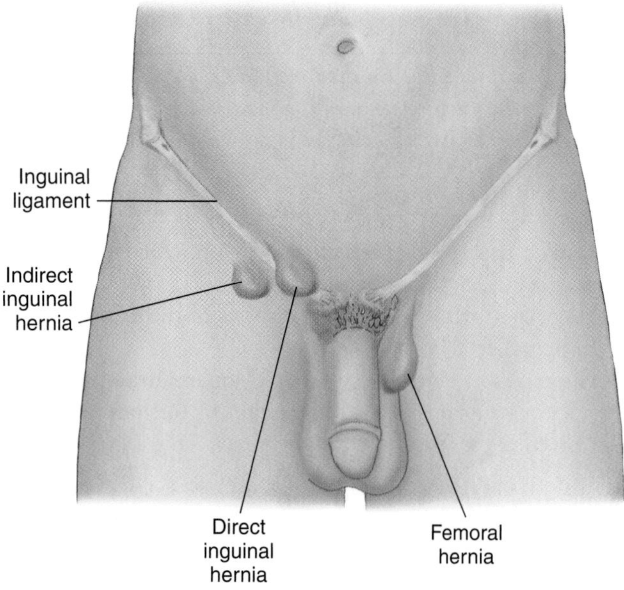

Figure 18–8 Hernia.

- One may acquire a groin hernia due to injury.
- Factors that increase the pressure in the abdomen may produce a groin hernia in susceptible adolescents: lifting heavy objects, obesity, pregnancy, constipation and resultant straining, and recurrent coughing or sneezing.
- Incarceration of hernia
  - *Refers to inability to reduce or push herniated tissue back through the opening; this is a surgical emergency and needs to be treated quickly.*
- Strangulation of hernia
  - *Refers to vascular compromise of the contents of an incarcerated hernia, caused by progressive edema from venous and lymphatic obstruction*
  - *Strangulation can occur within 2 hours of incarceration.*
  - *Children with hernias may present with a painless intermittent mass, a constant reducible mass, or pain with strangulation.*

Nursing Interventions

- Assess for signs and symptoms of infection after surgery.
- Provide adequate pain control and offer nonpharmacological methods for pain relief.
- Assess for bleeding at surgical site.
- Brace lower abdomen with pillow when coughing or deep breathing to prevent dehiscence of wound.

Child and Caregiver Education

- Discourage heavy lifting after repair.
- Watch for bleeding or drainage from surgical site.
- Notify physician if fever present.
- Provide pain medications as ordered by physician.
- Brace lower abdomen with a pillow when coughing or deep breathing.

SEXUALLY TRANSMITTED INFECTIONS (STIS)

Evidence-Based Practice Research: Adolescents at Highest Risk for Sexually Transmitted Infection

Centers for Disease Control and Prevention (CDC). (2010). *2010 STD treatment guidelines.* Retrieved from www.cdc.gov/std/treatment/2010/default.htm

Prevalence rates for sexually transmitted infections (previously called "sexually transmitted diseases") are highest among adolescents. Nearly 50% of STIs are estimated to occur in 15- to 24-year olds. STIs are among the highest of all racial/ethnic health disparities—71% of all gonorrhea, 48% of chlamydia, and 52% of syphilis infections occur in African Americans, according to the Centers for Disease Control and Prevention (CDC). Screening guidelines have been updated by the CDC for even asymptomatic persons in certain high-risk populations, including adolescent clinics, pregnant women, men who have sex with men, and teens in detention centers.

1. What questions should be included when obtaining a medical history from an adolescent?
2. What are some suggestions for anticipatory guidance for adolescents?

Risk Factors for STIs

Behavioral and biological factors play a role in the increased incidence of STIs in adolescence compared to adults.

- Behavioral issues
  - *Multiple partners*
  - *New partners*
  - *Partners with multiple other partners*
  - *Inconsistent use of condoms, especially with established partners*
  - *Alcohol and other drug consumption, often associated with inappropriate birth control and condom use*
- Biological issues
  - *Cervical ectopy or cervical immaturity, which refers to the area of ectocervix that is covered by columnar epithelium after puberty*
  - *Columnar epithelium is thought to be more susceptible than is squamous epithelium to sexually transmitted organisms:* Neisseria gonorrhoeae, C. trachomatis, *and human papilloma virus (HPV).*

Screening for STIs

- CDC and American College of Gynecology Recommendations (CDC, 2010)
- Annual *C. trachomatis* screen for all sexually active females aged ≤25 years
- Annual *N. gonorrhoeae* screen for all sexually active females at risk for infection
- Females aged <25 years are at highest risk for gonorrhea infection.
- All teens or young adults should have at least one HIV screen.

- Routinely screen adolescents who are asymptomatic for certain STIs (e.g., syphilis, trichomoniasis, bacterial vaginosis, herpes simplex virus).
- Young men who have sex with men and pregnant adolescent females might require more thorough evaluation and testing.
- Pap screens should be done on younger teens who engage in high-risk behavior, such as having multiple sexual partners.

PELVIC INFLAMMATORY DISEASE (PID)

- Acute infection of the upper genital tract structures in women
- Can involve the uterus, oviducts, and ovaries, or all of these
- Often accompanied by involvement of the neighboring pelvic organs
- Involvement of these structures may result in:
  - *Endometritis—infection of uterine lining*
  - *Salpingitis—infection of the fallopian tubes*
  - *Oophoritis—infection of the ovaries*
  - *Peritonitis—infection of the abdominal lining or peritoneum*
  - *Perihepatitis—inflammation of the hepatic area, and tubo-ovarian abscess*
- Caused most often by genital gonorrhea and the effect of other infections
- Douching may actually increase the risk of developing PID, especially when performed frequently.
- Health-care providers should maintain a low threshold for the diagnosis of PID.
- Sexually active young women with the combination of lower abdominal, ovarian or fallopian structures (adnexa), and cervical motion tenderness should receive empiric treatment (CDC, 2010).

Nursing Interventions

- Complete antibiotic regime as ordered.
- Educate child or adolescent to take medication as directed.
- Provide pain management.
- Teach signs and symptoms of infection.
- Educate about the prevention of STIs.
- Educate about condom use.
- Educate about abstinence.

Child and Caregiver Education

- Complete antibiotics as prescribed.
- Educate about the prevention of STIs.
- Educate about the use of condoms.
- Educate about abstinence.

TRICHOMONIASIS

- The responsible organism is the flagellated protozoan *Trichomonas vaginalis*, a single-celled organism with a tail (**Figure 18-9**).

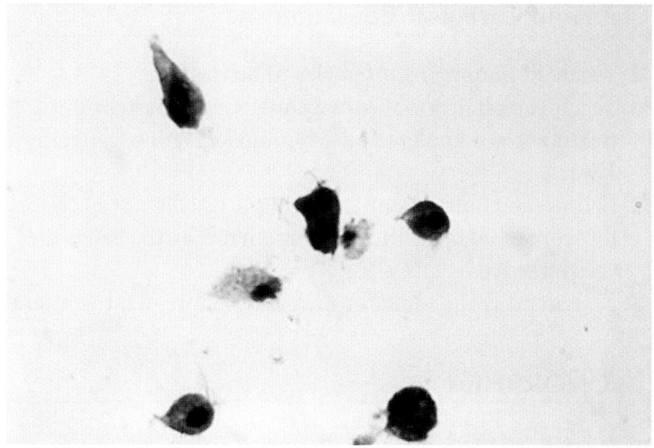

Figure 18-9 Trichomonas vaginalis. *(From Centers for Disease Control and Prevention, Department of Health and Human Services. [1986]. Retrieved from http://phil.cdc.gov/Phil/etails.asp—5237)*

- Humans are the only natural host; it is rarely cultured from surfaces.
- Transmission is nearly always through sexual contact.

Classic Signs and Symptoms in Females

- Purulent, malodorous, thin discharge (70% of cases)
- Burning, pruritus (itching)
- Dysuria (painful urination), frequency
- Dyspareunia (pain with intercourse)
- Postcoital bleeding can occur.
- Urethra is also infected in the majority of women.
- Symptoms may be worse during menstruation.
- Discharge classically described as green, frothy, and foul-smelling is found in fewer than 10% of symptomatic women.

Classic Signs and Symptoms in Males

- Symptoms in men are generally less severe; often affected men remain asymptomatic, and spontaneous resolution may occur.
- Less than 10% of men develop any symptoms.
- Symptoms are the same as those for urethritis from any cause and consist of a clear or mucoid, purulent urethral discharge and/or pain with urination.
- Potential complications include prostatitis, balanoposthitis, epididymitis, and infertility.
- The only reliable test to diagnose trichomonas in the male is PCR testing of urine, which is not widely available; other tests, such as saline microscopy of urethral swabs, have low sensitivity.

Nursing Interventions

- Complete antibiotic regime as ordered.
- Should avoid any alcohol consumption for at least 72 hours after treatment completed to avoid severe vomiting (medication interaction)

Child and Caregiver Education

- Teach all nonpregnant females to be treated.
- Teach to abstain from sexual contact with partner until treatment is complete and symptoms are gone, generally 1 week.
- Follow-up clinical exam or testing is usually not necessary for women who are then asymptomatic, as the drugs are very effective.
- Treatment is the same for men and nonpregnant women.

GONORRHEA

- Caused by *Neisseria gonorrheae.*
- Infection can occur in the cervix, vagina, and fallopian tubes in women, but also the eyes, throat, urethra, and anus of males and females.
- Gonorrhea may also spread to the blood or the joints, causing painful arthritis with red, swollen joints.
- Spread by contact with infected sites, most often through sexual contact in adolescents, and can signal sexual abuse in children.
- Can be spread from mother to infants during delivery
- Severe eye infection in infants can lead to blindness.

> **Medication**
>
> **Preventing Gonorrhea Eye Infections in Infants**
>
> All infants receive antibiotic eye ointments to prevent gonorrhea eye infections at the time of delivery.

- Often associated with co-infection of *Chlamydia trachomatis.*

Signs and Symptoms

- Pain with urination
- Yellow or white, sometimes green, urethral discharge, more often in men
- May be asymptomatic or mimic urinary tract infection
- Symptoms of rectal infection in both men and women may include discharge, anal itching, soreness, bleeding, or painful bowel movements.
- Rectal infection also may cause no symptoms.
- Infections in the throat may cause a sore throat, but usually cause no symptoms.

Nursing Interventions

- Obtain cultures prior to the start of antibiotics.
- Antibiotics as prescribed

Child and Caregiver Education

- Educate about the use of condoms.
- Educate about abstinence.
- Complete antibiotics as prescribed.

CHLAMYDIA

- Caused by the bacterium *Chlamydia trachomatis*
- Most common bacterial agent of sexually transmitted genital infections
- Significant numbers of patients are asymptomatic, providing an ongoing reservoir for infection; this includes men and women.
- Conjunctivitis and pneumonia can occur in infants born to mothers through an infected birth canal.

Nursing Interventions

- Complete antibiotic regime as ordered.
- Educate about the prevention of STIs.
- Educate about condom use.
- Educate about abstinence.

Child and Caregiver Education

- All females should be tested for pregnancy, and test of cured status is necessary in about 3 weeks for pregnant women only.
- Notify physician if infection is not appearing to improve.
- Test of cured status is not recommended for others, even HIV-positive persons.

SYPHILIS

- **Syphilis** is an STI caused by the bacterium *Treponema pallidum.*
- It has often been called "the great imitator" because so many of the signs and symptoms are indistinguishable from those of other diseases.
- *T. pallidum* is a very long, thin, and coiled bacterium, a spirochete.
- Syphilis is a chronic infection that occurs in several stages.
  - *Primary stage*
    - Marked by the appearance of a single sore (called a chancre), but there may be multiple sores.
    - The time between infection with syphilis and the start of the first symptom can range from 10 to 90 days (average 21 days).
    - The chancre is usually firm, round, small, and painless. It appears at the spot where syphilis entered the body.
    - The chancre lasts 3 to 6 weeks, and it heals without treatment. However, if adequate treatment is not administered, the infection progresses to the secondary stage.
  - *Secondary stage*
    - Skin rash and mucous membrane lesions characterize the secondary stage; starts with the development of a rash on one or more areas of the body.
    - Rashes associated with secondary syphilis can appear as the chancre is healing or several weeks after the chancre has healed.

- Characteristic rash of secondary syphilis may appear as rough, red, or reddish brown spots both on the palms of the hands and the bottoms of the feet.
- Rashes with a different appearance may occur on other parts of the body, sometimes resembling rashes caused by other diseases.
- Other symptoms of secondary syphilis may include fever, swollen lymph glands, sore throat, patchy hair loss, headaches, weight loss, muscle aches, and fatigue.
- The signs and symptoms will resolve with or without treatment.
- Without treatment, the infection will progress to the latent and possibly late stages of disease (Hicks & Sparling, 2011).

- *Late and latent stages*
  - The latent (hidden) stage of syphilis begins when primary and secondary symptoms disappear.
  - Without treatment, the infected person will continue to have and be contagious, even without active symptoms.
  - The late stages develop in about 15% of people who have not been treated for syphilis.
  - It can appear 10 to 20 years after infection was first acquired, and last for years, even decades.
  - The disease may subsequently damage the internal organs, including the brain, nerves, eyes, heart, blood vessels, liver, bones, and joints.
  - Signs and symptoms of the late stage of syphilis include difficulty coordinating muscle movements, paralysis, numbness, gradual blindness, and dementia. This damage may be serious enough to cause death.

- Congenital syphilis
  - *Occurs when the spirochete* T. pallidum *is transmitted from a pregnant woman to her fetus* (**Figure 18-10**).
  - *Infection can result in stillbirth, prematurity, or a wide spectrum of clinical manifestations; only severe cases are clinically apparent at birth.*
  - *All pregnant women should be tested.*
  - *Infants can be asymptomatic for up to 2 years after birth.*
  - *Symptoms in an infant can include chronic rhinitis or nasal congestion, "snuffles," enlarged liver and spleen, and development of a rash 1 to 2 weeks later.*
  - *Rash involves palms and soles; starts as pink or red and can turn dark or even coppery.*
  - *Long-bone abnormalities may occur, with possible fractures or pain, and may limit movement of the involved extremity, giving the appearance of paralysis ("pseudoparalysis of Parrot").*
  - *Central nervous system involvement can occur, and long term may cause seizures, hydrocephalus, developmental delay, or loss of developmental milestones.*

Nursing Interventions

- Assess for localized and systemic infection.
- Infants need to have long-term follow-up care to evaluate for chronic infections.
- A lumbar puncture is needed to evaluate cerebral spinal fluid.

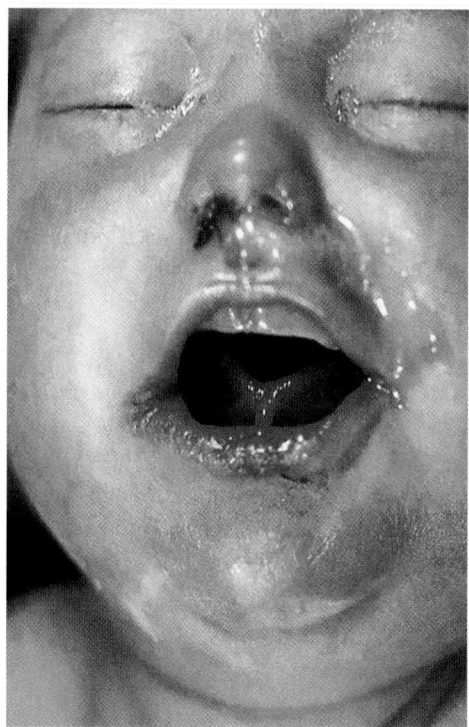

Figure 18-10 Infant with congenital syphilis. *(From Centers for Disease Control and Prevention, Department of Health and Human Services. [1963]. Retrieved from http://phil.cdc.gov/Phil/details.asp—2246)*

Child and Caregiver Education

- Antibiotics as ordered
- Assess for penicillin allergy, as this is the typical drug of choice.

GENETICS AND GENETIC DISORDERS

REVIEW OF HUMAN GENETICS

CRITICAL COMPONENT

Origin from a Single Cell

Humans are composed of almost a trillion cells, all of different types, but each derives from a single cell. This single cell then differentiates, or develops, into highly specific cell types. The cell is composed of a central enclosed core, or **nucleus**, and the outer area, or **cytoplasm**, that contains more fluid and other cell organelles. The nucleus houses the **chromosomes**, the highly organized structures that contain the genetic code, **deoxyribonucleic acid (DNA)**. The DNA is then organized into hundreds of units of heredity, or **genes**. The genes are responsible for determining our physical attributes, and biological functions. Under the direction of genes, the cell cytoplasm then produces products necessary for the organism's functions, such as growth, release of energy, and elimination of waste products at the cellular level.

Genetic Inheritance

- Human cells have a total of 46 chromosomes, organized into 23 complementary pairs. Each pair contains two copies, or two **alleles**.
- There are 22 pairs of **autosomes**, which both males and females have.
- There is one pair of sex chromosomes, again one from each parent.
  - *These are called X and Y; females have XX and males have XY.*
  - *The Y chromosome is only about one-third as large as the X, and contains many fewer genes*
  - *The presence of the Y chromosome determines "maleness."*

Genetic Errors

- Defects can occur with the ongoing processes of cell reproduction.
- **Mitosis**—cell division into identical sister cells, each with 46 chromosomes, or 23 pairs of alleles.
  - *Ongoing cell mitosis is essential throughout the life span to maintain proper body function; it takes place in nearly all cells of the body.*
  - *Different types of cells reproduce by mitosis at different rates.*
  - *Skin cells divide about every 10 hours, liver cells about once a year.*
  - *More highly differentiated cells, such as muscle and nerve cells, may take many years, and brain cells do not appear to reproduce or undergo mitosis after birth.*
  - *This accounts for the different rates in healing from injury.*
  - *As organisms age, the rate and ability for cells to divide decrease, limiting the body's capacity to recover.*
  - *Errors or changes in the process of mitosis account for diseases such as cancers, but do not contribute to inherited disorders.*

Meiosis

- Reproductive division, creating four daughter cells, each one containing only 23 single alleles.
- Can only take place in the germ cell, to create the reproductive **gametes**, the egg and sperm
- There are two meiotic divisions, and, unique to meiosis, both copies of the chromosomes match up and are then intertwined.
- The intertwined chromosomes may actually wrap around and then break and recombine so that portions of each are exchanged, a process called **recombination**.
- In the second meiotic division, the pairs are separated into the reproductive cells, or gametes, each with just 23 alleles.
- This process may result in disorders by some loss or gain of material—the reason for genetic variance.
- **Nondisjunction** occurs when chromosome pairs divide unequally, one daughter cell with 24 chromosomes and another with 22.

Oocyte

- The result of meiosis in females
- Commonly called the egg, the female reproductive cell
- All of the immature oocytes are produced during the fetal stage; the first meiotic division takes place at birth.
- Baby girls are born with a certain number of "pre-egg" cells that are arrested at an early stage of meiosis.
- In fact, the pre-egg cell does not complete meiosis until after fertilization has occurred.
- Fertilization itself triggers the culmination of the process.
- This means that meiosis in women typically takes decades and can take as long as 40 to 50 years.
- Increased maternal age can result in increased gene errors, as these oocytes have been present for the life span of the mother.

Spermatocyte

- The result of meiosis in males
  - *Spermatocytes are the immature sperm cells that contain 23 single chromosomes in the male.*
  - *Produced throughout the life span of the male*
  - *The average life span of a single sperm is about 1 week to maturation within the epididymis.*

Reproduction

- Egg and sperm unite, forming a **zygote**, or new cell, again with 46 chromosomes.
- The zygote undergoes rapid cell division to form the **embryo** and ultimately the fetus.
- Errors may occur during this rapid time of cell proliferation.
- Rarely, some of the cell's chromosome are normal and others abnormal, a condition called **mosaicism**.

ALTERATIONS IN CHROMOSOMES AND DEVELOPMENT

- In reproduction, the 23-chromosome, or **haploid**, egg and sperm unite to form a **diploid** cell with the full 46 chromosomes; this then rapidly divides by mitosis to form the embryo and ultimately the fetus.
- Additional errors or abnormalities can occur at any time during the process, from meiosis, to mitotic division after fertilization, to cell differentiation, and organ formation and development.

TRISOMY 21 (DOWN SYNDROME)

- In about 95% of those with Down syndrome, each cell has three copies of chromosome 21, or 47 chromosomes.

- Associated with advanced maternal age, over 35 years, with alteration in oocyte prior to reproduction
- Rarely, pieces of the long arm of chromosome 21 are attached to another chromosome, usually chromosome 14, 21, or 22; this is known as translocation Down syndrome and affects about 4% of persons with Down syndrome (American Academy of Pediatrics [AAP], 2001) (**Figure 18-11**)
- Mosaicism, noted earlier, is a condition where nondisjunction occurs in mitosis of the fertilized egg, resulting in a different makeup from cell to cell—some are normal and some are not—and affects about 1% of persons with Down syndrome (AAP, 2001).

Signs and Symptoms

Following are the features of Down syndrome (**Figure 18-12A, B**):

- Small head (microcephaly)
- Flattened, broad head with flat posterior areas
- Underdeveloped, flattened middle of face (mid-face hypoplasia)
- Almond-shaped, up-slanting eyes, with redundant tissue along inside
- Prominent epicanthal folds, with small downturned mouth
- Small oral opening with protruding tongue
- Small, low-set ears that may be cupped (**Figure 18-13**)
- Chest may be broad, with heart murmurs related to defects
- Short hands that may have a single crease (**Figure 18-14**)
- Congenital heart defects—very high incidence of about 44% (Alasdair, 2005)
- Endocardial cushion effect (atrioventricular, or AV, canal)—connection between the atria, upper chambers, and ventricle, lower chambers, most common
- Low tone; can be floppy, with breathing and feeding problems at birth

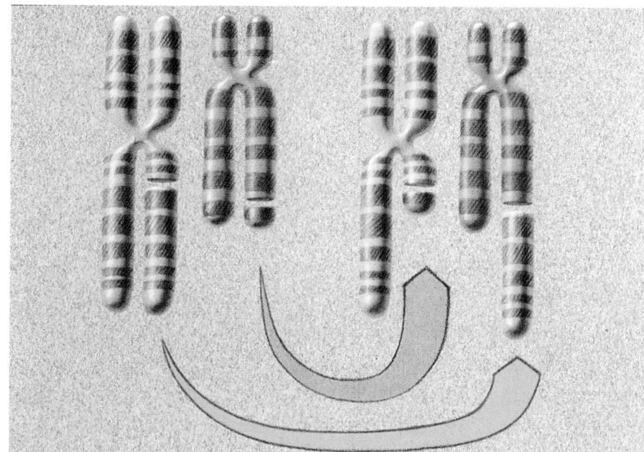

Figure 18-11 Translocation. *(From the National Cancer Institute, U.S. National Institutes of Health. [1988]. Retrieved from http://visualsonline.cancer.gov/details.cfm?imageid=2323)*

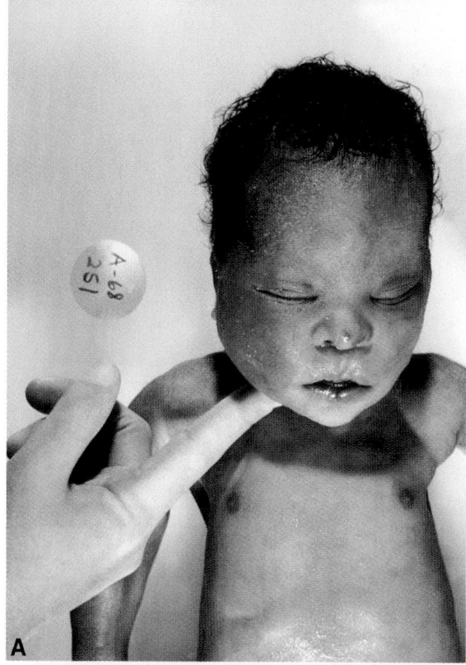

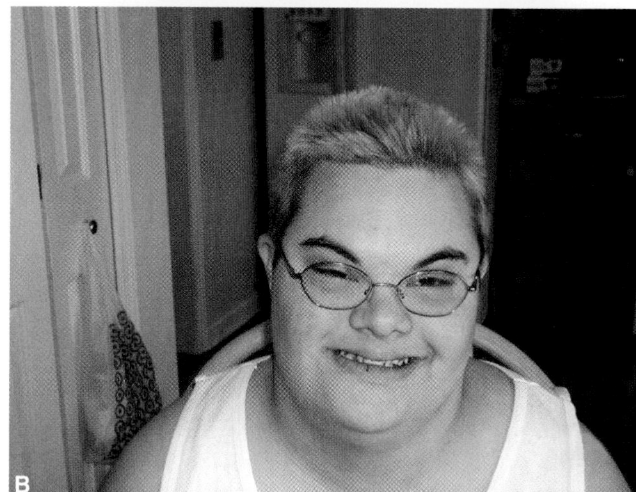

Figure 18-12 **A**, Infant with Down syndrome. *(From Centers for Disease Control and Prevention, Department of Health and Human Services, and Dr. Godfrey P. Oakley. [1974]. Retrieved from http://phil.cdc.gov/Phil/details.asp2634).* **B**, Adolescent with Down syndrome. *(Courtesy of D.M. Kocisko.)*

Nursing Interventions

- Health-care providers are a vital link in helping parents and families to adapt to the initial shock and disappointment in learning their child has Down syndrome.
- Diagnosis is usually suspected based on physical appearance, and specific testing should take place as soon as possible to avoid diagnostic error and instances of **translocation** or partial duplication of trisomy 21.
- Parents should ideally be informed as soon as possible of the definitive diagnosis, by someone known to the couple, and literature about Down syndrome as well as support groups and community supports should be made available before discharge.

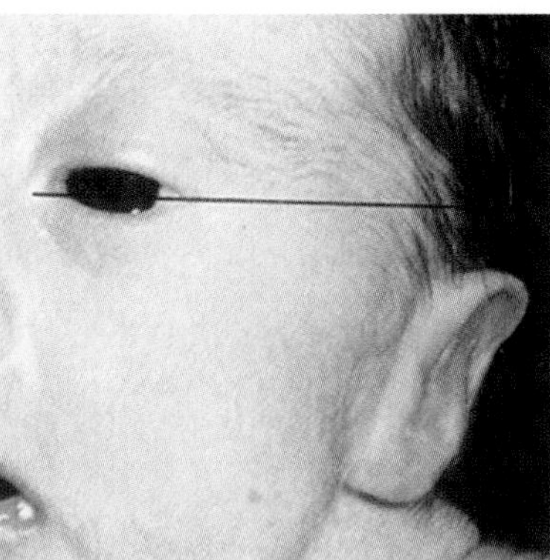

Figure 18–13 Low-set ears in Down syndrome.

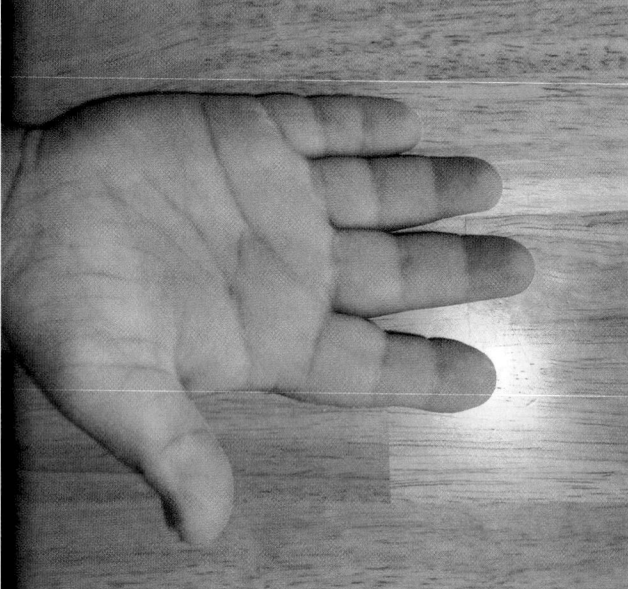

Figure 18–14 Hand of an adolescent with Down syndrome.

- Newborn can by hypotonic and hyperextensible, with poor feeding; the large protruding tongue produces tendency for mouth breathing

Promoting Safety

When feeding an infant with Down syndrome, in order to assess respirations do the following:

- Make sure the infant is well awake and mouth and nares are cleared of mucus.
- Position correctly and steady the chin.
- May need to be burped more frequently and offered smaller, more frequent feedings.
- Monitor color and respiratory patterns, as these may be clues for congenital heart defects.
- Infants with heart defects also tire easily at feeding.

- Need strict attention to feeding and elimination related to high association of malformations of the gut
  - *Atresia of the duodenum—may have a blind pouch, so feeding may result in immediate emesis*
  - *Annular pancreas—wraps around the gut to cause obstruction*
  - *Hirschsprung's disease—lack of ganglia that affects motility in the colon; can present as severe constipation or frank obstruction*
  - *Specific growth curves for children with Down syndrome need to be used to plot weight, height, and head circumference; overall these children are smaller, shorter, and have smaller heads, as well as increased obesity in the teen years.*
- Motor development takes about twice as long as in the usual child; about 90% can walk by age 3 years.
- All children with suspected delay and or known syndromes need to be referred to local early intervention services.
- Developmental delay, including intellectual disabilities, is common; IQs typically range from very low to near normal, and average around 55.
- Thyroid disease, especially hypothyroidism, is very common and needs to be monitored across the life span.
  - *Newborn screens are required in all 50 states for congenital hypothyroidism.*
  - *Thyroid studies need to be done several times in the first years of life, and then at a minimum of yearly, and considered related to poor growth velocity.*
- Immune dysfunction is common, such as abnormalities in immunoglobulin levels and other cellular types of immunity.
- The risk of pneumonia is high, although mortality is less frequent with modern antibiotics.
- Ear infections are more common, in part due to anatomy and known immune dysfunction, and the risk for both conductive and sensorineural hearing loss is higher as well.
- Musculoskeletal concerns related to joint laxity are common.
  - *Instability of the neck, specifically at the area between the first and second cervical vertebrae, or atlanto-axial joint, is also possible.*
  - *Routine films for this condition are felt to have poor sensitivity; regular and careful assessment of young children with Down syndrome and monitoring for signs and symptoms of cervical cord changes—such as in gait, flexion, and bladder or bowel function—are more sensitive.*
  - *Flexion and extension films of the neck with evaluation of the atlanto-odontoid distance and neural canal by a pediatric radiologist are recommended (magnetic resonance imaging [MRI]).*
- Malignancies are also more common with Down syndrome, and incidence of leukemia is about 18 times greater than in the general population (see Chapter 19).
- Skin problems, such as dry skin and allergic dermatitis, are also very common.

- Hair loss and thin hair may be evident.
- Sleep problems, including obstructive sleep apnea, are associated with a narrow posterior throat (hypopharynx) and hypotonia, even with a relatively normal size of the tonsils and adenoids.
- Suspicion should be raised if parents or caregivers note snoring or unusual sleeping positions, such as with the head hyperextended, looking up and back, or on the stomach with the knees drawn up, as well as restless, disturbed sleep.

> **Clinical Reasoning**
>
> **Snoring and Down Syndrome**
>
> The caregiver of a Down syndrome child reports that the child is restless when he sleeps and often snores very loudly. She is concerned that something is wrong.
>
> 1. Is there a logical reason for this report?
> 2. What should the caregiver do about this problem?

TRISOMY 18 (EDWARDS SYNDROME)

- Maternal nondisjunction during meiosis causes 95% of cases.
- Each chromosome has three copies of chromosome 18; this is the second most common **trisomy** after Down syndrome.
- Characterized by prenatal growth deficiency, craniofacial features, characteristic hand gestures with overriding fingers, nail hypoplasia, and short sternum.
- Internal anomalies and severe heart defects are common.
- A bedside scoring system has been developed to help clinicians without specialized training to make the diagnosis of trisomy 18 in the newborn period.

TRISOMY 13 (PATAU SYNDROME)

- The least common and most severe of the viable autosomal trisomies
- Average survival is fewer than 3 days.

Nursing Interventions (Trisomy 18 and Trisomy 13)

- A plan for minimal intervention can be initiated from the time of the delivery room on.
- Provide support and end-of-life care as necessary.

Caregiver Education (Trisomy 18 and Trisomy 13)

- Central apnea and its presence with other congenital malformations may result in death within a few weeks (see Chapter 5 for end-of-life issues).
- Although severe heart defects are noted, these alone do not account for early death, and some may be amenable to surgeries.
- At 1 year of age, 5% to 10% may be alive without any extraordinary means of support, and may exhibit very slow developmental gains in milestones (Carey, 2005).
- Some children do live to later childhood years, but this is rare.
- There are no factors in the 1- to 2-week-old infant who does not require a ventilator to help determine whether the child will live beyond the first year of life.

TURNER SYNDROME

- Result of chromosomal loss of entire X chromosome (45, X)
- Only known disorder where a fetus can survive despite loss of an entire chromosome
- Affects only girls; no known living males with 45,Y
- Usually the result of abnormal meiotic error in the sperm
- Girls receive no sex chromosome from the sperm of the father, and receive the X from the mother

Signs and Symptoms

- Prematurity
- Feeding difficulties, with spitting, emesis, and difficulty latching on
- Frank gastroesophageal reflux and failure to thrive

Physical Assessment Findings

- Girls often with webbed, thick short neck or nuchal folds
- Short stature
- Broad "shield-like" chest with wide-spaced nipples
- Nonfunctional ovaries
- Common to have thyroid dysfunction
- Common to find heart defects
  - *Obstruction of the left side of the heart*
  - *Coarctation or narrowing of the aorta*
- Most affected girls have normal intelligence, but many have visual-perceptual impairments that predispose them to develop nonverbal learning disabilities.
- Endocrine disorders result in short stature that can be improved with growth hormone injections.
- Absence of a single kidney (renal agenesis), horseshoe kidney, duplication of the collecting system, and aberrant renal arteries can occur.
- Approximately one-fifth to one-third of affected girls are identified at birth because of the presence of lymphedema, a notable swelling or puffiness of the hands and feet (Sybert, 2005).

Nursing Interventions

- Anticipate feeding difficulties and be patient when feeding.
- Lack of secondary sexual characteristic by mid-teens may be the first symptom noted.

- Assess for hypothyroidism.
- Assess for cardiovascular disorders.
- Baseline electrocardiograms and then monitoring on a regular basis are recommended.

Child and Caregiver Education

- Lack of pubertal development can be treated with estrogen supplementation so that girls can develop secondary sexual characteristics; however, they will remain infertile.
- Endocrine referral is recommended so that growth hormone treatment can be started early.
- Provide anticipatory guidance on obesity, which can become a problem in later childhood and adult life.
- Height and weight are usually within normal parameters at birth, and then deceleration of height velocity continues.

CRI-DU-CHAT SYNDROME

- "Cat cry" syndrome—the result of a **deletion** or loss of a portion of chromosome 5 (**Figure 18-15A, B**)

Assessment

- Distinctive high-pitched, cat-like cry
- Profound microcephaly, round face with widely spaced eyes, epicanthal folds, and low-set ears; significant intellectual disability

Nursing Interventions

- Supportive care—feeding issues and poor growth
- All children with this diagnosis need early referral to genetics and neurology.

Caregiver Education

- Severe central nervous system (CNS) irritability and minimal developmental progress of the child put family members at very high risk for depression.
- Provide education and information regarding family support groups.

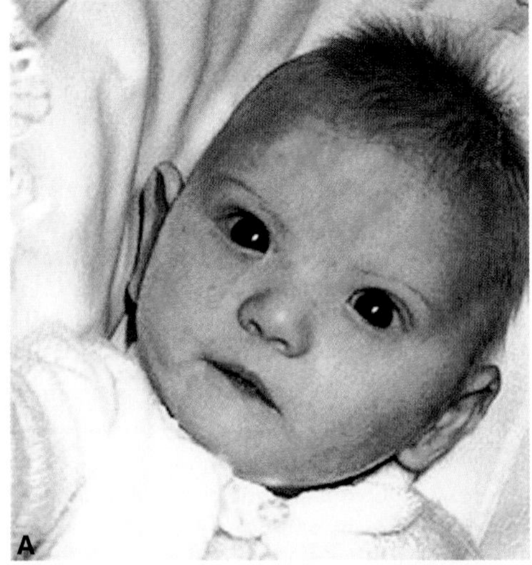

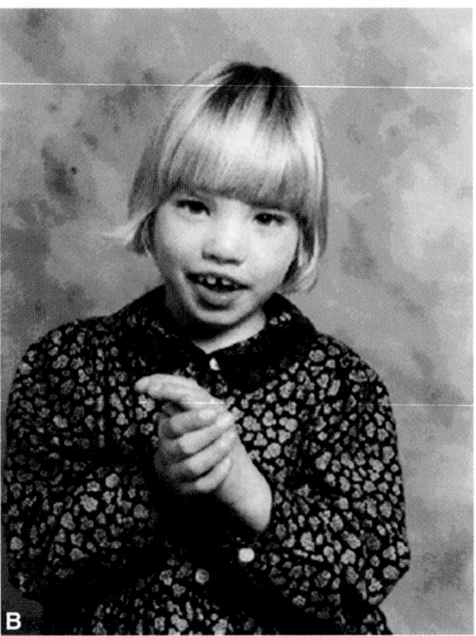

Figure 18-15 **A**, Infant with cri-du-chat. **B**, School-age child with cri-du-chat. (© www.genetic-diseases.net, with permission)

WILLIAMS SYNDROME

- Result of a microdeletion in the long arm of chromosome 7 (7q11.23)

Assessment

- Characteristic pattern of dysmorphic facial features:
  - *Broad forehead*
  - *Bitemporal narrowing*
  - *Low nasal root*
  - *Periorbital fullness*
  - *Stellate/lacy iris pattern*
  - *Bulbous nasal tip*
  - *Strabismus (crossed or wandering eyes)*
  - *Long philtrum, full lips, wide mouth*
  - *Full cheeks, small jaw*
  - *Prominent earlobe*
  - *Malocclusion of the teeth and a long neck in older children*
- Developmental delay
  - *IQ scores on standard tests range from severe intellectual delay to low normal.*
  - *Highly verbal and overly sociable, "cocktail personality"*
- Connective tissue abnormalities, including cardiovascular disease
  - *Hoarse and deep voice, hernias, soft and loose skin, joint laxity or limitation*
  - *Supravalvar aortic stenosis*

Nursing Interventions

- Affected children often have severe difficulties with feeding and short stature; growth and height should be plotted on Williams syndrome growth curve chart.
- Difficulty with gross motor function and depth perception; very difficult to negotiate uneven surfaces and stairs
- Attention deficit/hyperactivity disorder (ADHD) present in about 70%; overly friendly to others, especially adults; generalized anxiety (Morris, 2005)
- Elastin problems cause arterial defects, including supravalvula aortic stenosis, but can involve any artery and lead to morbidity and mortality

Child and Caregiver Education

- Puberty commonly occurs early (anticipatory guidance needed).
- Difficulty with handwriting, drawing, buttoning, and pattern construction; poor math skills; strong memory for auditory information, such as instructions read out loud

VELOCARDIAL FACIAL SYNDROME

- Result of a microdeletion in the q, or long arm, of chromosome 22 at the 11th position (22q11 deletion)

Assessment

- Variable physical presentations
- Because of the variability in the severity of defects, this deletion in the same gene has been described under many different names: VCF syndrome, DiGeorge syndrome, CATCH 22, Sphrintzen syndrome, Cayler syndrome, deletion 22q11 syndrome, conotruncal anomaly face syndrome.
- No specific criteria for diagnosis are noted because of variability, but presence of cleft palate and heart defects should indicate need for chromosomal testing.
- Right-sided heart defects or defects of the aortic arch, including:
  - *Right-sided, double or interrupted, ventriculoseptal defect*
  - *Pulmonary atresia*
  - *Tetralogy of Fallot*
  - *Aberrant subclavian arteries*
  - *Tracheal ring*
- Characteristic but subtle facial appearance
  - *Increased vertical length*
  - *Long cylindrical or tubular nose*
  - *Small posterior jaw (retrognathia)*
  - *Hooded upper eyelids*
- Mild developmental delays
  - *Learning disabilities*
  - *Social immaturity*
  - *Hypernasal speech*
  - *Impulsivity*
  - *Anxiety or phobias*
- Classic DiGeorge sequence includes absent thymus, hypocalcemia, and immune deficiency with characteristic facial features
- Cayler syndrome also known as asymmetric crying face syndrome, with unusual "crying" mouth and face asymmetry with movement, and heart defects

Nursing Interventions

- Vascular anomalies and heart defects can be noted in the newborn nursery as murmurs, feeding difficulties, color change, and stridor or breathing difficulty related to vascular rings.
- Seizures can occur related to hypocalcemia.
- Aspiration pneumonias may occur in relation to immune dysfunction and cleft palate.
- Hypotonia can lead to breathing problems.
- Low gut motility is also seen with constipation.
- Immune disorders can lead to chronic upper and lower respiratory infections.
- Hearing loss—sensorineural hearing loss in up to 15% (Shprintzen, 2005)

Caregiver Education

- Provide education on prevention of constipation.
- Provide education on prevention of chronic respiratory infections.
- Promote good hand hygiene.

PHENYKETONURIA (PKU)

- Result of a single **mutation** at a single site or base pair mutation
- Results in abnormality in the production of pheylalanine hydroxylase, the enzyme that breaks down the protein phenylalanine
- The result is accumulation of phenylalanine in the blood and brain, causing brain damage with progressive mental retardation/intellectual disability.
- Testing for PKU is performed during the newborn period (**Figure 18-16**).

Assessment

- Appear completely typical at birth, although commonly fair, blonde, and blue-eyed, then progressive intellectual disability

Nursing Interventions

- All 50 states now screen for PKU as part of standard newborn screening; need to ensure screen is performed when child has been fed full-strength formula or breast milk, ideally for 48 hours.

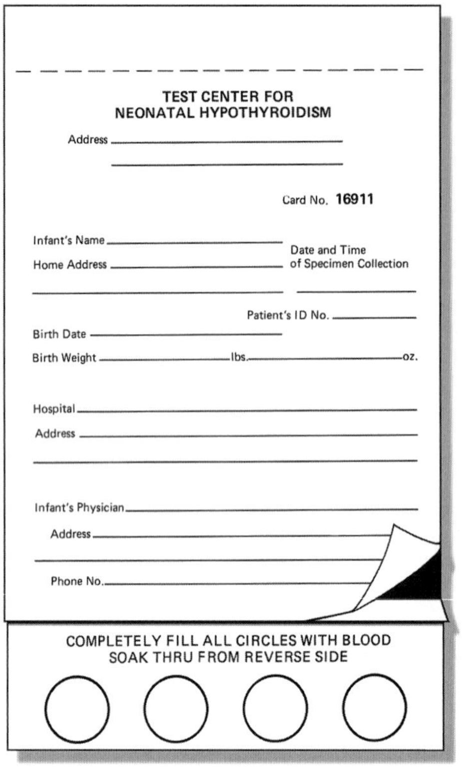

TEST CENTER FOR
NEONATAL HYPOTHYROIDISM

Address

Card No. 16911

Infant's Name
Date and Time of Specimen Collection
Home Address

Patient's ID No.

Birth Date
Birth Weight lbs. oz.

Hospital
Address

Infant's Physician
Address
Phone No.

COMPLETELY FILL ALL CIRCLES WITH BLOOD
SOAK THRU FROM REVERSE SIDE

Example of Specimen Card
with Essential Information Requested

Figure 18–16 Specimen card to test for PKU. *(From Centers for Disease Control and Prevention, Department of Health and Human Services. Retrieved from http://phil.cdc.gov/Phil/details.asp 2567)*

- Genetics department may need to measure phenylalanine level, as some individuals have a residual amount of the enzyme.
- Phenylalanine is an essential protein; it cannot be removed completely from the human diet, but caregivers need to provide a phenylalanine-free formula and low-protein diet.
- Fetus needs to have phenylalanine to develop

Child and Caregiver Education

- Women with PKU can become pregnant.
- Teens often want to disregard the diet; encourage compliance.
- Once brain injury occurs, it is irreversible, and thus the restrictive diet is recommended for life.
- Once screened as abnormal, individuals require immediate referral to a geneticist and a metabolic nutritionist for information on protein restriction and replacement formula.
- Cannot continue to breastfeed without risk for brain injury
- Pregnant women with PKU need referral to high-risk center with nutrition and genetics support, and ideally pregnancies should be planned.

NEUROFIBROMATOSIS, TYPE 1 (VON RECKLINGHAUSEN'S DISEASE)

- Also known as peripheral neurofibromatosis; the result of a single "nonsense" mutation on the long arm of chromosome 17, locus 11.2 (17q11.2)
- **Autosomal dominant inheritance** pattern—presence of just one copy of the abnormal 17q11.2 mutation, plus one normal allele, results in the disease syndrome.
- Males or females who have this mutated allele can pass it on to half of their offspring, a 50% chance for each pregnancy.

Assessment

- Wide range of variability
- Neurofibromin is a tumor-suppressor protein; absence of neurofibromin results in multiple tumors that form on the body and in the brain.
- Instead of neurofibromin, a useless protein is produced.
- Variable expression in different individuals; various physical presentations
- Age-related abnormal tissue proliferation due to lack of neurofibromin
- Diagnosis is usually clinical, and the presence of just two of seven characteristics is considered enough to make a clinical diagnosis.
- The presence or number of these physical characteristics does not, however, indicate the ultimate severity of the disease or long-term prognosis.
- Seven recognized cutaneous manifestations (change based on age; develop over time)

Seven Criteria for Diagnosing Neurofibromatosis Type 1 (NF-1; Viskochil, 2005)

1. Six or more café-au-lait macules, patches, or spots; pigmented birthmarks, >5 mm in greatest diameter in prepubertal children, or >15 mm in greatest diameter after puberty
   - *The name* café au lait *is French for "milky coffee" and refers to their light-brown color* (**Figure 18-17**).
   - *These can be present from birth but others may develop later.*
2. Two or more neurofibromas of any type or one or more plexiform neurofibroma
   - *Neurofibromas are benign nerve sheath tumors. They arise from the supportive tissue within the nerve itself.*
   - *As these neurofibroma tumors grow, they displace and compress important nerve fascicles within the nerve. This causes pain, weakness, and numbness.*
   - *Although neurofibromas are frequently solitary and occur at random, they can also occur in multiple locations in patients with neurofibromatosis.*

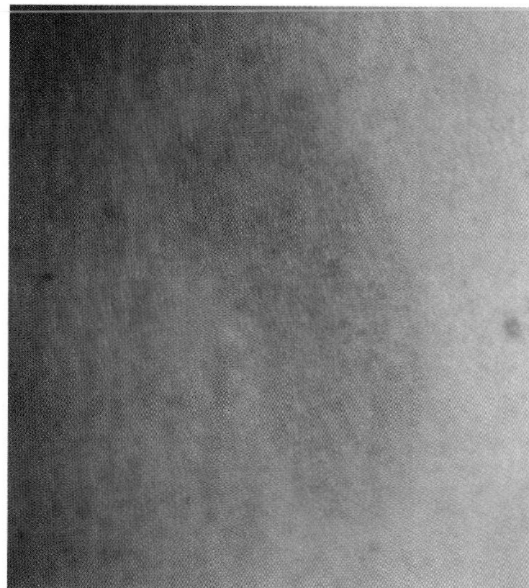

Figure 18–17 Café-au-lait spot on left arm.

3. "Freckling" in the axillary or inguinal regions—minute irregular, and sometimes raised areas
4. Optic glioma—enlargements of the optic nerve; symptomatic lesions usually seen after age 3 as progressive visual loss.
   - *Optic pathway gliomas (OPGs) occur in 15% of children younger than 6 years of age with NF-1 (Lewis, Gerson, Axelson, Riccardi, & Whitford, 1984); they may rarely occur in older children and adults.*
   - *Presence of optic gliomas is usually asymptomatic, but they can cause progressive visual loss, loss of color sensitivity, and possible bulging of the eyes as tumors become enlarged.*
   - *They are low-grade tumors; injury results from location along the optic pathways.*
   - *Incidence is enough to recommend serial eye exams by a pediatric ophthalmologist on a regular basis for children with known NF-1 up to age 6 years.*
   - *Once detected, very close supervision and MRI follow-up is necessary.*
   - *Screening MRI is not currently recommended unless presence is suspected by eye exam. Still, many clinicians often opt for a screening MRI of the brain and orbits at 1 to 2 and 2 to 3 years of age to detect optic pathway tumors before they become symptomatic, primarily because of the difficulty assessing vision in this age group.*
   - *Eye exams should be performed every 3 to 6 months until age 6 years and then yearly after that time.*
5. Two or more Lisch nodules (iris hamartomas)
   - *Lisch nodules characteristically are raised, often pigmented hamartomas of the iris and represent a relatively specific finding for NF-1.*
   - *These do not affect vision in any manner.*
   - *These are present in only about 10% of children with NF-1 at age 6, but in nearly 90% of adults (Lewis & Riccardi, 1981).*
   - *A slit lamp exam by an ophthalmologist is recommended, but may be seen without this exam in persons with light or blue iris color.*
6. A distinctive bony lesion such as sphenoid dysplasia or thinning of the long bone cortex with or without pseudoarthrosis
   - *A pseudoarthrosis, or false joint, is formed because of nonunion of bone fragments. Pseudoarthrosis in NF-1 results from impaired healing due to bone dysplasia, and may severely compromise the function of the limb.*
   - *Sphenoid dysplasia describes abnormalities of the sphenoid bone, commonly seen by computed tomography (CT) scan, and can result in asymmetry of the face.*
   - *Scoliosis, sideways curving, and kyphosis, anterior curvature, can be seen in 10% to 25% of children with NF-1, often presenting around 6 to 10 years of age or early adolescence (Friedman & Birch, 1997).*
7. A first-degree relative (parent, sibling, or offspring) with NF-1 based on the previous six criteria
   - *Genetic testing is increasingly being used in the diagnosis of NF-1 for patients who meet only the two criteria of café-au-lait spots and axillary freckling, as these can be seen in other conditions as well (see Figure 18-17).*
   - *If the child is the first identified case in the family, a clinician with experience with NF-1 needs to examine the parents; however, the criteria of a first-degree relative cannot be used for diagnosis in that parent, two of the other criteria must be met.*

Nursing Interventions

- Obtaining and plotting accurate growth parameters, including height, weight, and head circumference, at every visit is recommended. Children with NF-1 are almost always macrocephalic, or have increased head circumference, in comparison to typical peers.
- Blood pressure should also be checked yearly at minimum due to high incidence of hypertension.
- Infants can present with a single or a few café-au-lait spots in early childhood, and then other changes develop over time. Careful skin exams during bathing and diaper changing are always necessary.
- Initially children with NF-1 can grow normally, but there is a higher incidence of short stature related to less growth throughout the pubertal growth spurt.
- Scoliosis is also seen and should be screened for at every exam starting in early childhood.
- Growth curves specific for NF-1 have been published.
- Complications of NF-1 result from direct involvement of multiple organ systems by plexiform neurofibromas.
- The lifelong risk of malignancy in affected individuals is increased.
- Malignant peripheral nerve sheath tumors represent the most common neoplasm, occurring in approximately 5% to 10% of individuals with NF-1 (Plun, 2011).

Health Supervision for Children with Neurofibromatosis

- NF-1 is associated with an increased incidence of mental retardation (4% to 8%) compared to 3% of risk for all persons (North, 2000).
- Usually, overall intellectual abilities are in the average to low-average range.
- In contrast, specific learning disabilities are observed in as many as 40% to 60% of affected children, and impaired performance on at least one test of academic achievement is present in 65% of children with NF-1 (North et al., 1997).
- ADHD also occurs more frequently in children with NF-1.
- Children with NF-1 have a higher likelihood of being hypotonic and having subtle neurologic abnormalities that affect balance and gait.
- Speech problems also may occur.
- Because of these issues, and autosomal dominant inheritance, parents may have multiple children with learning and physical problems, and may also be affected themselves.
- Child psychology and referral for early intervention and then special education evaluation are recommended if there are any developmental delays or concerns.

NEUROFIBROMATOSIS, TYPE 2 (NF-2)

- Neurofibromatosis type 2 (NF-2) is less common.
- Symptoms usually appear in the teens or young adulthood.
- Tumors frequently occur on the auditory nerve, causing:
  - *Hearing loss*
  - *Ringing in the ears*
  - *Problems with balance*
- Problems with hearing and balance worsen over time, causing greater disability than children experience with NF-1 (NINDS, 2012b).

Assessment

- General physical examination
- Thorough skin examination
- Hearing evaluation

> **CLINICAL PEARL**
>
> **Comparing NF-1 and NF-2**
>
> Children with NF-2 do not have the café-au-lait spots or axillary freckling that is seen in NF-1, but they do exhibit similar tumors on the skin.

Diagnosis

- Diagnosis is based on clinical findings.
- MRI of the brain and auditory nerve should be performed.
- An EEG should be performed if seizures occur.
- A blood test can be performed to evaluate for a genetic marker.

Nursing Interventions

- The treatment focuses on managing the symptoms.
- Sometimes the neurofibromas are removed by surgery.
- Referral to an audiologist is necessary because of the problems with hearing.
- Physical therapy can be helpful in treating the problems with balance.
- Seizures can usually be controlled with medication.
- A child may need specialized educational plans, as learning problems are common.
- Psychological therapy may be needed for children and adolescents with self-esteem problems due to the visible tumors.

TUBEROUS SCLEROSIS

- *Tuberous sclerosis* causes benign growths called "tubers" to form on different body organs, including the brain, eyes, kidneys, heart, skin, and lungs (Behrman, Kliegman, Jenson, & Stanton, 2007; Feinichel, 2001).
- It occurs in approximately 1 in 6000 births.
- A child of a parent with tuberous sclerosis has a 50% chance of inheriting the disorder.
- Skin lesions are called *ash leaf lesions,* which are patches of skin with less color or pigment than other skin (Zitelli & Davis, 2007).
- Symptoms of tuberous sclerosis
  - *Mild skin abnormalities*
  - *Lung tumors*
  - *Heart tumors*
  - *Tumors in the retina or along the optic nerve*
  - *Kidney failure*
  - *Seizures*
  - *Mental retardation*

Assessment

- General physical examination
- Thorough skin examination
- Measurement and documentation of skin lesions

Diagnosis

- Diagnosis is based on clinical findings.
- A baseline MRI of the brain should be performed and then repeated as the child grows to monitor for tumors.
- Screening studies of the heart, lungs, kidneys, and eyes should be performed at regular intervals.
- An EEG should be performed if seizures occur.

Nursing Interventions

- The treatment focuses on managing the symptoms.
- Sometimes surgery is required to remove tumors from vital organs.
- Medication may be needed to treat seizures.

- A child may need specialized educational plans if learning is a problem.
- Genetic counseling is recommended.

STURGE-WEBER SYNDROME

- *Sturge-Weber syndrome* is a rare condition caused by a spontaneous genetic mutation that affects the skin and the brain.
- The cause of this genetic mutation is unknown. The symptoms vary widely and some patients are undiagnosed for many years.
- The most common symptom is a skin lesion called a *port-wine stain* that is present at birth (Volpe, 2001).
  - *This is so named for its distinctive purple-red color that gives the appearance of "spilled wine"; it usually covers at least one eyelid and a portion of the forehead.*
- Blood vessel growths, called *angiomas,* can occur on the brain.
  - *These lesions can cause seizures, usually occurring before the first birthday.*
  - *The seizures tend to worsen with age and may be convulsions on the opposite side of the body from the skin discoloration.*
  - *These angiomas may or may not be surgically repairable, depending on their size and location.*
- *Glaucoma* is also common, usually in the eye affected by the port-wine stain. The eye may sometimes become enlarged.
- Children with Sturge-Weber syndrome are also at higher risk for pediatric stroke.

Assessment

- General physical examination
- Careful skin examination

Diagnosis

- Diagnosis is based on physical findings.
- An MRI of the brain and the brain blood vessels should be performed to evaluate for angiomas.
- An EEG may be performed if the child develops seizures.

Nursing Interventions

- Treatment is aimed at symptom management.
- In some cases, laser surgery can be done for infants as young as 1 month of age to reduce the size (and therefore the long-term effects) of the port-wine stain lesion.
- Seizures and glaucoma can be managed with medications.
- Screening should be done for angiomas.
- Measures to prevent stroke should be instituted, such as weight management and control of blood pressure, blood glucose levels, and blood lipids.

CHARCOT–MARIE–TOOTH

- *Charcot–Marie–Tooth disease* is an inherited form of neuropathy that primarily affects the feet and legs, but can affect the arms and hands in advanced stages.
- Symptoms usually manifest in late childhood or adolescence and usually begin with *foot drop*, in which the child cannot dorsiflex the foot.
- Some children develop *hammer toes*, where the toes remain curled.
- Later wasting of the lower leg gives the appearance of an inverted champagne bottle or a stork's leg.
  - *The leg exhibits hypertrophy of the proximal muscles.*
  - *The peroneal muscles show marked atrophy.*
  - *The distal portion of the extremities is thin due to the atrophied muscles.*
- As the condition progresses, other weaknesses can occur in the pelvis and trunk (NINDSa, 2012).

Assessment

- Thorough physical examination
- Thorough history of the child's illness

Diagnosis

- Diagnosis is made based on symptoms.
- Blood can be tested for genetic markers for this disorder.
- Electromyography (EMG) is done to determine the extent of the disease.
- Nerve conduction velocity (NCV) studies are done to determine the speed of the electrical signal through the nerves. Delayed or weakened responses indicate a neuropathy such as Charcot–Marie–Tooth.
- Nerve biopsy is done to confirm the disease. A small piece of a peripheral nerve is taken from the calf of the leg.

Nursing Intervention

- Treatment is supportive care for the child and prevention of further disability.

ACHONDROPLASIA

- Achondroplasia is one of a group of disorders called *chondrodystrophies* or *osteochondrodysplasias*.
- Disorder of bone growth that causes the most common type of dwarfism
- Most common form of disproportionate short stature
- Occurs once in every 15,000 to 40,000 live births (Trotter & Hall, 2005)
- Achondroplasia is caused by a gene alteration (mutation) in the *FGFR3* gene on chromosome 4, short arm (4p16.3).
- The *FGFR3* gene makes a protein called fibroblast growth factor receptor 3 that is involved in converting cartilage to bone.

- *FGFR3* is the only gene known to be associated with achondroplasia.
- May be inherited as an autosomal dominant trait.
- Most cases appear as spontaneous mutations. Over 80% of individuals who have achondroplasia have parents with normal stature and are born with achondroplasia as a result of a new (*de novo*) mutation of parental gamete (Pauli, 2005).
- Infants born to two parents with achondroplasia have a 50% chance of having achondroplasia, but a 25% chance of inheriting the abnormal gene from both parents, resulting in "double dominant dwarfism"; these infants may be stillborn or do not often live beyond a few months.

Assessment

- The typical appearance of achondroplastic dwarfism can be seen at birth.
- Some cases are now identified prior to birth (*in utero*) by routine prenatal ultrasound.
- Prenatal ultrasound may show excessive amniotic fluid surrounding the unborn infant (polyhydramnios).
- There may be signs of hydrocephalus ("water on the brain").
- X-rays of the long bones can reveal achondroplasia in the newborn.
- Disproportionately large head-to-body-size difference (macrocephaly) with specific facial features, such as a prominent forehead (frontal bossing) and mid-face hypoplasia (flattening)
- Shortened arms and legs (especially the upper arm and thigh)
- Short stature
  - *Significantly below the average height for a person of the same age and sex*
  - *Adult height generally 4 feet for men and women (Trotter & Hall, 2005)*
  - *Rarely reach 5 feet (Trotter & Hall, 2005)*
- Decreased muscle tone (hypotonia)
- Spinal stenosis
  - *Narrowing of the spinal column that causes pressure on the spinal cord*
  - *Narrowing of the openings (called neural foramina) where spinal nerves leave the spinal column*
- Abnormal hand appearance with persistent space between the long and ring fingers—a "trident"-shaped hand
- Bowed legs (see Chapter 20)
- Defects of the joints at the knee that may later cause premature joint degeneration and pain
- Clubbed feet can also occur (see Chapter 20)

Nursing Interventions

- There is no specific treatment for achondroplasia.
- Intelligence and life span are normal for most persons with achondroplasia.
- Prenatal diagnosis
  - *Close, high-risk monitoring of a mother carrying a child with achondroplasia*
  - *Close monitoring for mothers with achondroplasia themselves*
- Children affected with achondroplasia commonly have delayed motor milestones related to tone.
- Should be referred for early intervention
- Growth curves
  - *Track appropriate head circumference, weight, and height with close attention to weight-for-height curves specific to achondroplasia.*
- Sudden death may occur.
  - *In the first year of life, central apnea related to abnormalities or narrowing of the foramen magnum and cord compression may occur.*
  - *Careful neurological exam, noting for any changes or loss of function, sleep study (polysomnogram), and CT/MRI of the craniocervical junction are recommended.*
- Great care needs to be taken with any neck manipulation, such as preparing for intubation.
- Upper airway obstruction can occur.
  - *Related to tone and relatively small posterior airway, the hypopharynx*
  - *About 5% of persons with achondroplasia may require tracheostomy (Pauli, 2005).*
- Related abnormalities
  - *Spinal stenosis and spinal cord compression, which should be treated by neurosurgery when they cause problems such as pain or change in gait*
  - *Obstructive sleep apnea due to decreased tone and obesity*
  - *Increased incidence of otitis media*

Caregiver Education

- Parents need to be instructed to use caution and care when I lifting the infant, and to use only infant carriers with a firm back that gives good neck support.
- Child should be placed in rear-facing car seat for as long as possible.
- Unsupported sitting should not be encouraged until the child has adequate trunk muscle strength, including discouraging the use of infant walkers or "excer-saucer"-type seating and infant swings that can cause excessive head movement and have poor trunk support.

X-LINKED HYDROCEPHALUS

- **X-linked** recessive disorder (Fishman, 2011)
- Due to mutation on the X chromosome, mapped to Xq28
- Because girls have one typical and one atypical X, they do not present with symptoms, but males are affected.
- The most common genetic form of congenital hydrocephalus with stenosis of the aqueduct of Sylvius (Schrander-Stumpel & Fryns, 1998)

- This disorder is due to mutations in the gene encoding L1, a neuronal cell adhesion molecule that belongs to the immunoglobulin "super family" and is essential in neurological development (Fransen, Van Camp, Vits, & Willems, 1997).

Assessment

- Approximately 50% of affected boys have adducted thumbs (held inward toward the palms), which is helpful in making the diagnosis.
- Some have other CNS abnormalities:
  - *Malformation of the corpus callosum*
  - *Small brainstem*
  - *Absence of the pyramidal tract*
- Mutations in L1 also result in other conditions, known as the L1 spectrum, which is characterized by neurologic abnormalities and mental retardation.
  - *These include MASA spectrum (mental retardation, aphasia, shuffling gait, adducted thumbs), X-linked spastic paraplegia type 1, and X-linked agenesis of the corpus callosum.*

Nursing Interventions

- Close monitoring of head circumference and then management of a CNS shunt if placed
- Assessment for age-appropriate developmental milestones

Caregiver Education

- Prenatal diagnosis may be made based on ultrasound and then amniocentesis.
- Referral to early intervention and neurosurgery, neurology, and developmental specialists is necessary.

FRAGILE X SYNDROME (FXS)

- Formerly known as fragile X mental retardation syndrome
- Result of decreased or absent levels of fragile X mental retardation protein (FMRP) due to a mutation in the fragile X mental retardation (*FMR1*) gene located at Xq27.3
- Males inherit a single X chromosome from their mother, and therefore show many more symptoms if there is a mutation present.
- Females have two copies of the X chromosome; they may inherit an abnormal X from one parent, but a typical X from the other. Only one X per cell is active; the other is said to be inactivated. Therefore, females can show varying symptoms, from only a few to very severe (Hagerman & McCandless, 2005).
- Fragile X is caused by an expansion, a series of repeats, in the DNA at Xq27.3. This number of repeats generally accounts for the severity of symptoms.
- Most individuals have between 5 and 40 repeats; 41 to 58 repeats is called an intermediate or gray-zone; 59 to 200 is called pre-mutation; and over 200 is referred to as full mutation.
- Repeats of more than 200 essentially turn off production of FMRP.
- Typically, mutated genes are passed on in a relatively stable fashion.
- In fragile X, when passed on from mother to children, the number of repeats tends to "expand," with more repeats at each generation. The greater the number of pre-mutation repeats a mother may have, the more likely the child will inherit a full mutation.
- An affected father will pass the mutation to his daughters, but they tend to contract, or have less repeats. Daughters do not inherit the full mutation from an affected father, but become carriers.
- Males that possess the full FMR1 mutation of more than 200 repeats are considered fully affected and have fragile X syndrome (FXS).

Assessment

- Males with over 200 repeats tend to have physical features such as:
  - *Long, narrow face*
  - *Prominent jaw and forehead*
  - *Large, protruding ears*
  - *High arched palate*
  - *Loose connective tissue*
- Loose connective tissue can cause:
  - *Hyperextensible joints*
  - *Flat feet*
  - *Mitral valve dysfunction (Visootsak, Warren, Anido, & Graham, 2005)*
- After puberty, men have remarkably enlarged testicles (macro-orchidism)
- Males with FXS often have intellectual disabilities, including:
  - *Issues with communication, generally speech and language delays*
  - *IQ in mild to moderate intellectual disability range*
  - *Hyperactivity*
- Stereotypic behaviors may also be displayed, such as the following:
  - *Hand flapping*
  - *Lack of eye contact and inattention*
  - *Aggression and anxiety*
  - *Higher incidence of meeting criteria of autistic spectrum disorder*
- Females with the full mutation often have the following characteristics:
  - *More subtle facial features*
  - *Less severe degrees of developmental delay and speech and language issues*
  - *Higher IQ than males with FXS*
- Females who are direct carriers are generally more typical; rarely a significant amount of shyness and anxiety is evident (Hagerman & McCandless, 2005).

Nursing Interventions

- Routine well-child care and immunizations should be performed.
- Seizures occur in about 20% (Berry-Kravis, 2002).
- Newborns can have feeding issues, and mild motor delays are common.
- Language delays tend to appear between 2 and 3 years of age, and autistic features such as hand flapping and hand biting, poor eye contact, and social anxiety and shyness may appear as well.
- Stimulants and parental guidance are necessary to address behaviors and hyperactivity.
- Complications include eye issues such as alignment errors (strabismus) and orthopedic issues with joint laxity and flat feet related to the connective tissue defects.
- Heart murmurs require echocardiograms and monitoring of the mitral valve.

Caregiver Education

- Daughters do not inherit the full mutation from an affected father, but become carriers.
- Genetic counseling concerning pregnancy for females affected by FXS is necessary.
- Girls with the full mutation may display early puberty, and women with direct effects may have early menopause (Hagerman & McCandless, 2005).
- Tantrum behavior and hyperactivity may begin by age 2 years.

PRADER-WILLI SYNDROME

- Another unique inheritance pattern genetic syndrome, caused by several different genetic alterations on chromosome 15's long arm (15q) (Cassidy & McCandless, 2005)
- In about 75% of individuals with Prader-Willi syndrome, there is a small deletion on chromosome 15 between q11 and q13.
- Additional cases can result from inheriting two maternal alleles of chromosome 15 and no paternal alleles, known as uniparental disomy.
- Inheritance of two paternal alleles results in Angelman's syndrome, a completely different syndrome.
- A third cause, in less than 5% of cases, is the result of a defect in the "imprinting process." These individuals do not have a notable deletion and have inherited alleles from each parent, but only the maternal allele is active.

Assessment

- Result of hypothalamic/pituitary gland dysfunction
  - *Although hypothalamus/pituitary is in fact structurally normal*
- Infants born with hypotonia:
  - *Often have feeding difficulties*
  - *Display early failure to thrive*
- Rapid onset of weight gain and large appetite presenting between 1 and 6 years of age (hyperphagia)
  - *May consume nonfood items*
- Characteristic facial features:
  - *Almond-shaped eyes*
  - *Narrow nasal bridge*
  - *Down-turned mouth*
  - *Thin upper lip*
- Small genitals (hypoplasia) and pubertal deficiency
- Developmental delay and intellectual disabilities:
  - *IQ median range is 60 to low 70s*
  - *Or may have mild intellectual delay, but may be within normal limits*
- Behavioral profile:
  - *Stubbornness*
  - *Can be manipulative*
  - *Obsessive-compulsive qualities*
  - *Great difficulties without routines*
- Physical traits:
  - *Hypopigmentation, fair hair and skin compared to family members (Butler, 1989)*
  - *Small hands and feet for height, tapered fingers*
  - *Overall short stature, genu varum (knock-knees; see Chapter 20)*
  - *Near sighted (myopia) and cross-eyed*
  - *Thick, viscous saliva*
  - *Speech articulation defects*
  - *Skin picking*
  - *High pain threshold*
  - *Temperature control problems*
  - *Scoliosis and kyphosis*
  - *Osteoporosis*

Nursing Interventions

- Feeding support and possible supplements in newborn period, rarely can breastfeed
- Endocrine involvement; improvement with growth hormone supplementation
- Early adrenarche but overall pubertal delay, and many are not sexually active as adults
- Infertility also common

Caregiver Education

- Feeding support and possible supplements in newborn period, rarely can breastfeed
- Early intervention for developmental delay
- Need to establish clear health routines early, with limited oral intake, daily exercise, and skin exam daily; treatment of picked skin areas with antibiotics
- Strict attention to feeding recommendations and dietary restriction; may eat to point of severe gastric distention without emesis
- Need to restrict access to items such as garbage, pet food, paste, glue

ANGELMAN SYNDROME

- Deletion on maternal chromosome 15
- Characteristic features:
  - *Developmental delay*
  - *Mental retardation*
  - *Severe speech and language impairment*
  - *Problems with movement, coordination, and balance*
  - *Happy, laughing demeanor*
  - *Hand-flapping behaviors*
  - *Hyperactivity with short attention span*
  - *Short sleep cycles*
  - *Epilepsy*
  - *Scoliosis is common (Behrman et al., 2007).*

Assessment

- General physical assessment
- Documentation of dysmorphic features or obvious abnormalities
- Assess presence or absence of developmental milestones
- Screening for other associated conditions

Diagnosis

- Children with chromosomal abnormalities are diagnosed by examination and documentation of characteristics seen with specific disorders.
- A blood test is necessary to evaluate the chromosomes and genetic codes.
- Because some chromosomal disorders may cause multiple malformations, such as heart defects or kidney defects as well as dysmorphic features, evaluations for other malformations should be performed.

Nursing Interventions

- Treatment is aimed at supportive care.
- Medications to treat medical disorders may be necessary, such as to control seizures.
- Physical, occupational, and speech therapies are often needed to help children progress in developmental milestones.
- Families require support because of added stressors, such as:
  - *Time to care for the child with special needs*
  - *Education of medical procedures that may be needed at home, such as tube feedings*
  - *Emotions*
  - *Grief*
  - *Finances*

FETAL ALCOHOL SPECTRUM DISORDER (FASD)

- The term *fetal alcohol spectrum disorder* (FASD) describes the broad range of adverse sequelae in alcohol-exposed offspring.
- FASD is an overall umbrella term that describes the spectrum of disorders caused by exposure to excessive maternal alcohol use.
- At one end of the spectrum are persons with typical FASD facial features and neuro-cognitive disorders, and at the other end are children with no physical features but behavioral and cognitive deficits.
- The exact amount of alcohol necessary to cause the full spectrum is unknown, so NO alcohol is to be consumed during pregnancy.
- Some persons seem to be at higher risk related to variance in the three different types of alleles for alcohol dehydrogenase that result in different levels of enzyme activity (Chudley & Longstaffe, 2005).

Four Subtypes of FASD

The spectrum can be divided into four subtypes (Hoyme et al., 2005):

1. **Fetal alcohol syndrome (FAS).** This is the most severe form of FASD and is defined by abnormalities in three domains: poor growth, abnormal brain growth or structure, and specific dysmorphic facial features. Prenatal alcohol exposure may or may not be confirmed.
2. **Partial fetal alcohol syndrome.** These children display the typical facial dysmorphic features associated with FAS, have abnormalities in only one of the other domains, and prenatal alcohol exposure is confirmed.
3. **Alcohol-related birth defects (ARBD).** These children have the typical facial features associated with FAS, normal growth, and normal brain function and structure, but have structural congenital anomalies in other organs (such as cardiac or renal abnormalities). Confirmation of prenatal alcohol exposure is required.
4. **Alcohol-related neurodevelopmental disorder (ARND).** These children have normal growth and lack the facial features of FASD but display a pattern of behavioral or cognitive abnormalities typical of prenatal alcohol exposure. These children are at risk for significant cognitive impairment, abnormalities on testing of verbal learning and memory skills, and low IQ scores (Mattson, Riley, Gramling, Delis, & Jones, 1997). Confirmation of prenatal alcohol exposure is required.

Assessment

- Typical facial features at birth:
  - *Flat midface*
  - *Thin upper lip*
  - *Small chin (micrognathia)*
  - *Short, upturned nose*
  - *Short palpebral fissures*
  - *Prominent epicanthal fold at inner portion of eyes*

- Growth deficiency, starting infancy and lasting throughout life
  - *Brain anomalies/defects can include abnormalities of the corpus callosum, cerebellum, and frank microcephaly (American Academy of Pediatrics, Committee on Substance Abuse and Committee on Children with Disabilities, 2000).*
  - *Sensory, motor, and regulatory behavior is also affected at the cellular level.*
  - *Communication and language can be affected.*
  - *Organ damage, including congenital heart defects, can occur (Hoyme et al., 2005).*

Nursing Interventions

- There may be difficulties with suck/swallow/breath coordination or aspiration.
- Gastrostomy feeding may be necessary.
- Sensory overreactivity to textures is often present.
- Behavioral management and environmental changes are necessary to address inattention.
- Co-morbidities must be recognized.

Caregiver Education

- No alcohol is to be consumed during pregnancy.
- Impulsivity, attention issues, and frank ADHD are common.
- Executive dysfunction is common.

Review Questions

1. During your clinical, the instructor describes a condition of one of the patients. She starts by saying this child has a history of "chronic urinary retention with ballooning that is only resolved with manual compression." You tell her the condition is known as
A. hydrocele.
B. pathologic phimosis.
C. urethrophyma.
D. urocele.

2. An accurate description of the vaginal discharge in bacterial vaginosis is
A. thin and brownish.
B. thick and green.
C. thick and yellow.
D. thin and whitish-grey.

3. Children with Down syndrome have specific features. Select the answer that describes the features of a child with Down syndrome.
A. Small head, round-shaped eyes, flattened middle face, and low-set ears
B. Small head, almond-shaped eyes, flattened middle face, and low-set ears
C. Small head, almond-shaped eyes, protruding middle face, and low-set ears
D. Small head, round-shaped eyes, protruding middle face, and low-set ears

4. There is one pair of sex chromosomes for both males and females. Which statement correctly identifies the sex chromosomes of the female and the male?
A. Females are XY and males XX.
B. Females are XY and males are YY.
C. Females are XX and males are XY.
D. Females are YY and males are XX.

5. Trisomy 13 is also known as
A. Down syndrome.
B. Edwards syndrome.
C. Patau syndrome.
D. Turner syndrome.

6. Ongoing cell mitosis is essential throughout the life span to maintain proper body function and takes place in nearly all cells of the body. Different cells reproduce by mitosis at different rates. Which cells can take years to reproduce? (select all that apply)
A. Brain cells
B. Liver cells
C. Nerve cells
D. Muscle cells
E. Skin cells

7. A mother presents to the clinic with her 10-year-old daughter, who has complaints of vaginal itching, pain during urination, vulva redness, and a thin vaginal discharge. The physician has diagnosed the child with vulvovaginitis. As a nurse, your education will include: (select all that apply)
A. causes of vulvovaginitis.
B. daily warm baths with gentle soap.
C. notify physician if the infection does not improve.
D. vulvovaginitis is sexually transmitted.
E. it is most common complaint in prepubescent girls.

8. Anatomy of the male reproductive system includes which of the following? (select all that apply)
A. Epididymis
B. Glans
C. Prepuce
D. Sulcus
E. Vas deferens

9. Gonorrhea is an infection that can occur in the cervix, vagina, and fallopian tube in women. It can also be present in the eyes, throat, urethra, and anus of both male and females. Other true statements include which of the following? (select all that apply)
A. Gonorrhea can spread to the blood and cause arthritis in the joints.
B. Symptoms are dependent on the part of the body that is infected.
C. Gonorrhea cannot be spread to infants during birth.
D. Females aged 25 and older have the highest risk for infection.
E. Gonorrhea in children can signal sexual abuse.

10. A common complication of neurofibromatosis type 2 is:
A. hearing loss.
B. memory loss.
C. speech loss.
D. drooling.
E. hair loss.

References

Alasdair, G. W. H. (2005). Down syndrome. In S. Cassidy & T. Allanson (Eds.), *Down syndrome in management of genetic syndromes* (2nd ed., pp. 191–210). Hoboken, NJ: John S. Wiley and Sons, Inc.

American Academy of Pediatrics (AAP). (2001). Committee on Genetics Health Supervision for Children with Down Syndrome. *Pediatrics*, *107*, 442–449. Retrieved from http://aappolicy.aappublications.org/cgi/content/full/pediatrics;107/2/442

American Academy of Pediatrics, Committee on Substance Abuse and Committee on Children with Disabilities. (2000). Fetal alcohol syndrome and alcohol related neurodevelopmental disorders. *Pediatrics*, *106*, 358–361. Retrieved from http://aappolicy.aappublications.org/cgi/content/full/pediatrics;106/2/358

Anderson, S. E., & Must, A. (2005). Interpreting the continued decline in the average age at menarche; results from two nationally representative surveys of U.S. girls studied 10 years apart. *Journal of Pediatrics*, *147*, 753. Retrieved from http://www.ncbi.nlm.nih.gov/pubmed/16356426

Behrman, R. E., Kliegman, R. M., Jenson, H. B., & Stanton, B. F. (2007). *Nelson textbook of pediatrics* (18th ed.). St. Louis, MO: W. B. Saunders.

Berry-Kravis, E. (2002). Epilepsy in fragile X syndrome. *Developmental Medicine and Child Neurology*, *44*, 724. doi: 10.1017/S0012162201002833

Butler, M. G. (1989). Hypopigmentation: A common feature of Prader-Labhart-Willi syndrome. *American Journal of Human Genetics*, *45*, 140. Retrieved from http://www.ncbi.nlm.nih.gov/pmc/articles/PMC1683374/

Carey, J. (2005). Trisomy 18 and trisomy 13 syndromes. In S. Cassidy & T. Allanson (Eds.), *Management of genetic syndromes* (2nd ed., pp. 555–568), Hoboken, NJ: John S. Wiley and Sons, Inc.

Cassidy, S. B., & McCandless, S. E. (2005). Prader-Willi syndrome. In S. B. Cassidy & J. E. Allanson (Eds.), *Management of genetic syndromes* (pp. 429–448). Hoboken, NJ: Wiley-Liss.

Centers for Disease Control and Prevention (CDC). (2010). *2010 STD treatment guidelines*. Retrieved from http://www.cdc.gov/std/treatment/2010/default.htm

Centers for Disease Control and Prevention (CDC). (2012). Male Circumcision. Retrieved from http://www.cdc.gov/hiv/malecircumcision/

Chudley, A., & Longstaffe, S. (2005). Fetal alcohol syndrome and fetal alcohol spectrum disorders in *Management of Genetic Syndromes* (2nd ed., pp. 369-384), S. Cassidy & T. Allanson (Eds.), Hoboken, NJ: John S. Wiley and Sons, Inc.

DeSilva, N., & Zurawin, R. (2011). *Definition and evaluation of abnormal uterine bleeding in adolescents*. Retrieved from http://www.uptodate.com

Feinichel, G. M. (2001). *Clinical pediatric neurology*. St. Louis, MO: W. B. Saunders.

Fishman, M. (2011). *Hydrocephalus*. Retrieved from http://www.uptodate.com

Fransen, E., Van Camp, G., Vits, L., & Willems, P. J. (1997). L1-associated diseases: Clinical geneticists divide, molecular geneticists unite. *Human Molecular Genetics*, *6*, 1625. doi: 10.1093/hmg/6.10.1625

Friedman, J. M., & Birch, P. H. (1997). Type 1 neurofibromatosis: A descriptive analysis of the disorder in 1,728 patients. *American Journal of Medical Genetics*, *70*, 138. doi: 10.1002/(SICI)1096-8628(19970516)70:2{138::AID-AJMG7>3.0.CO;2-U

Garcia, C. T. (2006). Genitourinary trauma. In G. R. Fleisher, S. Ludwig, & F. M. Henretig (Eds.), *Textbook of pediatric emergency medicine* (5th ed., pp. 1463). Philadelphia: Lippincott Williams and Wilkins.

Grosfeld, J. L. (1989). Current concepts in inguinal hernia in infants and children. *World Journal of Surgery*, *13*, 506. doi: 10.1007/BF01658863

Hagerman, R., & McCandless, S. (2005). *Fragile X syndrome*. In S. Cassidy & T. Allanson (Eds.), *Management of genetic syndromes* (2nd ed., pp. 251–264). Hoboken, NJ: John S. Wiley and Sons, Inc.

Hicks, C., & Sparling, P. F. (2011). *Pathogenesis, clinical manifestations, and treatment of early syphilis*. Retrieved from http://www.uptodate.com

Hoyme, H. E., May, P. A., Kalberg, W. O., Kodituwakku, P., Gossage, J. P., Trujillo, P. M., . . . Robinson, L. K. (2005). A practical clinical approach to diagnosis of fetal alcohol spectrum disorders: Clarification of the 1996 institute of medicine criteria. *Pediatrics*, *115*, 39. doi: 10.1542/peds.2005-0702

Hsieh, T. F., Chang, C. H., & Chang, S. S. (2006). Foreskin development before adolescence in 2149 schoolboys. *International Journal of Urology*, *13*, 968. doi: 10.1111/j.1442-2042.2006.01449.x

Joishy, M., Ashtekar, C. S., Jain, A., & Gonsalves, R. (2005). Do we need to treat vulvovaginitis in prepubertal girls? *British Medical Journal*, *330*, 186. doi: 10.1136/bmj.330.7484.186

Klebanoff, M. A., Schwebke, J. R., Zhang, J., Nansel, T. R., Yu, K. F., & Andrews, W. W. (2004). Vulvovaginal symptoms in women with bacterial vaginosis. *Obstetrics and Gynecolology*, *104*, 267. doi: 10.1097/01.AOG.0000134783.98382.b0

Laufner, M., & Emans, S. J. (2011). *Vulvovaginal complaint in the prepubertal child*. Retrieved from http://www.uptodate.com

Lewis, R. A., Gerson, L. P., Axelson, K. A., Riccardi, V. M., Whitford, R. P. (1984). Von Recklinghausen neurofibromatosis. II. Incidence of optic gliomata. *Ophthalmology*, *91*, 929. Retrieved from http://www.ncbi.nlm.nih.gov/pubmed/6436764

Lewis, R. A., & Riccardi, V. M. (1981). Von Recklinghausen neurofibromatosis. Incidence of iris hamartomata. *Ophthalmology*, *88*, 348. Retrieved from http://www.ncbi.nlm.nih.gov/pubmed/6789269

Marshall, W. A., & Tanner, J. M. (1969). Variations in pattern of pubertal changes in girls. *Archives of Disease in Childhood*, *44*, 291. doi: 10.1136/adc.44.235.291

Mattson, S. N., Riley, E. P., Gramling, L., Delis, D. C., & Jones, K. L. (1997). Heavy prenatal alcohol exposure with or without physical features of fetal alcohol syndrome leads to IQ deficits. *Journal of Pediatrics*, *131*, 718. Retrieved from http://www.ncbi.nlm.nih.gov/pubmed/9403652

Morris, C. (2005). Williams syndrome. In S. Cassidy & T. Allanson (Eds.), *Management of genetic syndromes* (2nd ed., pp. 665–665). Hoboken, NJ: John S. Wiley and Sons, Inc.

National Institute of Neurological Disorders (NIND). (2012a). Charcot Marie Tooth Fact Sheet. Retrieved from http://www.ninds.nih.gov/disorders/charcot_marie_tooth/detail_charcot_marie_tooth.htm#102833092

National Institute of Neurological Disorders (NIND). (2012b). NINDS Neurofibromatosis Information Page. Retrieved from http://www.ninds.nih.gov/disorders/neurofibromatosis/neurofibromatosis.htm

North, K. (2000). Neurofibromatosis type 1. *American Journal of Medical Genetics, 97*, 119. doi: 10.1002/1096-8628(200022)97:2{119::AID-AJMG3>3.0.CO;2-3

North, K. N., Riccardi V., Samango-Sprouse C., Ferner, R., Moore, B., Legius, E., . . . Denckla, M. B. (1997). Cognitive function and academic performance in neurofibromatosis 1: Consensus statement from the NF1 Cognitive Disorders Task Force. *Neurology, 48*, 112. Retrieved from http://www.ncbi.nlm.nih.gov/pubmed/9109916

Pauli, R. (2005). Achondroplasia. In S. Cassidy & T. Allanson (Eds.), *Management of genetic syndromes* (2nd ed., pp. 13–30). Hoboken, NJ: John S. Wiley and Sons, Inc.

Perron, C. E. (2006). Pain—scrotal. In G. R. Fleisher, S. Ludwig, & F. M. Henretig (Eds.), *Textbook of pediatric emergency medicine* (5th ed., p. 525). Philadelphia: Lippincott, Williams & Wilkins.

Plun, S. E. (2011). *Neurofibromatosis, von Recklinghausen's disease*. Retrieved from http://www.uptpdate.com

Reyes Mendez, D. (2011). *Straddle injuries*. Retrieved from http://www.uptodate.com

Schrander-Stumpel C., & Fryns, J. P. (1998). Congenital hydrocephalus: Nosology and guidelines for clinical approach and genetic counseling. *European Journal of Pediatrics, 157*, 355. doi: 10.1007/s004310050830

Shprintzen, R. (2005). Velo-cardio-facial syndrome. In S. Cassidy & T. Allanson (Eds.), *Management of genetic syndromes* (2nd ed., pp. 615–632). Hoboken, NJ: John S. Wiley and Sons, Inc.

Skoog, S. J., & Conlin, M. J. (1995). Pediatric hernias and hydroceles. The urologist's perspective. *Urologic Clinics of North America, 22*, 119. Retrieved from http://www.ncbi.nlm.nih.gov/pubmed/7855948

Skoog, S. J., Roberts, K. P., Goldstein M., & Pryor, J. L. (1997). The adolescent varicocele: What's new with an old problem in young patients? *Pediatrics, 100*, 112. doi: 10.1542/ peds.100.1.112

Sobal, J. (2011). *Bacterial vaginosis*. Retrieved from http://www.uptodate.com

Sybert, V. (2005). Turner syndrome. In S. Cassidy & T. Allanson (Eds.), *Management of genetic syndromes* (2nd ed., pp. 589–605). Hoboken, NJ: John S. Wiley and Sons, Inc.

Trotter, T. L., & Hall, J. G. (2005). Health supervision for children with achondroplasia. *Pediatrics, 116*, 771. doi: 10.1542/peds.2005-1440

Viskochil, D. (2005). Neurofibromatosis Type 1. In S. Cassidy and T. Allanson, (Eds.), *Management of Genetic Syndromes* (2nd Ed., pp. 369–384), Hoboken, NJ: John S. Wiley and Sons, Inc.

Visootsak, J., Warren, S. T., Anido, A., & Graham, J. M. (2005). Fragile X syndrome: An update and review for the primary pediatrician. *Clinical Pediatrics, 44*, 371. doi: 10.1177/ 000992280504400501

Volpe, J. (2001). *Neurology of the newborn* (4th ed.). St. Louis, MO: W. B. Saunders.

World Health Organization, Task Force on Adolescent Reproductive Health. (1986). Longitudinal study of menstrual patterns in the early postmenarcheal period, duration of bleeding episodes and menstrual cycles. *Journal of Adolescent Health Care, 7*, 236. Retrieved from http://www.ncbi.nlm.nih.gov/pubmed/3721946

Wu, T., Mendola, P., & Buck, G. M. (2002). Ethnic differences in the presence of secondary sex characteristics and menarche among US girls: The Third National Health and Nutrition Examination Survey, 1988–1994. *Pediatrics, 110*, 752. Retrieved from http://www.ncbi.nlm.nih.gov/pubmed/12359790

Zampieri, N., Corroppolo, M., Camoglio, F. S., Giacomello, L., & Ottolenghi, A. (2005). Phimosis: Stretching methods with or without application of topical steroids? *Journal of Pediatrics, 147*, 705. Retrieved from http://www.ncbi.nlm.nih.gov/pubmed/16291369

Zitelli, B. J., & Davis, H. W. (2007). *Atlas of pediatric physical diagnosis* (5th ed.). Philadelphia: Elsevier.

19

Hematologic, Immunologic, and Neoplastic Disorders

Sheryl Stuck, MSN, RN, CNS

OBJECTIVES

- ☐ Define key terms.
- ☐ Identify the classifications of anemia.
- ☐ Compare iron deficiency and sickle cell anemia.
- ☐ Identify the major pathophysiology associated with the care of the child with cancer.
- ☐ Identify nursing assessments and interventions that promote health during the care of children with leukemia and their families.
- ☐ Develop a nursing care plan for the child with cancer experiencing pain.
- ☐ Develop a caregiver education plan for high-risk oncology clients.
- ☐ Demonstrate an understanding of the pathophysiology of and nursing interventions for the child with immunodeficiency disorders.
- ☐ Identify the categories of hematopoietic stem cell transplant.

KEY TERMS

- Anemia
- Erythropoietin
- Petechiae
- Purpura
- Sickle cell disease (SCD)
- Hemophilia
- Blood coagulation
- Hemarthrosis
- Tumor
- Leukemia
- Oncology
- Hodgkin's lymphoma
- Non-Hodgkin's lymphoma
- Metastasis

HEMATOLOGIC DISORDERS

The process of hematopoiesis:

- Bone marrow produces blood cells and platelets.
- The flat bones of the sternum, ilium, ribs, and vertebrae differentiate cells.
- Erythropoiesis is the production of the red blood cells (RBCs) with erythropoietin and iron.
- An RBC's life span is 120 days.
- Hemolysis is the destruction of RBCs by phagocytes in the spleen and liver.

IRON DEFICIENCY ANEMIA

- Etiology is dietary deficiency, with infants consuming cow milk having a greater incidence
- Microcytic **anemia** is characterized by small, pale RBCs and depletion of iron stores with subsequent decrease in bone marrow erythropoiesis.

Assessment

- Screening hemogram at 9-month and 12-month health supervision visits recommended by the American Academy of Pediatrics (n.d.)
- Adequate intake of 0.27 mg/day for term infants through 6 months (Baker & Greer, 2010)
- Infants 7 to 12 months of age: recommended dietary allowance for iron is 11 mg/day (Baker & Greer, 2010)
- Irritability, anorexia, tachycardia, systolic murmur, brittle and concave nails
- Poor muscle tone
- Prone to infection

Don't have time to read this chapter? Want to reinforce your reading? Need to review for a test? Listen to this chapter on DavisPlus at davispl.us/rudd1.

- Skin may be described as porcelain-like
- Edematous
- Retarded growth
- Decreased serum concentration of the proteins albumin, gamma globulin, and transferrin
- Diminishing growth and learning in children

Diagnostic Testing

- Complete blood count (CBC) with RBC indexes normal, borderline, or moderately reduced
- RBCs small in size
- Low serum iron (serum iron concentration circulating; reference values 30–160 μg/dL) (Corbett, 2008)
- Serum ferritin (reference values 20400 ng/mL) (Corbett 2008)
- Total iron-binding capacity (TIBC; reference values 250–410 μg/dL) (Corbett, 2008)
- **Erythropoietin** assay (EPO) level of reference values of 5–20 m/U/mL (children may have higher values) (Corbett, 2008)
- Reticulocyte count (reference value of 3%–5% of the total RBC count for first week) normal (reference value of 0.5%–2.5%) or slightly reduced (Corbett, 2008)

Nursing Interventions

- Use commercial iron-fortified formula.
- Dietary therapeutics with oral elemental iron preparations (**Table 19-1**)
- Liquid dosage of iron sipped through a plastic straw to avoid colored tooth enamel
- Iron supplementation may be necessary in adolescence.
- Use Z track method for iron dextran (Imferon).

Caregiver Education

- Teaching to add iron-rich foods to diet (**Table 19-2**)

ACQUIRED THROMBOCYTOPENIA (ATP)

- Pathophysiology: causative agent may be drug or infection (e.g., Rocky Mountain spotted fever, Colorado tick fever, malaria, or bacterial)
- With removal of the causative agent, platelet count recovers.

Assessment

- Recent bleeding, nose epistaxis, blood in feces, blood in mucous membranes or gums, hematemesis
- Assess for **petechiae**, often over bony prominences.
- Recent exposure to chemicals, insecticides, paint, gasoline, kerosene, and lawn care supplies may be the causative agent
- Recent exposure to Rocky Mountain spotted fever, malaria, bacteremia, viral infection, measles, mumps, rubella, and chickenpox
- Petechiae, **purpura** on face, thorax, and extremities
- Bleeding from orifices, epistaxis, scabs, and bleeding gums

Diagnostic Testing

- Platelet count decreased (normal 150,000–450,000/mm^3) (Corbett, 2008)

Nursing Interventions

- Mouth care with soft toothettes
- Monitor stools for occult blood.
- Avoid intramuscular injections and suctioning.
- Avoid use of salicylates (aspirin), which interfere with platelet aggregation.
- Administer steroids to increase platelet production and decrease vascular fragility.

TABLE 19–1 IRON AND FOLIC ACID PREPARATIONS

Drug (Pregnancy Category)	Pharmacologic Class	Usual Dosage Range	Indications/Uses
ferric gluconate (B)	Parenteral iron salt	Older than 6 yr: 1.5 mg/kg/dose for 8 doses	Iron deficiency associated with hemodialysis
ferrous fumarate (A)	Oral iron salt	4–6 mg kg/day	Severe iron deficiency anemia Iron deficiency anemia
Folic acid (A)	Water-soluble B-complex vitamin	PO/IV/IM/subcut: 0.1–0.4 mg/day	Folate deficiency tropical sprue, nutritional and pregnancy-related supplementation
Iron dextran (C)	Parenteral iron salt	IM/IV: 5–10 kg: 25 mg/day; greater than 10 kg: 50 mg/day	Iron deficiency when oral iron therapy is unsatisfactory
Iron sucrose	Parenteral iron salt	Adult IM/IV: 100 mg/day (2 mL/day)	Iron deficiency in adult with chronic renal failure

Adapted from Lilley, L. L., Harrington, S., & Snyder, J. S. (2011). *Pharmacology and the nursing process* (6th ed.). St. Louis: Mosby.

TABLE 19–2	RECOMMENDATIONS FOR FOODS RICH IN IRON AND FOLATE
Iron	Organ meats, shellfish, poultry, legumes, molasses, fortified cereals
Folate (folic acid)	Legumes, liver, dark green or leafy vegetables, lean beef, potatoes

Adapted from Baker & Greer (2010).

- Modify age-appropriate activities to avoid injuries.
- Collaborate with physical therapist.
- Encourage a positive self-image and self-care.

Caregiver Education

- Teach about side effects of steroid therapy.
- Give steroids with food and limit sodium intake.
- Provide range of activity based on platelet count.
- Avoid exposure to causative agent.
- Encourage parent to support positive self-concept of child.
- Support appropriate activities for child.

SICKLE CELL DISEASE (SCD)

- Etiology: most commonly genetic and hereditary condition
- When both parents have the sickle cell trait, there is a one in four chance with each pregnancy that the child will have **sickle cell disease (SCD)**.
- Pathophysiology is characterized by partial or complete replacement of abnormal hemoglobin S for normal hemoglobin A. The deformed cell changes from round to sickle (crescent) shape (**Figure 19-1**).
- Tissue damage can occur all over the body, and complications relate to delayed growth and sexual maturation, acute and chronic pulmonary dysfunction, stroke, aseptic necrosis of the hip and shoulders, retinopathy, dermal ulcers, severe and chronic pain, psychosocial dysfunction.

Assessment

- Asymptomatic until 4 to 6 months due to presence of fetal hemoglobin, which resists sickling and suppresses symptoms
- Hemolytic anemia occurs with sickled RBC destruction.
- Vasoocclusive crisis (obstruction of blood flow causing tissue hypoxia and necrosis) is a painful episode with hand–foot syndrome (dactylitis) causing symmetrical infarct in the bones of the hands and feet and very painful swelling of soft tissue.

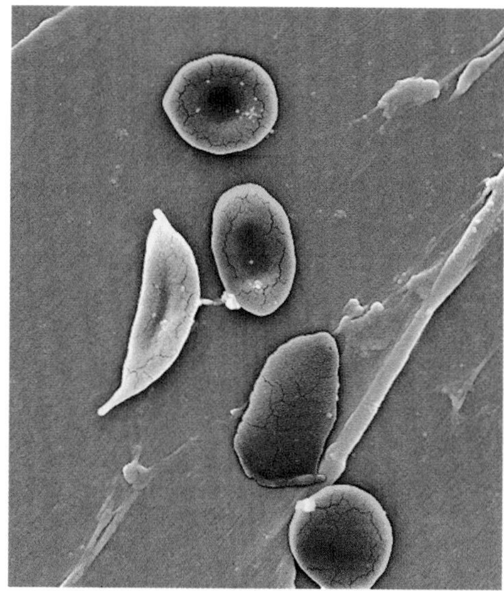

Figure 19–1 Example of a sickle cell.

- Acute chest syndrome occurs as new pulmonary infiltrate with chest pain, fever, cough, tachypnea, wheezing, and hypoxia.
- Sequestration crisis is the loss of spleen function as a result of frequent infarcts and the pooling of large amount of blood, causing enlargement.
- A cerebrovascular accident is a blocking of the blood vessels in the brain with impaired neurologic function; severe headache; twitching of the face, legs, or arms; seizures; change in speech; weakness in the hands, feet, or legs; abnormal behavior
- Assess for psychological adjustment, including emotional and behavioral problems related to long periods of hospitalization.

Diagnostic Testing

- Sickle-turbidity test (sickledex) with fingerstick blood yields results in 3 minutes to determine if Hgb S present.
- Hemoglobin electrophoresis is accurate and rapid; quantifies the percentages of various types of hemoglobin S and Hgb A.

Nursing Interventions

- Analgesics for the pain of vasoocclusion
- Pain distraction techniques, including self-hypnosis and negating/negative affect
- Activity rest cycling for periods of activity intolerance
- Hydration with IV therapy and oral fluids
- Antibiotics for infection treatment
- Penicillin prophylaxis significantly reduces the risk of pneumococcal infection starting at 2 months of age.
- Hydrourea is cytoxic and used to reduce the frequency of painful crises and reduce the need for blood transfusions

in patients with recurrent, moderate to severe crisis (Lilley, Harrington, & Snyder, 2011).
- Metabolic acidosis treatment with IV electrolyte replacement
- Physical therapy
- Complementary therapy, including cognitive-behavioral therapy approaches, controlled breathing, positive self-talk, behavioral rehearsal, transcutaneous electrical nerve stimulation, hand holding, humor, music, and memory reframing
- Splenectomy as a life-saving measure
- Hematopoietic stem cell transplantation (HSCT) may be an option
- Monitor for acute chest syndrome for possible severe chest, back, or abdominal pain; fever; congested cough; dyspnea; tachypnea; retractions; decreased oxygen saturation (≤92).

CULTURAL AWARENESS: Health Care Practices Involving Blood Transfusions

Culture is the pattern of assumptions, beliefs, and practices that frames the decisions of a group of people. Health practices are affected by culture, which should be considered in the plan of care. As a nurse advocate, look beyond preconceived notions and stereotypes to see the child underneath.

Arrange a translator for inpatient daily rounds and explanation of the plan of care. The culture of the caregiver may determine the response to a child's distress.

Nurses provide culturally competent care to communicate and negotiate mutually acceptable interventions. Children with cancer frequently need blood transfusions for an intervention. The beliefs of Jehovah's Witness children and their caregivers are to not accept blood products, and caregivers may refuse the administration of blood to the child. Hispanic culture and several others rely on the presence of extended family members at the bedside.

Caregiver Education

- Resources for the family, including genetic counseling
- Teach caregivers signs of infection.
- Seek medical care with temperature of 38.3°C (101°F) as directed by prescribing physician.
- May need prophylactic penicillin before dental procedures
- Immunizations against HIV, pneumococcal and meningococcal organisms
- Discuss feelings of altered self-concept manifested as poor academic performance, low social and interpersonal functioning, and withdrawal.
- Resulting pain contributes to depression, anxiety, and other psychiatric disturbances.
- Develop a relationship with the child and caregiver to work together to find the safest medical solution.
- Take the time to get to know the child and answer any questions.

APLASTIC ANEMIA

- Pathophysiology is a deficiency of the formation of blood elements; pancytopenia is decreased leukocytes, platelets, and erythrocytes.

Assessment

- Fatigue
- History of illness or injury that does not heal

Diagnostic Testing

- CBC with differential and platelet count to diagnose the specific type of anemia
- Reticulocytes are less mature RBCs, and an increase in the percentage of reticulocytes indicates that a release of RBCs is occurring more rapidly than usual to compensate for deficiency (reference value of 0.5%–2.5% of the total RBC count) (Corbet, 2008).
- Bone marrow aspiration confirms red bone marrow conversion to yellow, fatty bone marrow.

Nursing Interventions

- Monitor immunosuppressive therapy to remove functions that prolong aplasia.
- Monitor blood transfusions and IV infusion access care to decrease infection.
- Prevent infection with hand hygiene.

Caregiver Education

- Describe the possibility of bone marrow transplant prior to multiple transfusion making the child sensitive to human leukocyte antigens (HLAs), which decreases the successfulness of the transplant.
- Encourage caregiver participation in daily care.
- Support the balanced diet of the child, including meat and meat substitutes.

HEMOPHILIA

- **Hemophilia** pathophysiology: commonly a deficiency of factor VIII, which is produced by the liver and assists with thromboplastin formation in **blood coagulation**
- Both hemophilia A and B are inherited as X-linked recessive traits, which affect males. Females are the carriers and do not have the disease. The clotting factors are present, but in a diminished capacity. The defective factor is unable to do its job in the clotting cascade, so the cascade is halted and the fibrin clot is unable to form.

Assessment

- History of bleeding, nosebleeds, and bruising
- **Hemarthrosis** into the joint cavities of the knees, ankles, elbows

- Hematoma with pain, swelling, and limited motion
- Spontaneous hematuria

Diagnostic Testing

- Partial thromboplastin time (PTT) prolonged, indicating ineffective clotting factors except factor VII (reference value 22.1–34.1 seconds for activated and 60–90 seconds if not activated) (Corbett, 2008).
- Low level of factor VII or IX coagulant
- Spontaneous genetic mutations may occur because some males in the family tree do not have the disease (Corbett, 2008).
- Often no bleeding in first year of life, until child starts to walk and fall; common first injury is oral mucosal membrane bleeding

Nursing Interventions

- Administration of factor VIII concentrate from pooled plasma as prescribed by physician
- Administration of DDAVP (1-deamino-8D-arginine vasopressin), a synthetic form of vasopressin to increase plasma factor VIII in mild cases as prescribed by physician
- Corticosteriods for child with hematuria, hemarthrosis, and synovitis as prescribed by physician
- Nonsteroidal anti-inflammatory drugs (NSAIDs) for relieving pain; may interfere with platelet formation (Lilley et al., 2011)
- Avoid aspirin, which interferes with platelet function.
- Avoid chronic use of demerol or codeine.
- Avoid heat or ice.
- Supportive care with exercise and physical therapy.

Caregiver Education

- Prevent injury in the environment with supervision, helmet use, and activity restrictions. Avoid contact sports. Provide soft toothbrushes and venipuncture in place of fingersticks to decrease bleeding.
- Medical alert tag is important.
- Prophylaxis by administrating periodic factor replacement of factor VIII, including self-administration as child is capable **(Table 19-3)**
- Resources from the National Hemophilia Foundation publications
- Altered family dynamics and impact on financial resources

CLINICAL PEARL

Development of Independent Functioning

A child's recreational activities should include other children for socialization whenever possible. Alternatives should be fun and build self-esteem and positive body image. An adolescent focuses on egocentrism and has a feeling that "nothing will happen to me" and is unable to see consequences of actions. Encourage the adolescent's involvement in care, allowing as much control as possible over aspects of care. Isolation from school, work, and community may cause a loss of independent functioning.

TABLE 19–3 BLOOD TRANSFUSION PRODUCTS

Transfusion Products	Indications	Critical Nursing Actions
RED BLOOD CELLS	Hemoglobin <8 grams in a stable patient with chronic anemia Hypovolemia due to acute blood loss Evidence of impending heart failure secondary to severe anemia Patients on hyper-transfusion regimen for sickle cell disease and history of: Cerebral vascular accident Splenic sequestration Acute chest syndrome Recurrent priapism Preoperative preparation for surgery with general anesthesia Hypoxia Children requiring increased oxygen-carrying capacity (i.e., complex congenital heart, intracardiac shunting, severe pulmonary disease—ARDS): Shock states (decreased BP, increased peripheral vasoconstriction, pallor, cyanosis, diaphoresis,	Observe for clinical signs and symptoms of anemia: • Fatigue • Syncope • Pallor • Tachycardia • Diaphoretic • Shortness of breath • Inability to perform activities of daily living Don appropriate personal protective equipment (PPE) for all blood product transfusions Monitor vital signs per hospital policy and procedure Monitor hemoglobin and hematocrit During blood product infusions, observe for adverse reactions

Continued

TABLE 19–3 BLOOD TRANSFUSION PRODUCTS—cont'd

Transfusion Products	Indications	Critical Nursing Actions
	clamminess, mottled skin, increased oxygen requirement, decreased urinary output) Cardiac failure Respiratory failure requiring significant ventilatory support Postoperative anemia	Blood can be stored only in a designated blood refrigerator Generally 10–15 mL/kg of packed red blood cells are transfused (Khilnani, 2005)
AUTOLOGOUS BLOOD (SELF-DONATED BLOOD PRODUCT)	For general scheduled surgical procedures in which there are clinical indications that a blood transfusion may be necessary during the intraoperative or postoperative period, the patient may elect to self-donate; check with blood bank facilities for time criteria for this type of donation For general surgical procedures, the recommended hemoglobin is 10 grams or greater and for orthopedic surgery the recommendation is hemoglobin of 11.5 or greater	Verify with parents that self-donation has occurred Patient identification and administration process is the same as for all other blood products
WHOLE BLOOD OR PACKED RED BLOOD CELLS (PRBCs) RECONSTITUTED WITH FRESH FROZEN PLASMA (FFP)	Hypovolemia due to acute blood loss nonresponsive to crystalloids Hct <35% Hypovolemia due to acute massive blood loss (i.e., major trauma) History of blood loss at delivery or large amount of blood drawn for lab studies (10% blood volume) Cardiac patients Hct <40% (structural heart disease, cyanosis, or congestive heart failure) Drop in Hgb to below 10 gm intraoperatively Exchange transfusion	Same nursing actions applicable to red blood cell infusions In major trauma situations, patient may be transfused with O-negative blood, the universal donor Use blood warmer and rapid infuser if available
PLATELETS	Platelet count <20,000 Active bleeding with symptoms of DIC or other significant coagulopathies Platelet count <50,000 with planned invasive procedure (i.e., surgical procedure, central line insertion, does not include drawing blood or intramuscular injection of intravenous catheter insertion) Prevention or treatment of bleeding due to thrombocytopenia (secondary to chemotherapy, radiation, or bone marrow failure) Treatment of patients with severe thrombocytopenia secondary to increased platelet destruction or immune thrombocytopenia associated with complication of severe trauma Massive transfusion with platelet dilution	Know normal platelet count (150,000–400,000) Obtain CBC Assess bruising, petechiae, and bleeding
FRESH FROZEN PLASMA (FFP)	Replacement for deficiency of factors II, V, VII, IX, X, XII; protein C or protein S Bleeding, invasive procedure, or surgery with documented plasma clotting protein deficiency (i.e., liver failure, DIC, or septic shock)	Notify blood bank to thaw FFP; product must be used within 6 hours of thawing Don appropriate PPE for all blood product transfusions

TABLE 19–3 BLOOD TRANSFUSION PRODUCTS—cont'd

Transfusion Products	Indications	Critical Nursing Actions
	Prolonged PT and/or PTT without bleeding Significant intraoperative bleeding (10% blood volume/hr) in excess of normally anticipated blood loss that is at high risk of clotting-factor deficiency Massive transfusion Therapeutic plasma exchanges Warfarin anticoagulant overdose	Monitor vital signs per hospital policy and procedure Monitor coagulation studies During FFP infusions, observe for adverse reactions
CRYOPRECIPITATE (CRYO)	Fibrinogen levels below 150 mg/dL with active bleeding Bleeding or prophylaxis in von Willebrand's disease or in factor VIII (hemophilia A) deficiency unresponsive to or unsuitable for DDAVP or factor VII concentrates Replacement therapy, bleeding, or invasive procedure in patients with factor XIII deficiency Patients with active intraoperative hemorrhage in excess of normally anticipated blood loss who are at risk of clotting factor deficiency	Assess for signs and symptoms of bleeding Don appropriate PPE for all blood product transfusions Monitor vital signs per hospital policy and procedure Monitor coagulation studies During cryoprecipitate infusions, observe for adverse reactions
GRANULOCYTES (WHITE BLOOD CELL TRANSFUSION)	Bacterial or fungal sepsis (proven or strongly suspected) unresponsive to antimicrobial therapy Infection (proven or strongly suspected) unresponsive to antimicrobial therapy	Type and crossmatch required for all WBC transfusions Pre-medications may be ordered, such as antihistamines or acetaminophen
FACTOR VII	Treatment of factor VII deficiency Treatment of factor VIII inhibitors Treatment of factor IX inhibitors Idiopathic uncontrolled bleeding	Assess for signs and symptoms of bleeding Don appropriate PPE for all blood products, even recombinant Monitor coagulation studies If undiluted, dilute vial with indicated amount of sterile water and administer intravenously as per manufacturer's guidelines
FACTOR VIII CONCENTRATE	Hemophilia A (factor VIII deficiency) Patients with factor VIII inhibitors Patients with von Willebrand's disease	Assess for signs and symptoms of bleeding Don appropriate PPE for all blood products Monitor coagulation studies Check product to see if refrigeration necessary Record expiration date and lot number of product
FACTOR IX CONCENTRATE (PROTHROMBIN COMPLEX)	Treatment of hemophilia B Hemophilia A with factor VIII inhibitors Patients with congenital deficiency of prothrombin, factor VII, and factor X	Assess for signs and symptoms of bleeding Don appropriate PPE for all blood products Monitor coagulation studies Record expiration date and lot number of product

Continued

TABLE 19–3 BLOOD TRANSFUSION PRODUCTS—cont'd

Transfusion Products	Indications	Critical Nursing Actions
INTRAVENOUS IMMUNOGLOBULIN (IVIG)	Congenital or acquired antibody deficiency Immunological disorders such as idiopathic thrombocytopenia (ITP), Kawasaki disease Posttransplant patients used prophylactically, newborns with severe bacterial infections	Don appropriate PPE for all IVIG infusions Monitor vital signs per hospital policy and procedure Start infusion slowly and increase rate/titrate per physician orders During IVIG infusion, observe for adverse reactions such as fever, chills, and headache Product is obtained from pharmacy Record expiration date and lot number of product

From Ward, S. L., & Hisley, S. M. (2009). *Maternal-child nursing care: Optimizing outcomes for mothers, children, and families* (p. 1093). Philadelphia: F.A. Davis.

LEAD POISONING

- A condition caused by chronic ingestion or inhalation of materials containing lead characterized by physical and mental dysfunction. Children with iron deficiency absorb lead more readily than those with sufficient iron stores.

Assessment

- Inquire about sources of lead: interior and exterior paint, plaster, caulking on playgrounds, soil, foods or liquids, water from leaded pipes, cigarette butts and ashes, colored newsprint, unglazed pottery, painted lead crib rails and window ledges.
- Inhalation sources: sanding and scraping of lead-based pained surfaces, burning of automobile batteries, burning of colored newspaper, automobile exhaust, sniffing leaded gasoline, cigarette smoke, dust (**Figure 19-2**)
- Look for pica, eating of non-food items, during assessment.
- Signs of anemia: abdominal pain, vomiting, constipation, anorexia, headache, fever, lethargy
- Central nervous system signs: hyperactivity, impulsiveness, lethargy, irritability, loss of developmental progress, hearing impairment, learning difficulties

Diagnostic Testing

- Blood lead level (BLL)
- Erythrocyte protoporphyrin (EP) level above 35 mcg/dL (Corbett, 2008)

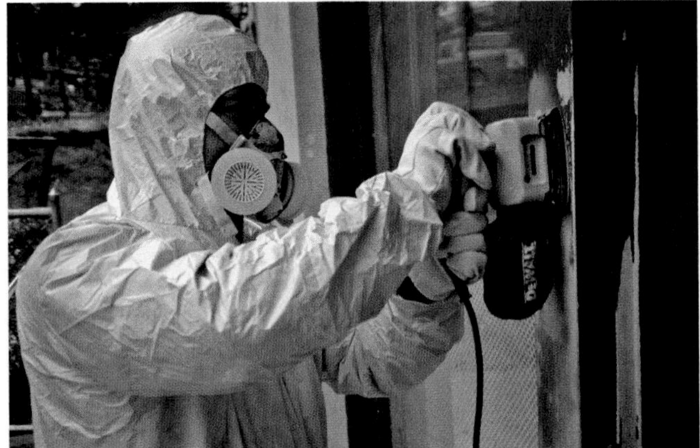

Figure 19–2 Man wearing protective clothing and mask to protect against lead-based paint dust.

- Bone radiography
- Urinalysis
- Hemoglobin and CBC

Nursing Interventions

- Prevent further exposure to lead.
- Chelation therapy with injections of calcium disodium edetate and succimer into a large muscle mass following administration of local anesthetic procaine

Caregiver Education

- Instruct about safety from lead hazards.
- Possible relocation of child until removal of lead

- Speech and child developmental specialist to evaluate child as needed

IMMUNOLOGICAL DISORDERS

ACQUIRED IMMUNODEFICIENCY SYNDROME (AIDS)

- Background includes human immunodeficiency virus (HIV) infection
  - *Transmission from mother to child has been controlled in the United States (Rivera & Steele, 2011).*
  - *Adolescent infection by engaging in high-risk behaviors, including unprotected intercourse, male homosexual intercourse, and intravenous (IV) drug use*
- Pathophysiology with AIDS development from HIV: This retrovirus infects specific T lymphocytes, the CD95+ T cells and monocytes found in blood, semen, vaginal secretions, and breast milk. Acute infection increases the viral load, which decreases slowly in infected children. It has an incubation period of months to years. Hematologic deficiencies including neutropenia increase the risk of complications.

Assessment

- Lymphadenopathy
- Mucocutaneous eruptions
- Failure to thrive and delayed development
- Hepatosplenomegaly
- Oral candidiasis
- Parotitis
- Chronic or recurrent diarrhea

Diagnostic Testing

- HIV enzyme-linked immunosorbent assay (ELISA) and Western blot immunoassay for children 18 months and older
- HIV polymerase chain reaction (PCR) for detection in infants born to HIV-infected mothers because of the presence of maternal antibodies transferred transplacentally; preferred virologic assays include HIV DNA PCR and HIV RNA assays (**Figure 19-3**).
- Virologic diagnostic testing is recommended at birth in infants at high risk of HIV infection (e.g., infants born to HIV-infected mothers who did not receive prenatal care or prenatal antiretroviral therapy)
- In children 18 months or older, HIV antibody assays are ordered.
- Rapid HIV testing may include oral specimen collection.

Nursing Interventions

- Administration of antiretroviral therapy drugs (ART) combination therapy (a strategy analogous to the treatment of infectious diseases) has improved efficacy, minimized toxicity, and delayed drug resistance (**Figure 19-4**).
- Immunization against common childhood illnesses is recommended if exposed to HIV.
- Nutritional management with high-calorie, nutrient-dense foods
- Maintain confidentiality
- Standard precautions followed in providing care
- Prevent and manage opportunistic infections (OPs) of children with severe immune suppressions. OPs include *Pneumocystis jiroveci* pneumonia (PCP) and tuberculosis (TB).

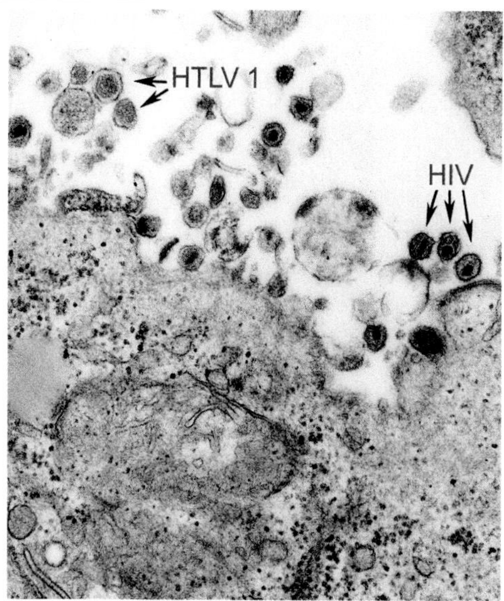

Figure 19-3 HIV cell.

> **Evidence-Based Practice: Medication Adherence with Pediatric AIDS**
>
> Naar-King, S., Montepiedra, G., Nichols, S., Farley, J., Garvie, P. A., Kammerer, B., . . . Storm, D. (2009). Allocation of family responsibility for illness management in pediatric HIV. *Journal of Pediatric Psychology, 34,* 187–194. doi:10.1093/jpepsy/jsn065
>
> In a research study conducted by Naar-King et al. (2009), 123 youth (ages 8–18) completed questionnaires as part of a sub-study of the Pediatric AIDS Clinical Trials Group protocol 219c. Results included approximately one-fourth of children being fully responsible for taking medications. Research supports caregivers' transitioning the medication responsibility to older children, but this transition was not always successful, as evidenced by poor medication adherence.
>
> 1. What age is appropriate for self-management of the multiple administration times of HIV medications?
> 2. What is the caregiver role in supporting youth and providing an environment to be responsible for self-medication?
> 3. What is the role of the nurse in medication teaching to prepare youth to adhere to the plan of care?

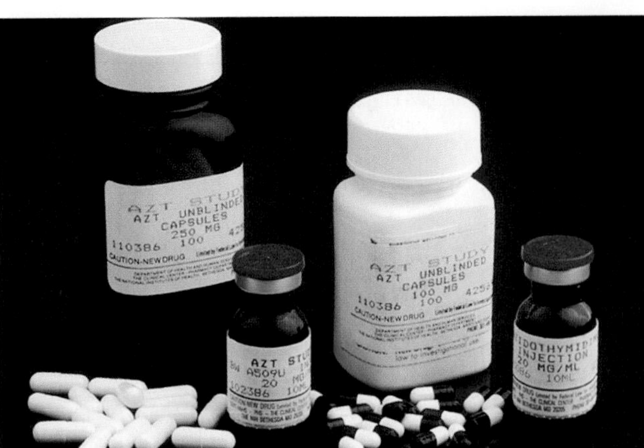

Figure 19–4 AZT is a common antiviral medication.

Caregiver Education

- Teach pain management techniques.
- Tolerance to opioids may indicate increased dosing.
- Encourage use of nonpharmacologic pain interventions.
- Emphasize time of administration of highly active antiviral therapy (ART) and its importance to maintain drug efficacy.
- Support caregivers with complex day-care arrangements or social/family problems.
- Educate day-care and school staff on current HIV information.
- Encourage positive self-concept and avoid the HIV-related stigma.
- Support of the child with a life-threatening illness

ONCOLOGIC DISORDERS

NEOPLASM

- Pathophysiology: uncontrolled abnormal cell growth usually arises from primitive embryonic tissue of the endoderm and ectoderm.
- Idiopathic causes of most cancers
- Chemical carcinogens and drugs
- Radiation exposure
- Viruses
- Genetic and hereditary conditions with oncogenes allow unregulated genetic activity and **tumor** growth (Wilms' tumor)
- Patterns of onset
  - *Infancy/early childhood (neuroblastoma, retinoblastoma) (**Figure 19-5**)*
    - Wilms' tumor of the kidney is discovered by caregivers noticing a lump in the abdominal area while dressing or bathing a child.
  - *Adolescence (Hodgkin's lymphoma, osteosarcoma)*
    - Treatable disease with cure as a realistic goal

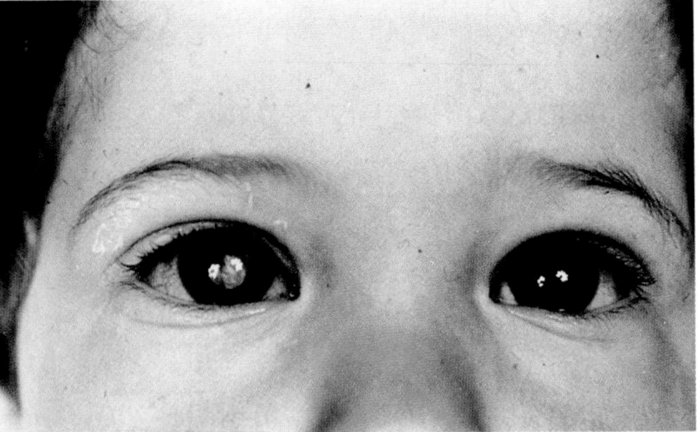

Figure 19–5 Young child with retinoblastoma.

Assessment

- Pain with neoplasm directly or indirectly affecting nerve receptors
- Cachexia with anorexia, weight loss, weakness
- Anemia due to chronic bleeding, iron deficiency, and limited RBCs in bone marrow
- Infection prevention due to an altered immune system
- Bruising from uncontrolled bleeding with decreased platelets
- Hematuria

> **CRITICAL COMPONENT**
>
> **Absolute Neutrophil Count (ANC) and Calculation**
>
> A nursing priority is the high risk of infection for the child with an oncologic disorder. Calculating the ANC requires three numbers from the CBC and differential. The following formula calculates the ANC:
>
> (% Bands + % Segmented cells) × Total WBC count = ANC
>
> Example:
>
> (3% Bands + 50% Segs) × 1500 = 795
>
> When the ANC is less than 500, the client is at high risk for infection.

Diagnostic Testing

- CBC, including absolute neutrophil count (ANC)
- Lumbar puncture (**Figure 19-6**)
- Computed tomography (CT), magnetic resonance imaging (MRI), ultrasound
- Biopsy to determine the type of benign or malignant tumor
- Bone marrow aspiration
- Surgery
- Chemotherapy following protocols based on research findings for type of cancer, staging of disease process, and cell type
- Radiation therapy as specific treatment protocol
- Bone marrow transplantation
- Biologic response modifiers stimulate the body's immune system to destroy cancerous cells.

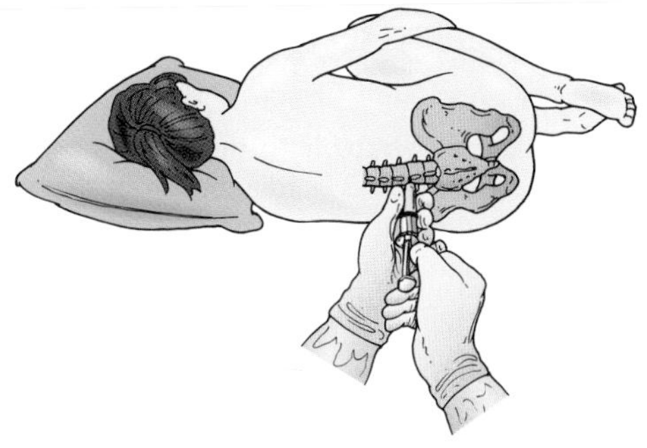

Figure 19-6 Lumbar puncture.

> **Medication**
>
> **Types of Antioncologic Medications**
>
> Classifications of medications include and are not limited to monoclonal antibodies, interleukins, interferon, tumor necrosis factors, and colony-stimulating factors to increase the production of blood cells using filgrastin and erythropoietin.

> **Clinical Reasoning**
>
> **Adolescence and Adherence to Medications**
>
> The 14-year-old male adolescent is receiving medications according to the research protocol in a regional medical center several miles from home. After weeks of hospitalization, the adolescent is experiencing the complications of fatigue and social isolation. Family members describe how the present changes of the body, progression to a new school building, and an additional group of friends have influenced his behavior. Goals agreed upon with the adolescent are to maximize immune function and maintain normal development.
>
> 1. What priority nursing assessment information does the nurse identify?
> 2. What nursing interventions would support the nursing goals?
> 3. When the adolescent develops boredom with the initial nursing interventions, what other activities are suggested?
> 4. How will the nurse evaluate these goals?

Nursing Interventions

- Management of pain
- Pharmacological management
- Nonpharmacological methods to decrease anxiety
- Administration of medications to prevent nausea and vomiting
- Hydration with IV fluid and replacement according to emesis loss
- Nutrition
- Prevent infection in peripheral intravenous central catheter (PICC) or implanted central venous access port (**Figure 19-7A and B**)

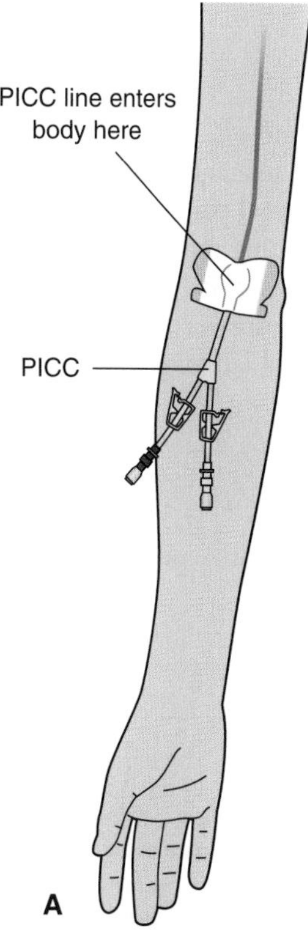

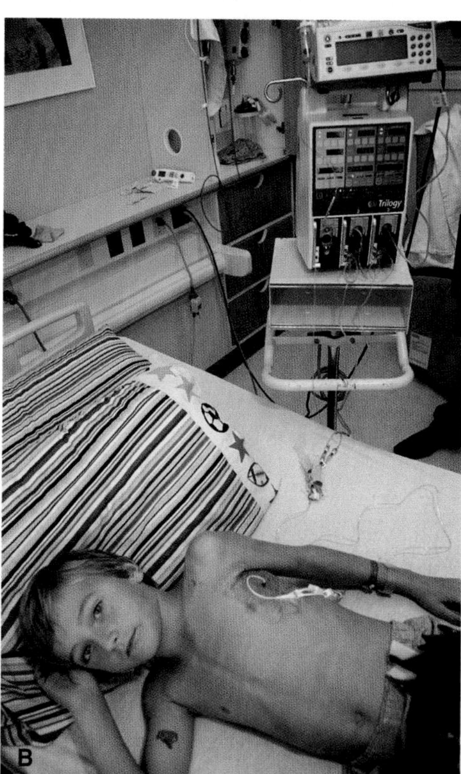

Figure 19-7 Peripheral intravenous central catheters in children.

- Provide knowledge and decrease fear of cancer relapse.
- Appropriate age and developmental stage nursing care for hospitalized child
- Listen, debrief, and offer support for daily care.
- Pharmacological management of pain
- Nonpharmacological pain management includes role-play with the child "acting out" the procedure on dolls; adolescents can observe a visual demonstration, video, or computer simulation. Answer questions as age appropriate and clarify medical language unfamiliar to caregivers.

Evidence-Based Practice: Accessing Central Line (CL) Catheters

Centers for Disease Control and Prevention. (2011). *Basic infection control and prevention plan for outpatient oncology settings.* Retrieved from http://www.cdc.gov/HAI/settings/outpatient/basic-infection-control-prevention-plan-2011/central-venous-catheters.html

- Maintain aseptic technique.
- Perform hand hygiene and assemble the necessary equipment.
- Wear clean gloves.
- Scrub the injection cap (e.g., needleless connector) with an appropriate antiseptic (e.g., chlorhexidine, povidone iodine, or 70% alcohol), and allow to dry (if povidone iodine is used, it should dry for at least 2 minutes).
- Access the injection cap with the syringe or IV tubing (opening the clamp, if necessary).
- Perform hand hygiene when done.
- Follow manufacturer instructions and labeled use for specific care and maintenance of the site, dressing, access, flushing, blood draws, and de-access of the CL.

- **Oncology** emergencies
- Tumor lysis syndrome: destruction of tumor cells releases uric acid, potassium, phosphates, calcium
- Septic shock from overwhelming infection
- Hyperleukocytosis is the infiltration of brain and lung tissue with blast cells.
- Increased intracranial pressure due to space-occupying lesions in brain

Caregiver Education

- Support a sense of control for child, family, and others.
- Encourage support system and coping with uncertainty of future.
- Potential loss of future of the child and future generations, including grieving the loss of their dreams and aspirations for the child (see Chapter 5)
- Grief and sadness may fade as hope grows.
- Hope gives strength to endure treatments and renewed appreciation for life.
- Identify financial support as needed.

Side Effects of Radiation Therapy

Caregivers should be made aware of the various possible side effects of radiation therapy, as follows:

- **Integumentary system**: skin erythema, ulceration, alopecia

CRITICAL COMPONENT

Radiation Types and Side Effects

The goal of radiation therapy is to target tumor destruction and spare surrounding tissues. Radiation is not dependent on cell cycle for maximum cell death. The principles of radiation exposure include duration of time of exposure and distance from the radiation to minimize exposure.

Types of Radiation Therapy

1. Conventional focal radiation is standard with a targeted tumor volume with a margin of 1–3 cm.
2. Three dimensional (3-D) conformal radiotherapy delivers a high dose of radiation while maintaining a tight margin to deliver only a low dose of radiation to the surrounding non-targeted tissues.
3. Hyperfractionated radiation therapy delivers two radiation treatments per day to treat aggressive, fast-growing tumors
4. Intraoperative radiotherapy (IORT) delivers radiation to the tumor bed during surgery.
5. Brachytherapy is the implantation of radioactive sources directly into the tumor bed under CT guidance.
6. Photon beam radiation is less likely to cause late effects of radiation because tissues are spared.

- **Nervous system**: learning disabilities, attention difficulties, headache, edema
- **Ophthalmologic:** dry eyes, cataracts, retinopathy, sclera melting
- **Cardiac:** pericarditis, valve dysfunction, cardiomyopathy
- **Pulmonary:** radiation pneumonitis, fibrosis
- **Gastrointestinal:** mucositis, esophagitis, nausea, vomiting, diarrhea, abdominal cramping, rectal ulceration, proctitis, anorexia, dysphagia, obstruction of small bowel
- **Genitourinary:** radiation nephritis, radiation cystitis, amenorrhea, decrease in sperm production, sterility
- **Hematologic:** myelosuppression
- **Skeletal:** slow bone growth at epiphyseal plates, growth arrest with high doses
- **Miscellaneous:** lethargy, headache, increased need for sleep, fatigue

LEUKEMIA

Leukemia pathophysiology: a group of malignant diseases of the bone marrow and lymphatic system. White blood cell (WBC) overproduction occurs, although the count is actually low. Immature cells do not deliberately attack and destroy normal cells but are in competition for metabolic elements.

- Possible viral origin
- Possible irradiation from prior x-rays or exposure to chemicals
- Risk factors for developing acute lymphoblastic leukemia and acute myeloid leukemia (AML) include Down syndrome and other genetic conditions (National

Cancer Institute at the National Institute of Health, 2011).

- A common form of childhood cancer, with dramatic improvements in survival rates (**Table 19-4**)

Assessment

- Anemia with weakness, fatigue, pallor, dyspnea, cardiac dilation, and anorexia
- Cough, wheezing, tracheal/bronchial compression, respiratory distress/arrest related to mediastinal mass and compression of great vessels
- Neutropenia with infection of skin and lungs, fever, decreased wound healing
- Thrombocytopenia (low platelet count) with bruises, petechiae, purpura, large ecchymosis, epistaxis, gums and sclera hemorrhages
- Hematuria and melena occasionally
- Bone and joint pain due to infarction, bone destruction, and pressure caused by hyperplastic neoplastic tissue in medullary spaces; gait problems
- Liver and enlarged spleen with pain, gastrointestinal (GI) symptoms, urinary symptoms
- Enlarged lymph nodes greater than 1 centimeter and firm but not painful in regional areas, elbow, and supraclavicular nodes
- Necrotic, ulcerative rectal lesions
- Painless testicular enlargement
- Central nervous system signs: nausea, vomiting, lethargy, morning headache, irritability, convulsions, cranial nerve palsies, papilledema, pain upon neck flexion, hyperphagia, blindness, decreased coordination, growth deceleration, and precocious puberty

Diagnostic Testing

- Bone marrow test for a positive diagnosis of abnormal cells
- CBC screen for abnormal cells
- Low reticulocyte count
- Thrombocytopenia with platelet count less than 40,000/mm^3 (reference values 150,000–450,000/mm^3) (Corbett, 2008)
- WBC with differential
- Lumbar puncture to determine central nervous system (CNS) infiltration and increased pressure, leukemia cells, blast cells, negative cultures, increased protein, decreased sugar
- CT, MRI

Nursing Interventions

- Blood transfusion
- Chemotherapy to suppress production of abnormal cells
- Prevention of infection
- See **Table 19-5** for information on two common childhood cancers and the nursing care for each.

Clinical Reasoning

Discussion on Disease Diagnosis Between Nurse and Child

A child asks to speak to you about the current diagnosis of leukemia. The caregiver has momentarily left the room and the nurse is alone with the child. The child asks the nurse if she is going to die.

1. How would you respond to this patient?
2. Is your response age appropriate?
3. Will you give an honest answer?

Caregiver Education

- Teach hand hygiene.
- Protect from all sources of infection.
- Avoid plants to prevent exposure to fungus.

TABLE 19–4 TYPES OF LEUKEMIA (ACUTE AND CHRONIC)

Type of leukemia	Possible Cause	Symptoms	Treatment
Acute lymphocytic (ALL)	Chromosome problems, radiation, chemotherapy	Bone and joint pain, bruising, bleeding, fatigue, swollen glands, weight loss	Chemotherapy, transfusion of blood products, antibiotics, bone marrow transplant
Acute myeloblastic (AML)	Certain chemicals, chemotherapy drugs, radiation	Bleeding from nose and/or gums, fever, shortness of breath, skin rash	Antibiotics, bone marrow transplant, blood and platelet transfusion
Chronic myeloblastic (CML)	Philadelphia chromosome abnormality, radiation exposure	Fever without infection, bone pain, swollen spleen with pain, night sweats, fatigue, rash	Imatinib (Gleevec) oral pill associated with remission, bone marrow transplant
Chronic lymphocytic (CLL)	Cause unknown, common in adults age 70 and older	Bruising, enlarged lymph nodes, night sweats, fatigue, fever, infections that recur, weight loss	In early stages, no treatment; later stages, chemotherapy, radiation, bone marrow transplants

Adapted from Penn State Hershey (2011).

TABLE 19–5 TWO COMMON CHILDHOOD CANCERS AND THEIR NURSING CARE

Type of Cancer	Medical Treatment	Basic Nursing Care of the Child
ALL	Remission reduction post-induction with one of the following: Consolidation/intensification OR maintenance/continuation therapy	Prevent infection, including hand hygiene and reduction of environmental molds and organisms from plants and fresh fruits Prevent bleeding from mouth with use of a soft toothbrush, offer mouth care, and provide a safe environment
AML	Induction to attain remission with combination chemotherapy OR Post-remission consolidation/intensification	Use of personal protective equipment to reduce child exposure to infection Promote nutrition and monitor elimination patterns

LYMPHOMAS

- Pathophysiology: a group of neoplastic diseases divided into **Hodgkin's lymphoma** and **non-Hodgkin's lymphoma** (**Table 19-6**)
- Hodgkin's disease involves the lymph nodes with Reed-Sternberg cells
- Non-Hodgkin's lymphoma with 3 types (**Figure 19-8**)
- Mature B cell identified as Burkitt lymphoma
- Lymphoblastic lymphoma of precursor T cell and precursor B cell
- Anaplastic large-cell lymphoma
- **Metastasis** to spleen, liver, bone marrow, and lungs
- Staging system assigns a stage based on number of lymph nodes, presence of extranodal disease, history of any symptom

Assessment

- Enlarged cervical or supraclavicular lymphadenopathy
- Fever, weight loss, night sweats, cough, abdominal discomfort, anorexia, nausea, pruritus

Diagnostic Testing

See **Table 19-7** for the different diagnostic tests for lymphomas.

- CBC
- Erythrocyte sedimentation rate (ESR)
- Serum copper, ferritin level, fibrinogen, immunoglobulins, uric acid, liver function test, T-cell function studies, urinalysis
- CT scans of neck, chest, abdomen, pelvis, gallium
- Scan to identify metastatic or recurrent disease

TABLE 19–6 DIAGNOSTIC TESTS FOR HEMATOLOGIC, IMMUNOLOGIC, AND ONCOLOGIC DISORDERS

Test	Preparation	Time to Complete	Data Given	Risks Involved
Complete blood count	EMLA cream on skin surface to anesthetize Visual imagery	Time varies from time of collection from peripheral or central venous catheter Lab reports may be ordered STAT	Differential for rapid treatment of antibiotics or need for further diagnostic tests	Low due to blood loss and prevention of infection
Tissue sample biopsy	Pre-procedure informed consent and patient safety precautions per agency protocol	Surgical asepsis of patient prior to physician intervention Duration of 1–4 hours in post-anesthesia area	Type of cancer and staging of disease to determine treatment protocol	Moderate due to risk of infection and risk of cancer cell dissemination
Bone marrow aspiration	Informed consent prior to procedure and note lab values at risk for patient bleeding	Patient preparation for procedure	Removal of bone marrow demonstrates initial disease and progression of treatment protocol	Low due to care of needle insertion and prevention of bleeding

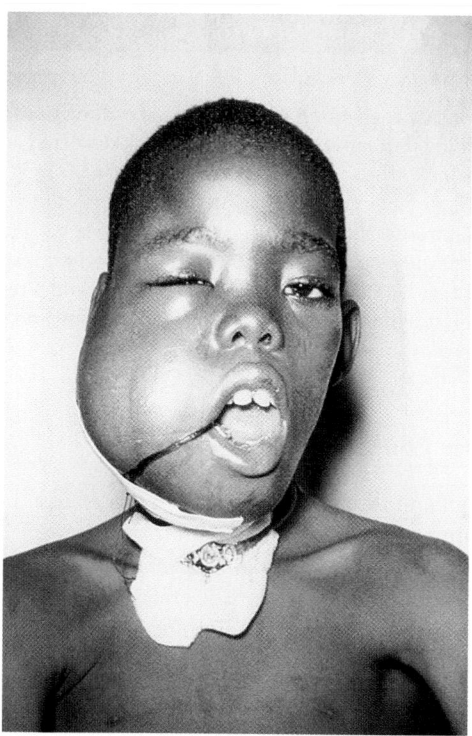

Figure 19–8 Child with non-Hodgkin's lymphoma.

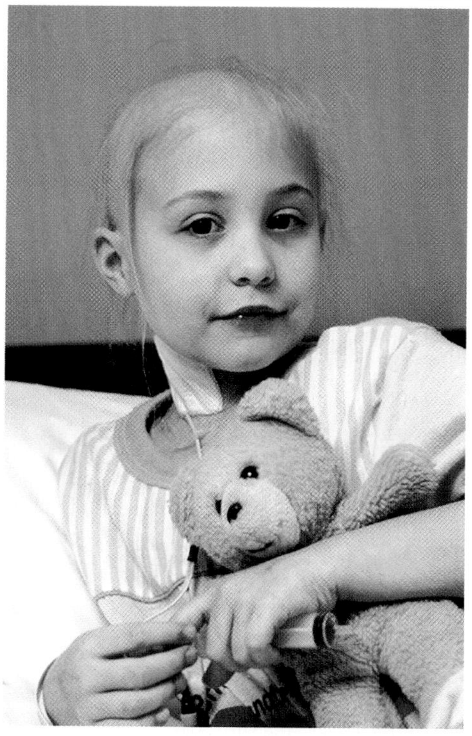

Figure 19–9 Girl with cancer using a syringe during medical play.

- Chest x-ray
- Bone scan if needed to identify metastatic disease

Nursing Interventions

- Administer chemotherapy.
- Prepare child for radiation and decrease activity intolerance.
- Allow for medical play when age appropriate (**Figure 19-9**).
- Administer pneumococcal and meningococcal immunizations.
- Prevent infection using Standard Precautions and isolation as required (**Figure 19-10**).

Medication

Special Considerations in Chemotherapy and Biotherapy Administration

- The priority is to assess child and caregiver understanding of the disease and treatment.
- Anticipate need for anti-emetic medication.
- Provide child and family safety.
- Intervene with education and support.
- Assess, collect data, document treatment, and evaluate outcomes.
- Prompt identification of adverse effects of medication is critical. (Andam & Silva 2008)

TABLE 19–7 CHARACTERISTICS OF HODGKIN'S AND NON-HODGKIN'S LYMPHOMA

	Pathophysiology	Staging	Nursing Assessment	Nursing Interventions
HODGKIN'S	Reed-Sternberg cells Metastasis (spleen, liver, lungs)	Stages I–IV	Enlarged cervical or supraclavicular nodes	Administer chemotherapy Monitor for effects of irradiation
NON-HODGKIN'S	Group of malignancies of lymphoid cells Undifferentiated or poorly differentiated cells, mediastinal and meninges involved Waldeyer's ring has lymphoid tissue encircling the tonsils	Revised European-American lymphoma system	Enlargement of lymph nodes causes airway and intestinal obstruction, cranial nerve palsies, spinal paralysis	Administer chemotherapy and prepare child for radiation Prevent infection

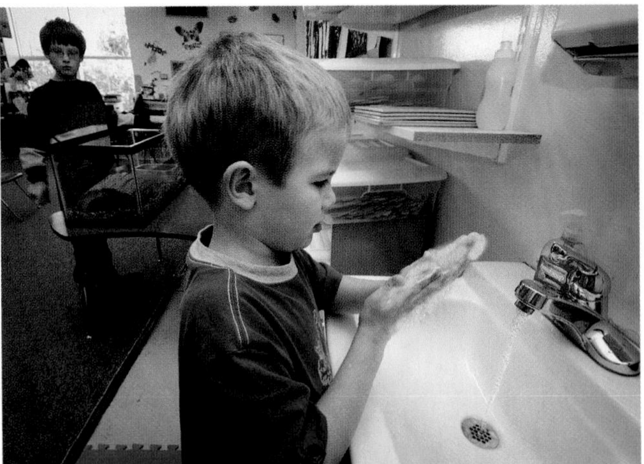

Figure 19–10 Encourage good hand hygiene to prevent infection.

Caregiver Education

- Activity level to provide for rest
- High risk of sterilization; sperm banking possible

NON-HODGKIN'S LYMPHOMA

- Pathophysiology: a group of malignant tumors involving lymphoid tissue
- Non-Hodgkin's in children more frequent than Hodgkin's
- Diffuse disease rather than nodular
- Cell type is either undifferentiated or poorly differentiated.
- Dissemination occurs early, more often, and rapidly.
- Mediastinal involvement and invasion of meninges are common.

Assessment

- Monitor for symptoms related to pressure for enlargement of adjacent lymph nodes, including airway obstruction, intestinal instruction, cranial nerve palsies, and spinal paralysis.

Diagnostic Testing

- Surgical biopsy of an enlarged node
- Confirmation of disease by histopathology
- Bone marrow examination
- CT scans of the lungs and GI organs
- Lumbar puncture

Nursing Intervention

- Monitor for effects of irradiation and chemotherapy.

> **CRITICAL COMPONENT**
>
> **Chemotherapy Precautions**
>
> - Assure that the written policies and procedures are followed regarding protective equipment required, restricted access to hazardous drug spills, and posted signs.
> - Cleanup of a large spill is handled by workers trained in handling hazardous materials.
> - Locate spill kits in the immediate area where exposures may occur. (Centers for Disease Control and Prevention and National Institute for Occupational Safety and Health, 2004)

Caregiver Education

- Teach about disease, and explain all procedures.
- Explain expected side effects and toxicities.
- Drug reactions may be complications of treatment.
- Describe what to do when side effects occur.
- Encourage discussion of feelings regarding disease.

HEMATOPOIETIC STEM CELL TRANSPLANTATION (HSCT)

- Conditions considered for HSCT are aplastic anemia, malignant disorders, nonmalignant hematologic disorders (sickle cell anemia), and immunodeficiency disorders.
- A lethal dose of chemotherapy is administered to kill the cancer and suppress bone marrow production.
- The body is resupplied with stem cells (autologous, allogeneic, umbilical cord blood).
- Disease-free marrow replaces cancerous marrow.
- Peripheral stem cell transplant (PSCT): autologous collection of stem cells with an apheresis machine; frozen until needed

Assessment

- Malignancy is life threatening, and family are supported in the decision to agree to HSCT.
- Prepare child for isolation to undergo intensive ablative therapy.

Diagnostic Testing

- Human leukocyte antigen (HLA) system complex matching is completed to prevent graft versus host disease (GVHD).
  - *GVHD is incompatibility of the donor bone marrow with the intended recipient related to the immunologic response of the recipient.*
  - *Histocompatibility testing for allogeneic transplantation decreases risk for rejection.*
  - *The most common complication of a transplant is when the donor is mismatched with two to three antigens using HLA tissue matching.*

- *Signs and symptoms of acute GVHD occur 7 to 30 days following transplant and affect the gut, liver, lungs, and skin.*
- *Signs and symptoms of chronic GVHD occur about 100 days after transplant and affect the liver, GI system, oral mucosa, and lungs. The skin has scleroderma-like skin and the oral mucosa is abnormally dry.*
- *Therapy for GVHD is high doses of methylprednisolone, antithymocyte globulin, antilymphocyte globulin, cyclosporine, and anti-T-cell immunotoxins as ordered by the physician.*

Nursing Interventions

- Administer high-dose chemotherapy with or without total body irradiation to suppress rejection of the transplanted marrow.
- IV transfusion of stem cells harvested from bone marrow, peripheral blood, or umbilical vein of the placenta
- Strict asepsis with central venous catheter care
- Monitor intake and output of fluids.
- Monitor nutritional intake.

Caregiver Education

- Inform caregivers about medications and the use of nonpharmacologic techniques.
- Teach the procedure for care of the venous access device.
- Caregiver should continue to participate in the child's care as much as possible to empower the caregiver and maintain a sense of control.
- Encourage siblings to be involved by bringing toys or food items.
- Normalization of caregiver processes

BRAIN TUMORS

- Pathophysiology: a tumor that arises from any cell within the cranium; its origin identifies the classification
- Neuroblastoma is the most common and originates from embryonic neural crest cells.
- Neuroblastoma is discovered after metastasis occurs in 70% of the cases with tumors in the head, neck, chest, or pelvis.

Assessment

- Increased head size in infants is a sign of increased intracranial pressure (ICP).
- Headache on awakening
- Vomiting is a sign of ICP.
- Monitor pulse pressure (difference between systolic and diastolic pressure).
- Pupils sluggish, dilated, or unequal and weak hand grasp

Diagnostic Testing

- MRI to determine extent of tumor and location
- CT, angiography, electroencephalography
- Lumbar puncture without increased ICP to prevent herniation
- Brain tissue removal during surgery to diagnose tumor type
- Single photon emission tomography (SPECT) scan to differentiate between brain cells, tumor cells, and scars
- Positron emission tomography (PET) scans used to study the biochemical and physiologic effects of tumor

CRITICAL COMPONENT

Preparing Children Before Diagnostic Testing

- The upcoming test/surgery details should be explained to the child by the nurse and/or the child life specialist.
- Consider the developmental level of the child.
- Use words that the child can understand.
- State what the child will hear, see, feel, touch, and smell.
- Tell child it is okay to cry.
- Give the child any equipment or pictures of equipment to play with prior to the procedure.
- Tell the child what can be done to encourage cooperation during the procedure.
- Distract with songs, listening to music, counting aloud.
- Explain how caregiver will be present before, during, and after the procedure. Anesthesia may put the child to sleep with a mask or intravenous medication. Medication will be given for any pain, including headache, as needed.
- State the positive aftercare for the child following the procedure.
- Provide a special box of toys to have a treat to look forward to after the procedure.

Nursing Interventions

- Care of child during radiotherapy to shrink tumor
- Assess postsurgical wound, including estimate of dressing drainage.
- Chemotherapy administration according to protocol
- Assess mouth for soreness and open areas of stomatitis.
- Monitor for seizures and changes in posturing.
- Monitor temperature increases, pulse, respirations, blood pressure, and visual disturbances.
- Monitor blood pressure and pulse pressure, which is the difference between systolic and diastolic pressures, and report variations immediately.
- Assess pupil equality, size, reactivity, accommodation, reaction to light, extraocular eye movements, and cranial nerve function.
- Monitor level of consciousness and sleep patterns.
- Monitor movement of all extremities, gag reflex, and blink or swallowing reflex.

- Elevate head of bed 30 degrees in a supratentorial craniotomy; avoid Trendelenburg position due to increases in ICP.
- Align the body with pillows so neck and head are in midline.
- With infratentorial craniotomy, give fluids with return of gag and swallowing reflex.
- Prevent vomiting to prevent aspiration and increased ICP.
- Monitor intravenous fluid to prevent cerebral edema and increased ICP.
- Pain management

CRITICAL COMPONENT

Nursing Interventions for Promoting Nutrition and Hydration in Children with Cancer

- Frequently offer any tolerated food and drink.
- Allow child to be involved in food and drink selection.
- Families can bring favorite foods from home or foods with appealing packaging.
- Culture-specific foods commonly served at home may comfort child.
- Fortify food with nutritious supplements, including liquids.
- Monitor child's weight.

Caregiver Education

- Encourage discussion of feelings of guilt caused by parents ignoring initial complaints.
- Explain plan of care and survival rates (**Table 19-8**).
- Encourage emotional support of the child with a life-threatening illness (**Figure 19-11**).

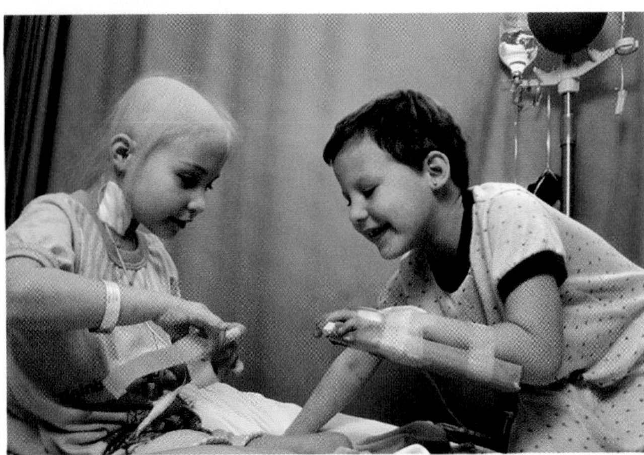

Figure 19–11 Children with cancer playing in the hospital.

TABLE 19–8 COMMON CHILDHOOD CANCERS AND SURVIVAL RATES

Common Childhood Cancers and Usual Age at Diagnosis	Common Percentage of Occurrence	Five-Year Survival Rates (1999–2005)
Leukemia	31%	82%
Brain cancer and other nervous system cancers	21%	71%
Neuroblastoma, <1 year of age	7%	74%
Wilms' tumor, 3 to 6 years of age	5%	88%
Lymphoma		
Hodgkin's cancer, ages 15–40	4%	94%
Non-Hodgkin's	4%	86%
Soft tissue sarcoma		
Rhabdomyosarcoma	3%	66%
Eye cancer, <4 years of age	3%	74%
Bone cancer		
Osteosarcoma	3%	69%
Ewing sarcoma	2%	

From American Cancer Society, http://www.cancer.org/.

Review Questions

1. What is the most frequently reported initial concern of the caregiver for a child with a Wilms' tumor?
   A. Dyspnea during playtime
   B. Abdominal mass noticed during removing of clothes
   C. Hematuria after a fall
   D. Frothy urine in the morning
2. In a child with leukemia, how can the nausea and vomiting associated with chemotherapy be minimized?
   A. Give the drug immediately after meals.
   B. Instruct the child to take shallow, deep breaths.
   C. Limit the child's intake to clear liquids.
   D. Provide music as a distraction.
   E. Administer an antiemetic before the onset of symptoms.
3. Children at high risk for iron deficiency anemia include
   A. vegetarians who eat large amount of raisins, nuts, and legumes.
   B. toddlers who eat few solids and drink large amounts of milk.
   C. school-age children who eat poultry but no beef.
   D. adolescents who refuse to eat vegetables.
   E. infants who eat rice cereal.
4. In preparing a 4-year-old child for diagnostic testing, which of the following would be appropriate for participation in medical play?
   A. Listening to a book read aloud
   B. Telling exaggerated stories
   C. Following directional commands in a song
   D. Thinking about future events
5. The nurse has received laboratory results for clients on the hematology unit. Which client would warrant intervention by the nurse?
   A. The client whose platelet count is 50,000 mm
   B. The client whose WBC count is 16,000/mm3
   C. The client whose serum ferritin is 200 ng/mL
   D. The client whose erythropoietin assay is 20 m/U/mL
6. Which of the following is a condition in which the normal hemoglobin is partially or completely replaced by abnormal hemoglobin?
   A. Sickle cell anemia
   B. Leukemia
   C. Aplastic anemia
   D. Iron deficiency anemia
7. When performing care to prevent infection during hospitalization for cancer treatments, what is most important for the nurse to consider?
   A. Ask the caregivers to bring familiar environmental items from home, including plants.
   B. Perform hand hygiene at the time of contamination, not during client assessment.
   C. Don mask and gown when the child has an elevated absolute neutrophil count.
   D. Follow aseptic techniques when drawing blood.
8. The nurse is talking to an adolescent who is concerned about hair loss secondary to radiation for non-Hodgkin's lymphoma. What is the most appropriate response to the adolescent?
   A. "Your hair will grow back in 12 months."
   B. "You have nice hair. Why are you asking this question?"
   C. "What do you know about the effects of radiation and your hair growing back?"
   D. "Other children have worn hats during the time of hair loss."
9. A child with sickle cell anemia comes to the emergency department with a complaint of joint pain after playing games at school. What is the priority nursing intervention?
   A. Assess behavioral concerns related to chronic illness.
   B. Administer analgesics for the pain.
   C. Check the pulse oximeter reading.
   D. Administer intravenous therapy.
10. An infant is hospitalized with a diagnosis of HIV and dehydration. A nurse determines understanding by the caregiver when the caregiver states which of the following?
    A. "I should put on a mask, gown, and gloves when I enter the room."
    B. "I should put on gloves when I am holding the baby."
    C. "I should keep the baby in the room unless instructed otherwise."
    D. "I should keep the door to the baby's room closed most of the time."
    E. "I should perform hand hygiene each time I change the baby's diaper."

References

American Academy of Pediatrics. (n.d.). *Bright future medical screening reference table 12 month*. Retrieved from http://brightfutures.aap.org/pdfs/Visit%20Forms%20by%20Age%20110/12%20Month/B.ECh.MST.12month.pdf

Andam, R., & Silva, M. (2008). A journey to pediatric chemotherapy competence. *Journal of Pediatric Nursing, 23*, 257–268. doi: 10.1016/j.pedn.2006.12.005

Baker, R. D., & Greer, F. R. (2010). Clinical report diagnosis and prevention of iron deficiency and iron-deficiency anemia in infants and young children (0–3 years of age). *Pediatrics, 126*, 1040–1050. doi:10.1542/peds.2010-2576.

Centers for Disease Control and Prevention. (2011). *Basic infection control and prevention plan for outpatient oncology settings*. Retrieved from http://www.cdc.gov/HAI/settings/outpatient/basic-infection-control-prevention-plan-2011/central-venous-catheters.html

Centers for Disease Control and Prevention and National Institute for Occupational Safety and Health. (2004). *Preventing occupational exposure to Antineoplastic and other hazardous drugs in health care settings* (Publication No. 2004-165). Retrieved from http://www.cdc.gov/niosh/docs/2004-165/2004-165b.html

Corbett, J. (2008). *Laboratory tests and diagnostic procedures with nursing diagnoses* (7th ed.). Upper Saddle River, NJ: Pearson Prentice Hall.

Lilley, L. L., Harrington, S., & Snyder, J. S. (2011). *Pharmacology and the nursing process* (6th ed.). St. Louis, MO: Mosby Elsevier.

Naar-King, S., Montepiedra, G., Nichols, S., Farley, J., Garvie, P. A., Kammerer, B., . . . Storm, D. (2009). Allocation of family responsibility for illness management in pediatric HIV. *Journal of Pediatric Psychology, 34*, 187–194. doi:10.1093/jpepsy/jsn065

National Cancer Institute at the National Institute of Health. (2011). *Childhood acute myeloid leukemia/other myeloid malignancies treatment (PDQ) health professional version*. Retrieved from http://www.cancer.gov/cancertopics/pdq/treatment/childAML/HealthProfessional/page1

Penn State Hershey. (2011). *Chronic lymphocytic leukemia (CLL)*. Retrieved from http://pennstatehershey.adam.com/content.aspx?productId=117&pid=1&gid=000532

Rivera, D. M., & Steele, R. W. (2011). *Pediatric HIV infection*. Retrieved from http://emedicine.medscape.com/article/965086-overview

Additional Resources

American Academy of Pediatrics. (n.d.). *Bright future medical screening reference table 12 month*. Retrieved from http://brightfutures.aap.org/pdfs/Visit%20Forms%20by%20Age%20110/12%20Month/B.ECh.MST.12month.pdf

American Cancer Society. (2011). *Cancer facts and figures*. Retrieved from http://www.cancer.org/Research/CancerFactsFigures/index

Andam, R., & Silva, M. (2008). A journey to pediatric chemotherapy competence. *Journal of Pediatric Nursing, 23*(4), 257–268.

Aukema, E., Last, B., Schouten-van Meeteren, A., & Grootenhuis, M. (2011). Explorative study on the aftercare of pediatric brain tumor survivors: A parents' perspective. *Supportive Care in Cancer, 19*, 1637–1646. doi:10.1007/s00520-010-0995-6

Baker, R. D., & Greer, F. R. (2010) Clinical report diagnosis and prevention of iron deficiency and iron-deficiency anemia in infant and young children (0–3 years of age). *Pediatrics, 126*(5), 1040–1050. doi:10.1542/peds.2010-2576. Retrieved from http://aappolicy.aappublications.org/cgi/content/full/pediatrics;126/5/1040

Bernstein, M. L. (2011). Targeted therapy in pediatric and adolescent oncology. *Cancer, 117*, 2268–2274. doi:10.1002/cncr.26050

Berry, J. G., Bloom, S., Foley, S., & Palfrey, J. S. (2010). Health inequity in children and youth with chronic health conditions. *Pediatrics, 126*, S111–S119. doi:10.1542/peds.2010-1466D

Burnette, M. (2009). Providing culturally competent sickle cell care. *Minority Nurse*, 28–31. Retrieved from http://www.minoritynurse.com/Providing-Culturally-Competent-Sickle-Cell-Care

Cantrell, M. A. (2007). The art of pediatric oncology nursing practice. *Journal of Pediatric Oncology Nursing, 24*, 132–138. doi: 10.1177/1043454206298842

Caudill, S., Goldman, T., & Marconi, K. (2003). Evaluation of pediatric HIV care provided in Ryan White CARE Act Title IV women, infants, children, and youth clinics. *AIDS Patient Care & STDs, 17*, 65–73. doi: 10.1089/108729103321150791

Centers for Disease Control and Prevention. (2011). *Basic infection control and prevention plan for outpatient oncology settings*. Retrieved from http://www.cdc.gov/HAI/settings/outpatient/basic-infection-control-prevention-plan-2011/central-venous-catheters.html.

Centers for Disease Control and Prevention and National Institute for Occupational Safety and Health. (2004). *Preventing occupational exposure to antineoplastic and other hazardous drugs in health care settings*. Publication # 2004-165. Retrieved from http://www.cdc.gov/niosh/docs/2004-165/2004-165b.html

Chandran, L., & Cataldo, R. (2010). Lead poisoning: Basics and new developments. *Pediatrics in Review, 31*, 399–406. doi:10.1542/pir.31-10-399

Cherry, L. (2011). Nutrition assessment of the pediatric oncology patient. *Oncology Nutrition Connection, 19*, 4–12. Retrieved from http://www.oncologynutrition.org/member-benefits/newsletters

Cleveland, L. M., Minter, M. L., Cobb, K. A., Scott, A. A., & German, V. F. (2008). Lead hazards for pregnant women and children: Part 1. *American Journal of Nursing, 108*, 40–50. doi: 10.1097/01.NAJ.0000337736.76730.66

Corbett, J. (2008). *Laboratory tests and diagnostic procedures with nursing diagnoses* (7th ed.). Upper Saddle River, New Jersey: Pearson Prentice Hall.

Freed, J., & Kelly, K. M. (2010). Current approaches to the management of pediatric Hodgkin lymphoma. *Pediatric Drugs, 12*, 85–98. doi: 10.2165/11316170-000000000-00000

Garfunkel, L. C., & Tanski, S. (YEAR). *Immunizations, newborn screening, and capillary blood tests*. Retrieved from http://brightfutures.aap.org/continuing_education.html

Janes-Hodder, H., & Keene, N. (2002). *Childhood cancer: A parent's guide to solid tumor cancers* (2nd ed.). Sebastopol, CA: O'Reilly Media, Inc.

Khan, D., & Lin E. (2011). *Lead poisoning imaging*. Retrieved from http://emedicine.medscape.com/article/410113-overview

Ladas, E. J., Sacks, N., Brophy, P., & Rogers, P. C. (2006). Standards of nutritional care in pediatric oncology: Results from a nationwide survey on the standards of practice in pediatric oncology. A children's oncology group study. *Pediatric Blood & Cancer, 46*, 339–344. doi: 10.1002/pbc.20435

Lallemant, M., Chang, S., Cohen, R., & Pecoul, B. (2011). Pediatric HIV—a neglected disease? *New England Journal of Medicine, 365*, 581–583. doi: 10.1056/NEJMp1107275

Landier, W., & Tse, A. M. (2010). Use of complementary and alternative medical interventions for the management of procedure-related pain, anxiety, and distress in pediatric oncology: An integrative review. *Journal of Pediatric Nursing, 25*, 566–579. doi: 10.1016/j.pedn.2010.01.009

Lilley, L. L., Harrington, S., & Snyder, J. S. (2011). *Pharmacology and the nursing process* (6th ed.). St. Louis: Mosby Elsevier.

MacKay, L., Jerusha, & Gregory, D. (2011). Exploring family-centered care among pediatric oncology nurses. *Journal of Pediatric Oncology Nursing, 28*, 43–52. doi: 10.1177/1043454210377179

Naar-King, S., Montepiedra, G., Nichols, S., Farley, J., Garvie, P. A., Kammerer, B., Malee, K., Sirois, P. A., & Storm, D. (2009). Allocation of family responsibility for illness management in pediatric HIV. *Journal of Pediatric Psychology, 34*(2), 187–194. doi:10.1093/jpepsy/jsn065

National Cancer Institute at the National Institute of Health. (2011). *Childhood acute myeloid leukemia/other myeloid malignancies treatment (PDQ) health professional version*. Last modified 12/09/2011. Retrieved from http://www.cancer.gov/cancertopics/pdq/treatment/childAML/HealthProfessional/page1

Pagana, K. (2009). What does the absolute neutrophil count tell you? *American Nurse Today 4*, 12–13. Retrieved from http://www.americannursetoday.com/article.aspx?id=4332&fid=4302

Penn State Hershey. (2011). *Chronic lymphocytic leukemia (CLL)*. Retrieved from http://pennstatehershey.adam.com/content.aspx?productId=117&pid=1&gid=000532

Peters, C., Cornish, J. M., Parikh, S. H., & Kurtzberg, J. (2010). Stem cell source and outcome after hematopoietic stem cell transplantation (HSCT) in children and adolescents with acute leukemia. *Pediatric Clinics of North America, 57*, 27–46. doi:10.1016/j.pcl.2010.01.004

Riis Olsen, P., & Harder, I. (2011). Caring for teenagers and young adults with cancer: A grounded theory study of network-focused nursing. *European Journal of Oncology Nursing, 15*, 152–159. doi:10.1016/j.ejon.2010.07.010

Ringnér, A., Jansson, L., & Graneheim, U. H. (2011). Parental experiences of information within pediatric oncology. *Journal of Pediatric Oncology Nursing, 28*, 244–251. doi: 10.1177/1043454211409587

Rivera, D. M., & Steele, R. W. (2011). *Pediatric HIV infection*. Retrieved from http://emedicine.medscape.com/article/965086-overview

Ruppert, R. (2011). Radiation 101. *American Nurse Today, 6*, 24–27. Retrieved from http://www.americannursetoday.com/article.aspx?id=7400&fid=7360

Sayed, H. A., Ali, A. M., Hamza, H. M., & Abdalla, M. A. (2011). Long-term follow-up of infantile Wilms' tumor treated according to International Society of Pediatric Oncology protocol: Seven years' follow-up. *Urology, 77*, 446–451. doi: 10.1016/j.urology.2010.05.049

Schulte, F., & Barrera, M. (2010). Social competence in childhood brain tumor survivors: A comprehensive review. *Supportive Care in Cancer, 18*, 1499–1513. doi:10.1007/s00520-010-0963-1

Shiminski-Maher, T., Cullen, P., & Sansalone, M. (2002). *Childhood brain & spinal cord tumors: A guide for families, friends & caregivers*. Sebastopol, CA: O'Reilly & Associates, Inc.

Unguru, Y. (2011). The successful integration of research and care: How pediatric oncology became the subspecialty in which research defines the standard of care. *Pediatric Blood & Cancer, 56*, 1019–1025. doi:10.1002/pbc.22976

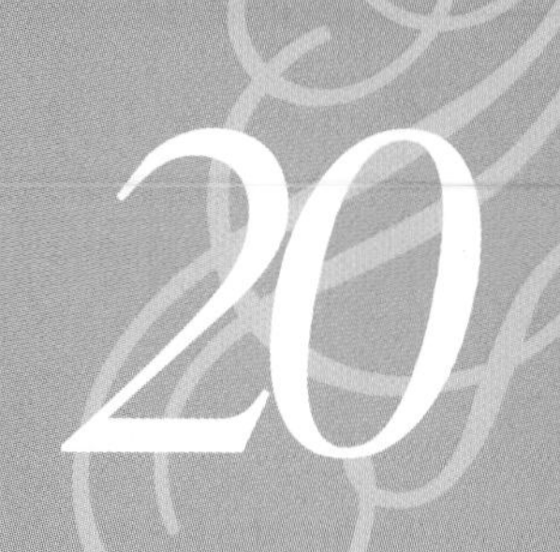

Musculoskeletal Disorders

Suzanne Fortuna, Post MSN, RN, CNS, FNP, APN-BC

OBJECTIVES

- ☐ Describe the anatomy and physiology of the musculoskeletal system.
- ☐ Describe the common disorders of the musculoskeletal system.
- ☐ Identify specific physical assessment skills for evaluation of the musculoskeletal system.
- ☐ Describe the diagnostic tests and lab values typically monitored in musculoskeletal disorders.
- ☐ Explain the applicable nursing interventions for musculoskeletal disorders.
- ☐ Integrate acute hospital care concepts for musculoskeletal disorders.
- ☐ Integrate chronic hospital care concepts for musculoskeletal disorders.
- ☐ Integrate emergency care or trauma concepts for musculoskeletal disorders.
- ☐ Describe strategies to support patient/caregiver education about musculoskeletal disorders.

KEY TERMS

- Bones
- Muscles
- Joints
- Tendons
- Ligaments
- PRICE
- Fractures
- Congenital
- Clubfoot
- Idiopathic
- Metatarsus adductus
- Internal tibial torsion
- Molding
- Ligament laxity
- Internal femoral torsion
- Varum (varus deformity)
- Physiologic
- Blount's disease
- Dysplasia
- Valgum (valgus deformity)
- Barlow test
- Ortolani test
- Galeazzi sign
- Legg-Calvé-Perthes (LCP) disease
- Slipped capital femoral epiphysis (SCFE)
- Transient monoarticular synovitis
- Synovitis
- Osteomyelitis
- Scoliosis
- Adolescent idiopathic scoliosis (AIS)
- Juvenile idiopathic arthritis
- Osteogenesis imperfecta
- Sprains and strains

ANATOMY AND PHYSIOLOGY

The musculoskeletal (MS) system is comprised of **bones, muscles, joints, tendons,** and **ligaments** that interconnect. Muscle contraction is innervated by the somatic nervous system. Fetal development of the musculoskeletal system begins with the formation of pure cartilage, which is then transformed by osteoclasts and osteoblast formation. The rapid formation of the skeletal structures makes abnormalities somewhat common (**Figure 20-1**).

- Several considerations in abnormalities include:
  - *Environment*
  - *Genetics*
  - *Trauma*
- Bones can be cartilaginous structures while children are growing and developing.
  - *Growth plates are open in children, making certain diagnoses more difficult at times due to age-specific qualities of bone and joint structures.*
  - *Once maturation occurs, bones are characteristically dense osseous structures typical of the description of a skeleton framework.*
  - *As a rule of thumb with children, skin, muscles, and ligaments protect the maturing bones; therefore, if these parts are weakened or not developed properly, the bones suffer.*

ASSESSMENT

Many clinical tools are used for the evaluation of musculoskeletal (MS) system abnormalities, and all require an understanding of MS system anatomy. The overall assessment of the

Don't have time to read this chapter? Want to reinforce your reading? Need to review for a test? Listen to this chapter on DavisPlus at davispl.us/rudd1.

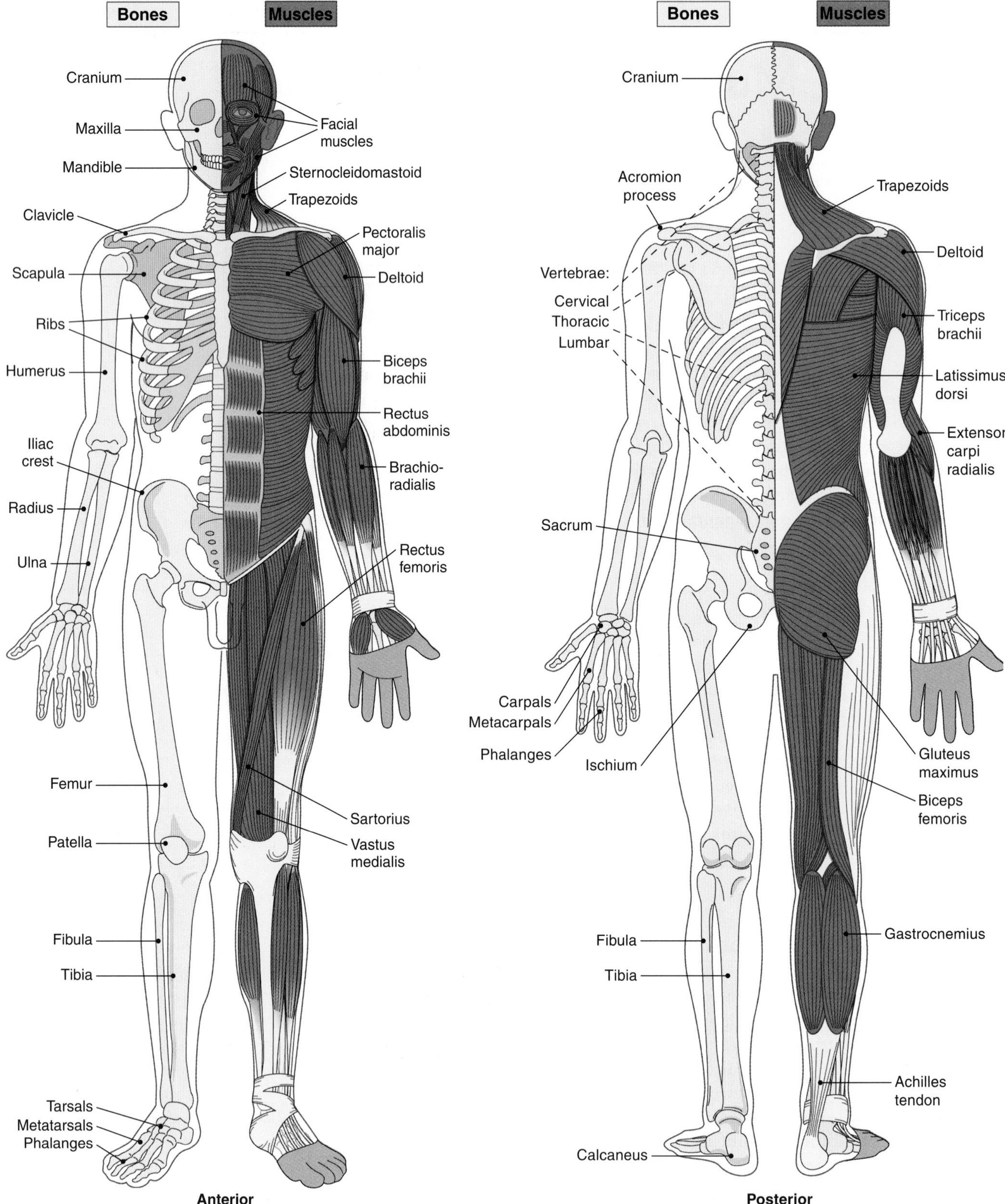

Figure 20–1 Cross section of musculoskeletal system.

MS system involves simple to complex physical tests to evaluate changes or deficits.

- Mainly, the evaluation involves:
  - *Inspection*
  - *Palpation*
  - *Range-of-motion (ROM) maneuvers*
  - *Laboratory tests if indicated (**Table 20-1**)*
  - *Radiographic tests: x-rays, computed tomography (CT) scans, magnetic resonance imaging (MRI), arthrograms (**Table 20-2**)*

TABLE 20–1 BLOOD AND BODY FLUID ANALYSIS FOR THE CHILD WITH ALTERATIONS IN MUSCULOSKELETAL CONDITIONS

Diagnostic Test	Function of the Test	Indications	Normal Values
COMPLETE BLOOD COUNT (CBC)	Blood sample evaluates many aspects	Platelets indicate a bleeding disorder >WBC indicates a bacterial infection or septic arthritis	Platelets: 150,000–400,000/μL WBC: 4500–10,000/μL
CBC DIFFERENTIAL	Breaks down WBC into various types (five total) Numbers indicate a percentage of total WBC Indicates the type of infection	Monocytes indicate a long-term infectious process Lymphocytes indicate an increase in viral illness Eosinophils indicate an allergic or parasitic condition Basophils indicate a chronic inflammatory condition Neutrophils (polys) Bands are immature neutrophils Segs are mature neutrophils (left-shift describes an increase in the band neutrophils) Suggests a severe bacterial infection such as sepsis	0% for bands and 31%–57% for segs Presence of bands is highly indicative of a bacterial infection
C-REACTIVE PROTEIN (CRP)	Measures a protein in blood that is released when an infection is present	>0.9 indicates an infection or septic arthritis	<1.0 mg/dL
CALCIUM AND PHOSPHATE	Measures the amount of these minerals	Low levels may indicate rickets	Calcium: 8.5–11 mg Phosphorus: 3.0–4.5 mg/dL
RHEUMATOID FACTOR (Rh FACTOR)	Measures the body's autoimmune response to an antigen	If positive, may indicate juvenile arthritis Not all children with juvenile arthritis have a positive Rh factor	Negative
ERYTHROCYTE SEDIMENTATION RATE (ESR)	Measures the speed at which RBCs settle out in solution	Elevated indicates septic arthritis May also indicate infection	0–10 mm/hr
BLOOD CULTURES	Measures whether microorganisms grow in the lab	Can identify an organism causing infection Forty percent of children with septic arthritis have a positive blood culture	No growth
BONE BIOPSIES	Diagnose tumor or infection of the bone	Osteomyelitis Bone tumor	Normal bone cells
FLUID ASPIRATION FROM JOINTS	Diagnose an infection of the joint or drain fluid from joint to relieve pressure	Drainage is purulent Culture of fluid is positive	Clear fluid No growth from culture

From Ward, S. L., & Hisley, S. M. (2009). *Maternal-child nursing care: Optimizing outcomes for mothers, children, & families* (p. 965). Philadelphia: F.A. Davis.

TABLE 20–2 ORTHOPEDIC DIAGNOSTIC TESTS

Diagnostic Imaging Test	Benefits	Limitations
RADIOGRAPH	Easily available Visualizes fractures well No sedation needed Inexpensive	Two-dimensional Does not visualize soft tissue such as cartilage Patient must be positioned properly Radiation exposure
FLUOROSCOPY	Guides many orthopedic procedures Can be used with contrast Real-time radiography Inexpensive	Radiation exposure
ARTHROGRAPHY	Provides visualization of joints Three-dimensional view	Risk of reaction to contrast Depends on the skill of the radiographer Radiation exposure
COMPUTED TOMOGRAPHY (CT) SCAN	Cross-sectional view of anatomy Clearer than radiographs Software programs can show reconstruction Can use contrast	Expensive May require sedation Risk of reaction to contrast
BONE SCAN (NUCLEAR MEDICINE)	Excellent at finding changes in bone as a result of infection, trauma, or tumor	Takes 4 hours Not always available on emergency basis Cannot distinguish benign from malignant tumors Radiation exposure to entire body IV access required
ULTRASOUND	Easily available No radiation No sedation needed Good for visualizing soft tissue masses and cysts Painless Inexpensive	Limited use Depends on the skill of the radiographer
MAGNETIC RESONANCE IMAGING (MRI)	Visualizes hard and soft tissue and bone marrow No radiation	Not readily available No metal can be present in the vicinity Sedation may be needed Need experienced radiologist to read MRI

From Ward, S. L., & Hisley, S. M. (2009). *Maternal-child nursing care: Optimizing outcomes for mothers, children, & families* (p. 964). Philadelphia: F.A. Davis.

Understanding normal motor development and screening tools also assists the health-care provider to determine problems or potential delays.

- "Motor development is the acquisition of the capability to move and interact with the environment" (Staheli, 2006).
- Although variability of motor development in children is common, it follows a developmental pattern.
- The common goal is for all children to master certain skills and improve in their efficiency, precision, and speed along the way.
- With abnormalities, however, typical skills may be delayed or nonexistent.
- History taking plays a great role in understanding how the child is growing and developing.
- Even the birth history and the degree of pre- and postnatal care can give us insights as to how the child potentially will master or become delayed in the attainment of certain skills.

General Assessment

Screening for appropriate growth and development includes the following:

- Physical examination
- History taking

- Height and weight
- Diagnostic imaging if applicable
- Laboratory testing if applicable
- Motor development evaluation
- Family expectations

Emergent and Initial Nursing Care of the Musculoskeletal System

The usual nursing care and positioning of the affected extremity involve:

- Elevation
- **PRICE** (protect, rest, ice, compression, and elevation)
- Neurovascular checks
- Natural alignment is best to prevent deformity, improve function.
- Keep splint/cast/brace application intact.
- Reinforcement as needed
- Maintenance of weight-bearing status
- Teach/monitor use of assistive aids as needed.
- Activity-level precautions can be age specific.

Promoting Safety

Typically, instruct patients and families in regard to the following activity limitations (if applicable):

- Keep two feet on the ground.
- No activities with balls or bikes
- Do not insert food, toys, or other objects into casts/ splints.
- Upper arms: use sling/brace if instructed.
- Lower extremities: use brace, crutches (over age 8), wheelchair (over age 4), or stroller (under age 3) as instructed.

- Pain medication usage, side effects, discontinuation
- Nonpharmacologic methods, especially distraction
- Problems or concerns that should prompt contact of health-care professional
- Postoperative coping and family support or community resources
- Ancillary team involvement, such as social work or rehab services
- School and gym class participation restrictions
- Toileting
- Follow-up visits

FRACTURES

Fractures in children are more complicated than in adults due to the nature of maturing bones or cartilaginous features and open growth plates.

- Some of the most common fractures in children are torus fractures, or buckle fractures.
- The mechanism of injury is usually a direct fall onto an outstretched arm or a fall from some height with a landing that compresses the bones.
- The compression can be at the growth plate or away from it.
- Many children, due to the process of growing or maturation, can have occult fractures.
- An occult fracture of the tibia commonly is called a toddler's fracture.
- An occult fracture is rarely seen on emergent x-rays, but the child may cry or refuse to bear weight on the affected extremity.
- Placing the child in either a walking boot or cast relieves the pressure and pain.
- Repeat films after 3 to 4 weeks note healing callus formation along the seam of the bone, proving occult fracture validity.
- Sometimes just symptom relief is the treatment for fractures.
- Advise families that new bone formation may or may not be visible, but clinical examination and immobilization are still recommended.

ANATOMY OF GROWING BONE

- Epiphysis
- Physis
- Metaphysis
- Diaphysis
- Periosteum

CRITICAL COMPONENT

Physis

What is so important about the physis?

- Children's bones are different from adult bones.
- Adult fractures have to be aligned perfectly.
- Children with open growth plates will remodel any deformity.
- Risk of physeal arrest with subsequent growth disturbance is present.

Skeleton

Children have an immature skeleton:

- Increased resiliency to stress
- Thicker periosteum
- Increased potential to remodel
- Shorter healing times
- Presence of a physis

Injury Pattern in Growing Bones

- Bones tend to *bow* rather than *break*.
- Compressive force = torus fracture/buckle fracture.
- Ligaments and tendons are stronger than young bone.
  - *Bone is more likely to be injured than soft tissue.*
  - *Periosteum is biologically active in children.*
    - Stabilizes fracture
    - Promotes healing

Unique Properties of the Immature Skeleton

- Children tend to heal fractures faster than adults.
- Advantage: shorter immobilization times

- Disadvantage: misaligned fragments become "solid" sooner
- Anticipate remodeling if child has >2 years of growing left.
- Mild angulation deformities often correct themselves.
- Rotational deformities require reduction (won't remodel).
- Fractures in children may stimulate longitudinal bone growth.
- Some degree of bone overlap is acceptable and may even be helpful.
- Children don't tend to get as stiff as adults after immobilization.
- After casting, a callus is formed but still may be fibrous.
- Children should avoid contact activities for 2 to 4 weeks once out of cast.

Physeal Injuries

- Many childhood fractures involve the physis.
- Account for 27% of all skeletal injuries in children (Kunes, 2011)
- Can disrupt growth of bone
- Injury near but not at the physis can stimulate bone growth

Incidence of Pediatric Fractures

- Approximately 20% of children who seek attention for injury have a fracture (Kunes, 2011).
- From birth to 16 years, chance of fracture:
  - *Boys: 42% (Kunes, 2011)*
  - *Girls: 27% (Kunes, 2011)*
- Most commonly involved sites:
  - *Distal radius*
  - *Hand*
  - *Elbow*
  - *Clavicle*
  - *Radius*
  - *Tibia*
- Most common fracture is of the distal radius
- Clavicle is second most common

Classification of Fractures

Fractures in general can be classified in several different categories: (**See Figure 20-2 A–E**)

- Greenstick, buckle or torus, and plastic deformation fractures
- Simple fractures
- Comminuted fractures
- Complex fractures
- Physeal fractures are classified as Salter Harris I through IV based on the level of growth plate involvement.
- The level of severity and the child's age may direct treatment modalities and outcomes.

Salter Harris Classification System

- System to delineate risk of growth disturbance:
  - *Higher-grade fractures are more likely to cause growth disturbance.*

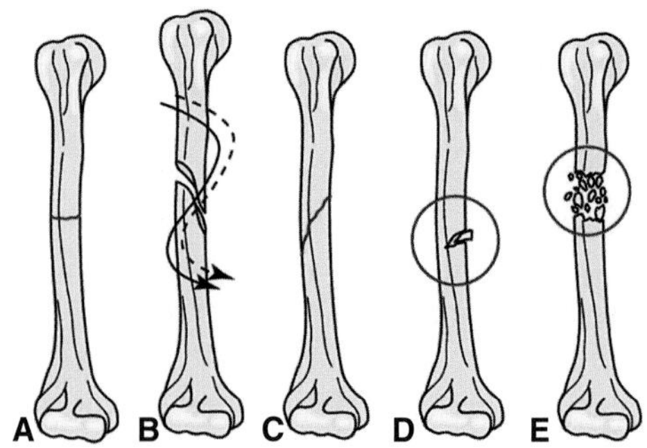

Figure 20-2 Different classes of fractures. A. Transverse B. Spiral C. Oblique D. Greenstick E. Comminuted.

- *Growth disturbance can happen with ANY physeal injury.*
- *Type I*
  - Fracture passes transversely through physis, separating epiphysis from metaphysis.
- *Type II*
  - Fracture passes transversely through physis but exits through metaphysis.
  - Triangular fragment
- *Type III*
  - Fracture crosses physis and exits through epiphysis at joint space.
- *Type IV*
  - Fracture extends upward from the joint line, through the physis, and out the metaphysis.
- *Type V*
  - Crush injury to growth plate

TORUS FRACTURES

Treatment

- Goals of treatment
  - *Prevent pain.*
  - *Prevent further deformity.*
- Many diagnosed days after injury
- No reduction needed, if anatomically aligned
- If >24 hours old
  - *Cast at first visit*
- Otherwise splint
  - *Cast at 5 to 7 days*
- Short arm cast for 3 to 4 weeks

GREENSTICK FRACTURES

Treatment

- If nondisplaced
  - *Short arm cast*
- If displaced >15 degrees
  - *Reduce and immobilize in long arm*
- Cast for 4 weeks, removable splint for 2 weeks

DISTAL RADIUS PHYSIS FRACTURE

Treatment

- A nondisplaced Salter I can appear normal on plain films.
- If tenderness over physis, treat as a fracture.

DISTAL RADIUS FRACTURES

Treatment

- Displaced fractures
  - *Reduce as soon as possible.*
- Nondisplaced fractures
  - *Short arm cast for 3 to 6 weeks*
- The older the child, the longer the immobilization.
- If x-rays are normal initially but tenderness is over growth plate:
  - *Immobilize for 2 weeks.*
  - *Bring child back to reexamine and follow-up x-ray.*
  - *If no callus, fracture is unlikely.*

ELBOW FRACTURES

Treatment

- Account for 10% of all fractures in children (Kunes, 2011)
- Diagnosis and management are complex.
- Early recognition and referral will provide best outcome.
- Most are supracondylar fractures.

SUPRACONDYLAR FRACTURES

Treatment

- Weakest part of the elbow joint where humerus flattens and flares
- Most common fracture is extension type
- Olecranon driven into humerus with hyperextension
- Marked pain and swelling of elbow
- Potential for vascular compromise:
  - *5 P's—pain, pulse, pallor, paresthesia, paralysis*
- Check pulse!
  - *Reduce fracture if pulse is compromised.*
- Check nerve function in hand.
- Most are displaced and need surgery
- Nondisplaced fractures can be managed with long arm cast, forearm neutral, elbow at 90 degrees for 3 weeks.
- Follow-up x-rays taken 3 to 7 days later to document alignment.
- X-rays taken at 3 weeks to document callus.
- Once callus noted at 3 weeks, discontinue cast, pull out pins in the office, and start active ROM slowly over the next 1 to 2 weeks.
- If no ROM improvement in 2 to 3 weeks, can recheck in office or send to occupational therapy as needed.

LATERAL CONDYLAR FRACTURES

Treatment

- Second most common elbow fracture
- Most common physeal elbow injury
- FOOSH (fall on outstretched hand) + Varus force = lateral condyle avulsion
- Exam: focal swelling at lateral distal humerus
- Most require surgery but not urgent
- If displaced
  - *Surgically pinned*
- If nondisplaced
  - *Treated with casting*
- Posterior splint acutely, elbow at 90 degrees
- At follow-up (weekly), check for late displacement.
- If stable for 2 weeks, long arm cast for another 4 weeks
- Complications: growth arrest, nonunion

CLAVICLE FRACTURES

- Most, 80%, occur in the middle third of the bone (Kunes, 2011)
- Of the remaining, 15% distal third, 5% proximal third (Kunes, 2011)
- Result from FOOSH, fall on shoulder, direct trauma
- Clinical: pain with any shoulder movement, holds arm to chest
- Point tender over fracture, subcutaneous crepitus
- Often obvious deformity

Treatment

- Sling versus figure-of-eight bandage
- If fracture fully healed
  - *Painless ROM at shoulder*
- Nontender
- Generally back to pain-free activity by 4 weeks
- No contact sports for 6 weeks
- Warn of the healed "bump" if enough growth remaining—will smooth out but may not disappear.

TIBIA FRACTURE

- Mechanism: falls and twisting injury of the foot
- Low force, intact periosteum, and support from fibula commonly prevent displacement.

Treatment

- Posterior lower leg splint if acute
- Nondisplaced fractures: long leg cast for 6 to 8 weeks
- Repeat radiographs weekly to check position
- Surgery if angulates more than 15 degrees

TODDLER'S FRACTURES

- Children younger than 2 years old learning to walk
- No specific injury notable most of the time
- Child refuses to bear weight on leg.
- Examine hip, thigh, and knee to rule out (r/o) other causes of limping.
- Consider and r/o abuse.
- Examine for soft tissue injury to buttocks, back of legs, head, and neck.
- Transverse fractures of the midshaft are more suspicious for child abuse.
- Management: long leg cast for 3 to 4 weeks
- Weight bearing as tolerated
- Heals completely in 6 to 8 weeks

CLINICAL PEARL

- Nearly 20% of children with injury have a fracture (Kunes, 2011).
- Consider bilateral x-rays in children if unsure of or difficulty visualizing fracture lines.
- Physeal injuries are common and may have no radiographic findings–treat as fracture!
- Remember to tell caregivers about possible growth problems.

FEMUR FRACTURES

- Most commonly fractured long bone, 19 per 100,00 fractures
- Represent 1.4% to 1.7% of all pediatric fractures (Kocher et al., 2009)
- Usually diaphyseal
- Males more common than females
- Children over age 3 mostly affected
- Seasonal—highest in summer months (Staheli & Hensinger, 2001)
- Predominantly due to trauma such as falls and car accidents
- Rule out child abuse in nonambulator, <2 year old, or when story doesn't match fracture pattern, especially in "spiral fractures" or "corner fractures."

Mechanism of Injury

- Rule out nonaccidental trauma in child <3 years of age (Kocher et al., 2009).
- Falls—young children/toddlers
- Motor vehicle accidents (pedestrian struck by a car)—juveniles
- Recreational sports/activities such as BMX biking, snowboarding, and so on—adolescents
- Motor vehicle crashes—all age groups

Treatment Goals

Restore

- Length
- Alignment
- Rotation

Avoid

- Osteonecrosis—disruption of blood supply to femoral head
- Physeal injury—preserve future growth potential

Treatment Options

Nonoperative

- Traction
- Casting

Operative

- Plate and screw fixation—open-reduction internal fixation (ORIF)
- External fixation
- Flexible nailing
- Rigid nailing
- Traction pre-surgery if needs to be reduced, usually skin traction (**Figure 20-3**)
  - *Older child may need skeletal traction depending on fracture and amount of translation. Traction is often not required due to the increased ability to use femoral rods or sliding plates with minimally invasive surgery options.*

Medication

Medication for Muscle Spasms

Children will have muscle spasms while in traction. The use of IV Ativan every 4 to 6 hours, as needed, may be ordered. The child may need oral Ativan at home for 1 to 3 days. Spasms typically subside once a spica cast has been placed.

Care of Child in Spica Cast (**Figure 20-4**)

- Turn and reposition every 2 to 4 hours while awake to prevent pressure sores at heals or sacrum
- Neurovascular checks every 2 hours 24 hours postoperative (post-op)
- Be sure can insert 2 fingers along abdomen of cast to verify not too tight, especially with position changes such as side lying or from side to back
- Toileting—use diapers in incontinent child, urinal or bedpan in continent child.

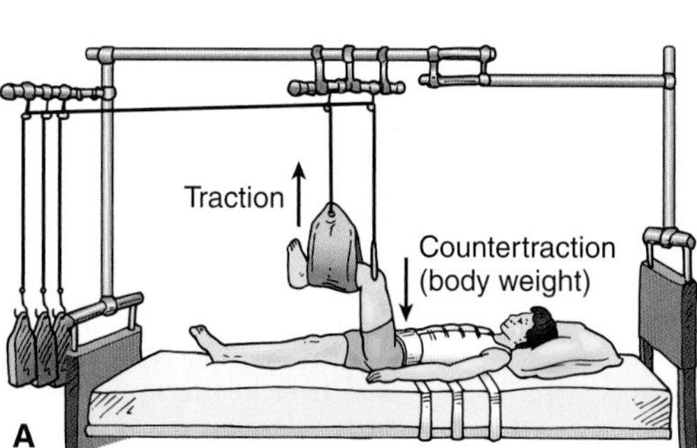

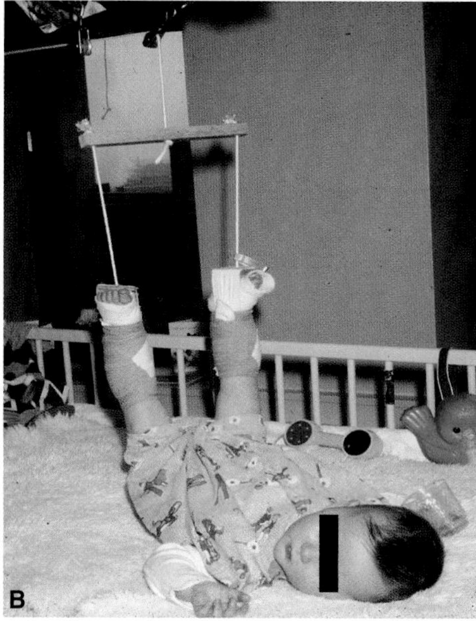

Figure 20-3 **A**, The 90/90 femoral traction is most commonly used to treat femur fractures and complicated femur fractures. **B**, Example of baby in traction.

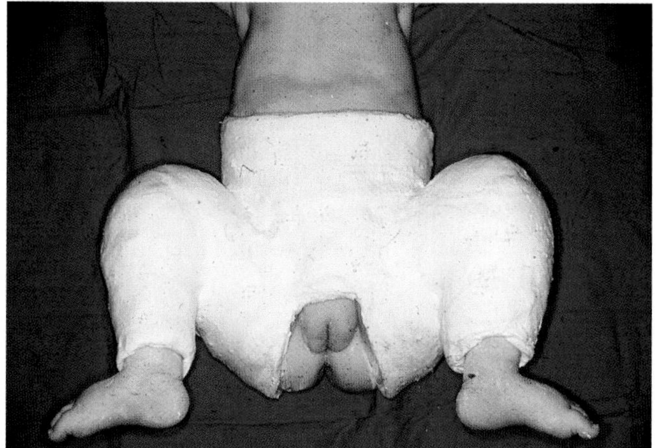

Figure 20-4 Child in spica cast.

- Padding protects the cast from urine and feces; use chux pads with absorbent side placed next to skin.
- Tylenol with codeine every 4 to 6 hours as needed, around the clock (ATC) for initial 24 to 48 hours, then before bed for up to 1 week post-op; may encourage Motrin or Tylenol during the day as needed.
- Constipation prevention
    - *Increase consumption of clear fluids.*
    - *Increase consumption of fresh fruits and veggies.*
    - *Decrease consumption of fried foods and constipation triggers such as cheese and milk until off narcotics.*
    - *Explain decreased physical activity's association with gastric motility.*
    - *Regulate consumption of high-fat and high-carbohydrate foods and encourage more lean and green types of foods.*
    - *Decrease intake of sweet, sugary food and drink until cast is off and normal activity is resumed.*

CONGENITAL MUSCULOSKELETAL ABNORMALITIES

Congenital refers to a condition that a child is born with, that develops in utero, or that involves hereditary considerations.

- Many congenital abnormalities or birth defects are apparent either in utero or shortly after birth.
- Some abnormalities are due to packaging—that is, the size and amount of amniotic fluid in the womb.
- Many disorders are not known or readily recognized until the child reaches a later stage of growth and development.

CLUBFOOT

Clubfoot is a congenital abnormality (**Figure 20-5**); it may also be neurogenic or **idiopathic** (no known reason).

- Syndrome development
- Teratologic (myelodysplasia and arthrogryposis)
- Positional (in utero malposition)

Risk Factors and Incidence

The incidence in infants occurs with the following considerations:

- Bilateral presentation in 50% of cases (Kliegman, Stanton, St. Geme, Schor, & Behrman, 2011)
- Family history increases incidence
- Males more affected, 2:1 (Kliegman et al., 2011)
- Presentation may be unilateral or bilateral.
- Affects the entire lower extremity from the knee down
- The calf looks smaller and has less ability to develop muscle strength than a typical lower extremity limb.

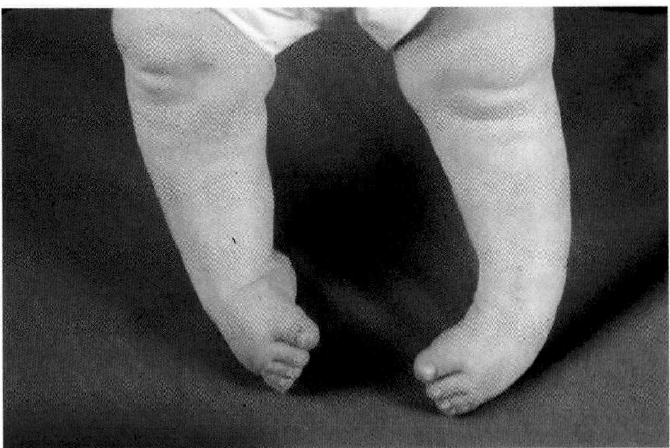

Figure 20–5 Clubfoot.

- The affected foot may be smaller in dorsal height and length.
- The foot itself is fixed and rigid in a plantar-flexed and pronated position that cannot be dorsiflexed or manually stretched into a neutral position.
- The Achilles tendon is extremely tight or shortened, with the inability to have the talus and calcaneus lowered into the neutral equinus position.

Treatment

Treatment options include both nonsurgical and surgical modalities.

Nonsurgical Modalities

- The first approach is to start the Ponseti technique of serial casting within the first week of life. Refer to Google images for online pictures of serial casting.
- This is a very time-consuming but successful treatment option.
- The casts are changed weekly for up to 12 weeks.

> **CLINICAL PEARL**
>
> **Casting Material**
>
> The casting material is always plaster because of its ability to be molded, whereas fiberglass is more rigid.

- The goal is to first re-create the deformity, then slowly progress to full correction in an abducted fully dorsiflexed turned-outward presentation.
- The casting is followed by maintaining the correction either in ankle-foot orthotics (AFOs) or with the use of a Denis-Browne bar or Dobb's bar for at least 23 hours a day full time for 3 months, then nighttime and naptime use for up to 3 years of age.
- The deformity wants to recur, so strict adherence to follow-up regimen is required or the failure rate is high.
- The deformity is harder to correct in failures and with lack of follow-up.
- Thus, it is essential to teach symptom monitoring so that caregivers can recognize an acute need to return to the clinic.

> **CRITICAL COMPONENT**
>
> **Alerts for Caregivers**
>
> Symptoms that indicate an acute need to return to a health-care setting
>
> - Feet appear to turn inward
> - Walking on the lateral border of foot
> - Tip-toe walking
> - Rocker-bottom foot

Other nonsurgical treatment options include:

- Physical therapy—stretching heel cords
- Serial splinting at age 12 weeks
- Splints
- Taping
- Orthoses

Surgical Modalities

Indications to use surgical treatments are:

- Failed conservative treatment (serial casting)
- Late referrals (seen well after first 7 to 10 days of life)
- Failure to follow up and/or early discontinuation of treatment options
- Recurrent deformity

Surgical treatment options include:

- Soft tissue releases
- Tendon transfers
- Bony procedures

METATARSUS ADDUCTUS

Metatarsus adductus is another common foot deformity involving the forefoot only (**Figure 20-6**). The patient still presents with "foot turned inward," but it is not the whole foot that is involved.

Risk Factors and Incidence

- Males greater than females
- Usually bilateral
- Inheritance factor minimal
- In utero molding—petite mother, prima gravida

Clinical Presentation

- Abducted forefoot
- Normal hind foot
- Prominent fifth metatarsus tuberosity
- Variable rigidity

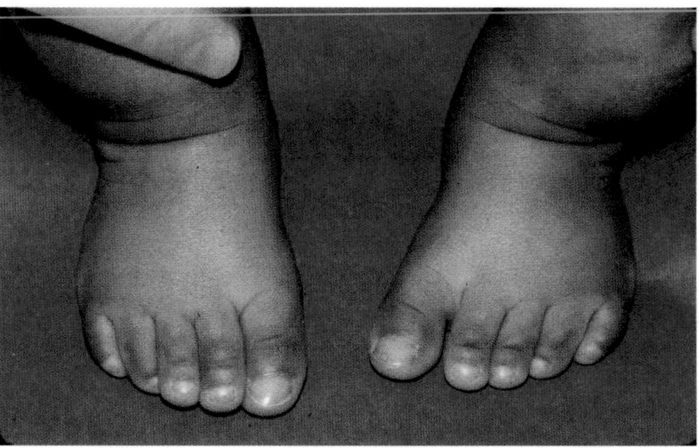

Figure 20-6 Metatarsus adductus.

Treatment

Treatment options are dependent on the flexibility of the forefoot:

- Flexible
  - *No treatment required*
  - *Resolves spontaneously*
- Moderately flexible
  - *Passive stretching (with infants, apply gentle stretch at every diaper change)*
  - *Corrective shoes/splinting (reverse last shoes)*
- Rigid
  - *Serial casting (0–3 years of age)*
  - *Surgery (4 years of age and older)*

INTERNAL TIBIAL TORSION

Internal tibial torsion is the most common cause of in-toeing in children less than 3 years of age (Lincoln & Suen, 2003). In the orthopedic outpatient clinic, it is the most common cause for parental referral to a specialist (**Figure 20-7**).

- The usual cause is in utero positioning or intrauterine **molding**.
- *Molding* refers to when in utero forces cause positional deformities.
- If unilateral, left sided (Lincoln & Suen, 2003)
- Patients generally have **ligament laxity**.
- They are very comfortable sitting on their feet.
- Often, parents report that the child sleeps on his or her stomach with the feet tucked up underneath, as well as excessive tripping and falling.
- The shin is twisted, making the feet appear to be turned inward.
- Parents report multiple bumps and bruises and the child tripping and falling a lot.
- Treatment is conservative.
- Spontaneous resolution is the norm, usually following aggressive ambulation and vigorous-paced running.
- Most cases resolve by the age of 3 or 4 years.

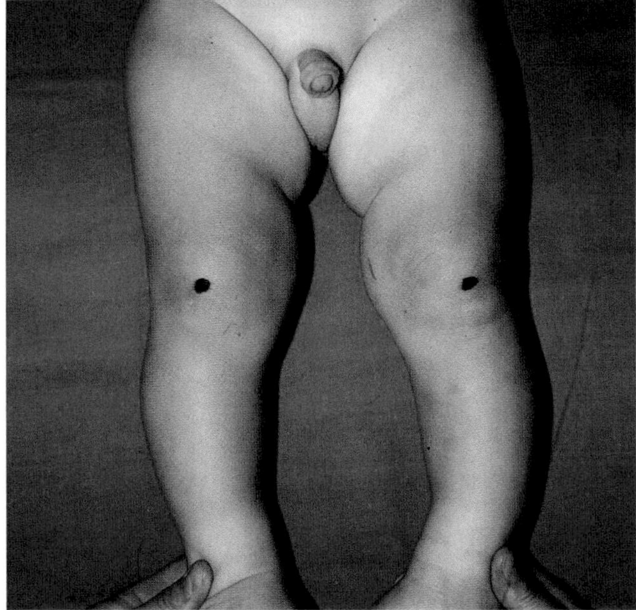

Figure 20-7 Internal tibial torsion.

- Teach the family to speak to daycare centers and church/school personnel about having the child avoid sitting on the heels or feet.
- Explain preferred sitting posture: with feet in front or in "Indian style."

INTERNAL FEMORAL TORSION

Internal femoral torsion is the most common cause of in-toeing in children over the age of 2 years (**Figure 20-8**).

- Incidence is greater in females (Lincoln & Suen, 2003)
- Classified as either medial femoral torsion or femoral anteversion

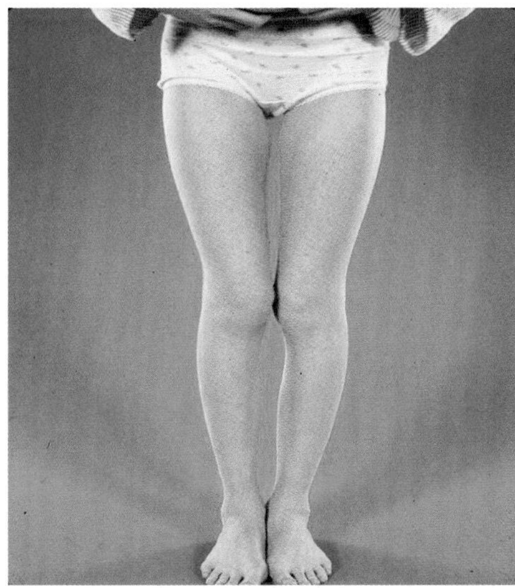

Figure 20-8 Internal femoral torsion.

- Clinical presentation of generalized ligament laxity and abnormal seating; preference of "W" sitting is classic (**Figure 20-9**).
- Excessive medial rotation and limited lateral rotation
- Children typically spontaneously correct this deformity with correction of sitting habits.
- If the deformity is present and severe by 8 or 9 years of age, it will not correct without surgical intervention.
- Most spontaneously resolve; of the few that do not, either a proximal femoral or tibial osteotomy is performed (Lincoln & Suen, 2003).
- Non-weight-bearing long leg casts for 6 to 8 weeks
- This intervention is offered as a last resort and for very severe cases.

GENU VARUM (BOWLEGS)

Genu **varum (varus deformity),** or bowlegs, is a lower leg deformity often seen in children between 18 months and 3 years of age.

- The typical clinical presentation is in-toeing, and a bowling ball could be placed between the legs (**Figure 20-10**).

Classification and Symptoms

Classification includes:

- **Physiologic**
- Tibial vara or **Blount's disease**
- Metabolic disorders—vitamin-D-resistant rickets or hypophosphatasia
- Skeletal dysplasia—achondroplasia, or dwarfism
- Focal fibrocartilaginous **dysplasia**
- Physeal abnormality—tumor, infection, or trauma

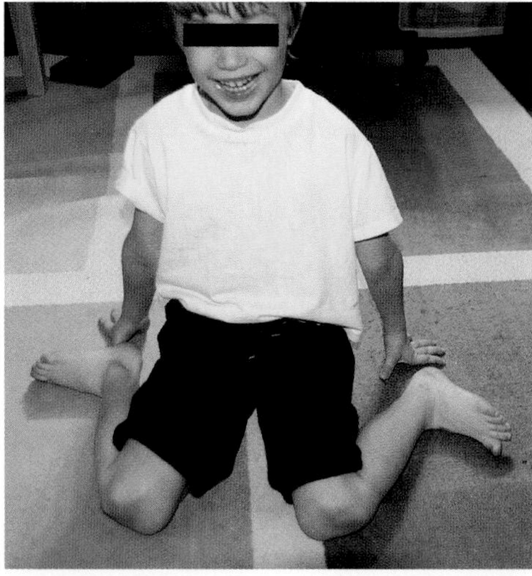

Figure 20-9 Ligament laxity and "W" sitting position.

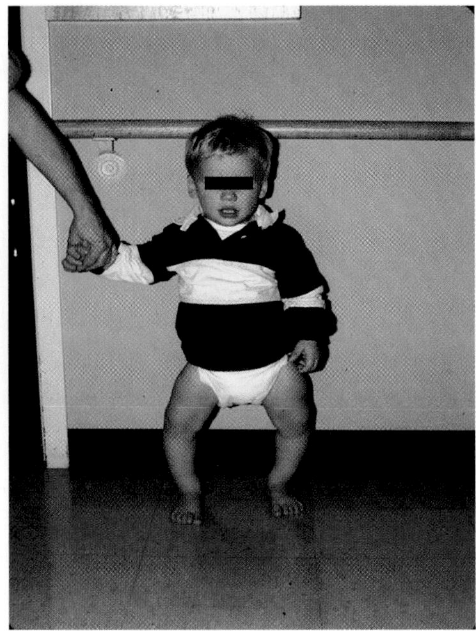

Figure 20-10 Genu varum.

Differences Between Normal Bowing and Deformity

Features differentiating between normal physiologic bowing versus deformity:

- Usually symmetrical
- No worsening with growth
- No lateral knee thrust
- No radiographic changes in severity
- Occurrence before 2 years of age
- Physiologic bowing is present in infancy but is outgrown by the time the child is about 2 years of age.
- The normal progression of limb development is physiologic bowing, then the lower legs straighten out, then physiologic knock-knees, then the legs again straighten out, and by the time a child is 7 or so, the limbs should be straight and not change throughout their remaining growth.
- Deformities occur outside the normal pattern of development.
- Blount's disease can be infantile or in the adolescent stages. In infantile Blount's disease, the deformity may be related to the following risk factors:
  - *Ambulation or full independent weight bearing before or between the ages of 9 and 12 months*
  - *Heavy children—greater than 95th percentile in early years—with early ambulation*
- In adolescent Blount's disease, the deformity occurs during growth maturation. The risk factors are similar to those seen in infantile cases:
  - *Morbidly obese children greater than 95th percentile for weight but average height or less than average height*
- Adolescent Blount's disease causes premature closure of the lateral epiphysis in unilateral or bilateral tibias.

Treatment

- The deformity must be observed and treated before the age of 4 years.
- Otherwise, the deformity is more difficult to correct and the risks of damage to the growth plates of the knees is more severe.
- Bracing in cumbersome long leg orthoses is a treatment option, but compliance is often difficult.
- The bracing slows down the progression of the deformity but it does not reverse it.
- The surgical correction for adolescent Blount's disease is tibial derotational osteotomies.
    - *Patients are placed in either long leg casts for the first 4 to 6 weeks followed by short leg non-weight-bearing casts for 6 to 12 weeks total, or in short leg non-weight-bearing casts for 6 to 12 weeks total.*
    - *It is highly recommended to do one side at a time to allow for assisted ambulation and activities of daily living (ADLs), with 6 to 8 weeks or more between procedures.*
    - *It is also customary to encourage lifestyle changes before the surgery to decrease the risk of complications such as bone nonunion or deep vein thrombosis (DVT) post-surgery.*
    - *This is a challenging population because most present with a history of teasing due to obesity compounded by ridicule due to bowed legs—the condition is quite eye-catching.*
    - *Therefore not only are patients emotionally scarred, but the families are emotionally charged, and family members rarely feel that the obesity is due to family dynamics.*
    - *Nutritionists, physical therapists, nursing staff, and social workers all need to meet with family members to discuss the rationales and expected outcomes for doing this complicated procedure; otherwise recurrence and/or failure to return to correct the opposite side is more likely.*

GENU VALGUM (KNOCK KNEES)

Genu **valgum (valgus deformity)**, or "knock knees," is the opposite of genu varum (**Figure 20-11**).

- Affected children present with "knees kissing."
- Affected children often run with an abnormal gait.

Classification

- Physiologic
- Asymmetric growth, such as that following trauma or infection
- Metabolic disorders
- Skeletal dysplasia
- Neuromuscular deformity, such as due to cerebral palsy

Treatment

The treatment modalities are both nonsurgical and surgical.

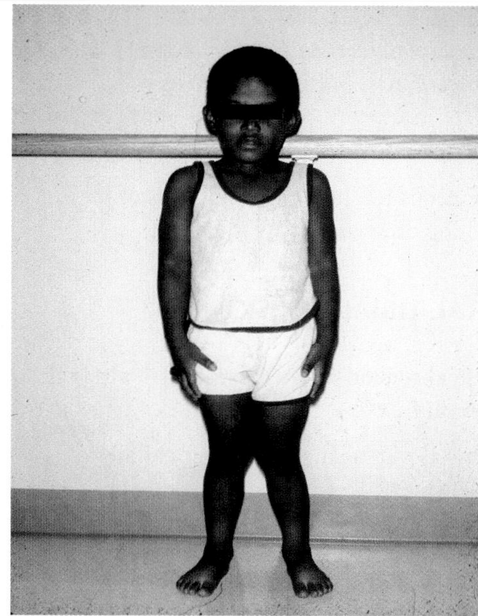

Figure 20-11 Genu valgum.

Nonsurgical Options

- Nonsurgical treatment options for children ages 2–10 include:
    - *Observation*
    - *Orthosis (controversial)*

Surgical Options

- Surgical treatment options for children ages 11–13 include:
    - *Medial physeal stapling*
    - *Medial physeal hemiepiphysiodesis*
    - *Osteotomy*

Differences Between Normal Knock Knees and Deformity

The following features differentiate between normal physiologic knock knees versus deformity:

- Normal variant (2–7 years)
- Asymptomatic
- Treatment rarely indicated in physiologic

CALCANEOVALGUS FOOT

Calcaneovalgus foot is one of the most common causes of foot deformity involving out-toeing.

- Clinically, this deformity is not classically considered as problematic in terms of growth and development, but to children and families it may hinder sports performance and cause untoward sociological concern.
- It is most often attributed to in utero positioning variants:
    - *One foot against the wall of the uterus*

- *Dorsiflexed, everted foot*
- *Lateral tibial torsion (usually flexible) (see* ***Figure 20-12****)*
- *Spontaneous resolution after delivery*

Treatment

- Spontaneous resolution (2–6 months of life)
- Stretching exercises (rarely indicated)

LATERAL TIBIAL TORSION

Lateral tibial torsion is often associated with calcaneovalgus foot deformity.

- Presents as out-toeing in younger children.
- The deformity does not cause lifelong problems.
- It usually resolves once the children reach walking age at about 18 to 24 months.
- The treatment in older children is a tibial osteotomy to derotate the limb into the correct neutral alignment.
- The condition does not change an individual's performance abilities or cause problems later in life, such as arthritis.

HIP DYSPLASIA

Hip dysplasia can be either congenital in nature (hereditary) or due to in utero positioning.

- It also has been called developmental dislocating hips (DDH) and congenital dislocating hips (CDH) (*see* **Figure 20-13**).
- The etiology of hip dysplasia development is multifactorial.
- Some features can result from a combination of mechanical factors, physiologic factors, and postnatal positioning.
- Therefore, the condition can be subtle and is often missed or misdiagnosed because initially infants are symptom free.

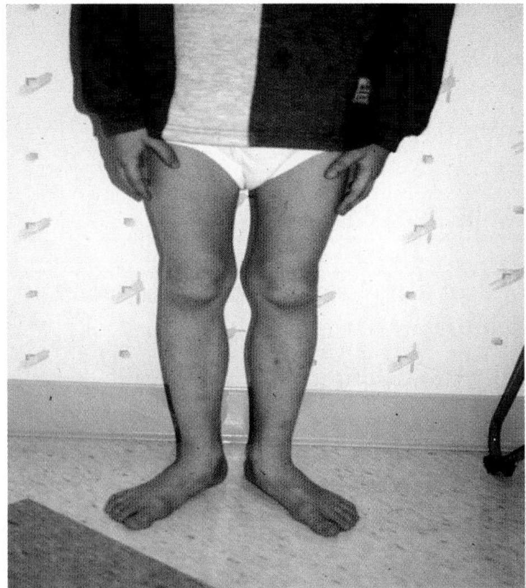

Figure 20-12 External tibial toeing.

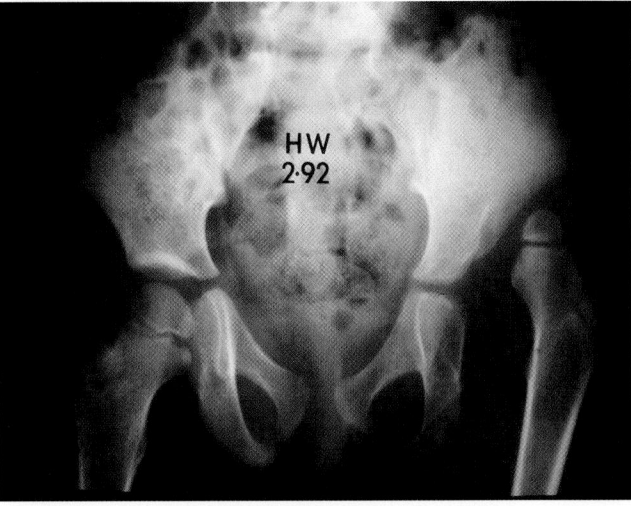

Figure 20-13 X-ray of dislocated hip.

- Pelvic x-rays after age 6 weeks assist with diagnoses.
- Dynamic ultrasound used for diagnosis <6 weeks of age.

Risk Factors

- The following are several risk factors that may be related to the development of hip dysplasia (Guille, Pizzutillo, & MacEwen, 1999):
  - *Firstborn child*
  - *Female gender (ratio of 6:1 to 8:1); 80% of affected children are female.*
  - *Left side affected*
  - *Breech presentation*
  - *Limited hip motion*
  - *Petite-sized mother with or without low amniotic fluid or gestation of multiples; maternal hormones and additional estrogen secretion of the female infant's uterus*
  - *Family history*
  - *Generalized ligament laxity*
  - *Neuromuscular disorders*
  - *Extension/adduction cradle boards*
  - *Geographical traditions (coastal)*
  - *Seasonal patterns (winter)*
- Neuromuscular conditions can cause gradual development of hip dysplasia.
  - *Children with neurologic conditions such as cerebral palsy or myelodysplasia could develop hip subluxation or dislocation.*
  - *The spasticity in children with cerebral palsy overpowers the muscles that keep the femoral head located in the socket.*
  - *Tone control is helpful, but patients may need more aggressive treatment options to slow down the progression.*
  - *Some may develop hip pain in the future or higher incidences of arthritis without treatment.*
  - *Surgical intervention is common before the hip dislocates in a growing child to prevent femoral head and acetabular deformities.*

- *Children with myelodysplasia may develop this disorder due to the inherent loss of muscle and nerve innervation caused by the condition.*
- *Children with certain levels of deformity are at higher risk.*
- *However, many may live either sedentary or ambulatory lives without any problems or procedural treatment interventions.*

Clinical Presentation

Clinical presentations most commonly observed in children with hip dysplasia include:

- Limited hip abduction
- Asymmetrical thigh skinfolds (number not size)
- Absence of knee flexion contractures (normal infants have some contraction)
- **Barlow test**—measures hip stability along with Ortolani test
- **Ortolani test**—dislocated
- **Galeazzi sign**—uneven knee heights in bent-knee position
- Infants must be calm to elicit tests.

Treatment

- Pavlik harness (**Figure 20-14**)
- Bryant's traction
- Spica cast
- Surgery

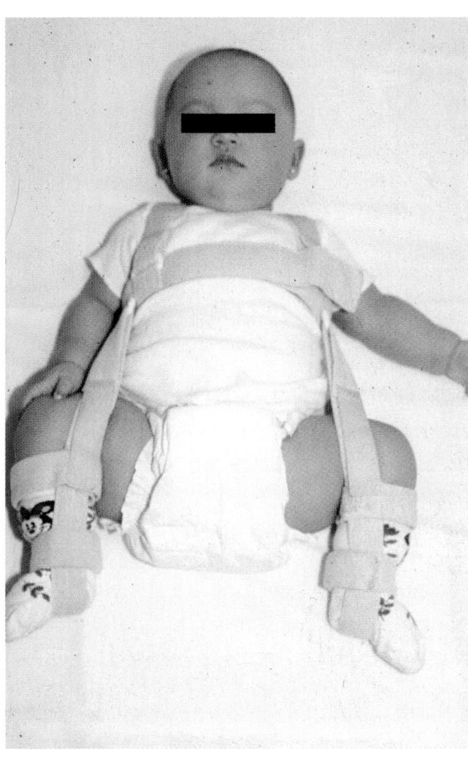

Figure 20-14 Example of the Pavlik harness.

LEGG-CALVÉ-PERTHES (LCP) DISEASE

Legg-Calvé-Perthes (LCP) disease is a loss of blood supply to the femoral head (**Figure 20-15**).

- Etiology is unknown.
- Most common cause of limping
- May or may not be painful
- Seen often in young boys aged 2 to 9

Incidence

- Male-to-female ratio of 5:1 (Mehlman & McCourt, 2010)
- Mean age 7 years; often children 4 to 8 years of age affected due to standard deviation from mean
- Unilateral, 90%; bilateral, 10%
- Family history, 3%
- Differences from one country to another
- Ethnicity most common: Caucasians, Orientals, Eskimos (Rowe et al., 2005)
- Ethnicity least common: Blacks, Indians, Polynesians (Rowe et al., 2005)

CULTURAL AWARENESS: Etiology

Multiple theories exist regarding causation of Legg-Calvé-Perthes disease. Incidence and geography are also widely varied. Some centers claim no causation; others note either thrombolytic components or trauma as causative factors. Geographical locations have noted higher and lower incidences of cases: "Rates that are four times higher than [in] Korea have consistently been noted in Great Britain" (Mehlman & McCourt, 2010).

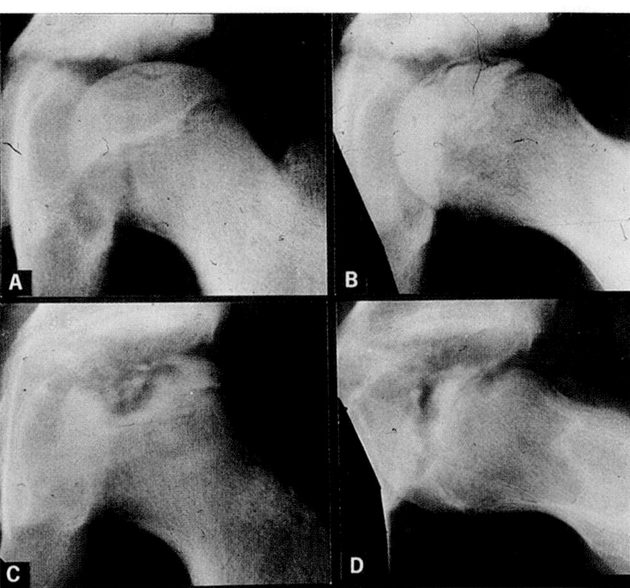

Figure 20-15 Legg-Calvé-Perthes disease.

Clinical Presentation

- Pain
  - *Sudden*
  - *Can be referred to groin, thigh, knee*
  - *Increases with movement*
  - *Decreases with rest*
  - *Not similar to pain of internal hip rotation*
  - *Limp*
- Decreased ROM
  - *Hip abduction*
  - *Hip internal rotation*

Avascular Necrosis (AVN)

The process of AVN may take up to 2 years to develop and then remodel.

- The end result may be dependent on severity based on the child's age of development.
- The femoral head sometimes appears as oddly shaped.
- The femur neck shaft is usually widened and the femoral head more ovoid in shape.
- The younger the child is at the time of diagnosis, the better the outcome.
- The AVN process occurs over approximately 1 to 4 years and has telltale stages of development and rebuilding (remodeling): prenecrosis, necrosis, and[space]revascularization.
  - *Prenecrosis*
    - Insult causing loss of blood supply
  - *Necrosis*
    - Femoral head without blood supply
    - Femoral head structurally intact
    - Asymptomatic
    - Radiographs may be normal.
  - *Revascularization (1- to 4-year process)*
    - New bone deposition
    - Dead bone reabsorption
    - Femoral head weak and susceptible to pathologic fracture
  - *Bone healing*
    - Reossification occurs gradually.
    - Reabsorption stops.
    - Bone returns to normal strength.
- Remodeling
  - *The younger the age of development, the greater the potential for remodeling.*
- The child usually presents with limping plus or minus hip, thigh, or knee pain.
- Patients have good days and bad days.
- The condition waxes and wanes for months to years.
- The goal is to keep the femoral head in the hip socket to maintain a good hip joint and decrease the risk of permanent deformity to the femoral head and acetabulum.
- The classification of LCP disease is Catterall and Salter/Thompson (Salter & Thompson, 1984).

Treatment

Treatment goals are:

- Eliminate hip irritation (pain).
- Restore and maintain ROM.
- Prevent collapse of the capital femoral epiphysis (proximal femur growth plate).
- Attain a spherical femoral head.
- Contain the femoral head in the rim of the acetabulum.

Treatment modalities include:

- Traction—Bryant's or Buck's
- Bracing is controversial (Hardesty, Liu, & Thompson, 2011).
- Casting—Petrie casts changed every 6 to 12 weeks
- Surgery—proximal femoral derotational osteotomy

SLIPPED CAPITAL FEMORAL EPIPHYSIS (SCFE)

- **Slipped capital femoral epiphysis (SCFE)** is a hip deformity of childhood (**Figure 20-16**).
- The epidemiology is widespread due to both environmental and neurologic factors.

Risk Factors and Incidence

The following factors increase the incidence:

- Adolescent onset
  - *Males 10 to 16 years old*
  - *Females 10 to 14 years old*
- Populations—African Americans and males
- Incidence is bilateral in 25% to 30% of cases (Gettys, Jackson, & Frick, 2011).
- Obesity
- Developmental delay

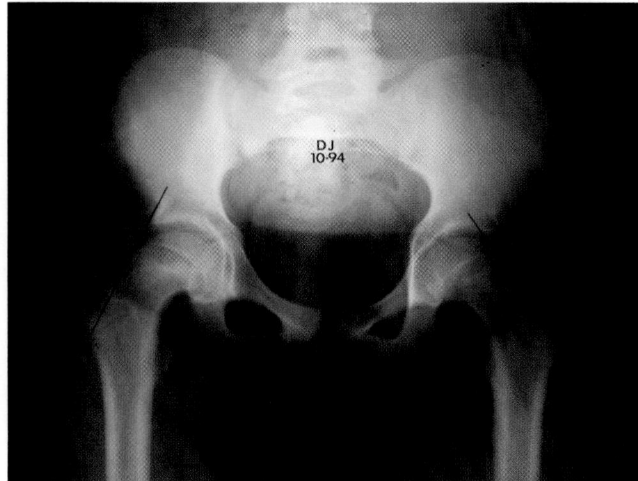

Figure 20-16 Slipped capital femoral epiphysis.

Etiology

- Idiopathic—most common
  - *Obesity*
  - *Juvenile hormonal changes*
- Endocrine problems
- Radiation exposure
- Chemotherapy

Clinical Presentation

- Anterior thigh and knee pain
- Antalgic gait
- Externally rotated lower leg
- Decreased ROM in hip(s)

Treatment

The treatment goals are:

- Stabilize the hip joint.
- Promote epiphysiodesis.
- Avoid complications.
- Improve hip function.

TRANSIENT MONOARTICULAR SYNOVITIS

Transient monoarticular synovitis is the most common cause of acute-onset short-duration limping in children.

- It is more common in males than females.
- The average age of onset is 6 years (can range from 2 to 12).
  - *The etiology is nonspecific* ***synovitis*** *or hip irritation.*
- Classified as
  - *Allergic*
  - *Viral-like—following an upper respiratory infection (URI) or other minor ailment*
  - *Result of a minor trauma*

Clinical Presentation

The following clinical presentations are indicative of typical toxic synovitis:

- Mild limp
- Low-grade fever (38°C)
- Anterior thigh or knee pain
- Irritable hip (positive roll test)
- Mild limb rotation (favored position is to hold the lower leg turned outward)

Different Disorders That May Cause Limping

- Septic arthritis
- Osteomyelitis
- Legg-Calvé-Perthes disease

Diagnostic Testing

- Normal complete blood count (CBC) and differential
- Elevated erythrocyte sedimentation rate (ESR)
- Negative arthrocentesis (negative cultures, no crystals)

Treatment

- Bedrest for 7 to 10 days
- Traction
- Bone scan

SEPTIC ARTHRITIS AND OSTEOMYELITIS OF THE HIP

Septic arthritis and **osteomyelitis** of the hip are acute orthopedic emergencies. Delay of treatment in both cases can cause severe deformity and even death. Both are primarily seen in infants and can follow an antecedent illness by several weeks.

Clinical Presentation

The following are clinical presentations in infants:

- Irritable; refuses to eat
- Hip flexion contracture
- Abduction and externally rotated position of comfort
- Pain with hip ROM
- Erythema, edema
- Minimal fever but may progressively get worse
- Child may look septic.
- Normal CBC

Clinical presentations in children:

- Limp—may refuse to walk or bear weight
- History of trauma, surgery, or infection
- Hip abnormality
  - *Flexed*
  - *Abducted*
  - *Externally rotated*
- Pain with hip ROM, especially internal rotation
- Febrile, toxic
- Positive leukocytosis

Treatment

Treatment of choice is to admit urgently to the hospital for care:

- Emergency surgery for incision and drainage (I&D)
- Drainage or repeat I&D every 1 to 3 days
- Systemic antibiotics coverage, usually via peripherally inserted central catheter (PICC) line for 3 to 12 weeks, depending on organism growth, followed by oral therapy
- Maintenance of hip motion

Prognosis is determined by several factors:

- Age of onset
- Site of initial infection

- Delay of diagnosis
- Organisms present
- "By far the most common bacterial pathogen causing osteomyelitis in children is *Staphylococcus aureus* in all age groups." While "Group A streptococcus (especially complicating varicella), *Streptococcus pneumoniae*, and the emerging pathogen *Kingella kingae* are the next most common organisms in infants and children. Group B streptococcus and gram-negative enterics are common causes of osteomyelitis in the neonatal period." (Kaplan, 2005).
- Patients are followed closely after hospital discharge, usually by both pediatric orthopedics and infectious disease, until lab levels have returned to normal and full restoration of pain-free ROM of the hip occurs.
- The length of antibiotic treatment both IV and then orally depends on the severity of the infection and the type of organisms involved.
- Most children need yearly follow-up after treatment to be sure the hip joint and bony anatomical features develop correctly.

SCOLIOSIS

Scoliosis is a term that describes curvature of the spine (**Figure 20-17**). It is a deviation from normal spinal alignment (Driscoll & Skinner, 2008).

- It can occur in several different groups:
  - *Congenital or infantile*
  - *Idiopathic or adolescent*
  - *Neuromuscular*

Scoliosis is predominantly considered idiopathic in origin, meaning it occurs for no known reason. Yet some other diagnoses, such as torticollis and hip dysplasia, occur with spinal curves, such that some experts feel this can be a result of the intrauterine molding relationships seen in many other musculoskeletal disorders.

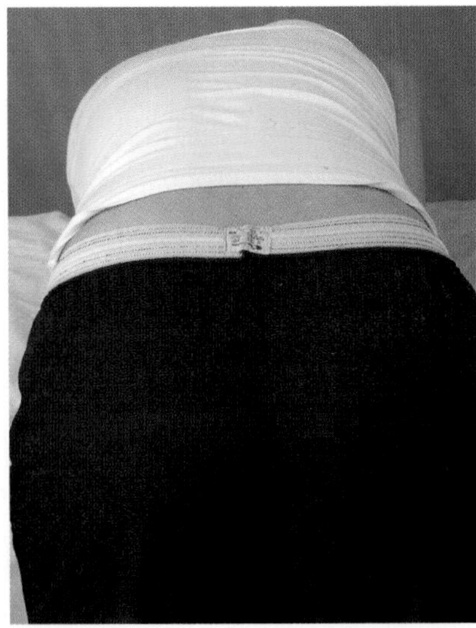

Figure 20-17 Adolescent with obvious scoliosis.

CONGENITAL OR INFANTILE SCOLIOSIS

Congenital or infantile scoliosis is described as occurring before age 6 months.

- It can be either genetic or due to the intrauterine or external uterine forces applied to infants during growth and development.
- Clinical evaluation at well-infant checkups by a health-care professional or parent observation usually detects deviation from normal infant anatomy.
- X-rays determine the level of severity of the curvature.
- A complete neurologic exam is crucial to rule out other deformities or conditions.
- Severe cases are evaluated with MRI scans, especially left-sided curves.
- The curvature is measured using the Cobb Method of angles to the deformity, usually in an S-shaped curve.
- Measured from the thoracic-to-lumbar curvature and lumbar-to-sacral curvature.

Clinical Presentation

Infantile scoliosis features (Larson, 2011):

- Idiopathic
- Rare condition
- More common in Europe versus United States
- Left sided—more common in infants
- Girls with right sided—worse prognosis

Treatment

- Bracing—thoracolumbosacral orthosis (TLSO)
- Casting—Risser cast
- Surgical instrumentation—growing rods, changed every 6 months
- Definitive spinal fusion

JUVENILE SCOLIOSIS

Juvenile scoliosis is a spinal curvature commonly diagnosed between ages 3 and 9.

Risk Factors and Incidence

Some identifying features include:

- Juvenile scoliosis is more common than infantile but less common than adolescent.
- Accounts for 10% to 15% of all idiopathic cases (Colliard, Circo, & Rivard, 2010)
- Occurs during a period of less significant growth pattern
- More common in adolescent females versus males
- In several periods of time, the female-to-male ratio is divided (Colliard et al., 2010).

- Tends to be right sided, but children with left-sided curves fare better than those with right-sided ones
- Not painful
- Common progression

Clinical Presentation

- Forward bend test; characteristic rib hump
- Asymmetrical shoulder heights
- Asymmetrical pelvic obliquity (first r/o scoliosis due to leg-length difference)
- Decreased ROM of upper trunk (e.g., leans forward and back and side to side or twists with difficulty)
- Radiographs reveal >10 degree curve, usually S or C shaped.

Treatment

Treatment options are based on the time of diagnosis, age of child, and likelihood of progression:

- Observation for minor curves of 15 to 25 degrees
- Bracing for flexible moderate curves of 25 degrees plus, such as with thoracic lumbar sacral orthotic (TLSO)
- Risser cast for rigid curves, changed every 6 to 12 weeks and followed by bracing
- Surgical intervention—instrumentation such as rods, or definitive fusion
- Generally speaking, with correct diagnosis and treatment options for juvenile scoliosis, good outcomes are the norm.
- Many children grow up without any limitations and are able to participate in active lifestyles.

ADOLESCENT IDIOPATHIC SCOLIOSIS (AIS)

Adolescent idiopathic scoliosis (AIS) is a condition that affects children age 9 through young adulthood.

- This curvature can be S or C shaped laterally to either side, left or right.
- Most common type of scoliosis
- Accounts for 80% of all idiopathic scoliosis; prevalence of 2% to 4% of adolescents aged 10 to 16 (Arlet & Reddi, 2007)
- Usually undetected, as affected children are very active and it is a pain-free condition.
- May be detected early on in puberty or during periods of rapid growth such as a growth spurt.
- It occurs more commonly in girls than boys (Arlet & Reddi, 2007).

NEUROMUSCULAR SCOLIOSIS

Neuromuscular scoliosis can occur in children with neurologic conditions at any age and at any stage of growth and development.

- The potential for curve progression is less accurately defined.
- It is especially increased in children with cerebral palsy (CP) or myelodysplasia.

JUVENILE IDIOPATHIC ARTHRITIS

Juvenile idiopathic arthritis (JIA, formerly JRA) is a common diagnosis for pain and inflammation in multiple joints.

- Presentation can be seen as early as 2 years old.
- The most common reason to be seeking care is on-and-off joint pain in several different joints for many months.
- It may involve only one joint at initial presentation.
- The most common first areas of complaints of pain are the ankles, knees, and hips.
- It can present unilateral but often bilateral is the chief complaint.
- Weiss and Ilowite (2007) note that "JIA is the most common chronic rheumatic illness in children and is a significant cause of short- and long-term disability."
- It is regarded as a complex genetic trait, with multiple genes causing inflammation and immune response.
- Some literature has implied that certain people are more genetically prone to develop JIA by triggers of stress, abnormal hormone levels, trauma to a joint, or infections (Lang & Shore, 1990; Weiss & Ilowite, 2007).

Diagnostic Testing

Laboratory tests common in evaluation of rheumatic conditions are:

- CBC with differential
- Antinuclear Antibody (ANA) titer
- Rheumatoid factor
- Human Leukocyte Antigen (HLA B27)
- Compliment Component 3 (C3) and Compliment Component 4 (C4)
- Epstein-Barr Virus (EBV) titer
- ESR

Children with JIA should be monitored for:

- Nutritional deficits
- Uveitis
- Growth disturbances, including delayed puberty
- Psychological concerns due to the chronicity of the disease and active disease causing functional limitations

Clinical Reasoning

Physical Activity and JIA

A 17-year-old female wants to participate in tennis but has frequent elbow effusions and chronic pain, causing her to feel powerless and isolated. She is depressed and wants to quit the team that she has been on for several years.

1. How can the nurse assist the teenager with full activity participation and safely protect her bones and joints?

Treatment

Treatment goals include:

- Controlling pain and inflammation
- Preserving function
- Promoting normal growth and development
- Promoting psychological well-being

Evidence-Based Practice: Treatment Options for JIA

Weiss, J. E., & Ilowite, N. T. (2007). Juvenile idiopathic arthritis. *Rheumatic Disease Clinics of North America, 33,* 441–470. doi: 10.1016/j.rdc.2007.07.006

Weiss and Ilowite (2007) categorized the following treatment options:

- Therapeutic modalities
  - Physical therapy and occupational therapy as vital adjuncts to all medical treatment options
  - Splints
  - Arthroplasty
- Nonsteroidal anti-inflammatory medications (NSAIDs)
- Glucocorticoids
- Disease-modifying antirheumatic agents (DMARDs)
- Sulfasalazine
- Methotrexate
- Leflunomide
- Biologic agents
- EtanerceptInfliximab
- Adalimumab
- Anakinra
- Humanized anti-interleukin-6 receptor antibody
- Autologous stem cell transplantation (ASCT)

1. If a child is poorly controlled on NSAIDs, is ASCT a viable option?
2. Is ASCT therapy safe?

OSTEOGENESIS IMPERFECTA

Osteogenesis imperfecta (OI), also called brittle bone disease, is an inherited disorder. It is considered to be the result of a collagen defect or dominant gene mutation.

- The disorder is classified into types I through VI, denoting mild to severe in its symptomatology.
- Some children diagnosed with OI have no known hereditary linkage.
- Fractures commonly are noted at birth via the birth canal, such as fractures of the shoulder or humerus, clavicle, and femur.
- The fractures occur although very little external trauma is present.
- Often, infants are sent home and then present in the emergency department with the chief complaint of inability to move an upper extremity or a swollen and painful lower extremity.
- This often prompts social work to get involved and/or a child protection team to rule out physical child abuse before a diagnosis of OI.
- Many families are traumatized by the negative social implication and then are shocked by the diagnosis of a chronic genetic disorder.
- The infant can also present with "blue sclera" that is harder to detect in some infants.
- Without a known family history, the diagnosis is sometimes made later in infancy or even at toddler age if the OI is a very mild case.
- OI can also be very severe.
- Children with severe OI have multiple fractures of the long bones of the body multiple times, often in short time periods.
- These multiple fractures can lead to growth plate deformities or unusual bowing of the extremities, especially in all four extremities.
- Labwork can assist in the diagnosis of OI.
- Sometimes the diagnosis is exhibited in utero as displayed by ultrasound, with identification of bowing or unusual shortness of the long bones.
- Specific types are diagnosed at certain gestational weeks.
- The more severe the type, the more identifiable the clinical presentation may be, but trained ultrasonographers may be the caveat.

Nursing Intervention

Promoting Safety

Nursing interventions to promote the safety of a child with OI include:

- Use noninvasive blood pressure measures when appropriate.
- Use caution when repositioning.
- Alert ancillary staff about precautions to prevent injury, such as during phlebotomy procedures.
- Fall-prevention education for all age groups.

- Nursing care in the hospital should be directed at demonstrating to the families gentle holding positions and, if severe OI, avoiding or limiting procedures that could "squeeze" extremities and induce fractures.
- Procedures can be minimally invasive, as manual and automatic blood pressure readings, or more invasive, such as placing IVs or obtaining radiographs.
- The OI Foundation's website, http://www.oif.org, has wonderful and detailed brochures for parents, health-care providers, and daycare centers/schools.
- The OI Foundation is a champion for people living with OI, providing advocacy in research, education, awareness, and family support.

SPORTS-RELATED INJURIES

More children are getting involved in competitive sports at younger ages. The number of children involved in year-round sports has also increased due to the availability of indoor arenas such as those for soccer and baseball.

- Common orthopedic injuries in children are:
  - **Sprains and strains**
  - *Dislocations and subluxations*
  - *Tears*
  - *Fractures*
  - *Hematomas*
  - *Overuse injuries—Little Leaguer's elbow, tendonitis, and growth plate fractures*

Clinical Presentation

- Swelling
- Pain
- Ecchymosis
- Mechanism of injury often rolled the ankle into inversion
- Treatment options—splint, cast, boot; graduate to sports lace-up ankle brace
- Prevention—physical therapy and more physical therapy

Dislocations and Subluxations

- Mechanism of injury—hyperextension or pulling, or varus/valgus stress
- Pain
- Swelling
- Nursemaid's elbow versus Ehlers–Danlos Syndrome; toddler versus adolescent
- Treatment usually requires sedation in emergency room for true dislocation to be relocated.
- Prevention—occupational therapy and physical therapy to strengthen and prevent recurrence
- Surgical intervention for repeated dislocation or subluxation—either bony or soft tissue procedures

Tears and Contusions

- Mechanism of injury—usually foot planted and body continues moving forward or some type of twisting injury
- Usually hear or feel "pop"
- Pain
- Swelling
- Diagnostic testing: x-rays and MRI
- Treatment (surgical vs. nonsurgical)
- Prevention
- Continued sports participation dependent on injury and severity

Overuse Injuries

- Mechanism of injury—repetitive forces such as in pitching, tennis, diving, gymnastics
- Evaluate for intensity, duration, and magnitude of training
- Proper coaching
- Occur when activity levels exceed the body's ability to recover
- Prevention
  - *Tips for prevention of overuse injuries in pediatric and adolescent athletes:*
    - Do warm-up exercises before you play any sport.
    - Always stretch before play or exercise.
    - Do not overdo it.
    - Cool down after hard sports or workouts.
    - Wear shoes and equipment that fit properly, are stable, and have good shock absorption.
    - Learn to do your sport right; use proper form; if unsure, ask coach or trainer for help.
    - Know your body's limits.
    - Build up your exercise level gradually.
    - Do a total-body workout consisting of cardiovascular, strength-training, and flexibility exercises.
    - Get a physical exam before you start playing competitive sports.
    - Follow the rules of the game.
    - Don't play if you're tired or in pain.
    - Resource: Fast Facts: An Easy-to-Read Series of Publications for the Public, available at http://www.niams.nih.gov

■ ■ ■ Review Questions ■ ■ ■

1. A firstborn female infant is brought into the primary physician's office for a well-child visit. The physician has difficulty abducting the left hip and notes asymmetrical thigh skinfolds. The physical exam demonstrates a "clunk" with abduction. The mother is concerned that upon diapering, she feels like the "hip is not right." The infant is most likely diagnosed with

A. slipped capital femoral epiphysis (SCFE).
B. developmental dislocated hip (DDH).
C. Legg-Calvé-Perthes (LCP) disease.
D. femoral anteversion.

2. You are seeing a 2 ½-year-old male child. The parent tells you that the boy has in-toeing and is bowlegged. The grandparents in the room insist the father had the same thing and was treated with a "bar and boots" from ages 1 to 4. They all are anxious about the problem. As the nurse with knowledge of normal growth and development, you would consider that this is

A. normal for a toddler, and no treatment is needed.
B. genu valgus.
C. a hereditary birth defect, and bracing should begin immediately.
D. a developmental dislocated hip (DDH)

3. A 6-year-old boy who comes to the clinic has been limping off and on for several months. The limping lasts several hours to several days, and the leg stops hurting once he sits down. He is an active soccer player and loves to run around. His mother is concerned because he stops playing soccer when it hurts. She is concerned that he may have "broke something." Physical examination demonstrates limited internal rotation. X-ray examination reveals avascular necrosis (AVN). Therefore you know the diagnosis is
   A. developmental dislocated hip (DDH).
   B. slipped capital femoral epiphysis (SCFE).
   C. Legg-Calvé-Perthes (LCP) syndrome.
   D. toxic synovitis.

4. A 1-week-old infant with a fetal ultrasound report describing clubfeet is in the clinic. The family history is positive for father with unilateral clubfoot treated as an infant. The mother is crying and anxious because the infant's grandmother told her terrible things about the treatment when her husband was a baby. You want to calm the mother down and allow her time to grieve and then explain which of the following about clubfoot?
   A. There is a hereditary component in 50% of cases.
   B. Clubfoot is easily treated with serial casting and possibly minor surgical repair to lengthen the Achilles tendon.
   C. The infant will be fully functional by walking age.
   D. The infant will not remember the treatment provided.
   E. All of the above

5. An 8-year-old female is seen in the emergency room with pain and swelling to her right wrist. She claims she fell off the monkey bars and landed on an outstretched arm (FOOSH injury). She is holding her arm carefully and crying. X-rays reveal no abnormality but she is tender on palpation at her distal physis. Your understanding of children with open growth plates and cartilaginous bone qualities makes you realize which of the following?
   A. She probably has strained her wrist.
   B. She probably sustained a Salter Harris I growth plate fracture.
   C. She probably wants a doll and her mother said no.
   D. Children heal their bones quickly; therefore another x-ray in a few weeks may reveal the healing bone.
   E. Both B and D

6. A 2-year-old child presents to the specialist's office with parental concern of gross motor delays. He is not yet walking. As an infant, the child underwent a difficult labor/delivery and required oxygen for several days postpartum. Apgar scores were 2 and 4, then 8 and 10. Mother reports baby looked "blue" upon delivery. She also reports that the infant sat up at 9 months and stood up at 18 months, but that he stands with his feet "scissored" and throws his head back when startled or laughing. She reports that he clenches his fists a lot too, especially when she plays "peek-a-boo." The nurse anticipates a diagnosis of
   A. femoral torsion.
   B. developmental dislocated hip (DDH).
   C. cerebral palsy (CP).
   D. meningocele.

7. A 14-year-old morbidly obese male presents to the emergency room with acute onset of severe left hip pain. He reports no trauma. He has had mild pain for the last few months. He limps into the room with his left leg turned outward. On physical exam he has pain with internal rotation. His vital signs are stable. There is no fever. X-rays are done of his pelvis. Based on his age and presenting symptoms, the most likely diagnosis for this patient is which of the following?
   A. Developmental dislocated hip (DDH)
   B. Osteomyelitis
   C. Acute stable slipped capital femoral epiphysis (SCFE)
   D. Tibial torsion

8. An 11-year-old female presents to the clinic with a chief complaint of back pain. She is pre-menarchal. Her mother started her menses around age 13. Her mother noticed that her daughter's ribs looked a little different on one side this summer in her bathing suit. Family history is negative for any bone or joint problems. She has a 19-year-old sibling who was treated for back pain a year ago with physical therapy. Understanding the physiology of bone and joint disorders, what diagnosis would you reasonably expect?
   A. Idiopathic juvenile scoliosis
   B. Compression fracture L5
   C. Leg-length discrepancy
   D. Ligament strain
   E. Both A and C

9. An 11-year-old female presents to the clinic with a chief complaint of back pain. She is pre-menarchal. Her mother started her menses around age 13. Her mother noticed that her daughter's ribs looked a little different on one side this summer in her bathing suit. Family history is negative for any bone or joint problems. She has a 19-year-old sibling who was treated for back pain a year ago with physical therapy. The x-rays demonstrate a 32-degree scoliotic curve. The physician recommends bracing. After the brace is fitted, the following statement by the child demonstrates her correct understanding of scoliosis:
   A. "If I wear the brace as instructed, I will never need surgery."
   B. "If I wear the brace as instructed, my curve will never increase."
   C. "If I wear the brace as instructed, my surgery will fail."
   D. "If I wear the brace as instructed, my curve will stabilize and I won't need surgery right away."

10. A 4-year-old female presents to the emergency room with a history of ear infection 2 weeks ago, which was treated with oral antibiotics. She now has severe right knee pain and swelling. She cannot walk on that leg. She is febrile at 39°C. Her mother tried ibuprofen and acetaminophen, but neither is working. The little girl woke up this morning in extreme pain and has been inconsolable all day. Her labs are: ESR 60, CRP 13, and WBC >13,000. Her clinical and laboratory picture are consistent with the diagnosis of which of the following?
   A. Slipped capital femoral epiphysis (SCFE)
   B. Anterior cruciate ligament (ACL) tear
   C. Septic arthritis
   D. Fever of unknown origin

References

Arlet, V., & Reddi, V. (2007). Adolescent idiopathic scoliosis. *Neurosurgery Clinics of North America, 18*, 255–259. doi: 10.1016/j.nec.2007.02.002

Colliard, C., Circo, A., & Rivard, C. (2010). SpinCor treatment for juvenile idiopathic scoliosis: SOSORT award 2010 winner. *Scoliosis Journal, 5*, 25. doi: 10.1186/1748-7161-5-25

Driscoll, S. W., & Skinner, J. (2008). Musculoskeletal complications of neuromuscular disease in children. *Physical Medicine and Rehabilitation Clinics of North America, 19*, 163–194. doi: 10.1016/j.pmr.2007.10.003

Gettys, F., Jackson, J., & Frick, S. (2011). Obesity in pediatric orthopaedics. *Orthopaedic Clinics of North America, 42*, 95–105. doi: 10.1016/j.ocl.2010.08.005

Guille, J., Pizzutillo, P., & MacEwen, D. (1999). Developmental dysplasia of the hip from birth to six months. *Journal of the American Academy of Orthopaedic Surgeons, 8*, 232–242. Retrieved from http://jaaos.org/content/8/4/232.abstract

Hardesty, C. K., Liu, R. W., & Thompson, G. H. (2011). The role of bracing in Legg-Calvé-Perthes disease. *Journal of Pediatric Orthopaedics, 31*, S178-S181. doi: 10.1097/BPO.0b013e318223b5b1

Kaplan, S. L. (2005). Osteomyelitis in children. *Infectious Disease Clinics of North America, 19*, 787–797. doi: 10.1016/j.idc.2005.07.006

Kliegman, R. M., Stanton, B. M. D., St. Geme, J., Schor, N., & Behrman, R. E. (2011). *Nelson textbook of pediatrics* (19th ed.). Philadelphia, PA: W. B. Saunders.

Kocher, M., Sink, E., Blasier, R., Luhmann, S. J., Mehlman, C. T., Scher, D. M., . . . Hitchcock, K. (2009). Treatment of pediatric diaphyseal femur fractures. *Journal of the American Academy of Orthopaedic Surgeons, 17*, 718–725. Retrieved from http://www.jaaos.org/content/17/11/718.abstract

Kunes, J. (2011). Pitfalls in assessing common pediatric fractures. *Journal of Urgent Care Medicine, 1*. Retrieved from http://www.jucm.com/

Lang, B. A., & Shore, A. (1990). A review of current concepts on the pathogenesis of juvenile rheumatoid arthritis. *Journal of Rheumatology; 21*, 1–15. Retrieved from http://www.ncbi.nlm.nih.gov/pubmed/2185362

Larson, N. (2011). Early onset scoliosis: What the primary care provider needs to know and implications for practice. *Journal of the American Academy of Nurse Practitioners, 23*, 392–403. doi: 10.1111/j.1745-7599.2011.00634.x

Lincoln, T. L., & Suen, P. W. (2003). Common rotational variations in children. *Journal of the American Academy of Orthopaedic Surgeons, 11*, 312–320. Retrieved from http://jaaos.org/content/11/5/312.abstract

Mehlman, C., & McCourt, J. (2010). Legg-Calvé-Perthes disease: Where are we 100 years later? *The Orthopod, 18*, 30–35. Retrieved from http://www.jaaos.org/content/18/11/643.citation

Rowe, S. M., Jung, S. T., Lee, K. B., Bai, B. H., Cheon, S, Y., & Kang, K. D. (2005). The incidence of Perthes' disease in Korea. A focus on differences among races. *Journal of Bone and Joint Surgery, 87-B*, 1666-1668. doi: 10.1302/0301-620X.87B12.16808

Salter, R. B., & Thompson, G. H. (1984). Legg-Calvé-Perthes disease: The prognostic significance of the subchondral fracture and a two-group classification of the femoral head involvement. *Journal of Bone Joint Surgery, 66*, 479–489. Retrieved from http://www.ncbi.nlm.nih.gov/pubmed/6707027

Staheli, L. T. (2006). *Practice of pediatric orthopedics* (2nd ed., pp. 8–10). Philadelphia, PA: Lippincott Williams and Wilkins.

Staheli, L. T., & Hensinger, R. N. (2001). Fractures in children. *Journal of Pediatric Orthopedics, 21*, 1. Retrieved from http://journals.lww.com/pedorthopaedics/Citation/2001/01000/From_the_Editors.1.aspx

Weiss, J. E., & Ilowite, N. T. (2007). Juvenile idiopathic arthritis. *Rheumatic Disease Clinics of North America, 33*, 441–470. doi: 10.1016/j.rdc.2007.07.006

Additional Resources

Herring, J. A., & Tachdjian, M. O. (2002.) *Tachdjian's pediatric orthopaedics. Texas Scottish Rite Hospital for Children* (4th ed., Vols. 1–3). Philadelphia: Saunders.

National Association of the Osteogenesis Imperfecta Foundation (1-800-981-2663), www.oif.org

National Scoliosis Foundation, www.scoliosis.org

Scoliosis Research Society, www.srs.org

Spina Bifida Association of America, www.sbaa.org

United Cerebral Palsy Foundation, www.ucp.org

National Association of Orthopaedic Nurses, www.orthonurse.org

Pediatric Orthopaedic Practitioners Society, www.pops.org

American Academy of Pediatrics, www.aap.org

National Institute of Arthritis and Musculoskeletal and Skin Diseases, www.niams.nih.gov

21 Dermatologic Diseases

Anita Mitchell, PhD, APN, FNP

OBJECTIVES

- ☐ Define key terms.
- ☐ Identify causes and precipitating factors of skin conditions and skin injuries seen in children and adolescents.
- ☐ Outline critical components of skin assessment in children and adolescents.
- ☐ Describe the clinical presentation of acquired skin diseases, skin infections and infestations, and various injuries to the skin.
- ☐ Explain diagnostic and laboratory studies used for skin conditions.
- ☐ Describe emergency care given for acute infections, bites, and burns to the skin.
- ☐ Describe care in the hospital for a child or adolescent with an acute or chronic skin condition or with an injury to the skin.
- ☐ Develop a home-based plan of care for a child or adolescent with a chronic skin condition.
- ☐ Discuss alternate therapies used for various skin conditions or injuries to the skin.
- ☐ Develop a teaching plan for caregivers of children or adolescents with skin conditions or injuries to the skin.

KEY TERMS

- Epidermis
- Papules
- Vesicles
- Pustules
- Dermis
- Nodules
- Macules
- Wheals
- Braden Q Scale
- Dermatitis
- Erythema
- Intertriginous
- Pruritus

ASSESSMENT

General History

Ask about the following issues:

- General health of child
- Date or time of onset of symptoms
- Growth or changes in rash or lesions
- Presence of itching
- Recent immunizations or medications
- Allergies
- Recent illness
- Similar rash or lesions in family members

Physical Examination

- Distribution or pattern of rash over body
- Are lesions on flexural or extensor surfaces of the body?
- Are lesions clustered (herpetiform) or scattered (diffuse)?
- Do lesions follow a dermatomal (nerve) pattern?
- Are lesions in a straight line (linear), serpiginous (wavy), annular (ring-shaped), circular, or reticulated (lacy)?
- Is the **epidermis** involved? These lesions include scales, **papules**, **vesicles**, and **pustules**.
- Is the **dermis** involved? If markings on the epidermis are normal, but there is an elevated area, this points to the dermis (examples: **nodule**, tumor).
- What color are the lesions?
- Primary lesions arise from the skin itself. These include **macules**, papules, plaques, vesicles, pustules, **wheals**, and nodules.
- Secondary lesions grow out of primary lesions or occur when a primary lesion becomes irritated or injured by scratching. Secondary lesions include crusts, ulcers, fissures, and scars.
- Check for any systemic signs and symptoms such as fever, headache, decreased responsiveness, and pain (Cohen, 2005)

CLINICAL PEARL

Purpura

Purple or blue lesions that do not blanch suggest purpura.

CULTURAL AWARENESS: Assessing Pallor, Cyanosis, and Jaundice in Dark Skin

When assessing pallor, cyanosis, or jaundice in a child with dark skin, examine the palpebral conjunctivae (lower eyelids) and the oral mucosa. Jaundice may also be observed in the sclera.

CRITICAL COMPONENT

Skin Integrity and the Hospitalized Child

Skillful nursing care of a hospitalized infant or child includes constant skin assessment, prevention of skin breakdown, and management of impaired skin integrity. Noonan, Quigley, and Curley (2006) outline several areas that must be addressed when caring for a hospitalized child. These include:

- Care of surgical incisions
- Maintenance of intravenous catheters with careful monitoring for infiltration
- Maintenance of invasive tubes or probes that must be taped. Common equipment such as urinary catheters, pulse oximeter probes, and nasal tubes must be taped in place, and skin integrity is threatened when the tape is in place and when it is removed. Tape removal may damage the epithelium.
- Tracheostomies, gastrostomies, and colostomies all put the child at risk for skin breakdown due to leakage of fluids and body secretions.
- Children who are acutely or chronically ill are at risk for pressure ulcers. The most common sites for pressure ulcers in children are the ears, occiput, sacrum, and scapula.
- Diaper rash with or without candidiasis is very common in the hospitalized infant, and is made worse by antibiotics, gastrointestinal surgery, and changes in the content of urine or stool.

CLINICAL PEARL

Braden Q Scale

The **Braden Q Scale** (Curley, Razmus, Roberts, & Wypij, 2003), used for children over 1 year of age, outlines seven factors that predict the likelihood that a child will develop a pressure ulcer (**Figure 21-1**): mobility or the likelihood that a child can change his or her own body position, the degree of activity, the ability to respond in a developmentally appropriate way to uncomfortable sensations of pressure, the degree of moisture on the skin, the degree of friction or shear from moving across bed linens or other surfaces, whether or not the child is well nourished, and whether or not the child is well oxygenated and the tissues are well perfused.

CRITICAL COMPONENT

Skin Integrity in the Hospital

Nursing care to maintain skin integrity in the hospitalized infant or child:

- Change diapers and linens frequently in order to keep the skin dry.
- Use barrier creams containing zinc oxide as needed on the diaper area. It is not necessary or therapeutic to completely remove all barrier cream with each diaper change. Remove soiled areas only.
- Use water-based moisturizers for dry skin.
- Bathe the child with mild, nonalkaline, pH-balanced cleansing agents. Avoid vigorous cleaning or scrubbing.
- Pay special attention to skin around tracheostomies and other ostomies. Keep the skin clean and dry. Foam dressings may help absorb exudates around tracheostomies and gastrostomies.
- Keep the child well oxygenated and well nourished.
- If the child is confined to bed or chair, turn or change position at least every 2 hours. Elevate the head of the bed no more than 30 degrees. Lower the head of the bed before repositioning the child. Keep the heels from rubbing on surfaces, and place the child on an egg crate or air flotation mattress as needed. Pay special attention to the back of the head and ears.
- Place foam dressings over boney prominences that are at risk for breakdown.
- Minimizing taping and use gauze as an alternative when possible. Tape without tension. Use barriers such as skin preps under tape to protect the skin. Remove tape carefully to avoid stripping the epithelium.
- Monitor carefully all probes, tubes, and intravenous catheters for skin irritation or breakdown at the site. Change pulse oximeter probes every 2 hours.

Clinical Reasoning

Impaired Skin Integrity

Meticulous skin care is critical when caring for infants and children in the hospital. These children are at high risk for impaired skin integrity. For example, the nurse is caring for a 1-year-old infant who is confined to the crib. She is not able to take oral feedings, and is receiving IV fluids and IV antibiotics. She has a tracheostomy. She also has a pulse oximeter on her foot.

1. What are risk factors for impaired skin integrity for this infant?
2. How can skin breakdown be prevented?
3. In areas where skin is not intact, how can healing be promoted?

The Braden Q Scale					
Intensity and Duration of Pressure					**Score**
Mobility The ability to change and control body position	**1. Completely immobile:** Does not make even slight changes in body or extremity position without assistance.	**2. Very Limited:** Makes occasional slight changes in body or extremity position but unable to completely turn self independently.	**3. Slightly Limited:** Makes frequent though slight changes in body or extremity position independently.	**4. No Limitations:** Makes major and frequent changes in position without assistance.	
Activity The degree of physical activity	**1. Bedfast:** Confined to bed	**2. Chair fast:** Ability to walk severely limited or nonexistent. Cannot bear own weight and/or must be assisted in to chair or wheelchair.	**3. Walks Occasionally:** Walks occasionally during day, but for very short distances, with or without assistance. Spends majority of each shift in bed or chair.	**4. All patients too young to ambulate OR walks frequently:** Walks outside the room at least twice a day and inside room at least once every 2 hours during waking hours.	
Sensory Perception The ability to respond in a **developmentally** appropriate way to pressure-related discomfort	**1. Completely Limited:** Unresponsive (does not moan, flinch, or grasp) to painful stimuli, due to diminished level of consciousness or sedation **OR** limited ability to feel pain over most of body surface.	**2. Very Limited:** Responds only to painful stimuli. Cannot communicate discomfort except by moaning or restlessness **OR** has sensory impairment which limits the ability to feel pain or discomfort over half of body.	**3. Slightly Limited:** Responds to verbal commands, but cannot always communicate discomfort or need to be turned **OR** has some sensory impairment which limits ability to feel pain or discomfort in 1 or 2 extremities.	**4. No Impairment:** Responds to verbal commands. Has no sensory deficit, which limits ability to feel or communicate pain or discomfort.	
Tolerance of the Skin and Supporting Structure					
Moisture Degree to which skin is exposed to moisture	**1. Constantly Moist:** Skin is kept moist almost constantly by perspiration, urine, drainage, etc. Dampness is detected every time patient is moved or turned.	**2. Very Moist:** Skin is often, but not always moist. Linen must be changed at least every 8 hours.	**3. Occasionally Moist:** Skin is occasionally moist, requiring linen change every 12 hours.	**4. Rarely Moist:** Skin is usually dry, routine diaper changes, linen only requires changing every 24 hours.	
Friction - Shear ***Friction:*** occurs when skin moves against support surfaces ***Shear***: occurs when skin and adjacent bony surface slide across one another	**1. Significant Problem**: Spasticity, contracture, itching or agitation leads to almost constant thrashing and friction.	**2. Problem:** Requires moderate to maximum assistance in moving. Complete lifting without sliding against sheets is impossible. Frequently slides down in bed or chair, requiring frequent repositioning with maximum assistance.	**3. Potential Problem:** Moves feebly or requires minimum assistance. During a move skin probably slides to some extent against sheets, chair, restraints, or other devices. Maintains relative good position in chair or bed most of the time but occasionally slides down.	**4. No Apparent Problem:** Able to completely lift patient during a position change; Moves in bed and in chair independently and has sufficient muscle strength to lift up completely during move. Maintains good position in bed or chair at all times.	
Nutrition *Usual* food intake pattern	**1. Very Poor**: NPO and/or maintained on clear liquids, or IVs for more than 5 days **OR** Albumin <2.5 mg/dl **OR** Never eats a complete meal. Rarely eats more than half of any food offered. Protein intake includes only 2 servings of meat or dairy products per day. Takes fluids poorly. Does not take a liquid dietary supplement.	**2. Inadequate:** Is on liquid diet or tube feedings/TPN which provide inadequate calories and minerals for age **OR** Albumin <3 mg/dl **OR** rarely eats a complete meal and generally eats only about half of any food offered. Protein intake includes only 3 servings of meat or dairy products per day. Occasionally will take a dietary supplement.	**3. Adequate:** Is on tube feedings or TPN, which provide adequate calories and minerals for age **OR** eats over half of most meals. Eats a total of 4 servings of protein (meat, dairy products) each day. Occasionally will refuse a meal, but will usually take a supplement if offered.	**4. Excellent:** Is on a normal diet providing adequate calories for age. For example: eats/drinks most of every meal/feeding. Never refuses a meal. Usually eats a total of 4 or more servings of meat and dairy products. Occasionally eats between meals. Does not require supplementation.	
Tissue Perfusion and Oxygenation	**1. Extremely Compromised:** Hypotensive (MAP <50mmHg; <40 in a newborn) **OR** the patient does not physiologically tolerate position changes.	**2. Compromised:** Normotensive; Oxygen saturation may be <95 % **OR** hemoglobin may be < 10 mg/dl **OR** capillary refill may be > 2 seconds; Serum pH is < 7.40.	**3. Adequate:** Normotensive; Oxygen saturation may be <95 % **OR** hemoglobin may be < 10 mg/dl **OR** capillary refill may be > 2 seconds; Serum pH is normal.	**4. Excellent:** Normotensive, Oxygen saturation >95%; Normal Hemoglobin ; & Capillary refill < 2 seconds.	
				Total:	

Figure 21–1 Braden Q Pressure Ulcer Risk Assessment Scale. *(Reprinted with permission from Curley, M. A. Q., Razmus, I. S., Roberts, K. E., & Wypij, D. [2003, January/February]. Predicting pressure ulcer risk in pediatric patients: The Braden Q Scale.* Nursing Research, *52[1], 22–33.)*

ACQUIRED DISORDERS

DERMATITIS

The three types of pediatric **dermatitis** are diaper, seborrheic, and contact.

Clinical Presentation of Diaper Dermatitis

- The skin around the diaper area becomes irritated from chemicals and enzymes in the urine or feces (**Figure 21-2**). Skin becomes erythematous, with possible small vesicles and shallow ulcerations. **Erythema** is worse in creases and folds.
- Infection with candida albicans, a yeast-like fungus, results in candidiasis of the diaper area. The skin becomes beefy-red and tender to touch. Papules and pustules may be present. Erythematous areas are well demarcated, and satellite lesions may be noted on the abdomen. These characteristics differentiate candidiasis from milder forms of diaper dermatitis (**Figure 21-3**).

Nursing Interventions

- Apply an ointment containing mycostatin as ordered for candidiasis in the diaper area.
- Hydrocortisone 1% cream may be ordered for severe diaper rash.
- Monitor for signs of bacterial infection with severe diaper rash: pustules, purulent discharge, increasing ulcerations, and erythema. Refer for medical treatment as needed.

Caregiver Education

Home Care

- For prevention and home care for diaper rash, keep diaper area dry; change diapers frequently.

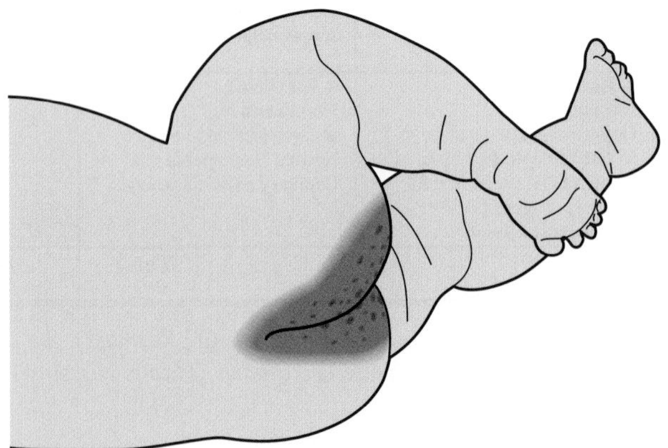

Figure 21-2 Diaper rash.

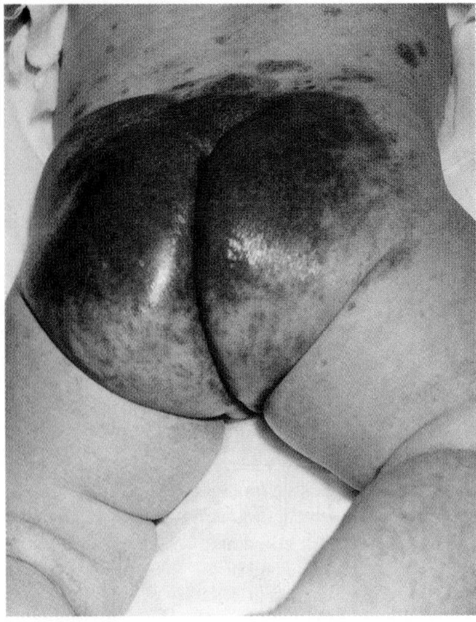

Figure 21-3 Candidiasis has a beefy-red appearance, different from the appearance of typical diaper rash.

- Clean diaper area with warm water each time diaper is changed. If soap is required, use a mild soap such as Cetaphil, Neutrogena, Dove, or Basic. Avoid vigorous scrubbing. Use caution with commercial wipes; some infants are sensitive to the chemicals in these wipes.
- Leave diaper area open to air when possible. Fifteen minutes four times daily is recommended.
- Do not use plastic pants. These hold in heat and moisture.
- Barrier ointments containing zinc oxide may be used. Examples are A&D ointment and Desitin ointment.
- Do not use baby powder.

Clinical Presentation of Seborrheic Dermatitis

- Seborrheic dermatitis (called cradle cap when it appears on scalp) appears greasy and scaly on the scalp and **intertriginous** (in body folds) areas. It may also appear on the face or behind the ears.

Diagnostic Studies

- Seborrheic dermatitis: caused by a yeast organism (pityrosporum ovale)

Caregiver Education

Home Care

- Daily shampoos with a mild pH-balanced infant shampoo will help to prevent seborrheic dermatitis (cradle cap) in infants.
- Avoid vigorous scrubbing of the scalp.
- An antiseborrheic shampoo may be recommended for cases of severe cradle cap.

Complementary and Alternative Therapies

- If cradle cap is present, apply warm olive oil or baby oil, wait 15 minutes, shampoo hair, and brush gently.

Clinical Presentation of Contact Dermatitis

- Contact dermatitis may be irritant or allergic.
- Irritant contact dermatitis is characterized by erythema, papules, vesicles, burning, and weeping. Causes include soaps and irritating chemicals.
- Allergic contact dermatitis is characterized by **pruritus** that is usually severe, erythema, papules, vesicles, and streaks or patches.
- Common causes of allergic contact dermatitis in children include poison oak, poison ivy, and poison sumac. Nickel found in buckles and jewelry can also be a problem.

Caregiver Education

Home Care

For prevention and home care of poison oak, ivy, or sumac:

- Wash area thoroughly with soap and water. This must be done within 15 minutes of exposure to remove the resin oils that cause the irritation.
- Apply cool wet compresses four times daily. Burrow's solution or Domeboro solution may be helpful as a wet compress.
- Apply lotions or creams to help control itching. Examples include Calamine lotion and pramoxine (Prax) or Sama with menthol, camphor, and phenol. Low-dose over-the-counter (1%) corticosteroid creams may also be applied in a thin coat to relieve inflammation and itching.
- Refer for medical help if the rash is extensive. Higher concentrations of topical corticosteroid creams may be prescribed.

Complementary and Alternative Therapies

- Bathe with powdered oatmeal bath such as Aveeno.

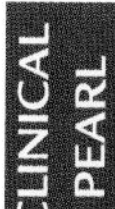

Latex and Contact Dermatitis

Latex allergies to gloves may produce contact dermatitis of the hands in health-care providers.

CRITICAL COMPONENT

Poison Oak, Poison Ivy, Poison Sumac

Plant resins are responsible for the skin lesions and intense itching associated with poison ivy and similar plants. Allergic dermatitis resulting from contact with poison ivy is not contagious. However, resins can be spread not only by direct contact with the plants, but by indirect contact, causing typical signs and symptoms of poison ivy. The resins may be spread indirectly through contact with clothing and pets. Resins may also be spread through the air if these plants are burned.

ATOPIC DERMATITIS (ECZEMA)

Clinical Presentation

- Eczema is an inflammatory disorder that is triggered by food allergies and topical irritants (**Figure 21-4**).
- Children from families with a history of asthma are at greater risk for developing atopic dermatitis or eczema.
- Eczema is characterized by skin scaling and intense itching. There may be patches of skin with erythema, papules, vesicles, crusting, and sometimes weeping. Patches of eczema may become infected. Scratching places the child at greater risk for infection.
- Infantile eczema involves mainly the extensor surfaces of the extremities and the face and scalp.
- Childhood eczema involves mainly the flexural surfaces of the extremities, the wrists, the neck, areas behind the ears, sometimes the hands.
- Adolescent eczema is more common on the hands and in skin creases.

Diagnostic Testing

- Cultures may be carried out if infection develops.

Caregiver Education

Home Care

- Wear loose, cotton clothing. Avoid wool clothing or blankets. Use mild, fragrance-free laundry detergents and fabric softeners.
- Apply moisturizers two or three times daily
- Use mild soaps such as Dove, Basic, Cetaphil, or Neutrogena.
- Keep the environment cool and humidified.
- Identify foods or irritants that trigger eczema or make it worse.
- Prevent scratching. Oral antihistamines may be given at night to promote sleep. Keep fingernails short.

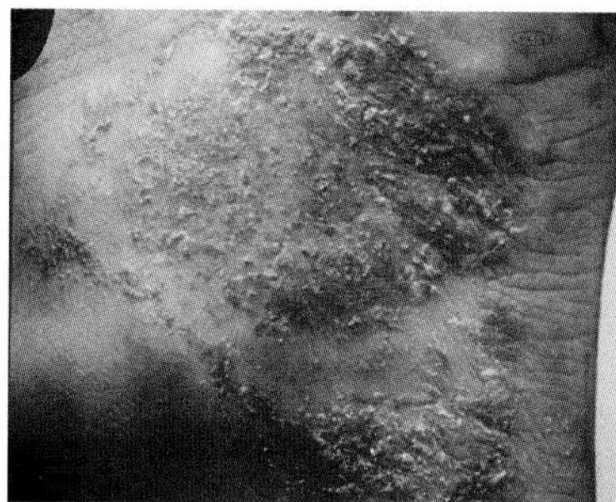

Figure 21-4 Child with atopic dermatitis (eczema).

- Apply topical steroids and immunomodulators as ordered (see Medication boxes).
- Carefully assess for signs of infection such as redness, swelling, pustules, and purulent drainage.

Complementary and Alternative Therapies

- Vitamin A (50,000 IU daily), vitamin E (400 IU daily), zinc (50 mg daily), omega 3 fatty acids, and evening primrose oil (3000 mg daily) may be used by adolescents and adults to treat eczema (Arcangelo & Peterson, 2006). However, it is important not to dose children with vitamins over and above their daily requirements.

CRITICAL COMPONENT

Dry Skin and Eczema

The key to successful treatment of atopic dermatitis (eczema) is hydration of the skin. Dry skin is a significant factor in the progression of eczema, and therefore moisturizers (emollients) are very effective in the management of this condition. Examples of moisturizers include Eucerin cream, Cetaphil cream, Aquaphor, and petroleum jelly. Moisturizers are applied to the skin two or three times daily immediately after bathing while the skin is still moist. The skin is patted dry instead of rubbed.

Evidence-Based Practice: Diet and Atopic Disease

Alm, B., Aberg, N., Erdes, L., Möllborg, P., Pettersson, R., Norvenius, S. G., . . . Wennergren, G. (2009). Early introduction of fish decreases the risk of eczema in Infants. *Archives of Disease in Childhood, 94,* 11–15. doi: 10.1136/adc.2008.140418

Greer, F. R., Sicherer, S. H., & Burks, A. W. (2008). Effects of early nutritional interventions on the development of atopic disease in infants and children: the role of maternal dietary restriction, breastfeeding, timing of introduction of complementary foods, and hydrolyzed formulas. Pediatrics, 121, 183–191. doi: 10.1542/peds.2007-3022

Thygarajan, A., & Burks, A. W. (2008). AAP recommendations on the effects of early nutritional interventions on the development of atopic disease. *Current Opinions in Pediatrics, 20,* 698–702. doi: 10.1097/MOP.0b013e3283154f88

A study of 8176 families found that introducing fish in the diet before 9 months of age reduces the risk of eczema in infants. Having a bird in the home was also found to be beneficial (Alm et al., 2009).

The American Academy of Pediatrics (AAP) recommendations state that there is little evidence that delaying introduction of complementary foods beyond 4 to 6 months of age has any protective effect on the development of atopic disease. Similarly, the AAP states that there is little evidence that any dietary intervention beyond 4 to 6 months of age has any protective effect on atopic disease (Greer, Sicherer, & Burks, 2008). However, exclusive breastfeeding of infants for at least 4 months may prevent or delay atopic dermatitis in high-risk infants (Thygarajan & Burks, 2008).

ACNE

Clinical Presentation

- The primary lesions of acne are comedones or plugged sebaceous follicles (**Figure 21-5**). The problem in mild acne is not inflammation but plugged sebaceous follicles in the skin that produce open comedones (blackheads) and closed comedones (whiteheads).
- The bacterium *Propionibacterium acnes* (P. acnes) may produce inflammation in individuals with more severe acne. The inflammation leads to pustules, cysts, and scarring (**Figure 21-6**).
- Acne lesions generally start on the face but also appear on the chest and back.

Medication

Medication to Treat Eczema

The two most effective medications for eczema are topical steroids and immunomodulators. Topical steroids may be applied at the same time as emollients. The steroid cream is applied in a thin layer first, and the emollient is applied over the steroid cream. Occlusive dressings such as a plastic wrap or damp towel may be placed over steroid creams for 10 minutes to promote absorption.

Topical immunomodulators such as tacrolimus (Protopic) or pimecrolimus (Elidel) may be used as alternates to topical steroid creams for children over 2 years of age. However, occlusive dressings should never be placed over topical immunomodulators.

Medication

Steroid Creams to Treat Eczema

Steroid creams come in three strengths: low, medium, and high. Low-strength creams are available over the counter, but medium- and high-strength creams may be obtained by prescription only and are used for the more severe cases. Special care must be taken not to apply medium- or high-strength steroid creams to the face or neck where the skin is thin, because they may produce skin atrophy. Steroid creams must be applied in a thin coat.

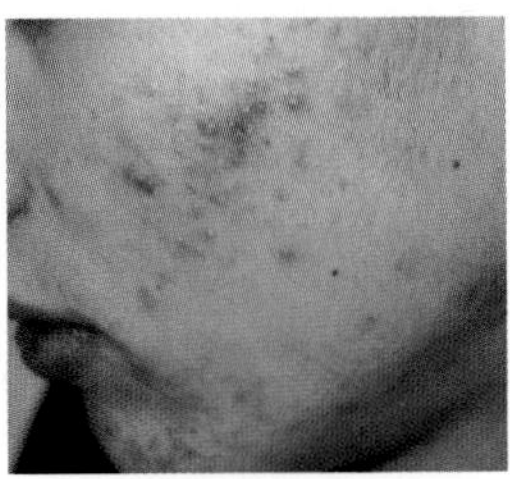

Figure 21–5 Adolescent acne (comedones).

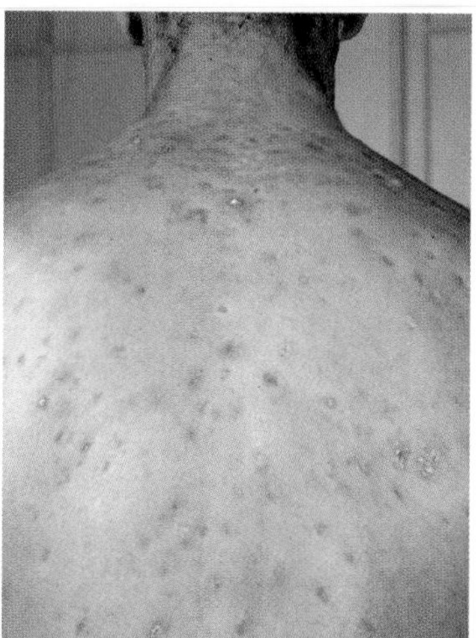

Figure 21-6 Adolescent with inflammatory acne (pustules, cysts).

Caregiver Education

Home Care

- Avoid touching the face or squeezing comedones.
- Avoid oil-based creams or cosmetics on the face. Make-up must be oil-free. Teach adolescents to read labels.
- Clean the face gently two or three times daily with a mild soap or cleanser such as Cetaphil, Basis, or Purpose. Harsh soaps and astringents are damaging to the skin.
- Keep hair clean and off the face.
- Administer topical comedolytic agents as ordered for noninflammatory acne (examples: tretinoin, azelaic acid, adapalene).
- Administer topical antibiotics as ordered for mild inflammatory acne (examples: benzoyl peroxide, erythromycin, clindamycin ointments).
- Administer oral antibiotics as ordered for inflammatory acne (minocycline or doxycycline).

CLINICAL PEARL

Management of Acne

The key to successful management of acne is skin care with gentle cleansing and avoidance of oil-based substances on the face. Dietary changes do not affect acne.

Medication

Skin Sensitivity with Comedolytic Creams

When comedolytic creams such as tretinoin, azelaic acid, or adapalene are ordered for the treatment of acne, it is important to teach patients to use sunscreen, as these creams make the skin more sensitive to the sun.

Evidence-Based Practice: Oral Contraception and Acne Reduction

Arowojolu, A. O., Gallo, M. F., Lopez, L. M., Grimes, D. A., & Garner, S. E. (2008). Combined oral contraceptive pills for treatment of acne. *Cochrane Database of Systematic Reviews, 4*. doi: 10.1002/14651858.CD004425.pub4

Combination oral contraceptives containing both an estrogen and a progestin have been shown effective in reducing acne lesions in women.

Promoting Safety

Isotretinoin (Accutane) may be prescribed for adolescents with severe inflammatory acne. This medication is known to be teratogenic: it causes birth defects in fetuses or even fetal death. Female adolescents taking this medication must be counseled to ensure that they are not pregnant and that pregnancy will not take place while the medication is being taken. The System to Manage Accutane Related Teratogenicity (SMART) program has been set up by the manufacturer of Accutane to ensure that the medication is taken safely. The SMART program requires that patients sign a consent, use two methods of contraception if sexually active or if there is a possibility of being sexually active, have two negative pregnancy tests before starting treatment, and undergo pregnancy testing monthly while receiving treatment (Food and Drug Administration, 2002).

BACTERIAL INFECTIONS

IMPETIGO

Clinical Presentation

- Papules turn into vesicles that crust over with a honey-colored crust (**Figure 21-7**).
- Lesions common around the nose and mouth
- Infection may develop in areas where skin has been damaged or area around nose has been irritated from nasal secretions.
- Contagious until the child has been on antibiotics for 24 hours

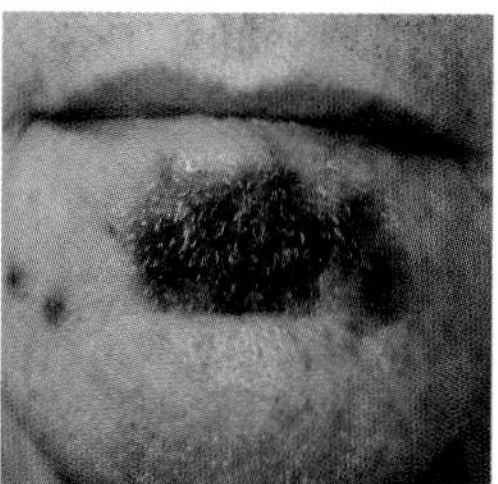

Figure 21-7 Child with impetigo.

Diagnostic Testing

- Caused by *Staphylococcus aureus* or group A B-hemolytic streptococcus

Nursing Interventions

Hospital Care

- Careful hand hygiene and contact isolation
- Administration of topical antibiotics as ordered for mild cases with small localized lesions
- Administration of oral antibiotics as ordered for more extensive infections

Caregiver Education

Home Care

- Careful hand hygiene after caring for child
- Teach hand hygiene to child.
- Keep fingernails clean and trimmed to prevent scratching.
- Disinfect surfaces such as sink, bathtub, and toys.
- Wash child's clothes daily.
- Cover impetigo lesions with loose, cotton clothing if possible.
- Administration of topical or oral antibiotics as ordered
- Complete all antibiotics.

METHICILLIN-RESISTANT STAPHYLOCOCCUS AUREUS SKIN INFECTIONS (MRSA)

Clinical Presentation

- Infections may develop where there has been a small break in the skin.
- The infection may begin as a red macule and progress to a warm, swollen, reddened area that is tender to touch. Purulent drainage may be present.
- The infection may present as a furuncle (boil), carbuncle (cluster of boils), or abscess.
- If the infection spreads to surrounding soft tissue, cellulitis will result. (Refer to section on cellulitis).

Diagnostic Testing

- Culture drainage to identify the bacteria involved.
- Sensitivity tests will also be performed to determine if the bacteria are resistant or susceptible to certain antibiotics.

Nursing Interventions

Outpatient Care

- Incision and drainage procedures are performed on skin lesions to release purulent material and promote healing.
- Culture any drainage present.
- Cover the lesion with a gauze dressing and give instructions on dressing the lesion at home.
- Administer antibiotics as ordered.

Hospital Care

- More severe infections that involve cellulitis may be treated in the hospital. Refer to the section on cellulitis.
- MRSA infections may complicate the healing of surgical wounds in the hospital. Meticulous hand hygiene, gloving, and sterile technique when changing dressings is essential.
- Complications of severe infections may include pneumonia, meningitis, and osteomyelitis.

Caregiver Education

Home Care

- Keep wound covered with sterile gauze and change as needed.
- Hand hygiene with soap for 30 seconds before and after changing dressing
- Disinfect shower, bathtub, and other surfaces used by the child.
- Complete course of antibiotics as ordered.
- Seek medical help for signs of cellulitis: increasing redness, streaks of red around lesion, increasing swelling or tenderness, fever.
- Seek medical advice for repeated infections. Nasal mupirocin or chlorhexidine baths may help to prevent infections in a colonized person.

CELLULITIS

Clinical Presentation

- Cellulitis may develop where there has been a small break in the skin or recent trauma. It may also follow sinusitis or otitis media.
- The organism may be *S. aureus*, MRSA, *Hemophilus influenzae*, or Group A Streptococcal (GAS) infection. Refer to section on MRSA for additional information on this common type of bacteria.
- GAS is responsible for common "strep throat" and impetigo. However, on rare occasions GAS may spread to the blood and then to the muscles or lungs. If it spreads to the soft tissues and muscles, it causes necrotizing fasciitis.
- Local clinical manifestations include redness, warmth, swelling, and tenderness. There may also be lymphangitis or red streaking in the area.
- Systemic clinical manifestations include fever, chills, and malaise.

Diagnostic Testing

- Culture and sensitivity tests on any drainage present
- Blood cultures if fever and systemic signs and symptoms are present

- Complete blood count (CBC) with white blood count (WBC) differential to assess for bacterial infection

Nursing Interventions

Hospital Care

- Assess temperature, heart and respiratory rate, and blood pressure at regular intervals (every 2–4 hours as needed).
- Assess local clinical manifestations and monitor site for increasing redness, swelling, warmth, tenderness, drainage, or streaking.
- Assess perfusion (color, warmth, capillary refill) of affected extremity or body part (every 2–4 hours as indicated).
- Assess hydration status and maintain intake and output records.
- Monitor child's behavior and level of consciousness.
- Apply warm, wet compresses to affected area as ordered.
- Elevate affected extremity or body part.
- Use contact isolation and meticulous hand hygiene.
- Administer acetaminophen or ibuprofen as ordered for pain and fever.
- Encourage oral fluids and administer IV fluids as ordered.
- Administer IV antibiotics as ordered.
- Provide for quiet play according to child's activity level.

Caregiver Education

Home Care

- Seek medical help for increased fever or for increasing redness, streaking, and pain and swelling at the infection site.
- Complete course of antibiotics as ordered.
- Administration of acetaminophen or ibuprofen for pain or fever.
- Application of warm, wet compresses or dressings if indicated.
- Careful hand hygiene before and after dressing changes or touching infected area
- Refer to home care instructions for MRSA.

CRITICAL COMPONENT

Hospital-Acquired and Community-Acquired MRSA

Methicillin-resistant *Staphylococcus aureus* (MRSA) infections may present as health hazards in the hospital (hospital-acquired MRSA) or in the community (community-acquired MRSA). Community-acquired MRSA (CA-MRSA) infections develop in otherwise healthy people who have not been in the hospital or other health-care organizations. Most CA-MRSA infections involve the skin or soft tissues. Hospital-based MRSA infections are more likely to affect people who are already ill, and tend to be more serious and affect internal organs such as the lungs.

CLINICAL PEARL

Colonization

An individual may be colonized with MRSA from an old infection. This person will not have any sign of infection, but can carry the bacteria on his or her body and pass the bacteria on to others. Careful hand hygiene is essential, as CA-MRSA may also be carried in the nose. Nasal mupirocin two or three times daily for 3 weeks may prevent nasal carriage (Nolt, 2007; So & Farrington, 2008).

Medication

Resistance to Antibiotics

MRSA developed because some *S. aureus* bacteria became resistant to penicillin-based antibiotics. Three common practices may be contributing to the development of resistant bacteria: (1) taking antibiotics unnecessarily for viral infections, (2) failing to complete the entire dose of antibiotics as ordered, and (3) saving left-over antibiotics for self-medication at a later date. An important part of the nurse's role is to teach proper administration of antibiotics.

Medication

Antibiotics for Treatment of MRSA

Vancomycin, linezolid, clindamycin, sulfamethoxazole-trimethoprim, and rifampin are all used to treat CA-MRSA infections in children. However, health-care providers must be alert for development of resistance. For example, some resistance has been shown to vancomycin and clindamycin (So & Farrington, 2008). Clindamycin is foul-tasting and may be difficult for children to take. Consider mixing this antibiotic with flavored syrup.

CLINICAL PEARL

Insect Bite or MRSA?

A MRSA infection of the skin may begin as a small red bump that may be mistaken for an insect bite.

Promoting Safety

To prevent MRSA infections, follow these guidelines:

- Careful hand hygiene after touching infected skin or changing bandages: wash hands with soap, and rub hands for 30 seconds.
- Avoid touching the nose.
- Disinfect sports equipment.
- Do not share towels and other personal equipment.
- Avoid line drying of clothes; use a clothes dryer.
- Keep any wound, boils, and draining sores covered.

Clinical Reasoning

Young Athletes and MRSA

Community-acquired methicillin-resistant *S. aureus* (CA-MRSA) skin infections are common in locker rooms used by athletes. Children who attend day care and camp are also at risk.

1. Scenario: you are approached by the coach of your local high school football team, who asks you for advice on how to reduce the incidence of CA-MRSA among his athletes. What recommendations would you give?

CLINICAL PEARL

Disinfectants

Disinfectants are used to clean surfaces such as showers and locker-room benches that have been in contact with bare skin. When purchasing a disinfectant, check the label to ensure that it is effective against MRSA and that the label includes an Environmental Protection Agency (EPA) registration number.

VIRAL INFECTIONS

PAPILLOMAVIRUS (VERRUCA OR WARTS)

Clinical Presentation

- Caused by human papillomavirus (HPV)
- Plantar warts on the soles of the feet or the palms of the hands are caused by HPV-1.
- Common warts or verruca vulgaris are caused by HPV-2. In children, these commonly appear on the hands and appear as rough, scaly papules.
- Refer to the chapter covering reproduction for a discussion of genital warts.

Caregiver Education

Home Care

- May be mildly contagious. Perform hand hygiene after touching warts.
- Do not scratch or pick at warts. This may lead to a secondary bacterial infection and scarring.
- Do not share towels.
- Many warts heal spontaneously and disappear without treatment within 2 to 3 years.
- Treatments such as liquid nitrogen stimulate the body's immune system and help it to fight against the papillomavirus.
- Cryosurgery may be required for warts that are resistant to other therapy.

Complementary and Alternative Therapies

- Salicylic acid in the form of liquid, gel, or a patch (Duofilm) may be effective in removing warts.

CLINICAL PEARL

Nail Biting

Children who constantly bite fingernails or pick at cuticles are at higher risk for developing warts under the nails. Use adhesive tape to wrap the finger(s).

HERPES SIMPLE 1 (COLD SORES OR FEVER BLISTERS)

Clinical Presentation

- Present as small vesicles on the lips, in the mouth, and/or on the gums (**Figure 21-8**). These vesicles are painful and may leak clear fluid or bleed slightly. Vesicles eventually crust over.
- Incubation period of 2 days to 2 weeks
- Contagious for at least 1 week and sometimes longer after initial infections; most contagious 3 to 4 days after recurrent infections, although viral shedding may continue after lesions have cleared
- Transmission by direct contact or contact with toys that have been put in the mouth
- Systemic signs and symptoms include fever, irritability, and enlarged, tender lymph nodes

Nursing Interventions

Acute Hospital Care

- Contact isolation with gown and gloves.
- Careful hand hygiene and sanitizing of surfaces
- Cool, bland liquids with careful attention to hydration status because mouth becomes very sore
- In severe cases, child or adolescent may be unable to tolerate oral liquids and may require total parenteral nutrition (TPN).
- Intravenous acyclovir is required for severe cases.

Caregiver Education

Home Care

- Careful hand hygiene
- Do not share cups or utensils between family members.

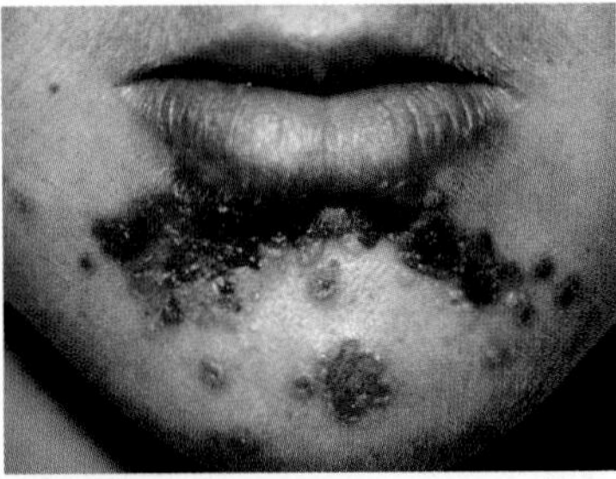

Figure 21-8 Child with herpes simplex (cold sore) on lips.

- Sanitize toys between children.
- Avoid touching sores on the mouth.
- Prescription creams may provide relief and facilitate healing in small, localized lesions. Examples are docosanol cream 10% (Abreva) and penciclovir cream 1% (Denavir).
- Administration of oral acyclovir as ordered for widespread or recurrent infections

Complementary and Alternative Therapies

- Cool water compresses to lips
- Use a lip balm with sun-blocking agents to prevent additional injury to lips.
- Over-the-counter creams such as those containing tetracaine cream 1% may be helpful.
- A mouthwash with 1 teaspoon Benadryl or 1/2 teaspoon sodium bicarbonate in a cup of slightly warm water may be soothing. The child must be taught to swish the medication in the mouth and then spit it out.

> **CRITICAL COMPONENT**
>
> **Signs and Symptoms of Herpes Simplex Virus**
>
> The herpes simplex virus can be shed by people who exhibit no signs or symptoms of illness.

FUNGAL INFECTIONS

TINEA INFECTIONS

Clinical Presentation

- Spread by direct contact, contact with personal items, and in some cases by pets (cats and dogs)
- Tinea corporis: fungal infection (ringworm) on the body (**Figure 21-9**). These appear as circular lesions with raised edges and central clearing. Itching is common.
- Tinea capitis: fungal infection (ringworm) on the scalp. There are circular patches with scaling and erythema. There may be patches with hair loss or broken hair.
- Tinea pedis: fungal infection of the foot (athlete's foot); more common in adolescents. Lesions may be scaly or made up of vesicles and pustules. Itching is common.
- Tinea cruris: fungal infection of the groin (jock itch); more common in adolescent males. There are scaling patches in the folds of the groin and upper thighs that are sharply demarcated. Itching can be intense.

Diagnostic Testing

- A Wood's lamp will cause some types of tinea to fluoresce and show as green. However, not all types of fungi will fluoresce under a Wood's lamp.
- The lesion can be scraped, and the tissue mixed with potassium hydroxide (KOH) before examining under a microscope. If fungi are present, branching strands (hyphae) may be seen under a microscope.

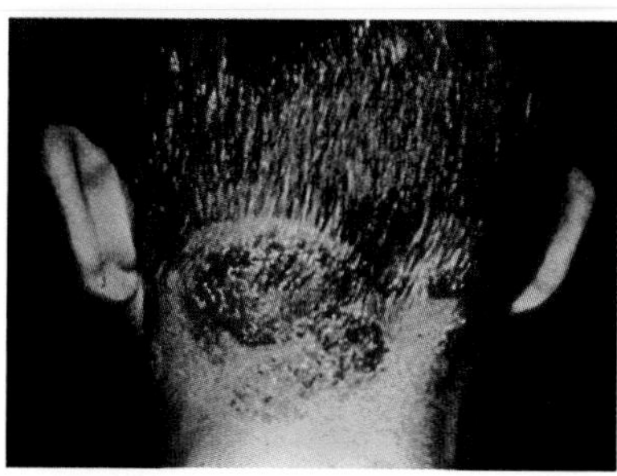

Figure 21-9 Child with ringworm (tinea capitis or tinea corporis).

Caregiver Education

Home Care

- Apply an antifungal cream such as miconazole to the lesion twice daily.
- If lesions are moist, such as in the groin area or between toes, apply wet compresses using Burrow's solution twice daily to dry the area.
- Do not share hats, combs, brushes, ribbons, scarves, clothing, or bedding.
- Cover skin lesions.
- For tinea pedis (athlete's foot), air the feet as much as possible. Sandals are recommended for airing the feet. Change socks daily, and alternate shoes in order to give them a chance to air out.
- For tinea capitis (ringworm on the scalp), shampoo the hair twice daily for 2 weeks. Shampoos such as selenium sulfide 2.5% or ketoconazole 2% are effective. Systemic oral medications are also required. Refer to the box on medication administration.

Complementary and Alternative Therapies

- Cornstarch is used by some to treat or prevent athlete's foot. However, cornstarch may promote growth of fungi.

> **Medication**
>
> **Medication for Tinea Capitis**
>
> Systemic oral medication is required for children with tinea capitis. Griseofulvin is given once or twice daily for 4 to 6 weeks or up to 8 to 12 weeks as needed. This medication must be given with high-fat foods such as ice cream or peanut butter to enhance absorption. Side effects of griseofulvin include nausea and sensitivity to the sun. Educate caregivers on the importance of using a sunscreen with an SPF of 15 or greater. Children must be reevaluated monthly, and the renal, hematologic, and hepatic systems must be monitored during administration of this medication (Tschudy & Arcara, 2012).

DISORDERS RELATED TO CONTACT WITH INSECTS

PEDICULOSIS CAPITIS (HEAD LICE)

Clinical Presentation

- Nits or lice eggs appear as very small white, translucent, or yellow dots that are firmly attached near the base of the hair shaft (**Figure 21-10**). Nits hatch in 7 to 10 days.
- An adult louse is approximately the size and shape of a sesame seed. Lice feed on blood from the scalp and cannot live more than 48 hours away from the scalp.
- Lice may cause a tickling sensation as they move through the hair. They may also cause intense itching. Scratching the scalp may result in excoriation and bacterial infection.
- Lice move by crawling and do not fly or hop. They are usually spread by direct contact between persons, but may be spread less commonly by sharing hats, combs, brushes, towels, and bedding.

Diagnostic Testing

- Examination of the hair under a bright light.
- A magnifying glass and fine-toothed comb may be helpful in finding the lice.
- It is helpful to divide the hair into sections and examine one section or strand at a time.
- Nits are usually found within ¼ inch of the base of the hair shaft.

Caregiver Education

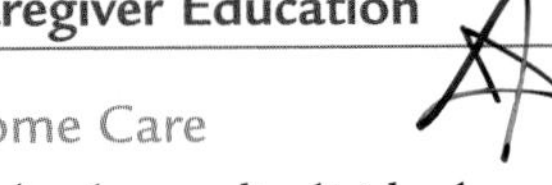

Home Care

- Apply a pediculicide shampoo to hair that has been shampooed and towel dried. Recommended pediculicides for children include permethrin 1% (Nix) and pyrethrin (RID, Clear Lice, Pronto). Leave medication on hair for 10 minutes and then rinse off. Repeat treatment in 7 to 10 days.
- A fine-toothed comb may be used to remove nits from wet hair.

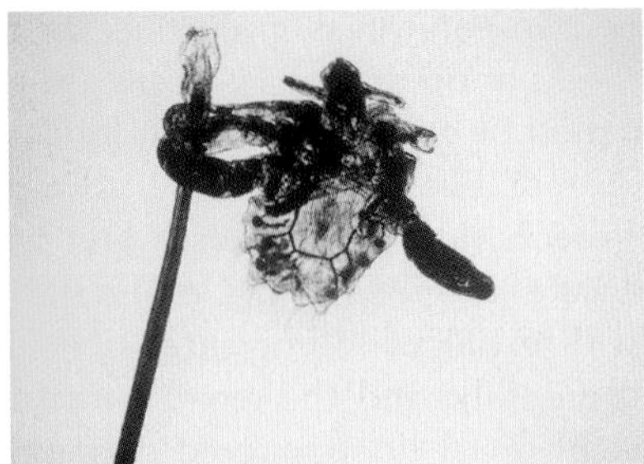

Figure 21–10 Nits and lice in hair.

- Soak combs and brushes in hot water with one of the pediculicide shampoos for 15 minutes.
- Wash clothing and bedding in hot, soapy water and dry on hot cycle. Alternately, dry clean items that cannot be washed.
- Vacuum the floor, mattresses, and soft/stuffed furniture.
- Toys, personal items, and other objects that cannot be laundered can be tied up in a plastic bag for more than 2 weeks.
- Examine the scalps of close contacts and family members.
- Do not spray the floor or other surfaces of the house and furniture with pesticides. These chemicals are toxic and may cause serious adverse effects.

Complementary and Alternative Therapies

- Application of mayonnaise, petroleum jelly, or Vaseline has been recommended to suffocate the lice. Parents are instructed to cover the child's hair with the oil-based product, cover with a shower cap overnight, and shampoo the next morning. This treatment has not been proved to be effective, but is widely used.

> CLINICAL PEARL
>
> **Identifying Nits**
>
> It may be difficult to distinguish nits (lice eggs) from dandruff or flaking skin. Note whether the white, translucent, or yellow spot adheres firmly to the hair shaft. If it is firmly attached, it is likely a nit. If it moves freely, it probably originates from dandruff or dry skin (Leung, Fong, & Pinto-Rojas, 2005).

> **CRITICAL COMPONENT**
>
> **Contraindications for Pediculicide Shampoos**
>
> Assess for history of asthma or allergies before recommending pediculicide shampoos. Permethrin or pyrethrin is contraindicated for children with ragweed allergies. These products may cause an allergic reaction or an exacerbation of asthma.

SCABIES (MITE INFESTATION)

Clinical Presentation

- Mites burrow under the skin, leaving tracks or lines of macules, vesicles, and pustules.
- Itching is severe, especially at night
- Children under age 2 are most likely to be affected on the head and neck, or on the palms and soles of the feet (**Figure 21-11**). Older children are most likely to be affected on skin folds between the fingers and toes, wrists, elbows, armpits, waist line, thighs, buttocks, and abdomen (Aronson & Shope, 2009).

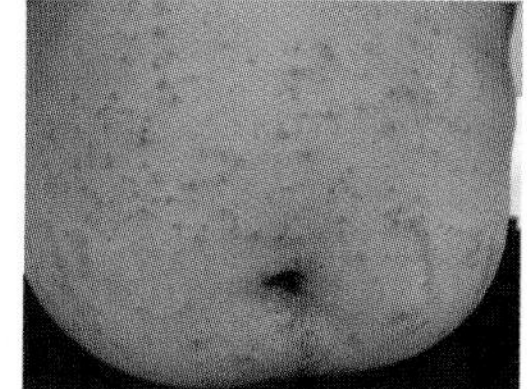

Figure 21-11 Child with scabies.

Caregiver Education

Home Care

- Wash clothing and bedding with hot water and dry on the hot cycle.
- Tie items that cannot be laundered in a plastic bag for more than 5 days.
- Apply permethrin 5% cream to the entire body from the neck down. Apply at bedtime and leave for 8 to 14 hours. Bathe the child the next morning. The treatment may be repeated in 7 days.
- Over-the-counter creams to relieve itching may be applied to the skin. Examples include Sama and Prax lotion.
- Close contacts of the child also need to be treated.

INSECT BITES AND STINGS

These include bites and stings from bees, wasps, hornets, fire ants, and the brown recluse spider.

Clinical Presentation

- Local presentation of stings includes redness, swelling, and pain.
- Systemic presentation due to an allergic reaction to the insect sting may include emesis, headache, syncope, hives, wheezing, and anaphylactic shock.
- Delayed reactions to stings may occur as long as 1 week later and include hives, fever, joint pain, and vasculitis.
- A brown recluse spider bite may range from mild to severe. In severe bites, the area becomes reddened and painful with a central vesicle or pustule that drains after 3 to 4 days, leaving an ulcer or a necrotic area. There may be systemic responses such as fever, chills, weakness, nausea, and vomiting approximately 12 hours after the bite. Systemic responses do not always occur.

Nursing Interventions

Emergency Care for Anaphylaxis

- Assess the skin at the local site and check for hives in other parts of the body.
- Assess for stridor or wheezing, indicating laryngeal edema or bronchospasm.
- Assess for hypotension and tachycardia, indicating anaphylactic shock. Assess level of consciousness.
- Administer epinephrine 0.01 mg/kg subcutaneously or intravenously as ordered. Repeat every 15 to 20 minutes as needed. Maximum dose is 0.5 mg (refer to medication administration box).
- Give 100% oxygen via nasal cannula or mask.
- Gain IV access, start IV fluids as ordered.
- Albuterol nebulizer treatments as ordered for wheezing
- Methylprednisolone (corticosteroid) or diphenyhydramine (Benadryl) IV as ordered to counteract the allergic reaction

Caregiver Education

Emergency Care

- If a child is known to be allergic to an insect sting, caregivers must keep an Epi-Pen available at all times and be able to inject it IM according to directions. Refer to the Clinical Pearl feature for Epi-Pen dosages.
- Give oral antihistamine if child is alert and able to swallow.
- Seek follow-up medical care immediately for any systemic reactions to stings or bites, including spider bites.

Home Care

- Wash the wound, apply ice to the sting or bite, and elevate the extremity. Use ice for 8 to 12 hours as needed to reduce pain and swelling.
- Do not squeeze the stinger. Use tweezers or a scraper to remove the stinger without crushing it.
- Give an antihistamine such as Benadryl orally, dosing according to child's weight and age, or apply it topically as a cream.
- If the child is allergic to insect stings, carry an Epi-Pen kit with the child; keep one at home and one in the car. Use a medical alert bracelet.
- Wounds that are draining or have a necrotic center must always be assessed and not assumed to be a spider bite. Many "spider bites" diagnosed by caregivers turn out to be staphylococcal infections, and spider bites.
- If a spider bite is confirmed, check on whether tetanus immunizations are up to date.

Complementary and Alternative Therapies

- A baking soda paste, made by mixing baking soda with cold water, may be soothing to a sting site.

Medication

Administration of Epinephrine

Epinephrine 0.01 mg/kg may be given subcutaneously with 0.01 mL/kg of 1:1000 solution or intravenously with 0.1 mL/kg of 1:10.000 solution (Tschudy & Arcara, 2012). Always check the concentration of epinephrine when calculating the volume of medication to administer. For example, to receive a dose of 0.01 mg/kg, a 10-kg child would receive 0.1 mL of 1:1000 solution or 1 mL of 1:10,000 solution.

CLINICAL PEARL

Epi-Pen

Use an Epi-Pen for children >30 kg and an Epi-Pen Jr for children <30 kg. The Epi-Pen delivers 0.3 mg in 2 mL of 1:1000 solution IM. The Epi-Pen Jr delivers 0.15 mg in 2 mL of 1:2000 solution (Tschudy & Arcara, 2012). Check the expiration on the Epi-Pen carefully. Most expire in 2 year. Instructions for Epi-Pen auto-injector use:

- Remove pen from plastic carrying tube.
- Remove grey cap from wider end of pen. This "arms" the pen for use.
- Grasp the pen in the fist. Do not touch either end.
- The active end of the pen is narrower and black. No needle will be visible. Press the black end at a 90-degree angle into the thigh. Press the black end harder into the thigh until a click or "pop" is heard. This activates the pen and starts the injection of epinephrine.
- Count for 10 to 15 seconds while the epinephrine is being injected.
- Remove the pen at a 90-degree angle. Massage the area.
- There will be a visible needle at this time. Dispose of equipment safely. Place pen back in plastic carrying tube.
- Seek continued medical help.

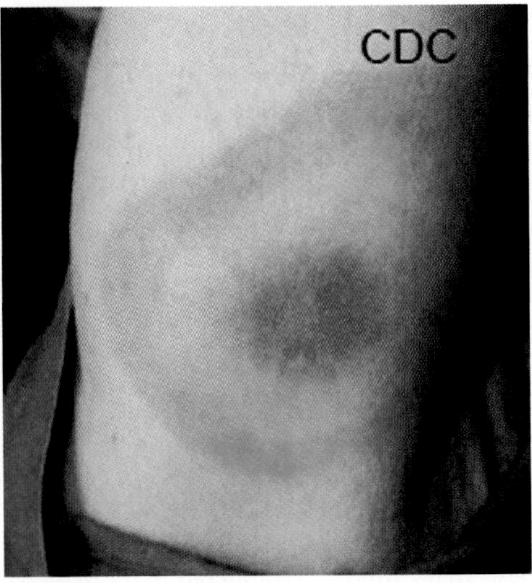

Figure 21-12 Lyme disease rash.

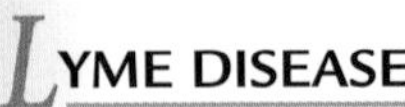

LYME DISEASE

Clinical Presentation

- Lyme disease is caused by the bite of a deer tick that transmits an infective spirochete. Signs and symptoms may appear 3 to 32 days following tick bite (Tschudy & Arcara, 2012).
- Characteristic skin rash: large circular rash with central clearing (**Figure 21-12**)
- Signs and symptoms include fever, headache, aching, and satellite rash.
- Later clinical manifestations include arthritis and neurological symptoms.

Diagnostic Testing

- Increased erythrocyte sedimentation rate
- Increased white blood count
- Positive IgM cryoglobulins, rising IgG titers, positive ELISA

Caregiver Education

Prevention

- When walking outdoors, avoid areas with tall grass or bushes. Wear light-colored clothing with long sleeves and long pants in the woods. Wear closed shoes and tuck pants legs into socks.
- Spray permethrin on clothing before walking outdoors in wooded areas.
- Use DEET to spray on skin. Refer to box on promoting safety.

Home Care

- First aid for tick removal (refer to Clinical Pearl box)
- Teach caregivers to be aware of signs and symptoms of Lyme disease following tick bites.
- Administration of antibiotics such as amoxicillin for younger children or doxycycline for children over 8 years of age (Tschuday & Arcara, 2012)

Complementary and Alternative Therapies

- Citronella or lavender oils may be used to prevent tick and other insect bites in children over 2 years of age. The effectiveness of these oils is unknown.

CLINICAL PEARL

How to Remove Ticks

- Use tweezers to remove the tick directly from the skin.
- Do not squeeze or handle the tick or pull it with bare fingers because tick feces carry disease organisms.
- Use gloves or tissues if gloves are unavailable, and wash hands afterward.
- If part of the tick remains in the skin, soak the skin to soften it and then remove any tick parts in the same way that a splinter would be removed.

Promoting Safety

Using DEET safely as an insect repellant—caregiver instructions (Aronson & Shope, 2009):

- Avoid spraying DEET onto a child's skin. Apply the DEET to your hand first and then rub it on the child's skin.
- Do not apply DEET to young children's hands, as they may rub their eyes or place their hands in their mouths.
- Do not use DEET for infants less than 2 months of age (Aronson & Shope, 2009).
- Do not spray apply DEET over broken places in the skin.
- Do not spray DEET near food.
- DEET protection: 10% DEET offers protection for 2 hours, and 30% DEET offers protection for 5 hours. These concentrations may be used safely in children. Choose the strength of DEET based on the length of time the child will spend outdoors.
- Use DEET once daily. Do not use DEET products that are combined with sunscreen, because frequent application may lead to toxicity.
- Wash skin to remove DEET following time outdoors, and wash clothing that may have been exposed to DEET.

DISORDERS RELATED TO INJURIES

Clinical Reasoning

Assessing the Cause of Injury

When a child presents with an injury, determine the cause of the injury and what the child was doing when the injury occurred. Most injuries are accidental, but some may be nonaccidental or intentional.

1. What are some signs that a child may have undergone physical abuse?
2. What is your responsibility?

LACERATIONS

Clinical Presentation

- Assess the size and location of the laceration, determine what type of material broke the skin and whether there are foreign objects remaining in the skin, determine whether the injury took place indoors or outdoors, determine how long ago the injury occurred, and determine what first aid was given when the injury occurred.
- Assess for bleeding.
- Assess the neurovascular status of any extremity involved. Determine whether there is limitation in movement. Check color, warmth, capillary refill, and pulses of the extremities involved.

Nursing Interventions

Emergency Care

- Use sterile gauze to apply pressure to the wound if bleeding is present.
- When bleeding is under control, irrigate the wound with normal saline and a syringe.
- Check whether the child's tetanus immunizations are up to date.
- Assist with application of steri strips or suturing as required. Refer to box on evidence-based practice for pain management during suturing.
- Apply sterile dressing and antibiotic ointment such as bacitracin or polysporin as ordered over suture site.
- Cyanoacrylate tissue adhesives may be used to close lacerations that are clean and straight. The adhesive seals the edges of the laceration and forms its own dressing.
- Wounds with a high risk of infection are not sutured initially. These include wounds that are contaminated with dirt or saliva from a bite and wounds that demonstrate a large amount of tissue damage.

Caregiver Education

Home Care

- Give instructions for application of bacitracin or polysporin ointments and sterile dressings as needed over suture sites. Dressings may range from a Band-Aid to gauze and tape. For sutured lacerations, keep sterile dressings over the wound for 24 to 48 hours. Keep the wound clean and dry.
- Steri strips are left in place until they fall off naturally or after 7 to 10 days. Keep the area clean and dry.
- If a tissue adhesive is used, an additional dressing is optional. Do not apply ointments over the adhesive. Gentle bathing is permissible, but swimming and scrubbing and pulling at the site are contraindicated.
- Perform hand hygiene carefully before and after caring for wounds.
- Teach caregivers signs of infection in the wound: erythema, tenderness, swelling, drainage, fever. Seek medical help if any of these signs are present.
- Give instructions on when to return for suture removal if applicable. The time needed for healing before sutures are removed depends on the site of the wound, but average length of time varies from 7 to 14 days.
- Pain management is essential during suturing.

CLINICAL PEARL

Wound Dressings for the Hospitalized Child

Tips for wound dressings for the hospitalized child include the following (Bookout, 2008):

- Foam dressings come in many shapes and sizes and may be useful in padding boney prominences or absorbing wound exudates.
- Transparent dressings are useful for securing tubes and intravenous catheters. They are also effective for covering incisions or dry, shallow wounds.
- Hydrogel sheet dressings are soothing and may be used for covering superficial abrasions or first- and second-degree burns.
- Hydrocolloid dressings are effective for wounds that are in the regeneration or maturation phase of healing.
- Alginate dressings are used to absorb wounds with moderate to heavy drainage.
- Any dressing can contain chemicals that are bactericidal or bacteriostatic. These are referred to as antimicrobial dressings and are used to reduce bacterial load in the wound.

CRITICAL COMPONENT

Process of Wound Healing

Injured tissue must progress through three stages to complete healing. These are:

- Inflammation or reaction phase: Damage to cells is brought under control and damaged cellular fragments are removed. Bleeding is controlled and barriers are formed to seal off bacteria
- Proliferative phase: New tissue is regenerated. The wound is filled with new connective tissue and new epithelium covers the wound
- Maturation phase: The area is remodeled and restructured and made stronger. This phase may take weeks or months (Bookout, 2008).

BITES (ANIMALS, HUMAN)

Clinical Presentation

- Bite wounds from animals or humans may involve punctures, lacerations, and crushed tissue. Cat bites are more likely to inflict puncture wounds that are difficult to clean, and large dogs or other large mammals are more likely to crush tissue or tear the skin.
- Signs of infection may follow the bite incident by a few hours. These include redness, pain, swelling, and subsequent purulent drainage.
- Bites on the hands and feet are most likely to develop infections. Infections are especially severe if the bite involves tendons or joints.
- Cat bites are the most likely to become infected. Human bites and other animal bites also transmit bacteria and a risk for infection.
- Muscles, tendons, blood vessels, and nerves may be damaged along with skin and subcutaneous tissue.

Diagnostic Testing

- The most common organism involved in dog and cat bites is *Pasteurella multocida*. However, a variety of organisms can be cultured from bite wounds. Staphylococcus and various strains of streptococcus may cause infections.
- Rabies may be transmitted from bites by carnivorous wild animals. The disease is occasionally transmitted by pets that have not been immunized. Refer to the Medication Administration box on rabies prophylaxis.

Nursing Interventions

Emergency Care

- Give immediate wound care. Wounds may be irrigated under pressure with large amounts of sterile saline.
- The wound may be left open and not sutured initially to allow drainage and reduce the chance of infection. Hand bites are not sutured because of the high risk of infection. Bites that are deep, involve puncture wounds, or are over 8 hours old are not sutured.
- Tissue adhesive dressings are not used for closing bite wounds because of reduced drainage and increased chance of infection.
- Check the child's immunization record to determine whether tetanus immunizations are up to date.
- Dress the wound with antibiotic ointment and a sterile dressing.
- Administer antibiotics as ordered.
- Bites and animal attacks may be very frightening. Provide emotional support for the child and family.

Caregiver Education

Home Care

- Teach caregivers to watch for signs of cellulitis or localized infection: erythema, warmth, red streaking, edema, purulent drainage, fever, increased pain.
- Teach hand hygiene and wound care with antibiotic ointment and gauze dressing.
- Teach importance of keeping tetanus immunizations up to date.
- Complete the course of oral antibiotics as ordered after bites.

Prevention

- Keep rabies vaccinations up to date for pets.
- Teach children to treat pets with respect and kindness.
- Do not tease animals or annoy them when they are eating.
- Do not leave young children alone with a pet.
- Keep dogs on leashes in public.
- Do not handle stray animals, especially if they are sick.
- Prevent aggressive or defensive biting on the part of children.

Medication

Rabies

Rabies can occur after bites from nonimmunized domestic animals, but is most likely to occur after bites from wild animals such as bats, skunks, raccoons, coyotes, foxes, and bobcats. Individuals who are bitten by these animals must receive rabies prophylaxis, and the incident must be reported to the Health Department. A domestic animal that is suspected of having rabies is confined for 10 days. If the animal develops signs of rabies, it is killed and the brain is examined. If the examination is positive, the individual who was bitten must receive rabies prophylaxis. Rabies prophylaxis includes passive immunization (rabies immune globulin) that is given initially into the wound and intramuscularly (IM). It also includes active immunization (rabies vaccine) that is given as a series of five IM injections over 28 days.

SUNBURNS

Clinical Presentation

- Erythema, tenderness, edema, blistering, itching
- First-degree sunburn: redness of the skin
- Second-degree sunburn: blistering of the skin

Nursing Interventions

- Assess skin for the presence of pediatric melanomas in children who have been exposed to the sun.

Caregiver Education

Prevention

- Infants less than 6 months of age should not be exposed to direct sunlight.
- Infants over 6 months of age and children should not be exposed to direct sunlight between 10 a.m. and 4 p.m. When children do play outdoors, indirect sunlight is recommended.
- Protective clothing such as broad-rimmed hats that protect the face are very effective in preventing sunburn.
- Shirts should be worn outdoors.
- Clothing items that contain SPF protection against UV rays are available.
- Apply sunscreen SPF 30 or greater 30 minutes before a child is exposed to the sun and every hour while outdoors. Apply the sunscreen all over the skin.
- Use water-resistant sunscreens for children who are swimming or playing in water.
- Remember that sunlight reflecting off of water or snow can damage the skin.
- Children with light complexions sunburn more easily, but children with darker complexions are also vulnerable to sunburn.

Home Care

- Cool baths and cool compresses
- Additional fluids to prevent dehydration
- Moisturizers to the skin
- Local anesthetic sprays and creams
- Acetaminophen or ibuprofen as needed for pain

CRITICAL COMPONENT

Damaging Ultraviolet Rays

There are three types of ultraviolet rays that are damaging to the skin. UVA rays penetrate the deepest and cause premature aging of the skin. UVB rays have a shorter wavelength but are damaging to outer layers of the skin, causing sunburn and skin cancer. SPF numbers refer to the protection that sunscreen has against UVB rays. Advise parents to use a sunscreen with an SPF of 30 or greater. UVC rays are potent, but are filtered by the ozone layer.

BURNS (MINOR AND MAJOR)

Clinical Presentation

- Superficial epidermis: red, painful, no blistering
- Superficial partial-thickness epidermis: red, painful, blisters, moist and weeping, blanches with pressure
- Deep partial-thickness epidermis: dry and white, red with blisters if the burn was caused by scalding, less pain experienced than with superficial partial-thickness, can feel pressure applied
- Full-thickness burn to epidermis and dermis: no blanching, no pain; white or charred appearance with contact burns
- Refer to Critical Components box on p. 494 on respiratory complications and assessments associated with burn injuries.
- Electrical burns are deep and may cause more damage to the body part internally than is apparent on the skin surface. Electrical burns may also trigger cardiac dysrhythmias up to 72 hours after the burn (Morgan, Bledsoe, & Barker, 2000).

Diagnostic Testing

- Arterial blood gases for severe burns or respiratory involvement
- Carboxyhemaglobin levels as indicated for carbon monoxide poisoning if child was in a confined space
- Electrocardiogram and cardiac monitoring as indicated for severe burns or electrical burns
- Wound cultures as needed
- Laboratory assessment may include CBC, basic metabolic panel, phosphorus, magnesium, albumin, serum myoglobin, zinc, PT, and PTT.

Nursing Intervention

Emergency Care

- Give 100% oxygen if the individual has been burned severely or if the fire was in a confined space. Use a pulse oximeter to monitor oxygen saturation levels. Assist with endotracheal intubation as needed.

- Refer to Critical Components box on p. 494 on airway obstruction and respiratory distress. Assess for signs of airway edema or pulmonary insufficiency.
- Place on a cardiac monitor if burns are severe or if the burn is electrical in origin.
- Obtain intravenous access for fluid replacement. Central venous access is required if burns are severe.
- Remove clothing that is burned, hot in temperature, or contaminated with chemicals. If necessary, cut the clothing away.
- Apply cool, sterile, normal saline compresses to cool and protect the skin.
- Monitor temperature; watch for hypothermia.
- Administer tetanus immunization if needed.
- Provide pain medication as needed.
- Provide emotional support to the child and family.

Acute Hospital Care

- Assess for signs of respiratory distress: dyspnea, wheezing, stridor, tachypnea, decreased breath sounds, retractions.
- Use a pulse oximeter to monitor oxygen saturation levels.
- Administer oxygen or assist with endotracheal intubation as needed.
- Keep head of bed elevated.
- Assess for changes in behavior or level of consciousness.
- Assess for signs of infection: fever; increased redness, swelling, pain; purulent drainage or foul odor.
- Maintain intravenous access.
- Monitor intake and output. Place Foley catheter to monitor hourly output with severe burns.
- Neurovascular checks every 1 to 4 hours as ordered: color, warmth, capillary refill of extremities, pulse or Doppler signals, ability to move fingers and toes, sensation. Report decreased movement, decreased Doppler signals, and increased pain in any extremity.
- Assess color of urine, monitoring for presence of myoglobinuria from damaged muscle.
- Assess pain levels frequently and administer pain medication as ordered before dressing changes and as needed.
- Use sterile technique to assist with dressing changes and application of topical creams or ointments.
- Partial- and full-thickness burns are covered with sterile, nonadherent dressings. Tubular net dressings may be used to anchor dressings onto extremities without tape.
- Insert feeding tube and administer tube feedings as ordered if the child cannot be fed orally or cannot maintain increased caloric requirement due to change in metabolic state.
- Maintain temperature between 37°C and 38.5°C. It is very important to maintain a normal body temperature. Monitor for hypothermia during dressing changes.

Chronic Hospital Care

- Obtain referrals as needed for the child and family: pastoral care according to cultural and spiritual beliefs, child life specialist, occupational therapy, physical therapy, social work, nutrition.
- Assist with manual debridement of necrotic tissue or whirlpool debridement as indicated. Escharotomy may be required to remove burned areas (eschar).
- Skin grafting is required for children with full-thickness burns. Refer to Critical Components box on p. 495 on grafting.
- Carry out dressing changes and wound care as ordered. Refer to the Evidence-Based Practice box for additional information on dressing changes and wound care.
- Monitor for hypertrophic scarring, which develops in 60% of children under 5 years of age (Papini, 2004). Silicone gel sheeting may reduce hypertrophic scars.
- Monitor for scar contractures. These contractures may be treated with silicone inserts, pressure, splinting, or surgery as needed.

Chronic Home Care

- Dressing changes are no longer required after new tissue grows over the wound (epithelialization).
- Continue to monitor for hypertrophic scarring and scar contractures (**Figure 21-13**).
- Therapy may be needed for the child and family to prevent post-traumatic stress disorder (PTSD) or to help the child and family cope with anxiety, guilt, and depression.

Caregiver Education

Emergency Care

- Note Critical Components box on first aid for minor burns.

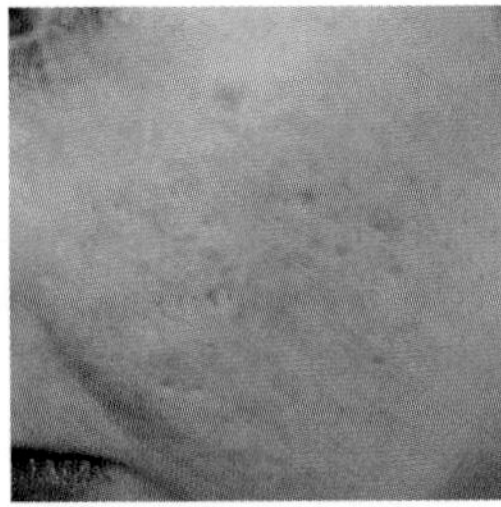

Figure 21-13 Child with hypertrophic scarring.

Evidence-Based Practice: Dressings for Burn Wound Healing

Wasiak, J., Cleland, H., & Campbell, F. (2008). *Dressings for superficial and partial thickness burns*. Retrieved from http://www.ncbi.nlm.nih.gov/pubmed/18843629

Jull, A. B., Rodgers, A., & Walker, N. (2009). *Honey as a topical treatment for wounds*. Retrieved from http://www.ncbi.nlm.nih.gov/pubmed/18843679

Hohlfeld, J., Roessingh, A., Hirt-Burri, N., Chaubert, P., Gerber, S., Scaletta, C., . . . Applegate, L. A. (2005). *Tissue engineered fetal skin constructs for pediatric burns. Lancet, 366,* 840–842. doi: 10.1016/S0140-6736(05)67107-3

Papini, R. (2004). Management of burn injuries of various depths. BMJ, 329, 158. doi: 10.1136/bmj.329.7458.158

A systematic review of dressings for superficial and partial-thickness burns was carried out by the Cochrane Wounds Group. They evaluated the effectiveness of hydrocolloid, silicon nylon, antimicrobial (containing silver), polyurethane film, and biosynthetic dressings. Outcome criteria included time to wound healing, number of dressing changes, and level of pain during dressing changes. The review found that biosynthetic dressings were effective in decreasing time to healing and reducing pain during dressing changes. More randomized trials are needed to provide guidelines for the most effective burn dressings (Wasiak, Cleland, & Campbell, 2009).

The Cochrane Wounds Group also carried out a systematic review on the effectiveness of honey in the care of superficial and partial-thickness burns. The review found that honey dressings improved healing times (Jull, Rodgers, & Walker, 2009).

Tissue engineered fetal skin constructs have been effective in healing deep partial-thickness and full-thickness burns. The fetal skin construct, which is developed from cultured fetal skin cells on horse collagen, may take the place of autologous skin grafts (Hohlfeld et al., 2005).

Transcyte, a tissue engineered dressing developed from human newborn fibroblast cells, is sutured into place and also promotes burn wound healing in children (Papini, 2004).

Hospital Care

- Teach the family infection control measures: hand hygiene, no stuffed toys, no live plants or flowers, visitor guidelines to prevent exposure to infection.
- Teach the family the plan for therapeutic management. Listen to concerns and answer questions. Include education on dressing changes and debridement, skin grafts, and any surgery required.
- Teach the family the plan for pain management and how often pain medication may be given.

Chronic Home Care

- Teach the family about complications such as infection, scar contractures, hypertrophic scarring, and post-traumatic stress disorder.
- Refer to home-based occupational or physical therapy as needed.
- Refer to counseling or therapy as needed.
- Teach family to plan and provide a nutritious, high-protein diet for the child.
- Care for the healing skin: use of moisturizing creams such as cocoa butter, Eucerin, Nivea, Neutrogena, or Vaseline Intensive Care lotion
- Management of itching while the skin is healing: antihistamines, loose cotton clothing, baking soda baths
- Use of sunscreen greater than 30 to prevent additional damage to the skin and to prevent hyperpigmentation of the healing skin
- Prevention of burn injuries in the future

Complementary and Alternative Therapies

- Aloe vera is an effective topical treatment for superficial and partial-thickness burns. Studies have shown that aloe vera products speed up the wound-healing process and the rate of epithelialization (Maenthaisong, Chaiyakunapruk, Niruntraporn, & Kongkaew, 2007). Note: Use commercial aloe vera products, not live plants.
- Products such as Burnaid that contain tea tree oil may be used as first aid for burns.

CRITICAL COMPONENT

Assessing Degree of Burn

- "Rule of Nines" estimates body surface area (BSA) burned: head = 9%, anterior trunk = 18%, posterior trunk = 18%, each upper extremity = 9%, each lower extremity = 18%, genitalia = 1% (**Figure 21-14**)
- Additional guidelines for assessing burns:
  - First- and second-degree burns covering <10% of body are considered minor burns.
  - Burns involving the face, eyes, ears, hands, feet, and genitalia are considered major burns.
  - Buns involving >30% of the body are considered major burns.

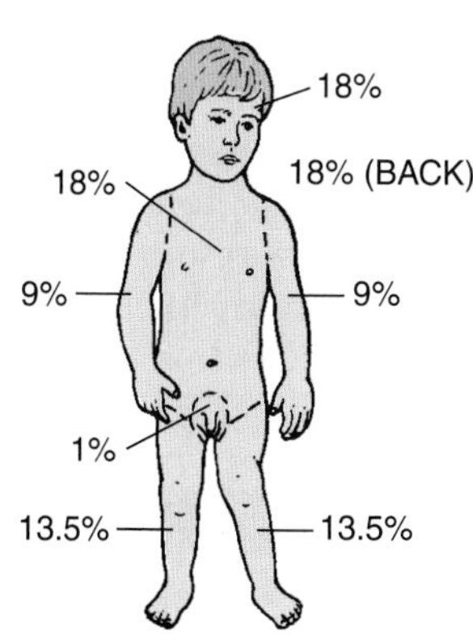

Figure 21–14 The Rule of Nines.

CLINICAL PEARL

Hospitalization for Burns

Children will require hospitalization if >10% BSA is burned, the burn was electrical or chemical in origin, there is evidence of smoke inhalation or carbon monoxide poisoning, there is evidence of abuse or an unsafe environment, or if one of the following body parts is burned: face, hands, feet, perineum, or joints (Tschudy & Arcara, 2012).

Evidence-Based Practice: Burn Injuries and Post-Traumatic Stress

Dyster-Aas, J., Willebrand, M., Wikehult, B., Gerdin, B., & Ekselius, L. (2008). Major depression and posttraumatic stress disorder symptoms following severe burn injury in relation to lifetime psychiatric morbidity. *Journal of Trauma, 64*, 1349–1356. doi:10.1097/TA.0b013e318047e005

Kenardy, J. A., Spence, S. H., & Macleod, A. C. (2006). Screening for posttraumatic stress disorder in children after accidental injury. *Pediatrics, 118*, 1002–1009. doi: 10.1542/peds.2006-0406

Stoddard, F. J., Ronfeldt, H., Kagan, J., Drake, J. E., Snidman, N., Murphy, J. M., . . . Sheridan, R. L. (2006). *American Journal of Psychiatry, 163*, 1084–1090. doi: 10.1176/appi.ajp.163.6.1084

Children and families who have suffered from burn injuries may experience anxiety, guilt, depression, and post-traumatic stress disorder. Two-thirds of burn patients may experience these long-term emotional problems (Dyster, Willebrand, Wikehult, Gerdin, & Ekselius, 2008).

Post-traumatic stress disorder (PTSD) has been validated in children 6 months after suffering from burns or other traumatic injuries (Kenardy, Spence, & Macleod, 2006). Toddlers 12 to 48 months of age have demonstrated signs of PTSD following hospitalization for burn injuries. PTSD in young children may be manifested as reduced smiling and vocalization (Stoddard et al., 2006). It is important for nurses to offer emotional support to children and their families following burn injuries and to refer both children and families to therapy or to support groups as part of their discharge planning.

Medication

Medications for Treatment of Burns

Bacitracin ointment is effective in the topical treatment of burns. Silver sulfadiazine (Silvadene) may still be used for topical treatment of burns but must never be used in pregnant women, infants less than 2 months of age, or children who are allergic to sulfonamides. Bismuth-impregnated petroleum gauze and Biobrane dressings are effective for children with superficial or partial-thickness burns (Morgan et al., 2000).

CRITICAL COMPONENT

Pain Management

Pain management is required when children need debridement and dressing changes with burn injuries. Superficial and partial-thickness burns are very painful. Opiates are effective analgesics for severe or extensive injuries. As healing takes place and the pain becomes less severe, acetaminophen or ibuprofen may offer adequate analgesia. Distraction techniques such as videos, therapeutic play, and virtual reality imaging may also help the child or adolescent to cope with the pain.

CULTURAL AWARENESS: Culture and Risk for Burns

The World Health Organization (2008) reports that there is a higher risk for burn injuries in developing countries. Using open fires for cooking and heating, cooking with pots on ground level, wearing loose-fitting clothing while cooking, and using kerosene appliances account for many burn injuries. Flammable materials used for buildings in developing countries and substandard wiring also lead to fires. The incidence of burns in developed countries has been decreased through smoke detectors, regulation of temperature settings in hot water heaters, and flame-retardant materials in children's clothing. Low-income countries do not have access to these burn-prevention strategies.

CRITICAL COMPONENT

First Aid for Burns

- Do not use butter, oils, or ice on the burn. These may cause additional injury.
- Perform hand hygiene before caring for burns.
- Superficial burns: soak the burn in cool water. Apply antibiotic ointment or aloe vera cream.
- Partial-thickness burns with blistering: soak the burn in cool water. Do not break blisters. Apply antibiotic ointment and nonstick dressing. Change the dressing daily.
- Watch for signs of infection: increased redness, swelling, pain, or drainage. Seek medical help if there are signs of infection.
- Make sure tetanus immunization is up to date.
- Chemical burns: wash with large amounts of water. Consult physician or poison control center.
- Electrical burns: seek medical help. The injury may be worse under the surface of the skin.

CLINICAL PEARL

Intentional Burn Injury

Some burn injuries in children are intentional. Consider whether the history or the story given is compatible with the severity or pattern of the injury. Also consider whether the injury is compatible with the child's age and development. Refer to child protection services if there is a concern.

CRITICAL COMPONENT

Airway Obstruction and Respiratory Distress with Burn Injury

Be aware of the possibility of airway obstruction if the child was exposed to smoke or to fire within a confined space, or if the child inhaled toxic chemicals. Airway obstruction may be immediate or may progress over 24 to 48 hours. If there is a burn on the face or neck, singed hair on the face, or the presence of carbon particles in the nose or mouth, the individual is at high risk for airway obstruction. Watch for coughing, wheezing, and dyspnea.

If the burn was severe or occurred in a confined space, assume that there may be carbon monoxide poisoning. These burn victims must always be given 100% humidified oxygen (Tschudy & Arcara, 2012).

Promoting Safety

To prevent burns:

- Be aware that burns may be chemical, electrical, or thermal.
- Install smoke detectors in homes and check expiration dates on batteries.
- Keep a fire extinguisher in the home.
- Infants are vulnerable to burns from scalding, direct contact with hot objects, and sunburn (Burlinson, Wood, & Rea, 2009).
- Do not hold infants when cooking or heating bottles.
- Keep curling irons and other hot objects out of infant reach.
- Be aware of infant seat buckles that become hot in the sun.
- Buy fire-retardant clothing for children.
- Cover electrical outlets.
- Keep matches and chemicals locked up.
- Keep pot handles turned inward. Supervise children around burners, hot plates, grills, and griddles. Keep hot objects pushed back on countertops.
- Protect children from stoves and heaters; keep guardrails in front of fireplaces.
- Check bathwater temperature before bathing children. Keep the hot water heater thermostat at 120 degrees.
- Educate children on fire safety and what to do in the event of a fire.
- Educate school-age children on playing safely with fireworks, cooking indoors and outdoors, and playing outdoors where electrical lines are present.
- Prevent sunburn. Refer to section on sunburn earlier in this chapter.

Clinical Reasoning

Severe Burns

Scenario: A child has been admitted to the hospital with severe burns over 30% of the body, including the face, trunk, and arms.

1. What are five top-priority physiological nursing diagnoses for this child?
2. What are five top-priority psychosocial nursing diagnoses for the child and family?

CRITICAL COMPONENT

Skin Grafts

- Burned skin is removed by excision or debridement before skin grafting takes place.
- Autografts: the child or adolescent's own skin is used for grafting onto the burned area (**Figure 21-15**).
- The donor skin may be split partial thickness or full thickness. A dermatome is used to shave off the skin that will be used for the graft.
- If the area to be grafted is large, the donor skin will be made into a mesh in order to cover a larger area.
- Allograft: skin from organ donors is kept preserved or frozen in a skin bank. This skin can be used as a temporary graft only because the body will reject it. It is useful to prevent infection or fluid loss and to allow time for autografting to take place.
- Cultured epithelial autograft (CEA): cells from the patient are used to grow thin sheets of tissue that may be grafted.
- Synthetic products such as the Integra dermal regeneration template may be used to cover the burn temporarily (Papini, 2004).

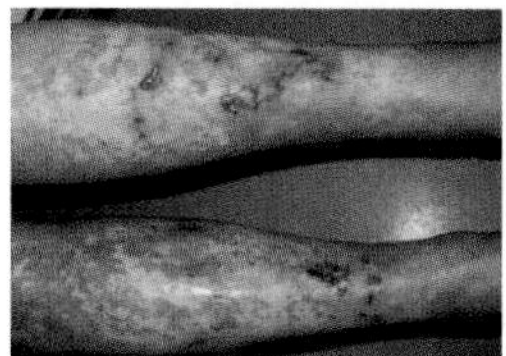

Figure 21-15 Child after skin grafting (graft versus host).

Review Questions

1. A 7-year-old child comes into the clinic with impetigo around his mouth and nose. Which of the following statements would indicate to the nurse that a caregiver understands the child's home care instructions?
   A. "After 2 days on antibiotic treatment, he can return to school."
   B. "He will be out of school for 6 weeks, and we need to plan homework."
   C. "He can return to school immediately if we apply the ointment now."
   D. "He will need intravenous antibiotics before he returns to school."

2. A 13-year-old athlete asks the nurse for advice on care of an "insect bite" on his leg. The nurse should give immediate consideration to which of the following symptoms? (select all that apply)
   A. Itching and slight swelling in the immediate area
   B. Erythema, red streaking, and purulent drainage
   C. Erythema, slight swelling, and warmth over the extremity
   D. Light crusting and itching around the lesion

3. A crying child arrives in the emergency room after being rescued from a burning house. There are minor burns on the arms, legs, and one side of the face. Upon arrival, which of the following parameters would be the initial focus of the nursing assessment?
   A. Capillary refill and pulses in the lower extremities, blood pressure
   B. Behavior, evidence of emotional trauma
   C. Breath sounds, oxygen saturation level
   D. Size and location of burns, presence of fluid loss from burns

4. A 2-year-old with scaly, itching patches on the face and arms has been diagnosed with atopic dermatitis (eczema). The nurse assessed that which of the following factors in the child's history most likely contributed to his condition?
   A. Has been playing outdoors among bushes and vines
   B. Has been playing with pet dogs
   C. Has history of asthma and food allergies
   D. Has history of scabies infections

5. An adolescent has been admitted to the hospital with cellulitis on the lower leg. Which finding would the nurse identify as consistent with the admitting diagnosis?
   A. Decreased pulses and coolness in the foot
   B. Pitting edema on the ankle
   C. An increasing area of pain and redness
   D. An increasing area of scaling and intense itching

6. A child has received an anti-lice shampoo treatment after lice were found at school. The nurse's teaching plan should reinforce which of the following concepts?
   A. The child's hair should be cut short to remove all nits.
   B. The carpet and couches at home should be sprayed with insecticide.
   C. Any pets in the home should also be treated with anti-lice shampoo.
   D. The shampoo treatment should be repeated in 1 week.

7. Soon after a child is admitted with burns to the lower extremities, the nurse observes diminished pulses and increased capillary refill time in one leg. The child cannot move the foot and complains of increasing pain. Which of the following actions would be most appropriate for the nurse to take at this time?
   A. Monitor closely, checking the extremity every 2 hours.
   B. Administer pain medication as ordered.
   C. Apply warm sterile compresses to the lower leg and foot.
   D. Notify the physician immediately.

8. A family is planning a noon picnic at the beach. To prevent sunburn in their infant, caregivers should carry out which of the following actions? (select all that apply)
   A. Apply a sunscreen with SPF 10.
   B. Change the time of their picnic to 5 PM.
   C. Dress the infant in loose cotton clothing.
   D. Dress the infant in clothing with built-in SPF protection.

9. The school nurse is consulted when a 5-year-old child is burned on the hand following an incident in which she inserted her hair clip into an electrical outlet. The burn is approximately 1 inch long, and the child is alert. Which nursing action would demonstrate an *unsafe* nursing judgment?
   A. Call the parents and refer the child to her health-care provider.
   B. Apply bacitracin ointment with gauze and arrange to transport the child.
   C. Monitor the child's vital signs while waiting for the parents.
   D. Apply a dressing to the hand and send the child back to class.

10. A child comes into the emergency room after being evacuated from a small room in a burning house. There is a partial-thickness burn on the side of the face, and full-thickness burns on the arms. Which nursing action receives the highest priority?
    A. Give pain medication as ordered.
    B. Give 100% humidified oxygen.
    C. Insert an intravenous catheter for fluid replacement.
    D. Cover burns with sterile gauze.

References

Alm, B., Aberg, N., Erdes, L., Möllborg, P., Pettersson, R., Norvenius, S. G., . . . Wennergren, G. (2009). Early introduction of fish decreases the risk of eczema in Infants. *Archives of Disease in Childhood, 94*, 11–15. doi: 10.1136/adc.2008.140418

Arcangelo, V. P., & Peterson, A. M. (2006). *Pharmacotherapeutics for advanced practice* (2nd ed.). Philadelphia, PA: Lippincott Williams & Wilkins.

Aronson, S. S., & Shope, T. R. (2009). *Managing infectious diseases in child care and schools* (2nd ed.). Elk Grove Village, IL: American Academy of Pediatrics.

Arowojolu, A. O., Gallo, M. F., Lopez, L. M., Grimes, D. A., & Garner, S. E. (2008). Combined oral contraceptive pills for treatment of acne. *Cochrane Database of Systematic Reviews, 4*. doi: 10.1002/14651858.CD004425.pub4

Bookout, K. (2008). Wound care product primer for the nurse practitioner: Part I. *Journal of Pediatric Health Care, 22*, 60–63. doi: 10.1016/j.pedhc.2007.09.009

Burlinson, C. E. G., Wood. F. M., & Rea, S. M. (2009). Patterns of burn injury in the preambulatory infant. *Burns, 35*, 118–122. doi: 10.1016/j.burns.2008.02.005

Cohen, B. A. (2005). *Pediatric dermatology* (3rd ed.). Baltimore, MD: Elsevier Mosby.

Curley, M. A. Q., Razmus, I. S., Roberts, K. E., & Wypij, D. (2003, January/February). Predicting pressure ulcer risk in pediatric patients: The Braden Q Scale. *Nursing Research, 52*(1), 22–33.

Dyster-Aas, J., Willebrand, M., Wikehult, B., Gerdin, B., & Ekselius, L. (2008). Major depression and posttraumatic stress disorder symptoms following severe burn injury in relation to lifetime psychiatric morbidity. *Journal of Trauma, 64*, 1349–1356. doi:10.1097/TA.0b013e318047e005

Food and Drug Administration. (2002). *Concerns regarding Accutane (isotretinoin).* Retrieved from http://www.fda.gov/newsevents/testimony/ucm115126.htm

Greer, F. R., Sicherer, S. H., & Burks, A. W. (2008). Effects of early nutritional interventions on the development of atopic disease in infants and children: the role of maternal dietary restriction, breastfeeding, timing of introduction of complementary foods, and hydrolyzed formulas. *Pediatrics, 121*, 183–191. doi: 10.1542/peds.2007-3022

Hohlfeld, J., Roessingh, A., Hirt-Burri, N., Chaubert, P., Gerber, S., Scaletta, C., . . . Applegate, L. A. (2005). Tissue engineered fetal skin constructs for pediatric burns. *Lancet, 366*, 840–842. doi: 10.1016/S0140-6736(05)67107-3

Jull, A. B., Rodgers, A., & Walker, N. (2009). *Honey as a topical treatment for wounds.* Retrieved from http://www.ncbi.nlm.nih.gov/pubmed/18843679

Kenardy, J. A., Spence, S. H., & Macleod, A. C. (2006). Screening for posttraumatic stress disorder in children after accidental injury. *Pediatrics, 118*, 1002–1009. doi: 10.1542/peds.2006-0406

Leung, A. K. C., Fong, J. H. S., & Pinto-Rojas, A. (2005). Pediculosis capitis. *Journal of Pediatric Health Care, 19*, 369–373. doi: 10.1016/j.pedhc.2005.07.002

Maenthaisong, R., Chaiyakunapruk, N., Niruntraporn, S., & Kongkaew, C. (2007). The efficacy of aloe vera used for burn wound healing: A systematic review. *Burns, 33*, 713–718. doi: 10.1016/j.burns.2006.10.384

Morgan, E. D., Bledsoe, S. C., & Barker, J. (2000). Ambulatory management of burns. *American Family Physician, 62*, 2015–2030. Retrieved from http://www.aafp.org/afp/20001101/2015.html

Nolt, J. D. (2007). Another mosquito bite . . . In the middle of winter? *Journal of Pediatric Health Care, 21*, 211–214. doi: 10.1016/j.pedhc.2007.02.007

Noonan, C., Quigley, S., & Curley, M. (2006). Skin integrity in hospitalized infants and children: A prevalence survey. *Journal of Pediatric Nursing, 21*, 445–453. doi:10.1016/j.pedn.2006.07.002

Papini, R. (2004). Management of burn injuries of various depths. *BMJ, 329*, 158. doi: 10.1136/bmj.329.7458.158

So, T., & Farrington, E. (2008). Community-acquired methicillin-resistant *Staphyloccus-aureus* in the pediatric population. *Journal of Pediatric Health Care, 22*, 211–217. doi:10.1016/j.pedhc.2008.04.010

Stoddard, F. J., Ronfeldt, H., Kagan, J., Drake, J. E., Snidman, N., Murphy, J. M., . . . Sheridan, R. L. (2006). *American Journal of Psychiatry, 163*, 1084–1090. doi: 10.1176/appi.ajp.163.6.1084

Thygarajan, A., & Burks, A. W. (2008). AAP recommendations on the effects of early nutritional interventions on the development of atopic disease. *Current Opinions in Pediatrics, 20*, 698–702. doi: 10.1097/MOP.0b013e3283154f88

Tschudy, M. M., & Arcara, K. M. (2012). *The Harriet Lane handbook* (19th ed.). Philadelphia, PA: Elsevier Mosby.

Wasiak, J., Cleland, H., & Campbell, F. (2009). *Dressings for superficial and partial thickness burns.* Retrieved from http://www.ncbi.nlm.nih.gov/pubmed/18843629

World Health Organization. (2008). *Burn prevention and care.* Retrieved from http://whqlibdoc.who.int/publications/2008/9789241596299_eng.pdf

Additional Resources

Brown, K. M. (2007). Dermatoses of summer. *Contemporary Pediatrics, 24*, 13–18. doi: 10.5172/conu.2007.26.2.238

Centers for Disease Control and Prevention. (2011). *Methicillin-resistant* Staphylococcus aureus *(MRSA) infections.* Retrieved from http://www.cdc.gov/mrsa/

Sondheimer, J. M. (2008). *Current essentials: Pediatrics.* New York: McGraw Hill.

Communicable Diseases

22

Anita Mitchell, PhD, APN, FNP

OBJECTIVES

- ☐ Define key terms.
- ☐ Describe the source and transmission of various communicable diseases.
- ☐ Outline critical components of a history for a child or adolescent with a communicable disease.
- ☐ Describe the clinical presentation of major communicable diseases.
- ☐ Explain diagnostic and laboratory studies used with communicable diseases.
- ☐ Outline immunizations that are recommended for infants, children, and adolescents.
- ☐ Describe care in the hospital for an infant, child, or adolescent with communicable disease.
- ☐ Plan appropriate isolation techniques to prevent the spread of communicable disease in the hospital.
- ☐ Provide emergency nursing care of children with complications of communicable disease.
- ☐ Develop a home-based plan of care for a child or adolescent with communicable disease.
- ☐ Discuss alternative and complementary therapies used with communicable diseases.
- ☐ Develop a teaching plan for caregivers of children and adolescents with communicable diseases.

KEY TERMS

- Active immunity
- Passive immunity
- Incubation period
- Prodromal
- Communicability
- Universal Precautions
- Transmission
- Standard Precautions

IMMUNIZATIONS FOR CHILDREN FROM BIRTH TO AGE 6

Immunizations for children from birth to age 6 are described by the Centers for Disease Control and Prevention (CDC, 2011a) as follows (**Figure 22-1**).

Hepatitis B

- The hepatitis B vaccine is administered to all newborns. If the mother is positive for hepatitis B surface antigen (HbsAg), 0.5 mL of hepatitis B immune globulin (HBIG) is also given.
- Three doses of hepatitis B are given before age 2: at birth, at 1 to 2 months of age, and after 24 weeks of age.

Hepatitis A

- The hepatitis A vaccine is not given before 12 months of age.
- Two doses are given, at least 6 months apart.
- The hepatitis A vaccine is given to children who are traveling or who are at risk for the disease.

Diphtheria, Tetanus, Pertussis (DTaP)

- Four doses are given for infants and toddlers: at 2, 4, and 6 months and 15 to 18 months.
- A final dose in the series is given between ages 4 and 6.
- The DTaP vaccine may cause irritability, loss of appetite, and localized swelling and tenderness at the injection site. Seizures are a rare side effect of the DTaP, due to the pertussis component of the vaccine. However, this vaccine is much safer now because only acellular components are used to manufacture the vaccine.

Hemophilus Influenzae Type B (Hib)

- Hemophilus influenzae type B is a bacterium that causes infection in various parts of the body.
- This organism was at one time a leading cause of meningitis in young children, and is a significant cause of conjunctivitis, otitis media, and sinusitis.

Recommended Immunization Schedule for Persons Aged 0 Through 6 Years—United States • 2011

For those who fall behind or start late, see the catch-up schedule

Vaccine ▼ Age ►	Birth	1 month	2 months	4 months	6 months	12 months	15 months	18 months	19–23 months	2–3 years	4–6 years
Hepatitis B[1]	HepB	HepB			HepB						
Rotavirus[2]			RV	RV	RV[2]						
Diphtheria, Tetanus, Pertussis[3]			DTaP	DTaP	DTaP	*see footnote[3]*	DTaP				DTaP
Haemophilus influenzae type b[4]			Hib	Hib	Hib[4]	Hib					
Pneumococcal[5]			PCV	PCV	PCV	PCV				PPSV	
Inactivated Poliovirus[6]			IPV	IPV	IPV						IPV
Influenza[7]					Influenza (Yearly)						
Measles, Mumps, Rubella[8]						MMR		see footnote[8]			MMR
Varicella[9]						Varicella		see footnote[9]			Varicella
Hepatitis A[10]						HepA (2 doses)				HepA Series	
Meningococcal[11]										MCV4	

Range of recommended ages for all children

Range of recommended ages for certain high-risk groups

This schedule includes recommendations in effect as of December 21, 2010. Any dose not administered at the recommended age should be administered at a subsequent visit, when indicated and feasible. The use of a combination vaccine generally is preferred over separate injections of its equivalent component vaccines. Considerations should include provider assessment, patient preference, and the potential for adverse events. Providers should consult the relevant Advisory Committee on Immunization Practices statement for detailed recommendations: **http://www.cdc.gov/vaccines/pubs/acip-list.htm.** Clinically significant adverse events that follow immunization should be reported to the Vaccine Adverse Event Reporting System (VAERS) at **http://www.vaers.hhs.gov** or by telephone, **800-822-7967.** Use of trade names and commercial sources is for identification only and does not imply endorsement by the U.S. Department of Health and Human Services.

1. **Hepatitis B vaccine (HepB).** (Minimum age: birth)
   At birth:
   - Administer monovalent HepB to all newborns before hospital discharge.
   - If mother is hepatitis B surface antigen (HBsAg)-positive, administer HepB and 0.5 mL of hepatitis B immune globulin (HBIG) within 12 hours of birth.
   - If mother's HBsAg status is unknown, administer HepB within 12 hours of birth. Determine mother's HBsAg status as soon as possible and, if HBsAg-positive, administer HBIG (no later than age 1 week).

   Doses following the birth dose:
   - The second dose should be administered at age 1 or 2 months. Monovalent HepB should be used for doses administered before age 6 weeks.
   - Infants born to HBsAg-positive mothers should be tested for HBsAg and antibody to HBsAg 1 to 2 months after completion of at least 3 doses of the HepB series, at age 9 through 18 months (generally at the next well-child visit).
   - Administration of 4 doses of HepB to infants is permissible when a combination vaccine containing HepB is administered after the birth dose.
   - Infants who did not receive a birth dose should receive 3 doses of HepB on a schedule of 0, 1, and 6 months.
   - The final (3rd or 4th) dose in the HepB series should be administered no earlier than age 24 weeks.
2. **Rotavirus vaccine (RV).** (Minimum age: 6 weeks)
   - Administer the first dose at age 6 through 14 weeks (maximum age: 14 weeks 6 days). Vaccination should not be initiated for infants aged 15 weeks 0 days or older.
   - The maximum age for the final dose in the series is 8 months 0 days
   - If Rotarix is administered at ages 2 and 4 months, a dose at 6 months is not indicated.
3. **Diphtheria and tetanus toxoids and acellular pertussis vaccine (DTaP).** (Minimum age: 6 weeks)
   - The fourth dose may be administered as early as age 12 months, provided at least 6 months have elapsed since the third dose.
4. ***Haemophilus influenzae* type b conjugate vaccine (Hib).** (Minimum age: 6 weeks)
   - If PRP-OMP (PedvaxHIB or Comvax [HepB-Hib]) is administered at ages 2 and 4 months, a dose at age 6 months is not indicated.
   - Hiberix should not be used for doses at ages 2, 4, or 6 months for the primary series but can be used as the final dose in children aged 12 months through 4 years.
5. **Pneumococcal vaccine.** (Minimum age: 6 weeks for pneumococcal conjugate vaccine [PCV]; 2 years for pneumococcal polysaccharide vaccine [PPSV])
   - PCV is recommended for all children aged younger than 5 years. Administer 1 dose of PCV to all healthy children aged 24 through 59 months who are not completely vaccinated for their age.
   - A PCV series begun with 7-valent PCV (PCV7) should be completed with 13-valent PCV (PCV13).
   - A single supplemental dose of PCV13 is recommended for all children aged 14 through 59 months who have received an age-appropriate series of PCV7.
   - A single supplemental dose of PCV13 is recommended for all children aged 60 through 71 months with underlying medical conditions who have received an age-appropriate series of PCV7.
   - The supplemental dose of PCV13 should be administered at least 8 weeks after the previous dose of PCV7. See *MMWR* 2010:59(No. RR-11).
   - Administer PPSV at least 8 weeks after last dose of PCV to children aged 2 years or older with certain underlying medical conditions, including a cochlear implant.
6. **Inactivated poliovirus vaccine (IPV).** (Minimum age: 6 weeks)
   - If 4 or more doses are administered prior to age 4 years an additional dose should be administered at age 4 through 6 years.
   - The final dose in the series should be administered on or after the fourth birthday and at least 6 months following the previous dose.
7. **Influenza vaccine (seasonal).** (Minimum age: 6 months for trivalent inactivated influenza vaccine [TIV]; 2 years for live, attenuated influenza vaccine [LAIV])
   - For healthy children aged 2 years and older (i.e., those who do not have underlying medical conditions that predispose them to influenza complications), either LAIV or TIV may be used, except LAIV should not be given to children aged 2 through 4 years who have had wheezing in the past 12 months.
   - Administer 2 doses (separated by at least 4 weeks) to children aged 6 months through 8 years who are receiving seasonal influenza vaccine for the first time or who were vaccinated for the first time during the previous influenza season but only received 1 dose.
   - Children aged 6 months through 8 years who received no doses of monovalent 2009 H1N1 vaccine should receive 2 doses of 2010–2011 seasonal influenza vaccine. See *MMWR* 2010;59(No. RR-8):33–34.
8. **Measles, mumps, and rubella vaccine (MMR).** (Minimum age: 12 months)
   - The second dose may be administered before age 4 years, provided at least 4 weeks have elapsed since the first dose.
9. **Varicella vaccine.** (Minimum age: 12 months)
   - The second dose may be administered before age 4 years, provided at least 3 months have elapsed since the first dose.
   - For children aged 12 months through 12 years the recommended minimum interval between doses is 3 months. However, if the second dose was administered at least 4 weeks after the first dose, it can be accepted as valid.
10. **Hepatitis A vaccine (HepA).** (Minimum age: 12 months)
    - Administer 2 doses at least 6 months apart.
    - HepA is recommended for children aged older than 23 months who live in areas where vaccination programs target older children, who are at increased risk for infection, or for whom immunity against hepatitis A is desired.
11. **Meningococcal conjugate vaccine, quadrivalent (MCV4).** (Minimum age: 2 years)
    - Administer 2 doses of MCV4 at least 8 weeks apart to children aged 2 through 10 years with persistent complement component deficiency and anatomic or functional asplenia, and 1 dose every 5 years thereafter.
    - Persons with human immunodeficiency virus (HIV) infection who are vaccinated with MCV4 should receive 2 doses at least 8 weeks apart.
    - Administer 1 dose of MCV4 to children aged 2 through 10 years who travel to countries with highly endemic or epidemic disease and during outbreaks caused by a vaccine serogroup.
    - Administer MCV4 to children at continued risk for meningococcal disease who were previously vaccinated with MCV4 or meningococcal polysaccharide vaccine after 3 years if the first dose was administered at age 2 through 6 years.

The Recommended Immunization Schedules for Persons Aged 0 Through 18 Years are approved by the Advisory Committee on Immunization Practices (**http://www.cdc.gov/vaccines/recs/acip**), the American Academy of Pediatrics (**http://www.aap.org**), and the American Academy of Family Physicians (**http://www.aafp.org**).

Department of Health and Human Services • Centers for Disease Control and Prevention

Figure 22–1 Immunization schedule for children from birth through age 6.

- The Hib vaccine is given in a series of four doses: at 2, 4, and 6 months and 12 to 15 months. No additional doses are given after this series.

Rotavirus

- Rotavirus causes severe diarrhea and dehydration.
- Two vaccinations available for rotavirus are RotaTeq and Rotarix. RotaTeq is licensed as a three-dose series. Rotarix is licensed as a two-dose series.
- The first immunization is given between 6 and 14 weeks. The series is not started if the infant is >14 weeks and 6 days.
- Three doses of RotaTeq vaccination are given orally at 2, 4, and 6 months.
- If Rotarix is given at 2 and 4 months, no additional doses are given.
- Avoid immunization if the child has a history of intussusception or other gastrointestinal disorder.

Pneumococcal (PCV13 and PPSV23)

- The pneumococcal conjugate vaccine (PCV13) is recommended for children under age 5 to protect against *Streptococcus pneumoniae* (pneumococcus).
- PCV13 replaces PCV7. A single additional dose of PCV13 is recommended for all children 14 to 59 months who have received an age-appropriate series of PCV7 and for all children 60 to 71 months with underlying specific medical conditions who have received an age-appropriate series of PCV7.
- Four doses of PCV13 are given in the series: at 2, 4, and 6 months and 12 to 15 months.
- The pneumococcal polysaccharide vaccine (PPSV23) is used for older children and adults, but may be used in children over 2 who have special medical conditions such as a cochlear implant.
- The pneumococcal vaccine protects children from meningitis, otitis media, and other infections.

Inactivated Poliovirus

- Inactivated poliovirus vaccine (IPV) has replaced the live, oral vaccine (OPV). IPV is safer to use because OPV contains live viruses and may cause paralysis in immunodeficient children or in close contacts who are immunodeficient.
- IPV is given in a series of four doses: at 2, 4, and 6 to 18 months, and 4 to 6 years

Influenza

- Children ages 6 months to 18 years should receive an influenza immunization annually.
- Children through 8 years of age who are receiving their first influenza immunization need two doses, at least 4 weeks apart.
- Children over the age of 2 have the option of receiving a live, attenuated influenza virus (LAIV) through a nasal spray as an alternative to the injection. The nasal spray vaccine is contraindicated for children with asthma and should not be given to children ages 2 to 4 who have been wheezing within the past 12 months.
- The influenza immunization is contraindicated for individuals who are allergic to eggs or egg products.
- The influenza nasal spray may cause symptoms of mild flu because it is manufactured from a weakened form of the live virus.

Measles, Mumps, Rubella (MMR)

- The minimum age for receiving this immunization is 12 months. Do not give before the first birthday.
- The second dose is generally given at 4 to 6 years of age but may be given before age 4 if at least 4 weeks have elapsed since the first dose.
- Children may experience maculopapular rash, fever, swollen cheeks, and mild joint pain following the MMR.
- MMR is contraindicated for persons who are allergic to neomycin or gelatin.

Varicella (Varivax)

- The minimum age for receiving this immunization is 12 months. Do not give before the first birthday.
- The second dose is generally given at 4 to 6 years of age but may be given before age 4 if at least 3 months have lapsed since the first dose.
- Side effects include erythema and soreness at the injection site. A few people may experience a varicella-type rash in the area of the injection site.
- Varivax is contraindicated for persons who are allergic to neomycin or gelatin.

Meningococcal (MCV4)

- The meningococcal conjugate vaccine (MCV4) is given as two doses 8 weeks apart to children ages 2 to 10 if they are high risk due to asplenia or immunodeficiency disorders. A booster is given every 5 years.
- Children with HIV receive two doses of MCV4 8 weeks apart.
- Children who travel to countries where meningococcal meningitis is endemic need one dose of MCV4.
- Avoid the immunization if the child is allergic to latex or has a history of Guillain–Barré syndrome.

General Considerations of Immunizations

- Some immunizations may cause mild fever, or soreness and redness at the injection site. Teach parents how to calculate appropriate doses of acetaminophen or ibuprofen to relieve any pain or fever following the immunization. Warm compresses may also be applied to the injection site.
- Children with mild signs and symptoms of a cold may receive immunizations. However, if they are febrile, it is better to hold the immunization until later.

- Caregivers must receive a Vaccine Information Statement (VIS) that explains the purpose of the vaccine, possible side effects, and how to care for the child. This statement also informs and questions the caregiver about possible contraindications and allergies to the vaccine. Caregivers must sign a permission form before the child receives the immunization.
- All adverse effects of immunizations must be reported. The physician or nurse practitioner may file a Vaccine Adverse Event Report (VAER) with the Centers for Disease Control and Prevention (VAERS, 2011).
- Documentation must include the lot number of the vaccine. The lot number is recorded on the vaccine label. Documentation also includes the route and site of vaccine administration and the date that the vaccine was given. Copies of permission forms must be kept on file.

CRITICAL COMPONENT

Immunization Success

Vaccines have significantly reduced the incidence of many communicable diseases. For example, diphtheria is now a rare disease in the United States, but was a major health problem in years past. Respiratory diphtheria causes severe illness and death as a result of airway obstruction from a membrane that covers the pharynx or nasal passages. Diphtheria remains a problem is some developing countries, and continued vigilance is needed. Similarly, polio crippled thousands of children until the 1950s when vaccinations became widespread. Today, the disease has been eliminated from most of the world. However, it is still endemic in several countries worldwide (CDC, 2011g).

IMMUNIZATIONS FOR CHILDREN AGES 7–18

Immunizations for children from ages 7 to 18 are described per the Centers for Disease Control and Prevention (CDC, 2011a) as follows (**Figure 22-2**).

Tetanus, Diphtheria, Pertussis (Tdap)

- The Tdap is given at age 11 to 12 to persons who have completed the childhood series of DTaP but have not received a Td booster. The minimum age for Boostrix is 10, and 11 for Adacef.
- The Tdap is given to all persons 13 to 18 years of age who have not received this immunization.
- The immunization adds pertussis immunity to the traditional Td dose (tetanus/diphtheria). Td boosters are given during adulthood.

Human Papillomavirus (HPV)

- The HPV vaccine is generally given to girls ages 11 to 18, but can be given as early as age 9. It protects against HPV infection that my lead to genital warts or cervical cancer.
- Check for pregnancy before giving the vaccine.
- Three doses are given, the second 2 months after the first dose, the third 6 months after the first dose.
- Dizziness, nausea, vomiting, and fainting may occur after the immunization.
- Best given before the girl becomes sexually active
- The vaccine may also be given to boys ages 9 to 18 to prevent genital warts.
- Do not give if allergic to yeast.

Meningococcal (MCV4)

- MCV4 is recommended for all persons age 11 to 12, with a booster dose given at age 16. It is also recommended for teens ages 13 to 18 if they have not already been vaccinated. If the first dose is given between ages 13 and 15, a booster dose is given at 16 to 18 years of age.
- MCV4 is given as two doses 8 weeks apart to children ages 2 to 10 if they are at high risk due to asplenia or immunodeficiency disorders. A booster is given every 5 years.
- Recommended for college students living in a dormitory

Influenza

- Annual immunization recommended
- Two doses at least 4 weeks apart are recommended for children through age 8 who are receiving their first immunization for influenza.

Pneumococcal (PPSV23)

- Recommended for children and adolescents with high-risk conditions such as cochlear implants, sickle cell anemia, congenital heart disease, or asplenia. The vaccination is repeated after 5 years.

Hepatitis A

- Two doses 6 months apart are recommended for persons who are at high risk or who are traveling.

Hepatitis B

- Three doses are recommended for persons who have not been previously immunized.

Measles, Mumps, Rubella (MMR)

- Catch-up immunizations are given to those who have not been previously vaccinated or who received only one dose.
- Do not vaccinate if the individual is pregnant or immunocompromised.

Varicella

- Catch-up immunizations are given to persons age 7 to 18 who have not been previously vaccinated or who received only one dose.
- Do not vaccinate if the individual is pregnant or immunocompromised.

2013 Recommended Immunizations for Children from 7 Through 18 Years Old

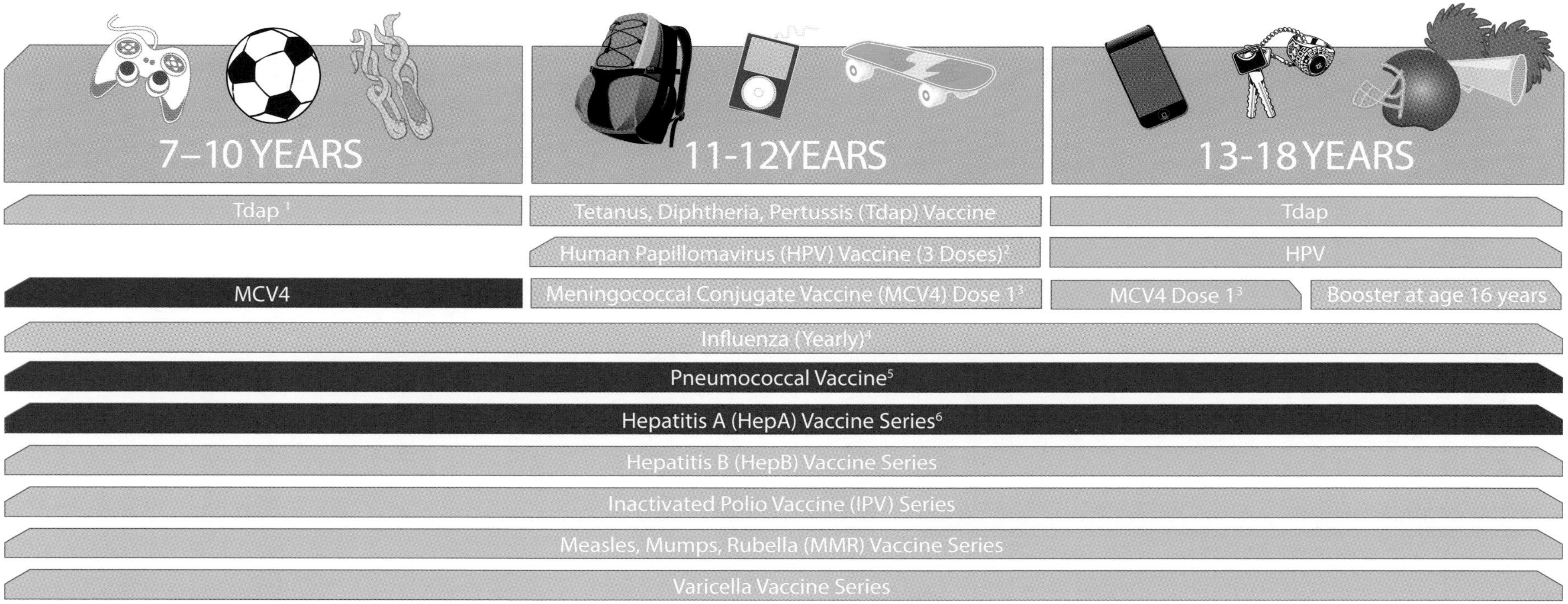

7–10 YEARS	11-12YEARS	13-18YEARS
Tdap [1]	Tetanus, Diphtheria, Pertussis (Tdap) Vaccine	Tdap
	Human Papillomavirus (HPV) Vaccine (3 Doses)[2]	HPV
MCV4	Meningococcal Conjugate Vaccine (MCV4) Dose 1[3]	MCV4 Dose 1[3] / Booster at age 16 years
Influenza (Yearly)[4]		
Pneumococcal Vaccine[5]		
Hepatitis A (HepA) Vaccine Series[6]		
Hepatitis B (HepB) Vaccine Series		
Inactivated Polio Vaccine (IPV) Series		
Measles, Mumps, Rubella (MMR) Vaccine Series		
Varicella Vaccine Series		

These shaded boxes indicate when the vaccine is recommended for all children unless your doctor tells you that your child cannot safely receive the vaccine.

These shaded boxes indicate the vaccine should be given if a child is catching-up on missed vaccines.

These shaded boxes indicate the vaccine is recommended for children with certain health conditions that put them at high risk for serious diseases. Note that healthy children **can** get the HepA series[6]. See vaccine-specific recommendations at www.cdc.gov/vaccines/pubs/ACIP-list.htm.

FOOTNOTES

[1] Tdap vaccine is combination vaccine that is recommended at age 11 or 12 to protect against tetanus, diphtheria and pertussis. If your child has not received any or all of the DTaP vaccine series, or if you don't know if your child has received these shots, your child needs a single dose of Tdap when they are 7 -10 years old. Talk to your child's health care provider to find out if they need additional catch-up vaccines.

[2] All 11 or 12 year olds – both girls *and* boys – should receive 3 doses of HPV vaccine to protect against HPV-related disease. Either HPV vaccine (Cervarix®) or Gardasil®) can be given to girls and young women; only one HPV vaccine (Gardasil®) can be given to boys and young men.

[3] Meningococcal conjugate vaccine (MCV) is recommended at age 11 or 12. A booster shot is recommended at age 16. Teens who received MCV for the first time at age 13 through 15 years will need a one-time booster dose between the ages of 16 and 18 years. If your teenager missed getting the vaccine altogether, ask their health care provider about getting it now, especially if your teenager is about to move into a college dorm or military barracks.

[4] Everyone 6 months of age and older—including preteens and teens—should get a flu vaccine every year. Children under the age of 9 years may require more than one dose. Talk to your child's health care provider to find out if they need more than one dose.

[5] A single dose of Pneumococcal Conjugate Vaccine (PCV13) is recommended for children who are 6 - 18 years old with certain medical conditions that place them at high risk. Talk to your healthcare provider about pneumococcal vaccine and what factors may place your child at high risk for pneumococcal disease.

[6] Hepatitis A vaccination is recommended for older children with certain medical conditions that place them at high risk. HepA vaccine is licensed, safe, and effective for all children of all ages. Even if your child is not at high risk, you may decide you want your child protected against HepA. Talk to your healthcare provider about HepA vaccine and what factors may place your child at high risk for HepA.

U.S. Department of Health and Human Services
Centers for Disease Control and Prevention

American Academy of Pediatrics
DEDICATED TO THE HEALTH OF ALL CHILDREN™

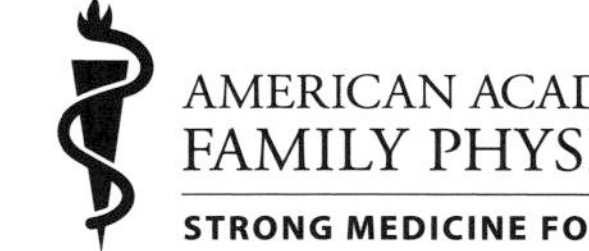

AMERICAN ACADEMY OF FAMILY PHYSICIANS
STRONG MEDICINE FOR AMERICA

For more information, call toll free 1-800-CDC-INFO (1-800-232-4636) or visit http://www.cdc.gov/vaccines/teens

Figure 22–2 Immunization schedule for children and adolescents ages 7–18. *(From the Centers for Disease Control and Prevention [CDC]. [2011].* 2011 child and adolescent immunization schedules. *Retrieved March, 2012, from http://www.cdc.gov/vaccines/recs/schedules/child-schedule.htm)*

CRITICAL COMPONENT

Types of Immunity

When a person carries antibodies to a disease, he or she has immunity to that disease. There are two types of immunity:

- **Active immunity**, when a person is exposed to the disease organism and makes his or her own antibodies. Active immunity is permanent or long-lasting.
  - Natural active immunity: a person actually has the infection and is then immune to the disease.
  - Vaccine-induced immunity: active immunity to a disease that comes from being immunized with a killed or weakened form of that disease.
- **Passive immunity**, when a person is given antibodies to a disease. This immunity is temporary and lasts for only a few weeks or months.
  - Natural passive immunity: antibodies are passed from mother to fetus by way of the placenta.
  - Passive immunity: given through immune globulins to provide immediate protection against a disease.

CRITICAL COMPONENT

Types of Vaccines

Types of vaccines (antigens that stimulate an immune response):

- Inactivated or killed organism (example–inactivated polio virus). The virus is disabled and unable to replicate itself, but it still contains enough of the original characteristics that it can stimulate an immune response.
- Live attenuated or weakened virus (examples–MMR and the varicella vaccine)
- Acellular vaccine (examples–pertussis and Hib). The vaccine contains fragments of cells that stimulate an immune response, but does not contain the whole cell.
- Toxoids (examples–tetanus and diphtheria). Toxins produced by the bacteria are inactivated so that they cannot cause harm but can still stimulate an immune response.
- Subunit of virus (example–hepatitis B). Small fragments of viral protein are used.

Evidence-Based Practice: Varicella and Vaccination

Macartney, K., & McIntyre, P. (2008). Vaccines for post-exposure prophylaxis against varicella (chickenpox) in children and adults. *Cochrane Database of Systematic Reviews 2008*. doi: 10.1002/14651858.CD001833.pub2.

The Cochrane Acute Respiratory Infections Group carried out a systematic review to determine whether chickenpox could be prevented by giving the varicella vaccine to children who had been exposed to the disease. Results suggested that giving the varicella vaccine to children within 3 days of exposure to chickenpox reduces the chance of developing the disease and also reduces the severity of the chickenpox if the child does develop the disease (Macartney & McIntyre, 2008).

CLINICAL PEARL

Routes of Vaccines

- **Intramuscular vaccines**
  - Diphtheria, tetanus, pertussis, (DTaP, DT, Tdap, Td)
  - *Haemophilus influenzae* type b (Hib)
  - Hepatitis A
  - Hepatitis B
  - Human papillomavirus (HPV)
  - Influenza, trivalent inactivated
  - Meningococcal—conjugate (MCV)
  - Pneumococcal conjugate (PCV)
- **Intramuscular or subcutaneous**
  - Pneumococcal polysaccharide (PPSV)
  - Polio, inactivated (IPV)
- **Subcutaneous**
  - Measles, mumps, rubella (MMR)
  - Varicella
  - Meningococcal—polysaccharide (MPSV)
- **Oral**
  - Rotavirus
- **Intranasal spray**
  - Influenza, live attenuated (LAIV)

CLINICAL PEARL

Reducing Fear of Immunizations

Children feel more in control and less fearful of receiving immunizations if they are allowed to sit up rather than lie down during the injection (Lacey, Finkelstein, & Thygeson, 2008).

Clinical Reasoning

Keeping Immunizations Current

Immunizations have significantly decreased the incidence of communicable diseases and have helped to keep children well. However, keeping immunization schedules up to date is an ongoing challenge for nurses.

1. What are some creative ways that nurses could promote immunizations among children and adolescents?
2. What are some barriers to keeping children immunized?
3. Could combination vaccines be one answer to keeping immunization schedules up-to-date? (Joyce, 2007; Koslap-Petrace & Judelsohn, 2008)

ASSESSMENT

General History

To assess the child who may be experiencing a communicable disease, the history is essential. It is important to ask about the following issues:

- Exposure to the disease. Has the child been around other children who have the communicable disease?

Evidence-Based Practice: Immunizations and Autism

Offit, P. A. (2006). *Thimersol and autism.* Retrieved from http://www.immunize.org/catg.d/p2066.pdf

There has been much concern and discussion over the presence of thimersol in some vaccines, linking it to autism. Thimersol is a preservative that contains ethyl mercury. Researchers have found no evidence that thimersol is linked to autism or other adverse effects. However, the Advisory Committee on Immunization Practices (ACIP) has recommended that thimersol be removed from all vaccines. Currently, this preservative is only found in very small amounts in some flu vaccines. Similarly, there is no evidence based on research that the MMR vaccine is associated with autism.

Is the child in close contact with other children at day cares or schools? Have family members been exposed to a communicable disease?

- Consider the **incubation period** of a disease and the length of time it takes for symptoms to appear from the time the child was exposed.
- Has the child had any communicable diseases in the past?
- What immunizations has the child had? Is he or she up to date with the immunization schedule?

Physical Examination

Physical assessment of a child with communicable disease includes assessing **prodromal** signs and symptoms that may appear before a rash or the main illness appears. The prodromal period is often associated with increased **communicability** of the disease. Prodromal signs and symptoms may include:

- Coryza (runny nose)
- Cough
- Fever
- Malaise

General signs and symptoms experienced by a child with communicable disease include the following:

- Changes in behavior—lethargy or irritability
- Skin rashes that may itch and may include macules, papules, pustules, and vesicles
- Enlarged lymph nodes that may vary in location based on the disease, but are predominately located in the anterior cervical, posterior cervical, and tonsillar areas
- Fever
- Vomiting and diarrhea
- Pain in any part of the body, but may be expressed as headache, abdominal pain, throat pain, or muscle aches

See **Table 22-1** for a list of common communicable diseases.

Promoting Safety

Universal Precautions prevent the **transmission** of human immunodeficiency virus, hepatitis B and C, and other blood-borne pathogens. Universal Precautions apply to blood, any body fluids containing blood, semen, and vaginal discharge. Universal Precautions provide guidelines for using protective barriers such as gloves, gowns, masks, and eyewear as needed to protect the health-care worker. Guidelines also prevent injuries from needle sticks and other sharp instruments (CDC, 1988).

Standard Precautions are more comprehensive than Universal Precautions and apply to all patients in any setting. Major components of Standard Precautions include careful hand hygiene, safe injection practices, safe handling of contaminated equipment, and appropriate isolation techniques based on possible exposure to pathogens. Isolation techniques may involve gloves only, or may call for gowns, masks (droplet precaution), or eye protection (invasive procedures). Standard Precautions also protect the patient by preventing spread of pathogens from health-care providers or equipment to the patient (CDC, 2007a). See **Table 22-2** for isolation guidelines in addition to Standard Precautions.

CRITICAL COMPONENT

Caregiver Education

Situations with an ill child that require emergency medical services include the following (Aronson & Shope, 2009):

- Difficulty breathing
- Blue, gray, or purple tinge on lips or skin
- Fever associated with difficulty breathing or abnormal skin color (pallor, bluish tinge, exceptionally pink)
- Fever with headache or stiff neck
- Behavior changes such as lethargy, acting withdrawn, or becoming more unresponsive
- Seizure activity in a child not known to have seizures and without a plan for managing seizures
- Purple or red rash that is spreading quickly, rash that does not blanch (petechiae)
- Dehydration accompanied by lethargy, sunken eyes, no tears, decreased urine output
- Vomiting blood, or blood in the stool

Clinical Reasoning

Infection Control in Schools and Day Care

When children are in close contact with each other at schools and day-care centers, infection is spread easily unless infection control measures are instituted.

1. What infection control measures would you set up in a day care to prevent the spread of disease?

TABLE 22–1 SUMMARY OF COMMON COMMUNICABLE DISEASES

Disease	Agent	Transmission	Incubation	Communicability
Erythema infectiosum (Fifth disease)	Human Parvovirus B19 (HPV)	Respiratory secretions	4–21 days	Contagious until rash appears
Hand-foot-mouth disease	Coxsackie or enterovirus	Direct contact	3–6 days	Virus may be shed for several weeks
Hepatitis A	HAV viral infection	Fecal–oral route Contaminated food	Approximately 30 days	2 weeks before symptoms until 1 week after symptoms
Hepatitis B	HBV viral infection	Blood or blood products Sexual contact	Average 90 days	Can be spread as long as virus is in the blood
Influenza	Influenza Type A or B virus	Coughing, sneezing Oral and nasal secretions	1–4 days	1 day before symptoms and 7 days after symptoms
Mononucleosis	Epstein-Barr virus	Saliva Person-to-person sharing of personal objects	30–50 days	Virus may be excreted for months after infection
Mumps (parotitis)	Paramyxovirus	Contact with oral and nasal secretions	16–18 days	2–3 days before swelling of glands to 5 days after swelling starts
Pertussis (whooping cough)	*Bordetella pertussis* bacteria	Oral and nasal secretions	6–21 days	Onset of symptoms for about 2 weeks Non-immunized infants 6 weeks
RSV bronchiolitis	Respiratory Syncytial Virus	Hands Oral and nasal secretions Lives on surfaces for hours	4–6 days	Viral shedding 3–4 weeks in infants, 3–8 days in older persons
Roseola (*Exanthem subitum*)	Human Herpesvirus 6	Saliva of persons who have the disease or who are carrying virus	9–10 days	Unknown
Rubella (German measles)	Rubella virus	Airborne through respiratory droplets Direct contact with respiratory secretions Found in blood, urine, stool	16–18 days	7 days before rash to 14 days after rash Most children contagious 3–4 days before rash to 7 days after rash
Rubeola (measles)	Rubeola virus	Airborne through respiratory droplets Direct contact with respiratory secretions	8–12 days	1–2 days before prodromal symptoms, 3–5 days before rash, 4 days after rash
Strep throat Scarlet fever	Group A beta-hemolytic streptococcus	Respiratory droplets Direct contact with secretions	2–5 days	Approximately 10 days 24 hours after antibiotics started
Chickenpox (Varicella zoster)	Varicella zoster virus	Fluid from vesicles Oral, nasal, eye secretions Coughing and sneezing	10–21 days	1 day before rash, while rash is spreading, until all vesicles have crusted

TABLE 22–2 ISOLATION GUIDELINES AND STANDARD PRECAUTIONS

Type of Isolation	Contact Precautions	Droplet Precautions	Airborne Precautions
DEFINITION	Prevents diseases spread by direct or indirect contact with the patient or patient's environment	Prevents diseases spread by close respiratory contact or respiratory secretions	Prevent diseases that remain infectious over long distances, organisms remain suspended in the air
SPECIAL EQUIPMENT	Gown and gloves for contact with patient or contaminated objects and areas in the room Patient-care equipment must be disposable or disinfected after use	Health-care providers must wear a mask The patient must wear a mask when being transported outside of room Teach patients to cover mouth with tissue when coughing, dispose of tissue in designated container, wash hands	Health-care providers must wear a mask or respirator depending on specific disease guidelines (refer to Appendix A of CDC isolation guidelines) Airborne infection isolation rooms (AIIRs) provide negative pressure, regular air exchanges, and air exhaustion to the outside or to HEPA filters
CONSIDERATIONS	Includes any patient condition with excess wound drainage, body discharges, or fecal incontinence	Pathogens do not remain infectious over long distances; therefore, special ventilation and air handling are not required	Nonimmune health-care providers should not care for these patients
SAMPLE DISEASES	Bronchiolitis, rotavirus, type A hepatitis in diapered or incontinent patients, impetigo, lice, scabies, poliomyelitis, staphylococcal and streptococcal skin infections Note: smallpox and varicella (chickenpox) require contact and airborne isolation	Influenza, pertussis (whooping cough), *Hemophilus influenzae* type B, epiglottitis or meningitis, meningococcal meningitis, mumps, parvovirus (erythema infectiosum), rubella (German measles), streptococcal group A infections for the first 24 hours, scarlet fever	Measles (rubeola), pulmonary tuberculosis Note: respirators required when caring for patients with tuberculosis Note: smallpox and varicella (chickenpox) require contact and airborne isolation

Source: Centers for Disease Control and Prevention (CDC). (2007). Isolation guidelines. Retrieved from http://www.cdc.gov/ncidod/dhqp/gl_isolation.html.

VIRAL COMMUNICABLE DISEASES

ERYTHEMA INFECTIOSUM (FIFTH DISEASE)

Disease Process

- Agent: Human parvovirus B19 (HPV)
- Transmission: contact with respiratory secretions
- Incubation period: 4–21 days
- Communicability: contagious until the rash appears

Clinical Presentation

- Prodromal: fever, aches, headache
- Rash distribution: erythema of the cheeks, giving the appearance of "slapped cheeks." The rash appears after the red cheeks appear, and is characterized by a lacy pattern on the trunk and extremities. The rash may disappear and then reappear if the child becomes hot.
- Systemic signs and symptoms: no signs or symptoms after the rash has appeared. In adults, there may be pain and swelling of joints (CDC, 2011f).

Diagnostic Testing

- Blood testing will reveal the presence of immunoglobulin M antibody that indicates immunity to parvovirus B19.

Nursing Interventions

Emergency Care

- Sickle cell crisis may occur with HPV in susceptible persons.

Acute Hospital Care

- Fifth disease may be severe in individuals with immune deficiency disorders.
- A child with HPV who is hospitalized with aplastic crisis or because of immunodeficiency must be placed on respiratory isolation.
- A child in aplastic crisis may not have the typical rash, but complain of fever, nausea and vomiting, abdominal pain, malaise, and lethargy.

Caregiver Education

Emergency Care

- The disease may trigger a crisis in persons with sickle cell disease. It may also trigger aplastic crisis in children who are immunodeficient (**Figure 22-3**).

Home Care

- Acetaminophen or ibuprofen for fever or discomfort; adequate hydration

> **CRITICAL COMPONENT**
>
> **Transmission of Fifth Disease to the Fetus**
>
> Erythema infectiosum (Fifth disease) may be passed on to the fetus and cause severe anemia in the fetus or possible complications such as miscarriage.
>
> - Approximately 50% of pregnant women have had Fifth disease in the past and are already immune to parvovirus B19. Therefore, they are not affected.
> - Less than 5% of pregnant women who are exposed to parvovirus B19 may experience complications, and these usually occur during the first half of the pregnancy.
> - To prevent complications from Fifth disease, pregnant women who are in contact with children should practice careful hand hygiene.
> - Women of childbearing age can have a blood test to determine whether they have had Fifth disease and are therefore immune to this disease (CDC, 2005).

HAND-FOOT-AND-MOUTH DISEASE

Disease Process

- Agent: Coxsackie virus or enterovirus
- Transmission: direct contact, respiratory, fecal–oral
- Incubation period: 3–6 days
- Communicability: the virus may be shed for several weeks.

Clinical Presentation

- Signs and symptoms: cold symptoms, coryza, fever, sore throat. Small vesicles appear in the mouth and on the palms of the hands and soles of the feet, and may also appear on the genitalia and buttocks (**Figure 22-4**).

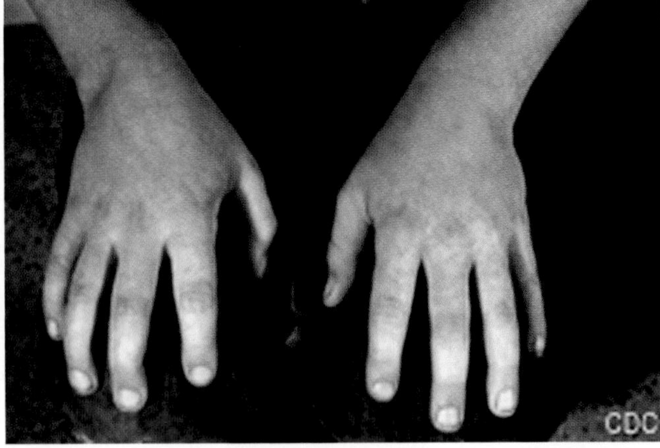

Figure 22-3 Child with Fifth disease.

Diagnostic Testing

- Stool samples and throat swabs can be tested for presence of a virus, but the disease is usually diagnosed clinically.

Caregiver Education

- Careful hand hygiene and disposal of tissues
- Clean surfaces and toys with soap and water, and disinfect with a solution of 1 tablespoon of bleach to 4 cups of water (CDC, 2011c).
- Give bland foods and drinks because the mouth may be sore. Make sure the child is well hydrated.
- Acetaminophen or ibuprofen for pain and fever
- Over-the-counter sprays and mouthwashes that contain local anesthetic to relieve pain in the mouth

HEPATITIS A (HAV)

Disease Process

- Agent: HAV viral infection
- Transmission: fecal–oral route, contaminated food
- Incubation period: approximately 30 days
- Communicability: most contagious for 2 weeks before onset of symptoms and for 1 week after onset of jaundice

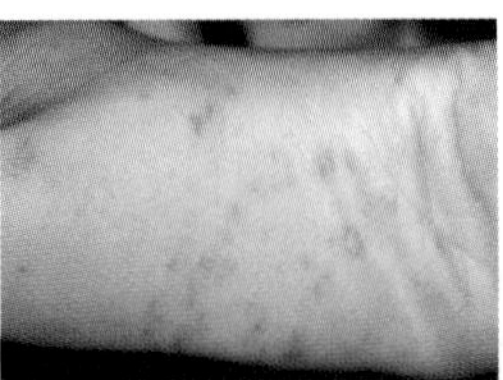
Figure 22-4 Blisters in hand-foot-and-mouth disease.

Clinical Presentation

- Fever, malaise, poor appetite, nausea, jaundice, abdominal pain, dark urine
- Children under age 6 may have mild or no symptoms. Therefore, they may play a significant role in the transmission of HAV.

Diagnostic Testing

- Blood test for presence of anti-HAV IgM in the serum
- Other abnormal lab work: presence of bilirubin in urine, elevated serum bilirubin, elevated liver enzymes (AST and ALT)

Nursing Intervention

Acute Hospital Care

- Contact isolation if the child is incontinent with feces
- Immune globulin can be given after exposure to prevent or reduce the severity of the disease.
- Report incidence to the local health department.

Caregiver Education

Home Care

- Strict hand hygiene and sanitizing of surfaces
- Appropriate rest and activity
- Nutritious, well-balanced diet

HEPATITIS B (HBV)

Disease Process

- Agent: HBV viral infection
- Transmission: blood or blood products, sexual contact
- Incubation period: average of 90 days
- Communicability: can be spread as long as the virus is in the blood of an individual. Some persons are chronic carriers and carry the disease for life.

Clinical Presentation

- Aching, malaise, joint pain, jaundice, dark urine, loss of appetite, mild right upper quadrant abdominal pain
- Children with chronic hepatitis B may be asymptomatic.
- Children with chronic hepatitis B are at risk for developing hepatocellular carcinoma later in life.
- Newborns may acquire HBV perinatally. The CDC (2011d) reports that 40% of infants who do not receive post-exposure prophylaxis will develop chronic hepatitis B. It is important to administer hepatitis B immune globulin (HBIG) in addition to the hepatitis B vaccine (HBV) if the mother is HbsAg positive.
- High-risk groups among children and adolescents include those living in institutions, those involved in IV drug use, those infected by sexual partners, and children who are hemophiliacs or receiving frequent blood transfusions. Individuals who have traveled to Africa or Asia are also at higher risk.

Diagnostic Testing

- Blood tests reveal the hepatitis B surface antigen (HbsAg) and the IGM anti-Hbc core antibody.
- In chronic hepatitis B, the positive HbsAg persists. Chronic carriers are those who have a positive HbsAg for more than 6 months. HBV DNA markers will also be present.

Nursing Intervention

Hospital Care

- Blood-borne precautions (Universal Precautions)

Caregiver Education

Home Care

- Teach family members not to share toothbrushes or razors.
- Lifestyle counseling if risky behaviors such as drug use or sexual activity are present
- Teach importance of treatment and follow-up.

Medication

Treatment for HBV

There are two medications that may be used for children with chronic HBV:

- Interferon-alpha (IFN) reduces replication of the HBV virus. It may be given as subcutaneous injection three times a week for 4 to 6 months. Side effects include fever, aching, joint pain, anorexia, and weight loss.
- Lamivudine inhibits replication of the HBV virus. This drug is given orally, and treatment may last for 1 year. There are fewer side effects than with IFN, but lamivudine may develop resistance (Sims & Woodgate, 2008).

CULTURAL AWARENESS: Hepatitis B Among Adoptive Immigrant Children

Hepatitis B remains a significant health problem, especially in countries such as Asia and Africa. Approximately 400 million people around the world have hepatitis B. Therefore, nurses and families must be aware that immigrant children and international children who are adopted into families in the United States may have been exposed to this disease. The health history is very important because children may be asymptomatic (Sims & Woodgate, 2008).

INFLUENZA

Disease Process

- Agent: influenza viruses. Influenza may be type A (H1N1), type A (H3N2), or type B, with type A being much more prevalent.
- Transmission: coughing and sneezing; contact with objects contaminated with oral or nasal secretions
- Incubation period: 1–4 days
- Communicability: 1 day before symptoms until approximately 7 days after child becomes ill

Clinical Presentation

- Fever, chills, headache, sneezing, cough, malaise, conjunctivitis, and myalgia (aching)

Diagnostic Testing

- Rapid screening for flu virus antigens in nasal secretions

Nursing Interventions

Emergency Care

- Influenza may trigger croup in infants.

Acute Hospital Care

- Pneumonia is a complication of influenza and may require hospitalization.
- Other complications include ear infections, sinus infections, dehydration, and increased severity of existing medical conditions such as diabetes and asthma.
- Isolation—droplet. Refer to box on isolation guidelines.

Caregiver Education

Home Care

- Tylenol or ibuprofen for fever (no aspirin due to risk of Reye syndrome)
- Careful hand washing and disposal of tissues
- Encourage fluids.
- Administration of medications within 48 hours of symptoms (see Medication box)
- Importance of annual influenza immunizations

Complementary and Alternative Therapies

- Traditional Chinese medicinal herbs may be effective in treating influenza (Chen et al., 2008).

> **Medication**
>
> **Treating Influenza**
>
> Medications for influenza must be given within 48 hours of the onset of symptoms. Two antiviral medications for influenza approved by the Food and Drug Administration (FDA) were recommended for the 2011-2012 influenza season: Oseltamivir (Tamiflu) and zanamivir (Relenza). These medications are effective for both influenza type A and influenza type B. Oseltamivir (Tamiflu) may be given to children over 1 year of age. Zanamivir (Relenza) is recommended for children over 7 years of age. It is administered as an inhalation medication and is not recommended for children with airway disease such as asthma (CDC, 2011b).

MONONUCLEOSIS

Disease Process

- Agent: Epstein-Barr virus
- Transmission: person-to-person contact, sharing personal objects such as cups or toothbrushes, through saliva
- Incubation period: 30–50 days
- Communicability: virus may be excreted for months following infection.

Clinical Presentation

- Fever, sore throat, malaise, pharyngitis, enlarged posterior cervical lymph nodes, with symptoms lasting 1 to 4 weeks (**Figure 22-5**)
- May develop splenomegaly or hepatomegaly
- Disease primarily affects adolescents and young adults. Children often have very mild symptoms and adults are usually immune due to previous exposure.

Diagnostic Testing

- Positive mono spot test, positive Paul-Bunnell heterophile antibody test, increased lymphocytes, greater than 10% atypical lymphocytes
- EBV antibody titers

Nursing Intervention

Acute Hospital Care

- Hospitalization may be needed if the child develops respiratory distress, abdominal pain with splenomegaly, or dehydration due to inability to swallow adequate fluids.

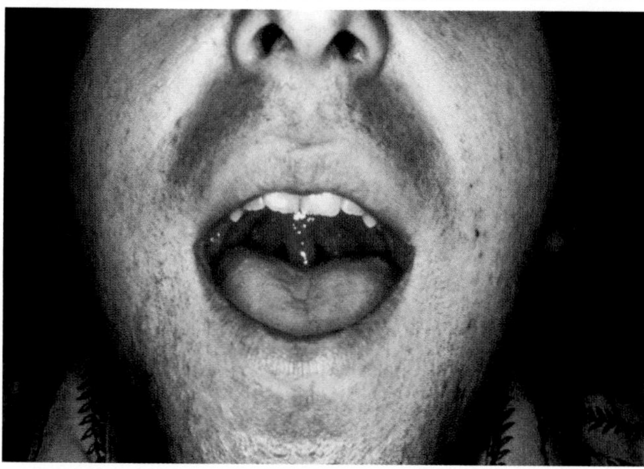

Figure 22-5 Pharyngitis in adolescent with mononucleosis.

Caregiver Education

Home Care

- To prevent injury to spleen, no contact sport for 6 to 8 weeks if spleen is enlarged. Examples of contact sports: basketball, football, soccer, rugby, baseball, boxing, ice hockey, rodeo, wrestling, martial arts, Lacrosse, water polo
- Rest, with appropriate quiet activities and play
- Fever management with acetaminophen or ibuprofen
- Hydration and nutrition
- Counseling and emotional support for adolescents who must be on bed rest

> **Medication**
>
> **Differentiating Between Mononucleosis and Streptococcal Disease**
>
> It may be difficult to distinguish mononucleosis from streptococcal sore throat or pharyngitis. However, health-care providers need to distinguish between the two infections. If ampicillin or amoxicillin is given to an individual with mononucleosis, a maculopapular rash will result.

MUMPS (PAROTITIS)

Disease Process

- Agent: paramyxovirus
- Transmission: contact with oral and nasal secretions
- Incubation period: 16–18 days
- Communicability: 2–3 days before swelling of salivary glands to 5 days after swelling starts

Clinical Presentation

- Location
  - *Swelling of parotid salivary glands in front of the ear, below the ear, under jaw* (**Figure 22-6**)
  - *Boys may have painful swelling of the testicles (orchitis).*
  - *Girls may have ovarian involvement with abdominal pain (oophritis) and breast inflammation (mastitis).*
- Systemic signs and symptoms: headache, fever, ear ache, muscle aches, malaise, loss of appetite

Diagnostic Testing

- Virus can be isolated from saliva.

Nursing Interventions

Emergency Care

- Complications may include meningitis, encephalitis, glomerulonephritis, permanent deafness, sterility, myocarditis, and joint inflammation. Infection during pregnancy may result in fetal death.
- Seek medical care immediately for complications.

Acute Hospital Care

- Respiratory isolation required

Caregiver Education

Home Care

- Acetaminophen or ibuprofen for fever and pain
- Bland, soft foods
- Bland liquids; avoid citrus juices. Keep well hydrated.
- Ice packs or warm compresses to neck for comfort and pain relief
- Snug-fitting underwear and warmth may provide comfort and pain relief for orchitis.

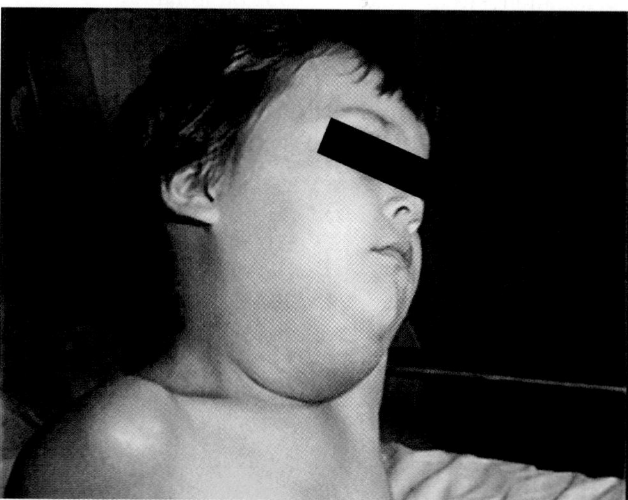

Figure 22-6 Child with mumps.

RESPIRATORY SYNCYTIAL VIRUS (RSV) BRONCHIOLITIS

Disease Process

- Agent: Respiratory Syncytial Virus (RSV)
- Transmission: contact with saliva and nasal secretions. The virus can live on surfaces for several hours and is readily transmitted by hands.
- Incubation period: usually 4–6 days
- Communicability: viral shedding may last as long as 3 to 4 weeks in infants. In older persons, it is shed for 3 to 8 days.

Clinical Presentation

- Symptoms of a cold in older children: cough, coryza (nasal congestion), fever
- As the disease progresses in infants, there may be respiratory distress with tachypnea, wheezing, retractions, severe coughing, and poor air exchange.
- Refer to the chapter on respiratory diseases for additional information on bronchiolitis.

Diagnostic Testing

- RSV screening

Nursing Interventions

Emergency Care

- The virus may cause respiratory distress in infants and toddlers.
- Emergency treatment may be needed.
- Infants who were born prematurely or who have medical problems such as congenital heart defects are especially vulnerable to the effects of RSV.

Acute Hospital Care

- Hospitalization may be needed for infants with bronchiolitis and pneumonia.
- Contact isolation with gowns and gloves
- Frequent assessments of respiratory status
- Schedule activities to allow rest time for infant.
- Cool humidified air at bedside
- Administer oxygen as needed.
- Hydration with intravenous fluids if needed
- Bronchodilator nebulizer treatments
- NOTE: Refer to Chapter 11 "Respiratory Disorders" for additional information on care of the infant or child with bronchiolitis.

Caregiver Education

Home Care

- Careful hand hygiene and disposal of tissues
- Cool mist humidifier, hydration
- Do not administer over-the-counter cough/cold products to children younger than 4 years.
- Teach parents signs of respiratory distress in an infant and when to seek medical care.
- Immunization: infants who are at risk and more vulnerable to RSV due to medical problems may require the Synagis (palivizumab) vaccine to prevent RSV.

Medication

Administration of Synagis (Palivizumab)

The Synagis (palivizumab) vaccine has significantly reduced the incidence of RSV bronchiolitis in infants. This immunization is needed for infants who were born at less than 35 weeks of gestational age or who have chronic lung or heart disease. The American Academy of Pediatrics (2009) has given specific guidelines based on gestational ages of infants and risk factors. The dose is given intramuscularly and repeated monthly (every 28–30 days) for 3 to 5 doses during RSV season. Specific RSV season varies from state to state, but it generally starts in the fall and ends in the spring.

ROSEOLA (EXANTHEM SUBITUM, HHV-6)

Disease Process

- Agent: human Herpesvirus 6
- Transmission: saliva of persons who have the disease or are carrying the virus; 75% of adults carry the virus in their saliva without having symptoms. Most people have had roseola by the time they are 4 years old.
- Incubation period: 9 or 10 days
- Communicability: unknown

Clinical Presentation

- Prodromal: fever above 103°F for 3 to 7 days. The high fever may trigger febrile seizures.
- Rash distribution: papular pink or red rash that appears on the day that the fever returns to normal (**Figure 22-7**)

Diagnostic Testing

Typically diagnosed based on the rash. A blood test may look for antibodies.

Nursing Intervention

- Emergency care may be needed for febrile seizures.

Caregiver Education

- Home care includes fever management, sponging with tepid water, and administration of acetaminophen or ibuprofen.

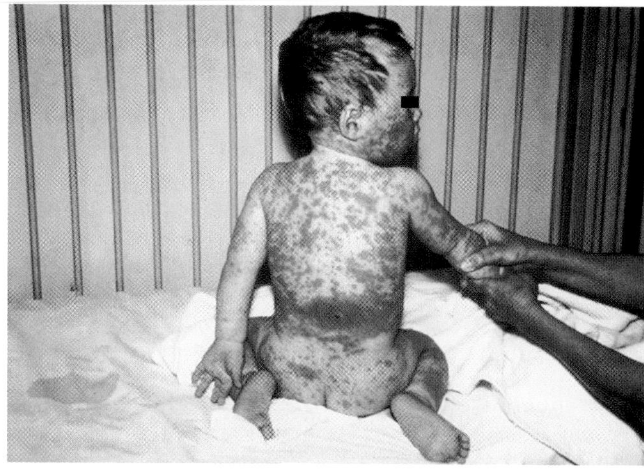

Figure 22-7 Child with roseola.

Figure 22-8 Child with rubella (German measles).

RUBELLA (GERMAN MEASLES)

Disease Process

- Agent: virus
- Transmission: airborne through respiratory droplets or direct contact with respiratory secretions; virus also found in blood, urine, and stool
- Incubation period: 16–18 days
- Communicability: 7 days before rash until 14 days after rash; most children contagious 3–4 days before rash to 7 days after rash

Clinical Presentation

- Prodromal: children do not have prodromal symptoms. Adolescents may experience mild fever, malaise, sore throat, and headache.
- Rash distribution: Fine red or pink rash that appears on the face first and then spreads downward. The rash lasts approximately 3 days and disappears in the same order that it appeared.
- Systemic signs and symptoms: fever, aching, posterior cervical lymph nodes tender and swollen (**Figure 22-8**)

Caregiver Education

- Home care includes fever management as needed.
- Teach the importance of the MMR vaccine before the childbearing years.

> **CRITICAL COMPONENT**
>
> **Rubella Infection During Pregnancy**
>
> Rubella infection during pregnancy may result in congenital heart defects, congenital cataracts, deafness, mental retardation, miscarriage, and fetal death. Infants who survive may be born with rubella syndrome. These infants may shed the virus and be contagious for 1 year.

RUBEOLA (MEASLES)

Disease Process

- Agent: measles virus
- Transmission: airborne through respiratory droplets or direct contact with respiratory secretions
- Incubation period: 8–12 days
- Communicability: 1 or 2 days before prodromal symptoms, 3–5 days before rash, 4 days after rash appears

Clinical Presentation

- Prodromal: coryza, cough, conjunctivitis, fever, malaise; small red spots in the mouth with a bluish white center (Koplik spots; **Figure 22-9**).
- Rash distribution: brownish red macular rash starts at hairline and spreads downward over body
- Systemic signs and symptoms: fever, cough, red, watery eyes, coryza (**Figure 22-10**)

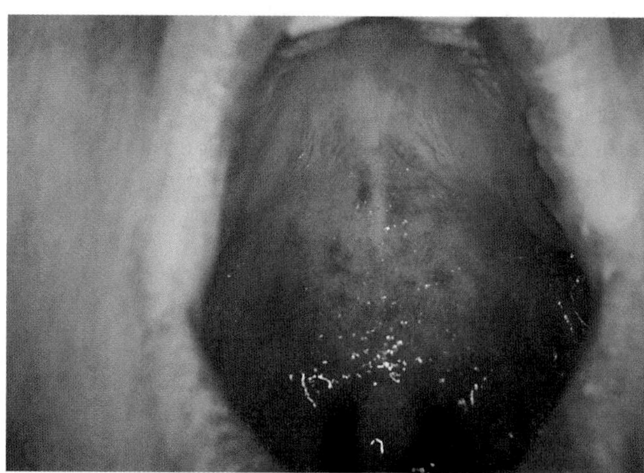

Figure 22-9 Koplik spots.

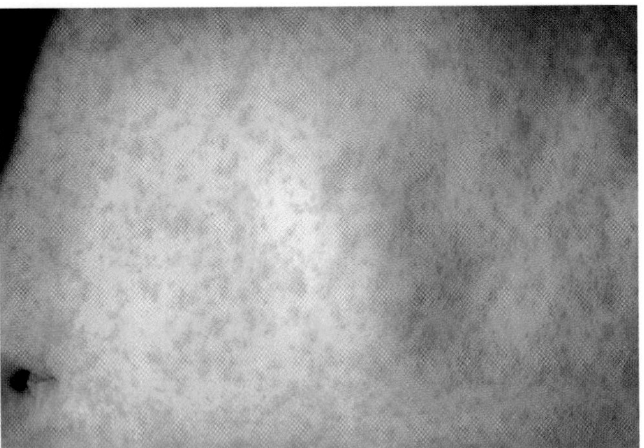

Figure 22-10 Child with rubeola (measles) rash.

Diagnostic Testing

Blood test to detect antibodies

Nursing Interventions

Emergency Care

- Complications include ear infections, diarrhea, encephalitis, pneumonia, seizures, deafness, mental retardation, and death. Seek medical care immediately for complications.

Acute Hospital Care

- Respiratory isolation required

Chronic Home Care

- Long-term care, including ventilator care, may be needed for children with brain damage resulting from measles encephalitis.

Caregiver Education

Home Care

- Fever management with acetaminophen or ibuprofen
- Keep child isolated for 5 days after rash appears.
- Dim lights if photophobia exists. Use warm compresses to remove crusting from eyes as needed.
- Give soft, bland foods.
- Keep child well hydrated with plenty of fluids.
- Use cool mist humidifier.

CULTURAL AWARENESS: Incidence of Measles Worldwide

The CDC (2011e) reports that there are 20 million cases of measles worldwide each year, with 197,000 of these cases resulting in death. Outbreaks of measles may occur in the United States when immigrants or travelers have not been immunized in their home countries. It is always important to check immunization records.

Medication

Use of Immune Globin after Exposure to Measles

- Immune globulin may prevent measles or lessen the severity of the case in unimmunized individuals if given within 6 days of exposure.
- This is especially helpful for infants less than 6 months of age, pregnant women, and those who are immunocompromised (Aronson & Shope, 2009).

Evidence-Based Practice: Measles and Vitamin A

Huiming, Y., Chaomin, W., & Meng, M. (2008). Vitamin A for treating measles in children. *The Cochrane Database of Systematic Reviews 2005*. doi: 10.1002/14651858.CD001479.pub3.

The World Health Organization has recommended two doses of vitamin A to reduce complications and death from measles in areas of the world where vitamin A deficiency may be present. The recommended dose is 100,000 IU daily × 2 for infants, and 200,000 IU daily × 2 for older children. A systematic review and meta-analysis by the Cochrane Database of Systematic Reviews found that vitamin A therapy reduced the risk of pneumonia and death in children under age 2.

VARICELLA-ZOSTER (CHICKENPOX)

Disease Process

- Agent: varicella-zoster
- Transmission: fluid from vesicles of an infected person; secretions from nose, mouth, and eyes; airborne from coughing and sneezing
- Incubation period: 10–21 days
- Communicability: 1 day before rash appears, while rash is spreading, and until all vesicles have crusted over

Clinical Presentation

- Prodromal: fever, malaise, coryza
- Rash distribution: the rash first appears on the trunk and face, and then spreads to other parts of the body. The rash goes through the stages of macule, papule, vesicle, and scab (crust). All stages are present at the same time. Severe itching may be present (**Figure 22-11**).
- Systemic signs and symptoms: fever, headache, dehydration

Diagnostic Testing

Typically diagnosed by visualizing rash.

Nursing Interventions

Emergency Care

- Complications may include bacterial infections of the skin, pneumonia, septicemia, encephalitis, and bleeding problems. Urgent medical care is needed for any complications.

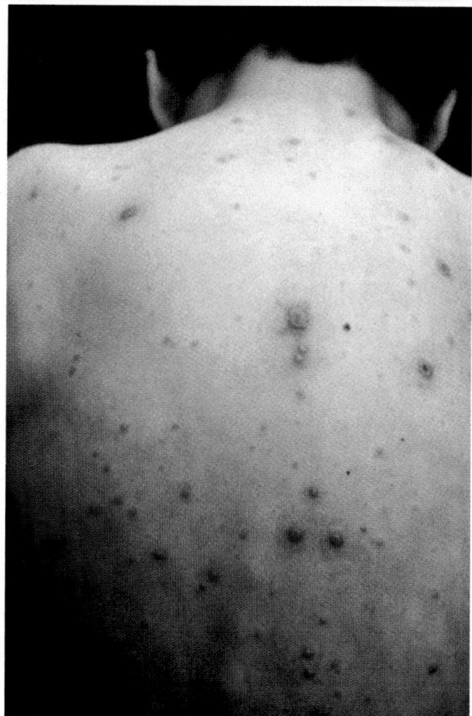

Figure 22-11 Child with chickenpox.

Acute Hospital Care

- Children with chickenpox are not generally hospitalized unless the child is immunocompromised or experiencing complications. Intravenous acyclovir may be given to children in these situations.
- Strict isolation for the hospitalized child, including contact and respiratory isolation

Special Considerations

- It is possible to get chickenpox twice. These are usually mild cases the second time with less fever and few vesicles. Care is the same as for the first case of chickenpox.
- The CDC (2009) reports that 15% to 20% of people who receive the chickenpox vaccine get chickenpox, but the disease is mild.
- It is possible to have a mild rash with a few vesicles around the injection site following varicella immunization. These vesicles must be covered with clothing or a nonporous bandage to prevent spread to others. Isolation may be needed if the rash is more widespread (Aronson & Shope, 2009).

Caregiver Education

Home Care

- Avoid the use of aspirin. Use acetaminophen to relieve fever.
- Keep child isolated until all vesicles have crusted over.
- Keep the child well hydrated. Offer cool, bland liquids because the inside of the mouth may be affected.
- To help prevent itching, keep child cool, dressed in light cotton, and distracted with play activities. Apply gloves or mittens if necessary; keep fingernails clean and cut short.
- Aveeno (oatmeal powder) or baking soda baths may bring relief.
- Apply calamine or Cetaphil lotion to lesions.

Complementary and Alternative Therapies

- Capsaicin may be used to relieve the pain of shingles (herpes zoster). See the Critical Component box on herpes zoster.

Medication

Reye Syndrome

Reye syndrome is a life-threatening disease that primarily affects the brain and liver. It typically follows a viral infection such as chickenpox, influenza, or an upper respiratory infection. The ingestion of aspirin or other medication containing salicylates during a viral illness greatly increases the probability of developing Reye syndrome. It is important to teach caregivers not to give aspirin or salicylate products to any child or adolescent during a febrile illness.

Medication

Ibuprofen Administration

Ibuprofen should never be given to infants less than 6 months of age.

CRITICAL COMPONENT

Shingles (Herpes Zoster)

Shingles (herpes zoster) is a reactivation of the varicella-zoster virus that causes chickenpox. It becomes reactivated in the nervous system and causes a painful, blistering rash in the portion of skin supplied by a particular nerve fiber (dermatome). It occurs after someone has already completely recovered from chickenpox and the virus that was inactive (latent) becomes active. It may occur years after having chickenpox. Educate caregivers that a child cannot get shingles from someone with chickenpox. However, a child may contract chickenpox from an individual with shingles if there is direct contact with uncovered lesions. Shingles lesions must be covered to prevent spread. It is contagious until all lesions are crusted over (Aronson & Shope, 2009).

Promoting Safety

The key to preventing the spread of communicable disease is careful hand hygiene. Hands must always be washed before and after caring for infants and children. Caregivers and children must be taught to wash hands before eating and handling food, after using the bathroom or changing diapers, after handling animals, after playing in water or in the sand, and after using tissues to wipe eyes or noses.

Medication

Over-the-Counter Drugs

The American Academy of Pediatrics (AAP, 2008) is urging health-care providers and caregivers to use caution in administering over-the-counter (OTC) cough and cold medications to young children. Serious side effects have been observed, and studies indicate that cold medications are not effective for children under the age of 6. The AAP recommends the use of home remedies such as cool mist humidifiers, saline nose drops, and suctioning bulbs to clear the nares. The FDA (2008) reports that the Consumer Healthcare Products Association (CHPA) has volunteered to label OTC cough and cold medications as "do not use" for children under 4 years of age. In addition, manufacturers are introducing improved child-resistant packaging on cough and cold medicines to prevent children from overdosing on these medications.

BACTERIAL COMMUNICABLE DISEASES

CONJUNCTIVITIS (PINKEYE)

Disease Process

- Agent: virus or bacteria
- Transmission: contact with discharge from an infected eye, either direct contact or by touching contaminated surfaces
- Communicability: varies depending on organism

Clinical Presentation

- Viral infection: pink or red conjunctiva, edema, watery discharge (**Figure 22-12**); may affect only one eye
- Bacterial infection: pink or red conjunctiva, edema, purulent discharge, crusted eyelids in the morning, complaints of itching or pain

Nursing Interventions

- Teach administration of eyedrops as ordered for bacterial infections

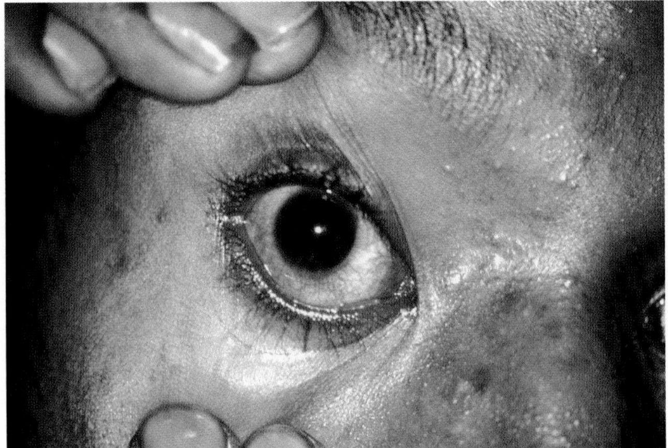

Figure 22-12 Child with conjunctivitis.

- If two or more children in the same setting (home or school) develop conjunctivitis, the cause may be adenovirus. This may cause epidemics in school or group settings.

Caregiver Education

Home Care

- Avoid touching eyes, wash hands carefully after touching eyes, sanitize objects that have been touched by eyes or hands, discard tissues that are used to wipe eyes, administer eyedrops as ordered.

Medication

Administering Eyedrops

- Perform hand hygiene.
- Draw the correct amount of medication into the dropper. Do not touch the dropper to the eye or any other surface. The dropper must remain sterile.
- Tilt the child's head back and pull down the lower eyelid.
- Squeeze the correct number of medication drops into the pouch formed by pulling down the lower eyelid.
- Allow the child to close the eye. Gently press the tear duct situated in the inner corner of the eye.
- Gently wipe off excess solution with a clean cotton ball or gauze pad.
- Perform hand hygiene.

PERTUSSIS (WHOOPING COUGH)

Disease Process

- Agent: *Bordetella pertussis*
- Transmission: oral and nasal secretions

- Incubation period: 6–21 days
- Communicability: contagious from the onset of symptoms and for about 2 weeks. Infants who have not been immunized may be contagious for at least 6 weeks.
- The disease is most dangerous to young infants.

Clinical Presentation

- Catarrhal phase that lasts 1 to 2 weeks: cold symptoms, including coryza, mild cough, and fever
- Paroxysmal phase that lasts 1 to 6 weeks or longer: cough ends with crowing (whooping) and may be severe enough to cause vomiting and cyanosis.
- Recovery phase when cough gradually becomes less severe
- In some children, adolescents, and adults, pertussis may present as a chronic cough that lasts for weeks. The crowing or whooping may not always be present.
- Pertussis is becoming more common among adolescents and adults.

Diagnostic Testing

- The polymerase chain reaction (PCR) test identifies genetic material of the *B. pertussis* bacteria in nasal secretions.

Nursing Intervention

Acute Hospital Care

- Infants have more severe cases of pertussis and may require hospitalization to manage respiratory distress and dehydration.

Caregiver Education

- Give small amounts of fluid frequently to keep the child hydrated, especially during bouts of vomiting. Refeed or give small amounts of fluid after episodes of coughing and vomiting.
- Teach signs of respiratory distress and dehydration and urge parents to seek medical care as needed (see boxes on teaching parents).
- Provide for rest and quiet activities and avoid stimuli that trigger coughing.
- Cool mist humidifier

Medication

Antibiotic Therapy

Pertussis must be treated with zithromax, erythromycin, or clarithromycin. Treatment should be started before 21 days into the illness.

STREP THROAT/SCARLET FEVER (GABHS)

Disease Process

- Agent: Group A beta-hemolytic streptococcus; causes GAS pharyngitis (**Figure 22-13**). This bacteria may also cause impetigo.
- Complications of Group A beta-hemolytic streptococcus include rheumatic fever and poststreptococcal glomerulonephritis. Please refer to chapters on cardiovascular and renal disease for additional information on these diseases.
- Transmission: respiratory droplets, direct contact with secretions
- Incubation period: 2–5 days
- Communicability: approximately 10 days without treatment; no longer contagious after 24 hours on antibiotics

Clinical Presentation

- Sore throat, fever, headache, enlarged and tender anterior cervical and tonsillar lymph nodes, abdominal pain, and decreased appetite
- Cough and coryza are not major signs of strep throat. If a child has nasal congestion, the sore throat is likely caused by another organism.
- Children under age 3 may have a streptococcal infection without complaining of a sore throat. Symptoms may include fever, irritability, and nasal discharge.
- Scarlet fever is strep throat with a fine, red rash (**Figure 22-14**) with the texture of sandpaper. The rash is more pronounced in the armpits and groin, in the creases of the elbows, and behind the knees. After the rash fades, the skin of the fingers and toes may peel. There may be pallor around the mouth and a white tongue with swollen, red papillae (strawberry tongue; **Figure 22-15**).

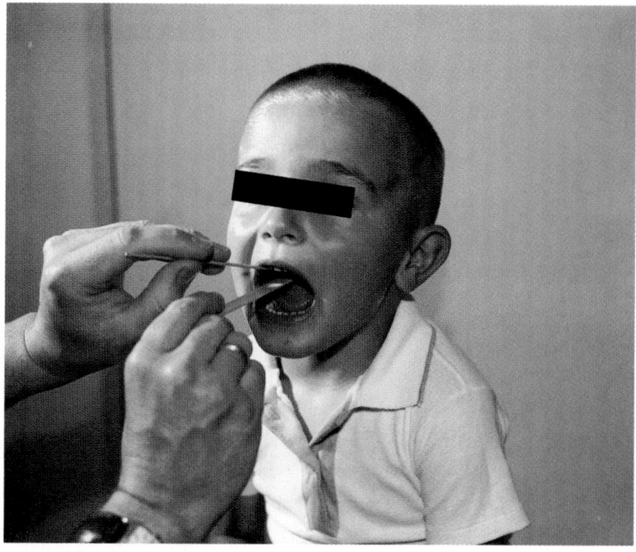

Figure 22-13 Child with streptococcal pharyngitis.

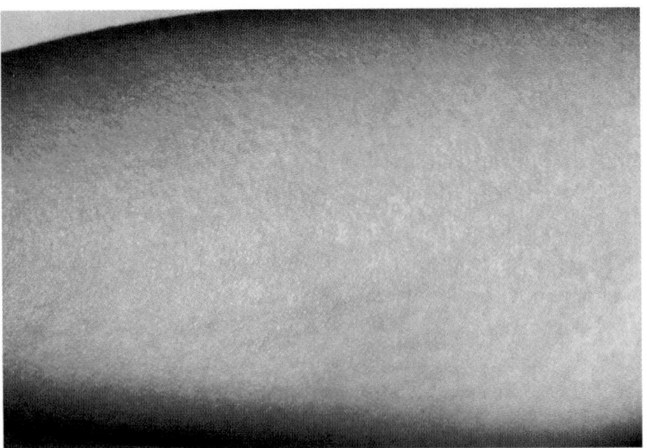

Figure 22-14 Child with rash from scarlet fever.

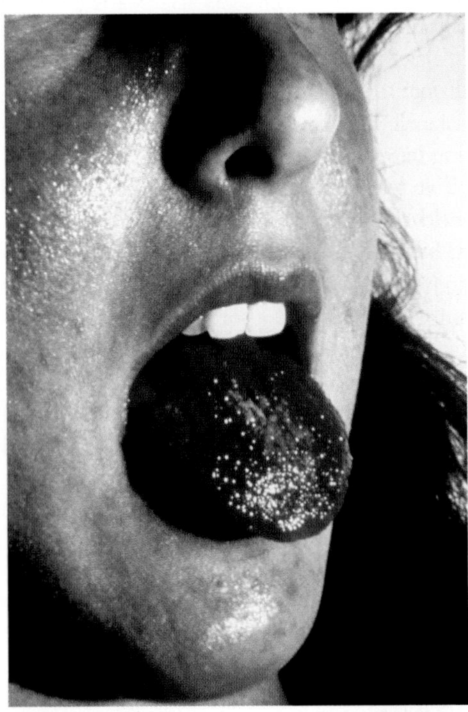

Figure 22-15 Child with strawberry tongue.

Diagnostic Testing

- Rapid strep test, throat culture

Nursing Intervention

Acute Hospital Care

- Complications of untreated strep throat include glomerulonephritis and rheumatic fever.

Caregiver Education

Home Care

- Administration of penicillin as ordered
- Fluids to keep the child hydrated—soups, popsicles, milkshakes
- Cool mist humidifier
- Acetaminophen or ibuprofen for pain and fever
- Replace toothbrush.
- Throat lozenges

Complementary and Alternative Therapies

- Saltwater gargles

CRITICAL COMPONENT

Signs of Respiratory Distress

Teach parents the signs of respiratory distress for seeking medical care:

- Restlessness, anxiety
- Respiratory rate over 60 in an infant, over 40 in a toddler
- Retractions
- Wheezing
- Distress that increases when lying down
- Breathlessness, gasping, continuous coughing
- Nasal flaring
- Color changes–duskiness around mouth, pallor
- Crowing sound when taking a breath
- Hoarse cry or barking cough

CRITICAL COMPONENT

Signs of Dehydration

Teach parents the signs of dehydration for seeking medical care:

- Lethargy
- No tears when crying
- For young infant, less than 5 or 6 wet diapers in 24 hours
- Eyes sunken
- Skin not elastic (poor skin turgor)

See **Table 22-1** or refer to Chapter 21 for information on communicable diseases of the skin, refer to Chapter 11 for additional information on bronchiolitis and tuberculosis, and refer to Chapter 18 for information on sexually transmitted infections.

Review Questions

1. A 3-year-old child with chickenpox is placed on Tylenol® as needed for fever. Which of the following comments by the caregiver would indicate to the nurse that he or she needs further instructions?
   A. "I can give the Tylenol® every 4 hours if needed."
   B. "I can give the Tylenol® with juice or ice cream."
   C. "I will draw up liquid Tylenol® in a syringe."
   D. "I can give baby aspirin instead of Tylenol®."

2. Which of the following statements would indicate to the nurse that a caregiver of a 1-year-old child understands the criteria for administering the influenza immunization?
   A. "It is especially important to use the nasal spray immunization because my child has asthma."
   B. "My child can have the nasal spray immunization because he has already had his first birthday."
   C. "My child needs the immunization now and again before he enters kindergarten."
   D. "My child cannot have the influenza immunization because he is allergic to eggs."

3. The nurse is teaching the caregiver of an infant about the Hib immunization. Which of the following statements by the caregiver would indicate to the nurse that the caregiver needs further instruction?
   A. "The immunization will protect my child from meningitis."
   B. "The immunization will protect my child from ear infections and conjunctivitis."
   C. "My child will need a booster before he goes to kindergarten."
   D. "My child may be a little sore after the shot."

4. The nurse should give immediate attention to which of the following symptoms in a child with mumps?
   A. Elevated temperature (>101.4°F)
   B. Swelling and tenderness below jaw
   C. Ear ache
   D. Lethargy, decreased responsiveness

5. A 6-month-old infant is in the paroxysmal stage of pertussis (whooping cough). The nurse should identify that the infant is at highest risk for which of the following nursing diagnoses?
   A. Deficient fluid volume
   B. Impaired physical mobility
   C. Impaired skin integrity
   D. Impaired parenting

6. A 5-year-old child has been diagnosed with scarlet fever. The nurse assessed that which of the following factors in the child's history most likely contributed to his condition?
   A. Recent mosquito bites
   B. Recent episode of pharyngitis
   C. History of repaired congenital heart defect
   D. History of frequent otitis media

7. Which of the following clinical signs should be included in a care plan for teaching parents when to call for emergency medical services? (select all that apply)
   A. Rash that spreads quickly and does not blanch
   B. Fever with stiff neck
   C. Tender, enlarged lymph nodes in the neck
   D. Lethargic and becoming more unresponsive

8. An admission nursing assessment of the child would reveal which of the following prodromal manifestations of rubeola?
   A. Vomiting, coryza, cough
   B. Koplik spots, maculopapular rash, malaise
   C. Coryza, cough, conjunctivitis
   D. Maculopapular rash, fever, enlarged cervical lymph nodes

9. A child has been diagnosed with varicella. Which of these nursing measures should be included in the child's care?
   A. Encourage hydration with cool citrus juices.
   B. Use elbow restraints to keep the child from scratching lesions.
   C. Give tepid Aveeno or baking soda baths to relieve itching.
   D. Give baby aspirin or Tylenol® to relieve fever.

10. An infant has been born to a mother who tests positive for hepatitis B. Which of the following treatment combinations will offer protection to the infant?
    A. HBV immunization plus HBIG (immunoglobulin)
    B. HBV immunization plus Ribavirin
    C. HBV immunization plus Acyclovir
    D. HBV immunization plus Bactrim

References

American Academy of Pediatrics (AAP). (2008). *American Academy of pediatrics urges caution in use of over-the-counter cough and cold medicines*. Retrieved from www.aap.org/advocacy/releases/jan08coughandcold.htm

American Academy of Pediatrics (AAP). (2009). Policy statements—modified recommendations for use of palivizumab for prevention of respiratory syncytial virus infections. *Pediatrics, 124*, 1694–1701. doi: 10.1542/peds.2009-2345

Aronson, S. S., & Shope, T. R. (2009). *Managing infectious diseases in child care and schools* (2nd ed.). Elk Grove Village, IL: American Academy of Pediatrics.

Centers for Disease Control and Prevention (CDC). (1988). Perspectives in disease prevention and health promotion update: Universal Precautions for prevention of transmission of human immunodeficiency virus, hepatitis B virus, and other bloodborne pathogens in health-care settings. *MMWR, 37*, 377–388. Retrieved from http://www.cdc.gov/niosh/topics/bbp/universal.html

Centers for Disease Control and Prevention (CDC). (2005). *Parvovirus B19 infection and pregnancy*. Retrieved from http://www.cdc.gov/ncidod/dvrd/revb/respiratory/B19&preg.htm

Centers for Disease Control and Prevention (CDC). (2007a). *Guideline for isolation precautions: Preventing transmission of infectious agents in healthcare settings*. Retrieved from www.cdc.gov/ncidod/dhqp/gl_isolation.html

Centers for Disease Control and Prevention (CDC). (2009). *Varicella disease questions and answers.* Retrieved from www.cdc.gov/vaccines/vpd-vac/varicella/dis-faqs-gen.htm

Centers for Disease Control and Prevention (CDC). (2011a). *2011 child and adolescent immunization schedules.* Retrieved from http://www.cdc.gov/vaccines/recs/schedules/child-schedule.htm

Centers for Disease Control and Prevention (CDC). (2011b). *2011–2012 Influenza antiviral medications: A summary for clinicians.* Retrieved from http://www.cdc.gov/flu/pdf/professionals/antivirals/clinician-antivirals-2011.pdf

Centers for Disease Control and Prevention (CDC). (2011c). *Hand, foot, and mouth disease.* Retrieved from http://www.cdc.gov/hand-foot-mouth/about/prevention-treatment.html

Centers for Disease Control and Prevention (CDC). (2011d). *Hepatitis B information for health professionals: Perinatal transmission.* Retrieved from http://www.cdc.gov/hepatitis/HBV/PerinatalXmtn.htm

Centers for Disease Control and Prevention (CDC). (2011e). *Overview of measles disease.* Retrieved from http://www.cdc.gov/measles/about/overview.html

Centers for Disease Control and Prevention (CDC). (2011f). *Parvovirus B19 (Fifth disease).* Retrieved from http://www.cdc.gov/ncidod/dvrd/revb/respiratory/parvo_b19.htm

Centers for Disease Control and Prevention (CDC). (2011g). *Update on the global status of polio.* Retrieved from http://wwwnc.cdc.gov/travel/notices/in-the-news/polio-outbreaks.htm

Chen, X., Wu, T., Liu, G., Wang, Q., Zheng, J., Wei, J., . . . Qiao, J. (2008). Chinese medicinal herbs for influenza. *Cochrane Database of Systematic Reviews 2007.* doi: 10.1002/14651858.CD004559.pub3.

Food and Drug Administration (FDA). (2008). *Using over-the-counter cough and cold products in Children.* Retrieved from http://www.fda.gov/consumer/updates/coughcold102208.htm

Huiming, Y., Chaomin, W., & Meng, M. (2008). Vitamin A for treating measles in children. *The Cochrane Database of Systematic Reviews 2005.* doi: 10.1002/14651858.CD001479.pub3

Joyce, C. (2007). Steps to success: Getting children vaccinated on time. *Pediatric Nursing, 33,* 491–495. Retrieved from http://www.pediatricnursing.net/issues/07novdec/abstr3.html

Koslap-Petraco, M. B., & Judelsohn, R. G. (2008). Societal impact of combination vaccines: Experiences of physicians, nurses, and parents. *Journal of Pediatric Health Care, 22,* 300–309. doi: 10.1016/j.pedhc.2007.09.004

Lacey, C. M., Finkelstein, M., & Thygeson, M. V. (2008). The impact of positioning on fear during immunizations: Supine versus sitting up. *Journal of Pediatric Nursing 23,* 195–200. doi: 10.1016/j.pedn.2007.09.007

Macartney, K., & McIntyre, P. (2008). Vaccines for post-exposure prophylaxis against varicella (chickenpox) in children and adults. *Cochrane Database of Systematic Reviews 2008.* doi: 10.1002/14651858.CD001833.pub2.

Offit, P. A. (2006). *Thimersol and autism.* Retrieved from http://www.immunize.org/catg.d/p2066.pdf

Sims, R. M., & Woodgate, R. L. (2008). Managing chronic hepatitis B in children. *Journal of Pediatric Health Care, 22,* 360–367. Retrieved from http://www.jpedhc.org/article/S0891-5245(07)00372-0/abstract

VAERS (Vaccine Adverse Event Reporting System). (2011). Retrieved from http://vaers.hhs.gov/index

Appendix

Dosage Calculation Problems

1. Order: Amoxil (amoxicillin) 70 mg PO q8h.
   Patient: Child weighs 22 lbs.
   Safe dose is 20–40 mg/kg/day in divided doses q8h.
   Available as: 125 mg/5 mL
   A. Is the dose safe? __________
   B. If safe, how much liquid will you give the child per dose? _____________
   C. If not safe, what is the range of safe doses for this child? _____________

2. Order: Phenobarbital 60 mg PO bid
   Patient: Infant weighs 12 lbs 8 oz.
   Safe dose is 4–8 mg/kg/day divided into two doses with maximum dose of 300 mg/day.
   Available as: Oral phenobarbital suspension of 30 mg/5 mL
   A. Is the dose safe? __________
   B. If safe, how much liquid will you give the child per dose? _____________
   C. If not safe, what is the range of safe doses for this child? _____________

3. Order: Benadryl (diphenhydramine hydrochloride) 25 mg IV q6h prn
   Patient: Child weighs 30 kg.
   Safe dose is 1.25–10.5 mg/kg but not to exceed 200 mg/day.
   Available as: Injection labeled 60 mg/mL
   A. Is the dose safe? __________
   B. If safe, how much will you draw up in the syringe for the child per dose? _____________
   C. If not safe, what is the safe dose for this child? _____________

4. Order: Zithromax (azithromycin) 320 mg PO for one dose on first day
   Patient: Child is 10 years old and weighs 32 kg.
   Safe dose for children 2–15 years is 10 mg/kg (but not more than 500 mg/dose) on day 1.
   Available as: Oral Zithromax suspension 100 mg/5 mL
   A. Is the dose safe? __________
   B. If safe, how much liquid will you give the child per dose? _____________
   C. If not safe, what is the safe dose for this child? _____________

5. Order: Augmentin (amoxicillin clavulanate) 175 mg PO q8h.
   Patient: Child weighs 29 lbs.
   Safe dose is 40 mg/kg/day in divided doses q8h.
   Available as: Oral suspension of 125 mg/5 mL
   A. Is the dose safe? _______________
   B. If safe, how much liquid will you give the child per dose? _____________
   C. If not safe, what is the safe dose for this child? _____________

6. Order: Lasix (furosemide) 15 mg PO bid
   Patient: The child weighs 16 lbs 8 oz.
   Safe dose for a child is 2 mg/kg/dose of furosemide as the initial dose.
   Available as: 10 mg/mL
   A. Is the dose safe?___________________
   B. If safe, how much in mL will you administer? ___________________

7. Order: Ampicillin 100 mg IV q 6 hrs
   Patient: Child is 4 months old and weighs 9 lbs 6 oz.
   Safe dose for this child's age and weight is 75–200 mg/kg/day.
   Available as: Vial of powder 500 mg/vial.
   Directions: Add 1.8 mL of sterile water; yields 250 mg/mL
   A. What are the safe ranges? low range ___________ high range______________
   B. What is the safe dose?______________________
   C. How much will you give? _____________

8. Order: Cefuroxime 185 mg IV q6h
   Patient: Infant is 6 months old and weighs 17 lbs 6 oz.
   Safe range is 50–100 mg/kg/day.
   Available as: Cefuroxime 90 mg/mL
   A. What are the safe ranges? low range ___________ high range_______________
   B. Is the dose safe? _________________________
   C. If safe, how much will you draw up? ___________________mL

9. Order: Epinephrine 0.3 mg sublingual
Patient: Child is 3 years old and weighs 66 lbs.
Safe dosage range is 0.01 mg/kg not to exceed 0.3 mg for any single dose.
Available: Epinephrine 1 mg/mL
A. What are the safe ranges? low range __________ high range __________
B. Is the dose safe? __________
C. If safe, how many mL do you draw up for this dose?__________

10. Order: Piperacillin 3375 mg IV q8h
Patient: Weighs 120 pounds.
Safe dosage range for adults is 4–8 grams per day.
Available: Piperacillin 3375 mg in 100 mL of normal saline to run over 30 minutes. You do not have a pump and need to run the medication by drop factor. You pick tubing that is 10 gtts/min.
A. Is the dose safe? __________
B. If safe, how many drops per minute will you regulate the tubing at __________/minute?

ANSWER KEY

1. Dosage of Amoxil is safe at 210 mg/day or 70 mg per dose tid for a child weighing 22 lbs or 10 kg. Range is 200–400 mg per 24 hours. For 70-mg dose, give 2.8 mL of medication.
A. Safe—yes
B. 2.8 mL of medication
C. n/a

2. Dosage of Phenobarbital is not safe at 30 mg PO bid for infant weighing 12 lbs 8 oz or 5.68 kg. Range of doses at 4–8 mg per kg day divided into two doses is 22.72–45.44 mg per day or 11.36–22.72 mg per dose. You cannot give the medication.
A. Not safe—30 mg is too high (11.36–22.72 mg is the safe dose range)
B. No medication
C. 22.72–45.44 mg per day in two divided doses of 11.36–22.72 mg is safe range

3. Dosage of Benadryl is safe at 25 mg IV q6h for a child weighing 30 kg based on dose of 1.25–10.5 mg/kg/day, not to exceed 200 mg per day. Daily dosage is 100 mg and does not exceed 300 mg per day. With 60 mg per mL, the dose is 0.42 mL of medication to be drawn into syringe.
A. Safe—yes
B. 0.42 mL of medication
C. n/a

4. Dosage of Zithromax is safe at 320 mg PO for one dose for a child weighing 32 kg. Safe dosage is based on 10 mg per kg per dose. This is not more than 500 mg per day. With 100 mg per 5 mL of medication, you would give 16 mL of medication.
A. Safe—yes
B. 16 mL of medication
C. n/a

5. Dosage is safe at 125 mg for a child who weighs 29 pounds or 13.18 kg. Dosage is based on 40 mg per kg per day in 3 doses q8h. Weight of 13.18 kg times 40 mg/kg is 527.27 mg per day with 3 doses of 175 mg equals 525 mg per day. For 175-mg dose, give 7 mL of medication (125 mg per 5 mL).
A. Safe—yes
B. 7 mL of medication
C. n/a

6. Child weighs 7.5 kg; 15 mg/kg is safe dose.
A. Safe—yes
B. Divide 15 mg/10 mg × 1 mL = 1.5 mL

7. Child weighs 4.3 kg.
A. 75 × 4.3 kg = 322.5 mg/day
200 × 4.3 kg = 860 mg/day
B. 400 mg/day
C. 100 mg/500 mg × 1.8 mL = 0.4 mL

8. Child weighs 7.9 kg.
A. 50 × 7.9 kg = 395 mg/day 100 × 7.9 kg = 790 mg/day
B. Child is receiving 185 mg × 4 doses = 740 mg/day.
C. Safe—yes
D. 185 mg/90 mg × 1 mL = 2.1 mL

9. Child weighs 30 kg.
A. 0.01 mg × 30 kg = 0.3 mg/day
0.3 mg × 30 kg = 9 mg/day
B. Safe—yes
C. 0.3 mg/1 mg = 0.3 mL

10. Child weighs 54.5 kg.
A. No, it is not safe
B. None; I would not give.

Answers to End of Chapter Review Questions

Chapter 1

1. C
2. B
3. D
4. D
5. B
6. A, C, E
7. D
8. A, B, E
9. A, B, C, E
10. A, B, C, E

Chapter 2

1. D
2. A
3. B
4. D
5. A
6. D
7. D
8. C
9. C
10. A

Chapter 3

1. B
2. B
3. A
4. B
5. D
6. D
7. A
8. B
9. C
10. D

Chapter 4

1. B
2. C
3. D
4. A
5. C
6. A
7. D
8. A
9. C
10. A

Chapter 5

1. D
2. B
3. A
4. C
5. B
6. A
7. D
8. B
9. B
10. D

Chapter 6

1. D
2. A
3. C
4. A
5. D
6. C
7. D
8. B
9. D
10. D

Chapter 7

1. A
2. C
3. C
4. D
5. C
6. C
7. A
8. D
9. B
10. C

Chapter 8

1. B
2. D
3. E
4. B
5. C
6. C
7. E
8. C
9. E
10. A, C

Chapter 9

1. D
2. A
3. C
4. E
5. C
6. E
7. B
8. A
9. D
10. E

Chapter 10

1. C
2. D
3. C
4. A
5. D
6. A
7. B
8. E
9. B
10. C

Chapter 11

1. E
2. C
3. E
4. E
5. B
6. C
7. E
8. E
9. A
10. B

Chapter 12

1. B
2. C
3. D
4. C
5. A
6. C
7. B
8. D
9. A
10. A

Chapter 13

1. D
2. D
3. B
4. B
5. D
6. C
7. A
8. A
9. C
10. D

Chapter 14

1. A
2. E
3. E
4. D
5. B
6. E
7. D
8. A
9. B
10. C

Chapter 15

1. A
2. C
3. D
4. D
5. A
6. C
7. B
8. C
9. B
10. B

Chapter 16

1. C
2. B
3. B
4. A
5. C
6. A
7. C
8. C
9. B
10. A

Chapter 17

1. B, C, D
2. C
3. A
4. False
5. True
6. Acanthosis nigricans
7. B
8. D
9. C
10. A

Chapter 18

1. B
2. D
3. B
4. C
5. C
6. C, D
7. A, B, C, E
8. A, B, C, E
9. A, B, E
10. A

Chapter 19

1. B
2. E
3. D
4. C
5. A
6. A
7. D
8. C
9. C
10. E

Chapter 20

1. B
2. A
3. C
4. E
5. E
6. C
7. C
8. E
9. D
10. C

Chapter 21

1. A
2. B, C
3. C
4. C
5. C
6. D
7. D
8. B, C, D
9. D
10. B

Chapter 22

1. D
2. D
3. C
4. D
5. A
6. B
7. A, B, D
8. C
9. C
10. A

Illustration Credits

Unless noted below, text credits appear with the figure.

Chapter 1

Figure 1-1: Courtesy of the National Institutes of Health, www.nih.gov

Chapter 3

Figure 3-1: © fotosearch.com

Figure 3-9: From Ward, S.L., & Hisley, S.M. [2009]. *Maternal-Child Nursing Care: Optimizing Outcomes for Mothers, Children, and Families:* Enhanced, revised revision. Philadelphia: F.A. Davis.

Chapter 5

Figures 5-2, 5-3, and 5-4: From Ward, S.L., & Hisley, S.M. [2009]. *Maternal-Child Nursing Care: Optimizing Outcomes for Mothers, Children, and Families*: Enhanced, revised revision. Philadelphia: F.A. Davis.

Chapter 7

Figures 7-1 through 7-4, 7-7, 7-9, 7-10 and 7-12: From Ward, S.L., & Hisley, S.M. [2009]. *Maternal-Child Nursing Care: Optimizing Outcomes for Mothers, Children, and Families*: Enhanced, revised revision. Philadelphia: F.A. Davis.

Figures 7-5, 7-6, 7-8, 7-11, 7-20, 7-21, 7-24 and 7-25: From Chapman, L., & Durham, R. [2010]. *Maternal-Newborn Nursing: The Critical Components of Nursing Care.* Philadelphia: F.A. Davis.

Chapter 8

Figures 8-2, 8-3, and 8-7: From Dillon, P.M. [2007]. *Nursing Health Assessment: A Critical Thinking, Case Studies Approach*, 2e. Philadelphia: F.A. Davis.

Figure 8-4: From National Institutes of Health. Retrieved from http://visualsonline.cancer.gov/details.cfm?imagineid=2097)

Chapter 9

Figures 9-1 through 9-4: From Centers for Disease Control and Prevention Public Health Library. *http://phil.cdc.gov*

Chapter 10

Figures 10-3 and 10-5: From Dillon, P.M. [2007]. *Nursing Health Assessment: A Critical Thinking Case Studies Approach*, 2e. Philadelphia: F.A. Davis.

Figure 10-4: From Chapman, L., & Durham, R. [2010]. *Maternal-Newborn Nursing: The Critical Components of Nursing Care.* Philadelphia: F.A. Davis.

Chapter 11

Figures 11-1, 11-3, 11-4: From Dillon, P.M. [2007]. *Nursing Health Assessment: A Critical Thinking Case Studies Approach*, 2e. Philadelphia: F.A. Davis.

Figure 11-2: From Centers for Disease Control and Prevention Public Health Library *http://phil.cdc.gov*

Chapter 12

Figures 12-1 through 12-4, 12-6 through 12-19: From Ward, S.L., & Hisley, S.M. [2009]. *Maternal-Child Nursing Care: Optimizing Outcomes for Mothers, Children, and Families:* Enhanced, revised revision. Philadelphia: F.A. Davis.

Chapter 13

Figures 13-1, 13-3, 13-7, 13-9: From Gilman, S., & Newman, S.W. [2003]. *Manter and Gatz's Essentials of Clinical Neuroanatomy and Neurophysiology,* 10e. Philadelphia: F.A. Davis.

Figure 13-2: From Scanlon V. & Sanders, T. [2011]. *Essentials of Anatomy and Physiology,* 6e. Philadelphia: F.A. Davis.

Chapter 15

Figures 15-1, 15-3 through 15-14: From the National Institute of Diabetes, Digestive and Kidney Disease, National Institute of Health.

Chapter 16

Figures 16-1, 16-2, 16-4: Adapted from National Institute of Diabetes and Digestive and Kidney Diseases [NIDDK]. [2006]. NIH Publications.

Figure 16-3: Adapted from the National Institutes of Health. Retrieved from http://kidney.niddk.nih.gov/kudiseases/pubs/nephrotic /.

Chapter 17

Figures 17-3 and 17-4: From Ward, S.L., & Hisley, S.M. [2009]. *Maternal-Child Nursing Care: Optimizing Outcomes for Mothers, Children, and Families*: Enhanced, revised revision. Philadelphia: F.A. Davis.

Chapter 18

Figure 18-1 and 18-7: From Chapman, L., & Durham, R. [2010]. *Maternal-Newborn Nursing: The Critical Components of Nursing Care.* Philadelphia: F.A. Davis.

Figure 18-2, figure 18-5, 18-8, 18-13: From Dillon, P.M. [2007]. *Nursing Health Assessment: A Critical Thinking Case Studies Aapproach,* 2e. Philadelphia: F.A. Davis.

Figure 18-6: From Ward, S.L., & Hisley, S.M. [2009]. *Maternal-Child Nursing Care: Optimizing Outcomes for Mothers, Children, and Families:* Enhanced, revised revision. Philadelphia: F.A. Davis.

Chapter 19

Figure 19-1: From the Centers for Disease Control and Prevention/Sickle Cell Foundation of Georgia, Jackie George, Beverly Sinclair, 2009. Photograph by Janice Haney Carr. Retrieved from http://phil.cdc.gov/Phil/details.asp, ID11690.

Figure 19-2: From the Centers for Disease Control and Prevention, Aaron L. Sussell. [1999]. Retrieved from http://phil.cdc.gov/phil/details.asp, ID73333.

Figure 19-3: From the Centers for Disease Control and Prevention, Cynthia Goldsmith. Retrieved from http://phil.cdc.gov/phil/details.asp, ID 8241.

Figures 19-6, 19-7A: From Ward, S.L., & Hisley, S.M. [2009]. *Maternal-Child Nursing Care: Optimizing Outcomes for Mothers, Children, and Families:* Enhanced, revised revision. Philadelphia: F.A. Davis.

Figures 19-7B, Figure 19-9 and 19-11: From the National Cancer Institute.

Figure 19-8: From the Centers for Disease Control and Prevention, Robert S. Craig. [1967]. Retrieved from http://phil.cdc.gov/Phil/details.asp, ID 6050.

Figure 19-10: From the Centers for Disease Control and Prevention, James Gathany. [2005]. Retrieved from http://phil.cdc.gov/Phil/details.asp, ID8277.

Chapter 20

Figure 20-1: From Dillon, P.M. [2007]. *Nursing Health Assessment: A Critical Thinking Case Studies Approach*, 2e. Philadelphia: F.A. Davis.

Figures 20-2 A-E, 20-3A, 20-17: From Ward, S.L., & Hisley, S.M. [2009]. *Maternal-Child Nursing Care: Optimizing Outcomes for Mothers, Children, and Families:* Enhanced, revised revision. Philadelphia: F.A. Davis.

Chapter 21

Figures 21-3 through 21-5, 21-8 through 21-10 : From Dillon, P.M. [2007]. *Nursing Health Assessment: A Critical Thinking Case Studies Approach*, 2e. Philadelphia: F.A. Davis.

Figures 21-6, 21-7, 21-11, 21-13 and 21-15: From Freiman, A., & Barankin, B. [2006]. *Derm Notes: Dermatology Clinical Pocket Guide*. Philadelphia: F.A. Davis.

Figure 21-12: From the Centers for Disease Control and Prevention, Department of Health and Human Services. [2007]. Retrieved from http://phil.cdc.gov/Phil/details.asp, ID #9875.

Figure 21-14: From Ward, S.L., & Hisley, S.M. [2009]. *Maternal-Child Nursing Care: Optimizing Outcomes for Mothers, Children, and Families:* Enhanced, revised revision. Philadelphia: F.A. Davis.

Chapter 22

Figures 22-1 and 22-2: From the Centers for Disease Control and Prevention [CDC]. [2011]. 2011 Child and Adolescent Immunization Schedules. Retrieved from http://www.cdc.gov/vaccines/recs/schedules/child-schedule.htm

Figure 22-3: From the Centers for Disease Control and Prevention, Department of Health and Human Services. [2007]. Retrieved from http://www.nlm.nih.gov/medlineplus/fifthdisease.html

Figure 22-4: From Freiman, A., & Barankin, B. [2006]. *Derm Notes: Dermatology Clinical Pocket Guide.* Philadelphia: F.A. Davis.

Figure 22-5: From the Centers for Disease Control and Prevention, Department of Health and Human Services. Retrieved from http://phil.cdc.gov/Phil/details.asp

Figure 22-6: From the Centers for Disease Control and Prevention, Department of Health and Human Services, NIP/Barbara Rice. Retrieved from http://phil.cdc.gov/phil/details.asp?pid=130

Figure 22-7: From the Centers for Disease Control and Prevention, Department of Health and Human Services. Retrieved from http://phil.cdc.gov/Phil/details.asp, ID #3318.

Figure 22-8: From the Centers for Disease Control and Prevention, Department of Health and Human Services. Retrieved from http://phil.cdc.gov/Phil/details.asp, ID #4514.

Figure 22-9: From the Centers for Disease Control and Prevention, Department of Health and Human Services, Dr. Heinz F. Eichenwald. [1958]. Retrieved from http://phil.cdc.gov/Phil/details.asp, ID #3187.

Figure 22-10: From the Centers for Disease Control and Prevention, Department of Health and Human Services, Dr. Heinz F. Eichenwald. [1958]. Retrieved from http://phil.cdc.gov/Phil/details.asp, ID #3168.

Figure 22-11: From the Centers for Disease Control and Prevention, Department of Health and Human Services. Retrieved from http://phil.cdc.gov/Phil/details.asp, ID #6121.

Figure 22-12: From the Centers for Disease Control and Prevention, Department of Health and Human Services, Joe Miller, V.D. [1976]. Retrieved from http://phil.cdc.gov/Phil/details.asp, ID #6784.

Figure 22-13: From the Centers for Disease Control and Prevention, Department of Health and Human Services, Dr. M. Moody [n.d]. Retrieved from http://phil.cdc.gov/Phil/details.asp, ID #10190.

Figure 22-14: From the Centers for Disease Control and Prevention, Department of Health and Human Services. Retrieved from http://phil.cdc.gov/Phil/details.asp, ID #5163.

Figure 22-15: From the Centers for Disease Control and Prevention, Department of Health and Human Services. Retrieved from http://phil.cdc.gov/Phil/details.asp, ID #5120.

Index

Note: A *b* indicates content appears in a boxed feature on the page. An *f* indicates a figure. A *t* indicates a table.

B

C

H

J

K

L

M

N

O

P

Q

R

S

T

U